Brief Contents

Unit I   General Principles, 1

1. Pharmacology and the Nursing Process in LPN Practice, 1
2. Legal, Regulatory, and Ethical Aspects of Drug Administration, 11
3. Principles of Pharmacology, 22

Unit II   Principles of Drug Administration, 35

4. Drug Calculation: Preparing and Giving Drugs, 35

Unit III   Drug Categories, 64

5. Anti-Infective Drugs: Antibacterial, Antitubercular, and Antifungal Agents, 64
6. Antivirals and Antiretrovirals, 93
7. Drugs for Allergy and Respiratory Problems, 106
8. Drugs Affecting the Renal/Urinary and Cardiovascular Systems, 125
9. Drug Therapy for Central Nervous System Problems, 158
10. Drug Therapy for Mental Health, 183
11. Drugs for Pain Management, 210
12. Anti-Inflammatory, Antiarthritis, and Antigout Drugs, 225
13. Drugs for Gastrointestinal Problems, 240
14. Drugs Affecting the Hematologic System, 265
15. Drugs for Immunization and Immunomodulation, 279
16. Hormones and Drugs for Osteoporosis, 292
17. Drug Therapy for Diabetes, 309
18. Drugs for Ear and Eye Problems, 329
19. Over-the-Counter Drugs, Herbal and Alternative Drugs, and Vitamins and Minerals, 346

Bibliography, 360
Glossary, 362

EDITION

9

Introduction to Clinical Pharmacology

Constance G. Visovsky, PhD, RN, ACNP, FAAN
Associate Professor and Director of Diversity
College of Nursing
University of South Florida
Tampa, Florida

Cheryl H. Zambroski, PhD, RN
Associate Professor
College of Nursing
University of South Florida
Tampa, Florida

Shirley Meier Hosler, RN, BSN, MSN
Adjunct Faculty
Santa Fe Community College
Santa Fe, New Mexico

SPECIAL EDITOR
M. Linda Workman,
PhD, RN, FAAN
Formerly, Gertrude Perkins
 Oliva Professor of
 Oncology
Frances Payne Bolton School
 of Nursing
Case Western Reserve
 University
Cleveland, Ohio

ELSEVIER

ELSEVIER

3251 Riverport Lane
St. Louis, Missouri 63043

INTRODUCTION TO CLINICAL PHARMACOLOGY,
NINTH EDITION

ISBN: 978-0-323-52911-2

Notices

Practitioners and researchers must always rely on their own experience and knowledge in evaluating and using any information, methods, compounds or experiments described herein. Because of rapid advances in the medical sciences, in particular, independent verification of diagnoses and drug dosages should be made. To the fullest extent of the law, no responsibility is assumed by Elsevier, authors, editors or contributors for any injury and/or damage to persons or property as a matter of products liability, negligence or otherwise, or from any use or operation of any methods, products, instructions, or ideas contained in the material herein.

Library of Congress Cataloging-in-Publication Data

Names: Visovsky, Constance G., editor. | Preceded by (work): Edmunds, Marilyn W. Introduction to clinical pharmacology.
Title: Introduction to clinical pharmacology / special editor, M. Linda Workman.
Description: 9th edition. | St. Louis, Missouri : Elsevier Inc., [2019] | Preceded by Introduction to clinical pharmacology / Marilyn Winterton Edmunds. 2016. | Includes bibliographical references and index.
Identifiers: LCCN 2017054727 | ISBN 9780323529112 (pbk. : alk. paper)
Subjects: | MESH: Pharmaceutical Preparations–administration & dosage | Drug Therapy | Nurses' Instruction
Classification: LCC RM300 | NLM QV 748 | DDC 615.5/8–dc23 LC record available at https://lccn.loc.gov/2017054727

Senior Content Strategist: Nancy O'Brien
Senior Content Development Specialist: Laura Goodrich
Publishing Services Manager: Jeff Patterson
Senior Project Manager: Tracey Schriefer
Design Direction: Renee Duenow

Printed in Canada

Last digit is the print number: 9 8 7 6 5 4 3

Reviewers

Linda Gambill, RN, MSN/Ed
LPN Instructor/Clinical Coordinator
Southwest Virginia Community College
Cedar Bluff, Virginia

James Graves, PharmD
Clinical Pharmacist
University of Missouri Hospital Inpatient Pharmacy
Columbia, Missouri

Teresa Peirce, RN, BSN
Nursing Instructor
Locklin Technical Center
Milton, Florida

Jackie Taylor-Wynkoop, RN, MSN, EMS-I, PHRN, FAEN
Coordinator
PITC Practical Nursing Program
Wyncote, Pennsylvania

Tiffany Vollmer, RN, BSN
Nursing Department Director
Locklin Technical Center
Milton, Florida

LPN/LVN Advisory Board

Preface

This ninth edition of *Introduction to Clinical Pharmacology* offers the fresh and exciting perspectives of authors who have years of experience teaching pharmacology. Most students believe that pharmacology is a very important part of their nursing education and one that is difficult to learn. The author team has strived to make the pharmacology learning experience one that combines updated information in an easy-to-remember format that promotes high levels of content retention.

This textbook is written using the second person throughout to engage students and help them understand the nursing responsibilities required for use in the clinical setting. The textbook's new organization and style are intended to engage students and help them develop an in-depth understanding of the "need to know" content that is critical for safely administering medications in all environments in which licensed practical nurses/vocational nurses (LPN/VNs) are employed. The components of the nursing process most important to this function are emphasized. The number of illustrations has been greatly expanded to explain drug actions and techniques for administration. The textbook uses current terminology for education and healthcare practice. For example, more settings include nurse practitioners and physician assistants as legal prescribers in addition to the physician. To reflect this change, the term *healthcare provider* is used throughout. Learning outcomes replace chapter objectives. These outcomes concisely and clearly let the student know which content represents the highest priority for safe medication administration. Drugs and drug categories no longer in common usage, or that do not apply to the LPN/VN role, have been eliminated. The textbook also helps students learn to make use of prevailing technology. Internet resources and references have been identified and highlighted with Bookmark This features.

Newly created drug tables are divided by drug category and organized to provide students with concise access to mechanisms, common adult drug dosages, and essential nursing implications for administration and patient teaching. Key terms critical for pharmacology are first listed at the beginning of the chapters and include phonetic pronunciations, definitions, and page numbers where each term is first used. This textbook takes advantage of the use of medical and nonpharmacologic terminology, with short definitions placed alongside the terms, as well in the Glossary, to aid student reading and retention.

Throughout this textbook, ensuring patient safety remains a major theme. The new safety features are the Top Tip for Safety boxes that highlight very specific precautions, unusual drug dosages, or critical nursing interventions. This author team deeply believes that it is critical to provide patient safety information to reduce drug errors. In addition, patients and families who understand the *why* of directions are more likely to adhere to them. Toward this purpose, nursing actions are accompanied by the appropriate rationale. In the discussion of each drug category, the sections on patient and family teaching provide direct examples of exactly what to teach patients and families, as well as the rationales for why these actions or precautions are necessary. Specific content on Lifespan Considerations for drug administration related to older adults and pediatric patients and for pregnancy and lactation are appropriately placed for maximum retention. A completely revised chapter covering herbals, vitamins, and supplements is included.

Other user-friendly learning techniques provided in this streamlined and updated edition include features such as Memory Jogger and mnemonics. All of the end-of-chapter review questions have been changed to reflect the latest NCLEX® format for critical thinking and application of content, including the "select all that apply" and multiple-choice questions. These formats help the student to think through responses rather than focus on rote memorization. All clinical chapters have newly developed case studies designed to help students learn to apply specific content.

The ancillary package has also been heavily revised. The Student Study Guide, written by a very experienced educator, is completely new. The instructor's TEACH resource is completely updated based on the revised Learning Outcomes for each chapter. The test bank is also heavily revised with new questions that require the student to apply knowledge, and they are in the latest question formats.

ORGANIZATION AND FEATURES

This textbook has been completely revised to include updated drugs, to remove drugs and terms that are no longer used in practice, and to add tables for each drug classification that list common drugs for each class and normal adult dosage ranges. Throughout this text, medications will be referred to as *drugs*, and the drug prescriber is called the *healthcare provider* because this can be a physician, advanced practice nurse, certified registered nurse anesthetist, or physician's assistant. The text has been reorganized into 3 units totaling 19 chapters to streamline access to specific content areas. Chapter-ending Get Ready for NCLEX® Examination questions have been updated and revised throughout the text, and use mostly application format questions to provide students with practice in answering these types of examination questions.

UNIT I

The first unit provides an overview of general content covering the nursing process as it relates to drug administration, the importance of safely giving drugs, and the principles of pharmacology that set the knowledge base for specified drug categories. For example, this completely revised textbook includes information on unique aspects of the contemporary LPN/VN practice environment, including working in teams with the registered nurse, healthcare provider, and other healthcare professionals. An overview of the nursing process as it applies to pharmacology is provided.

Safe practice is accentuated throughout Chapter 1, with a guide to planning and giving drugs to patients. The updated 9 Rights of Drug Administration is presented in detail and includes the right of the patient to refuse a drug. Although giving drugs properly is important, equally important are evaluating the expected drug response, understanding common side effects, and knowing how to handle adverse events from drugs.

The legal regulatory and ethical content related to giving drugs in the LPN/VN role has been updated to include a thorough discussion of schedule drugs, drug diversion, and a distinction between addiction and physical dependence in a patient. In Chapter 2, technology-associated patient identification, drug orders, and the giving and recording of drugs in either a standard Kardex or electronic health record are covered.

UNIT II

Unit II is concerned with drug calculation, preparation, and administration. LPN/VNs often practice in assisted nursing centers, nursing homes, and care centers where high-tech drug administration systems may not be used. Thus they need to be able to give medications safely and accurately, relying on their own ability to calculate the drug dosages accurately. Chapter 4 incudes the "need to know" content related to drug calculation and includes dimensional analysis, a mathematical technique that is being adopted by many nursing programs for drug calculation. Intravenous drugs, oral drugs, parenteral drugs, and intravenous infusion calculation are presented in an organized, step-by-step manner. The application of topical, transdermal, mucous membrane, and eye and ear drugs is also presented with accompanying illustrations to help the student visualize the process while reading the material.

UNIT III

Drug classification groups provide essential information on 15 specific drug classifications. Unit III focuses on content that has application to treatment purpose (i.e., anti-infective drugs) and are associated with body systems, such as renal, urinary, and cardiovascular systems. Drugs for the treatment of cancer have been removed because the LPN/VN does not administer or monitor these drugs, which are given by specially certified oncology nurses. By grouping drugs using the drug classification system, students quickly learn about individual drugs by understanding their drug class. The narrative content in the text focuses on major drug groups, and coverage of specific drugs appears in reference tables. All chapters have been updated in this edition to represent the latest clinical drug treatment information. Each drug class is presented in a consistent format with a separate Patient and Family Teaching section. Even though additional drug references may be used by students, the author team believes it is critical that students have a base knowledge of the potential dosage ranges for adult drugs to promote safe, effective practice. Thus drug dosage ranges are included in tables with each chapter in Unit III.

A chapter-ending Case Study requires the student to apply information gained for each chapter to address patient scenarios. Suggested answers to the Case Studies are provided online in the TEACH Instructor Resources on Evolve at http://evolve.elsevier.com/Visovsky/LPNpharmacology/.

TEACHING AND LEARNING PACKAGE FOR THE INSTRUCTOR

TEACH INSTRUCTOR RESOURCES

TEACH Instructor Resources on Evolve, available at http://evolve.elsevier.com/Visovsky/LPNpharmacology/, provide a wealth of material to help you make your pharmacology instruction a success.

In addition to all of the Student Resources, the following are provided for faculty:

The Exam View Test Bank has been *completely updated* with approximately 450 new application-style questions in multiple-choice and alternate-format for the NCLEX-PN® Examination. Each question is coded for correct answer, rationale, page reference, and cognitive level.

TEACH Lesson Plans, based on textbook chapter Learning Objectives, serve as ready-made, modifiable lesson plans and a complete roadmap to link all parts of the educational package. These concise and straightforward lesson plans can be modified or combined to meet your particular scheduling and teaching needs.

PowerPoint Presentations with incorporated Audience Response Questions provide approximately 550 text and image slides for classroom or online presentations.

Open-Book Quizzes for each chapter in the textbook help to ensure that your students are reading and comprehending their textbook reading assignments.

An Image Collection includes all the illustrations and photos from the textbook.

Suggestions for Working with Students Who Speak English as a Second Language help you promote the success of ESL learners.

Answer Keys to the Critical Thinking Questions, Case Studies, and Study Guide activities and exercises are available for your own use or for distribution to your students.

FOR THE STUDENT

Evolve Student Resources, available at http://evolve. elsevier.com/Visovsky/LPNpharmacology/, include more than 400 interactive Review Questions for the NCLEX-PN® Examination, Video Clips, an Audio Glossary with pronunciations for more than 150 Key Terms, 12 Interactive Drug Dosage Calculators, newly proposed

FDA Guidelines on Pregnancy and Lactation, and links to updated information on the Top 200 Prescription Drugs.

A comprehensive Study Guide, available separately, includes Worksheets and Review Sheets with an enhanced focus on critical thinking, prioritizing, care of older adults, and cultural considerations. The exercises focus on promoting medication safety and prevention of drug errors.

In working with patients, the nursing student will quickly learn that giving medications is one of the most challenging parts of the nursing role. A nurse who develops the knowledge and skills needed to correctly give medications will be noticed and recognized with respect by both patients and colleagues in the healthcare system. Both the responsibilities and the personal rewards are great.

Constance G. Visovsky, PhD, RN, ACNP, FAAN
Cheryl H. Zambroski, PhD, RN
Shirley Meier Hosler, RN, BSN, MSN

Acknowledgments

The ninth edition of *Introduction to Clinical Pharmacology* represents the first collaboration among three experienced educators and clinicians who have taught pharmacology to all levels of nursing students. Much thought and discourse took place among us regarding the content that students really need to know and the best way to present the material to maximize student use of the text, as well as comprehension and retention of the material. Thus I am truly grateful to my colleagues, Dr. Zambroski, Ms. Hosler, and Dr. Passmore, for their excellence and dedication to this work and for providing a textbook, test bank, and student study guide that will prove to be a critical resource for the LPN/VN student and faculty.

The author team is extremely grateful to our dear friend and mentor, Dr. M. Linda Workman, who served as a special editor to this author team. Dr. Workman freely shared her knowledge and expertise in pharmacology content, teaching, and publishing that surely impacted the success of this text and supplemental materials. She assisted us from the initial concept through the entire production of this textbook, study guide, and test bank. Her patience, guidance, and support to this author team can never be adequately repaid.

The author team is grateful for the Elsevier editorial, production, marketing, and design staff. Special thanks to Nancy O'Brien, Senior Content Strategist, for believing in this new author team; and to Laura Goodrich, Senior Content Development Specialist, and Tracey Schriefer, Senior Project Manager, who provided ongoing editorial guidance and support and worked tirelessly to keep the text production on track.

On behalf of the author team, I would like to express our eternal gratitude to our families and friends, who supported our endeavors on this project and were our cheerleaders throughout the process. I would like to acknowledge the love and support of my husband and soulmate, Bob Visovsky, that sustained me during this project. Thank you to my students, who inspire me every day to be a better teacher. Lastly, I would like to thank my God for presenting this opportunity to me and for providing the fortitude to take this textbook to completion.

**Constance (Connie) G. Visovsky,
PhD, RN, ACNP, FAAN**

A special thank you to my husband, James, for his ongoing love and support during this project.

Thanks to M. Linda Workman for her patience and guidance as we were writing this textbook.

Cheryl H. Zambroski, PhD, RN

Thank you to M. Linda Workman for your patient mentoring, and thank you to Connie Visovsky for being a colleague and an extraordinary forever friend.

To every student who has shared a path with me along the way: I could never have achieved the process of learning how to write if you hadn't first taught me how to teach.

To my hearts: Daniel, James, Crissy, and Emerald—never be afraid to step out of your comfort zone.

Shirley Meier Hosler, RN, BSN, MSN

About the Authors

CONSTANCE G. VISOVSKY, PHD, RN, ACNP, FAAN

Constance (Connie) G. Visovsky received her BN and MS degrees in nursing from the University of Rochester, Rochester, New York, and her PhD from Case Western Reserve University, Cleveland, Ohio. She is an acute care nurse practitioner, specializing in the treatment of patients with cancer. She is considered an expert in the area of chemotherapy-induced peripheral neuropathy and has many publications on this topic to her credit. Dr. Visovsky is an experienced nurse educator and scientist, and is currently an Associate Professor at the University of South Florida.

CHERYL H. ZAMBROSKI, PHD, RN

Cheryl H. Zambroski received her diploma in nursing from Rockford Memorial Hospital School of Nursing, her BS and MS in Nursing from the University of Illinois, and her PhD in Nursing from the University of Kentucky. Her clinical experiences focused on adult health in areas including emergency nursing, critical care, and medical-surgical nursing. She also worked as a clinical nurse specialist in cardiovascular and thoracic nursing. Her teaching career began at Jefferson Community College in Louisville, Kentucky. She later taught a variety of courses in the undergraduate program and clinical nurse specialist track at the University of Louisville. Currently, Dr. Zambroski teaches pharmacology, population health, and mental health nursing at the University of South Florida, where she serves as the Director of Undergraduate Student Success.

SHIRLEY MEIER HOSLER, RN, BSN, MSN

Shirley Meier Hosler received her AAS from Maria College in Albany, New York, later receiving her BSN from the University of New Mexico and MSN from the University of Illinois, Chicago. Shirley has more than 40 years of clinical, administrative, educational, and academic experience having worked as a staff nurse, held numerous administrative nursing positions, and served on the faculty of colleges and universities. Her educational accomplishments include the development of online and classroom programs for nursing, emergency medical personnel, and paramedic professionals. Shirley has a broad base of expertise with specific concentration in the areas of prehospital medicine, adult medicine, and critical care. She has received numerous awards for her unique and innovative educational accomplishments and has been particularly recognized for her ability to translate complex clinical principles to a diversity of audiences and students with varying degrees of training, experience, and expertise through her down-to-earth teaching approach and style. Shirley currently serves as Adjunct Faculty for National American University in Albuquerque, New Mexico, and Santa Fe Community College in Santa Fe, New Mexico.

To the Student

READING AND REVIEW TOOLS

Objectives introduce the chapter topics.

Key Terms are listed with page number references, and difficult medical, nursing, or scientific terms are accompanied by simple phonetic pronunciations. Key terms are considered essential to understanding the professional language and chapter content. Key terms are defined within the chapter, are in color the first time they appear in the narrative, and are briefly defined in the text, with complete definitions in the Glossary.

Each chapter ends with a **Get Ready for the NCLEX®
Examination!** section that includes: (1) **Key Points**
that reiterate the chapter objectives and serve as a
useful review of concepts, (2) an extensive set of
Review Questions for the NCLEX® Examination
with answers located on the Evolve site, (3) **Case
Studies** with answers located on the Evolve site, (4)
Drug Calculation Review Questions with answers
located on the Evolve site, and (5) **Critical Thinking
Questions** with answers located on the Evolve site.

A complete Bibliography section in the back of the text
cites evidence-based information and provides
resources for enhancing knowledge.

CHAPTER FEATURES

Procedures related to giving drugs are presented in a
logical format with a defined *purpose* and relevant
illustrations and are clearly defined and presented in
a logical set of *steps*.

Memory Jogger boxes restate key points from
anatomy, physiology, or pharmacology that are
important for students to remember and serve as
foundational information for giving and monitoring
drug therapy. Basic principles of drug calculation
are presented in easy-to-follow steps to reinforce
learning.

Top Tip for Safety boxes identify the important
knowledge that will aid students in giving particular
drugs and provide critical information and warnings
of adverse effects of drugs that are important to
patient safety.

Lifespan Considerations boxes draw attention to
information that would be especially important to
remember in giving a specific drug to older adults,
children, or pregnant/lactating women.

Safety Alerts indicate a particularly important
factor to remember about a specific drug or drug
class.

Canadian Drugs indicated within the tables point
out brands available only in Canada.

Video Clips located in the margins of the text
indicate available relevant videos located on the
Evolve site.

Bookmark This boxes list useful websites that
provide important resources for all nurses.

Contents

UNIT I GENERAL PRINCIPLES, 1

1 Pharmacology and the Nursing Process in LPN Practice, 1

The LPN/VN's Role and the Nursing Process, 1
Assessment, 2
Diagnosis, 4
Planning, 4
Drug Orders and the Nursing Care Plan, 4
Implementation, 5
The 9 Rights of Drug Administration, 5
Evaluation, 9

2 Legal, Regulatory, and Ethical Aspects of Drug Administration, 11

Introduction, 11
Regulation of Drug Administration, 12
Federal Laws, 12
Canadian Drug Legislation, 15
The Drug Order, 16
Legal Prescriptions, 16
Types of Drug Orders, 16
State Law and Healthcare Agency Policies, 16
Drug Administration Systems, 17
Kardex and Electronic Drug Systems, 18
Drug Errors, 18
Medication Reconciliation, 20
Protection of Healthcare Workers, 20

3 Principles of Pharmacology, 22

Drug Names, 23
Drug Attachment, 23
Basic Drug Processes, 24
Absorption, 24
Distribution, 25
Metabolism, 25
Excretion or Elimination, 26
Drug Actions, 27
Bioequivalence, 28
Drug Interactions, 28
Drug Therapy and Special Populations, 29
Pediatric Drug Therapy Considerations, 30
Older Adult Drug Therapy Considerations, 30
Patient Teaching Considerations, 31
Drug Therapy Considerations During Pregnancy and Lactation, 32
Drug Cards, 32

UNIT II PRINCIPLES OF DRUG ADMINISTRATION, 35

4 Drug Calculation: Preparing and Giving Drugs, 35

Calculating Drug Dosages, 36
Fraction Method, 36
Ratio and Proportion Method, 36
Dimensional Analysis Method, 36
Drug Calculation Using Units, 37
Calculating Drug Dosages for Infants and Children, 38
Calculations for IV Infusions, 39
Calculating IV Flow Rate, 39
Calculating IV Administration Time, 39
Calculating Total Infusion Time, 39
Factors That Influence IV Flow Rates, 40
Flow Rates for Infants and Children, 40
General Principles of Drug Administration, 40
Enteral Drugs, 41
Giving Oral Drugs, 41
Giving Drugs by Nasogastric or Percutaneous Endoscopic Gastrostomy Tube, 42
Parenteral Drugs, 43
General Principles, 43
Procedure for Preparing and Giving Parenteral Drugs, 45
Percutaneous Drugs, 56
Giving Topical and Transdermal Drugs, 56
Giving Drugs Through Mucous Membranes, 57

UNIT III DRUG CATEGORIES, 64

5 Anti-Infective Drugs: Antibacterial, Antitubercular, and Antifungal Agents, 64

Infection, 65
Normal Flora, 65
Pathogens, 65
Determination of Infection, 65
Anti-Infectives, 66
Drug Susceptibility and Resistance, 66
General Considerations for Anti-Infective (Antimicrobial) Drug Therapy, 66
Antibiotics, 66
Penicillins, 68
Cephalosporins, 72
Other Cell Wall Synthesis Inhibitors, 73
Tetracyclines, 73

Macrolides, 74
Aminoglycosides, 76
Miscellaneous Protein Synthesis Inhibitors, 76
Sulfonamides, 76
Fluoroquinolones, 77
Antitubercular Drugs, 78
Antifungal Drugs, 83
Antiparasitic Drugs, 87
Protozoa, 87
Antiprotozoal Drugs, 87
Anthelmintics, 90

6 Antivirals and Antiretrovirals, 93

Virus, 94
Antivirals, 94
Antiviral Drugs for Herpes Simplex Virus
Infections, 94
Antiviral Drugs for Influenza, 94
Antiviral Drugs for Cytomegalovirus and
Respiratory Syncytial Virus, 94
Antiviral Drugs for Hepatitis B and Hepatitis C
Viruses, 96
Retrovirus, 98
Antiretrovirals, 99
Actions of Drugs Used for Antiretroviral
Therapy, 102
Expected Side Effects of Antiretroviral
Drugs, 102
Adverse Reactions of Antiretroviral Drugs, 102
Pre-Exposure Prophylaxis, 103

7 Drugs for Allergy and Respiratory Problems, 106

Allergy, 107
Drug Therapy for Allergy, 107
Antihistamines, 107
Leukotriene Inhibitors, 111
Mast Cell Stabilizers (Cromones), 112
Decongestants, 112
Asthma and Chronic Obstructive Pulmonary
Disease, 114
Asthma, 114
Chronic Obstructive Pulmonary Disease, 114
Drug Therapy for Asthma and Chronic
Obstructive Pulmonary Disease, 114
Bronchodilators, 115
Anti-Inflammatory Drugs, 119
Mucolytics and Antitussives, 119
Mucolytics, 119
Antitussives, 121

8 Drugs Affecting the Renal/Urinary and Cardiovascular Systems, 125

DRUGS THAT AFFECT THE RENAL/URINARY
SYSTEM, 126
Diuretics, 126
Drugs for Benign Prostatic Hyperplasia, 130
Bladder Anesthetics, 130
Drugs for Overactive Bladder, 132

DRUGS THAT AFFECT THE
CARDIOVASCULAR SYSTEM, 132
Antihyperlipidemics, 134
HMG-CoA Reductase Inhibitors (Statins), 135
Nonstatin Antihyperlipidemic Drugs, 137
Antihypertensive Drugs, 138
Antihypertensive Drug Actions, 140
Antihypertensive Drug Uses, 145
Expected Side Effects of Antihypertensive
Drugs, 145
Adverse Reactions of Antihypertensive
Drugs, 146
Drug Interactions With Antihypertensive
Drugs, 146
Drugs Used for Angina and Myocardial
Infarction, 147
Antianginals, 147
Nitrates, 147
Antidysrhythmics, 149
Inotropic Drugs, 153

9 Drug Therapy for Central Nervous System Problems, 158

Central Nervous System Functions, 159
Drugs for Parkinson's Disease, 160
Dopamine Agonists, 161
Catechol-O-Methyltransferase Inhibitors, 165
Monoamine Oxidase Type B Inhibitors, 165
Drugs for Alzheimer's Disease, 166
Cholinesterase Inhibitors, 167
N-Methyl-D-Aspartate Blockers, 169
DRUGS FOR EPILEPSY, 169
Traditional Antiepileptic Drugs, 170
Newer Antiepileptic Drugs, 174
Oxcarbazepine, 174
Lamotrigine, 174
Lacosamide, 176
Topiramate, 177
Drugs for Multiple Sclerosis, 178
Nonspecific Anti-Inflammatory Drugs, 179
Specific Drugs for Multiple Sclerosis, 179

10 Drug Therapy for Mental Health, 183

Drug Therapy and Mental Illness, 184
Drugs for Sleep and Anxiety, 184
Sedatives-Hypnotics, 184
Antianxiety Drugs, 187
Antipsychotics, 189
Typical Antipsychotic Drugs, 190
Atypical Antipsychotic Drugs, 193
Antidepressants and Mood Stabilizers, 195
Antidepressants, 195
Selective Serotonin Reuptake Inhibitors, 196
Serotonin Norepinephrine Reuptake
Inhibitors, 201
Tricyclic Antidepressants, 202
Monoamine Oxidase Inhibitors, 203
Mood Stabilizers, 204

11 Drugs for Pain Management, 210

Pain, 210
 Pain Definition, 210
 How Pain Is Perceived, 211
 Principles of Pain Management, 212
Analgesic Drugs for Pain Management, 212
 Opioid Agonist Analgesics, 214
 Opioid Agonist-Antagonist Analgesics, 217
 Nonopioid Centrally Acting Analgesics, 218
 Acetaminophen, 219
Miscellaneous Drugs for Pain Management, 220
 Corticosteroids, 220
 NSAIDs, 221
 Skeletal Muscle Relaxants, 221
 Antidepressants, 222
 Anticonvulsants, 223

12 Anti-Inflammatory, Antiarthritis, and Antigout Drugs, 225

Inflammation Causes and Action, 225
Inflammation Management, 226
 NSAIDs, 227
 Corticosteroids, 230
 Disease-Modifying Antirheumatic Drugs, 235
Gout, 237
 Management of Inflammation and Gout Pain, 237
 Antigout Drugs, 237

13 Drugs for Gastrointestinal Problems, 240

The Digestive System, 241
Antiemetic Drugs, 242
 Serotonin (5-HT₃) Receptor Antagonists, 243
 Substance P/Neurokinin₁ Receptor Antagonists, 245
 Phenothiazines, 246
 Cannabinoids, 247
 Promotility Drugs, 248
Drugs for Peptic Ulcer Disease and Gastroesophageal Reflux Disease, 248
 Antacids, 251
 Histamine H₂ Receptor Antagonists, 252
 Proton Pump Inhibitors, 252
 Cytoprotective Drugs, 253
Drugs for Constipation and Diarrhea, 253
 Drugs for Constipation, 254
 Drugs for Diarrhea, 259

14 Drugs Affecting the Hematologic System, 265

Blood Clotting, 265
Anticoagulants, 266
 Platelet Inhibitors, 268
 Direct Thrombin Inhibitors, 270
 Indirect Thrombin Inhibitors, 271
 Vitamin K Antagonists, 273
Fibrinolytic Drugs, 275
Erythropoiesis-Stimulating Agents, 276

15 Drugs for Immunization and Immunomodulation, 279

Overview of Immunity, 280
 Innate Immunity, 280
Vaccination, 282
Immunomodulating Therapy, 287
 Selective Immunosuppressants for Autoimmune Diseases, 287
 Selective Immunosuppressants to Prevent Transplant Rejection, 287

16 Hormones and Drugs for Osteoporosis, 292

Overview of the Endocrine System, 292
Drugs for Thyroid Problems, 293
 Hypothyroidism, 293
 Thyroid Hormone Agonists, 294
 Hyperthyroidism, 296
 Antithyroid Drugs, 296
Drugs for Adrenal Gland Problems, 297
 Adrenal Gland Hypofunction, 297
 Adrenal Gland Hyperfunction, 298
Female Sex Hormones, 299
 Overview, 299
 Menopause, 300
 Drugs for Menopause Relief, 300
 Drugs for Hormonal Contraception, 302
Male Sex Hormones, 304
 Overview, 304
 Androgens, 304
Drugs for Osteoporosis, 305
 Bisphosphonates, 306
 Estrogen Agonists/Antagonists, 307
 Osteoclast Monoclonal Antibodies, 307

17 Drug Therapy for Diabetes, 309

Diabetes, 310
 Blood Glucose Control, 310
 Loss of Glucose Control, 310
 Classification of Diabetes Mellitus, 311
DRUG THERAPY FOR DIABETES MELLITUS, 311
Non-Insulin Antidiabetic Drugs, 311
 Insulin Stimulators (Secretogogues), 312
 Biguanides, 314
 Insulin Sensitizers, 314
 Alpha-Glucosidase Inhibitors, 315
 Incretin Mimetics, 316
 Amylin Analogs, 317
 DPP-4 Inhibitors, 318
 Sodium-Glucose Co-Transport Inhibitors, 320
 Insulin, 320

18 Drugs for Ear and Eye Problems, 329

EAR PROBLEMS, 329
Ear Structure and Function, 329
Drugs to Manage Ear Problems, 330
EYE PROBLEMS, 331

Eye Structure and Function, 332
Glaucoma, 334
    Prostaglandin Agonists, 335
    Beta-Adrenergic Antagonists, 336
    Alpha-Adrenergic Agonists, 340
    Cholinergic Drugs, 341
    Carbonic Anhydrase Inhibitors, 342

19　Over-the-Counter Drugs, Herbal and Alternative Drugs, and Vitamins and Minerals, 346

Overview, 346
    Documenting Patient Healthcare Practices, 346
Over-the-Counter Drugs, 347
    Product Labeling, 347
    Patient Teaching, 347
Herbal Products and Complementary and Alternative Medicine, 348
    Product Labeling, 349
    Pros and Cons, 349
Vitamins, 350
    Vitamin A, 351
    Vitamin B_1 (Thiamine), 352

    Vitamin B_2 (Riboflavin), 352
    Niacin, 352
    Vitamin B_6, 352
    Folic Acid, 353
    Vitamin B_{12}, 353
    Vitamin C, 354
    Vitamin D, 354
    Vitamin E, 355
    Vitamin K, 355
Minerals, 356
    Calcium, 356
    Iron, 356
    Magnesium, 357
    Potassium, 357
    Zinc, 358

Bibliography, 360

Glossary, 362

Pharmacology and the Nursing Process in LPN Practice

1

http://evolve.elsevier.com/Visovsky/LPNpharmacology/

Learning Outcomes

1. Explain how licensed practical or vocational nurses (LPNs/VNs) use the nursing process in practicing safe drug administration.
2. Compare the differences between subjective and objective data relating to drug administration.
3. Describe the specific actions involved in using the nursing process to safely give drugs.
4. List specific nursing activities related to assessing, planning, implementing, and evaluating the patient's response to drugs.
5. Describe each of the nine rights of administration as essential components of safe drug administration.

Key Terms

9 Rights of Drug Administration (p. 5) A series of nursing actions to protect the patient from drug error.

adverse effect (advurs' ē-fekt, p. 9) A drug effect that is more severe than expected and has the potential to damage tissue or cause serious health problems. It may also be called adverse effect, toxic effect, or toxicity and usually requires an intervention by the prescriber.

assessment (ă-SĔS-mĕnt, p. 2) The first step of the nursing process that involves gathering information about the patient that will be used in planning care.

contraindication (con-tra-in′dikā′shən, p. 5) A health-related reason for not giving a specific drug to a patient or a group of patients.

diagnosis (dǐ-ăg-NŌ-sǐs, p. 4) A name (or label) for the patient's disease or condition.

expected side effects (p. 9) Unintended but not unusual effects of the drug that occur in many people taking the drug; they are usually mild and do not require that the drug be stopped.

evaluation (ǐ-văl-ū-Ā-shŭn, p. 9) The process of determining the right response looking at what happens to the patient when the nursing care plan is put into action. It is an appraisal of the treatment effectiveness.

healthcare setting (HĔLTH-kār SĔT-tǐng, p. 2) Any setting in which the LPN/VN practices nursing.

identifiers (ī-DĚN-tǐ-fī-rz, p. 6) Information used to reliably prove an individual is the person for whom the drug treatment is intended. Identifiers may be person's full name, their medical record identification number, birth date, or even the telephone number.

implementation (ǐm-plě-měn-TĀ-shŭn, p. 5) The act of carrying out the planned interventions.

nursing process (NŬR-sǐng PRŎ-sěs, p. 2) A system to guide the nurse's work in a logical way. Consists of five major steps: (1) assessment; (2) diagnosis; (3) planning; (4) implementation; and (5) evaluation.

objective data (ŏb-JĔK-tǐv DĀT-ă, p. 3) Information that can be seen, heard, felt, or measured by someone other than the patient.

planning (p. 4) Using information gathered in the nursing assessment about the patient to set short-term and long-term goals.

subjective data (sŭb-JĔK-tǐv DAT-ă, p. 2) Reports of what the patient says he or she is feeling or thinks.

therapeutic effect (thěr-ă-PŬ-tǐk, p. 9) The intended action of the drug, also known as a drug's beneficial outcome.

THE LPN/VN'S ROLE AND THE NURSING PROCESS

Licensed practical or vocational nurses (LPNs/VNs) play a vitally important role in providing nursing care for patients and families. In fact, the need for a well-educated LPN/VN workforce is predicted to grow even faster than the average rate of all other occupations. The factors that increase the demand for LPNs/VNs include an aging nursing workforce reaching retirement age, an aging population in general, and an increased number of people who are living with chronic (and complex) illnesses.

LPN/VN practice has shifted quite dramatically over the past decades from the time when most graduates practiced in acute care settings (hospital-based care) to today when graduates practice in a wide variety of long-term and community-based settings. LPNs/VNs practice in nursing homes, assisted living agencies, outpatient clinics, home health agencies, hospices, and rehabilitation centers, to name just a few. No matter the setting, as an LPN/VN, you will share a responsibility with registered nurses (RNs) and other members of the healthcare team to provide safe, quality, and cost-effective care.

Wherever you choose to practice, it is likely that drug administration will be a significant part of your role. In fact, a recent survey of new LPN/VNs revealed that about 40% of work hours were related to providing care relating to giving drugs and to monitoring patients who are receiving drugs, including parenteral therapies.

Before we begin discussing specific drugs, we will review the nursing process as it relates to drug administration. Although you may be familiar with the nursing process, we are going to focus on how you will use the nursing process as you safely give drugs to patients in a variety of settings. To review, the nursing process is a system that guides the nurse's work in a logical way (Fig. 1.1). The nursing process consists of the following five major steps: (1) assessment, (2) diagnosis, (3) planning, (4) implementation, and (5) evaluation.

ASSESSMENT

Assessment is the first step in the nursing process and involves gathering information (also called "data") about the patient that will be used in planning care. An RN is typically assigned as the staff member who must perform the initial full assessment for each patient. As an LPN/VN, you will often make vital contributions to this assessment. This step of the nursing process is important because it gives you initial information as you begin to make a record for developing the plan of care.

The first part of assessment relating to drug administration involves gathering information about the patient and the patient's health condition before you give the drugs. When the patient is admitted to the healthcare setting (any setting in which LPN/VNs practice nursing), you can obtain that information by talking to the patient (or his or her caregiver if necessary), checking the patient closely for signs and symptoms of illness, viewing past medical records, or reviewing information the patient may bring with him or her. Ask carefully about any current health problems, a history of illnesses and/or surgeries, and drugs (including over-the-counter and herbals) taken both now and in the past. This information is important for all team members and helps everyone to plan the patient's care. Information in the patient's history often directs the nurse and the physician to look for certain physical signs of illness that may be present.

Information you gather through assessment falls into two groups: subjective data and objective data. Subjective data are reports of what the patient says he or she is feeling or thinks. For example, if a patient reports feeling nauseated after taking a drug, you must accept the patient's word. You cannot see, hear, or feel the patient's nausea—that is why it is subjective. A patient may state that he or she has trouble breathing. Although you may observe rapid breathing, the degree of difficulty the patient feels cannot be measured. Information is subjective if you have to rely on the patient's words or

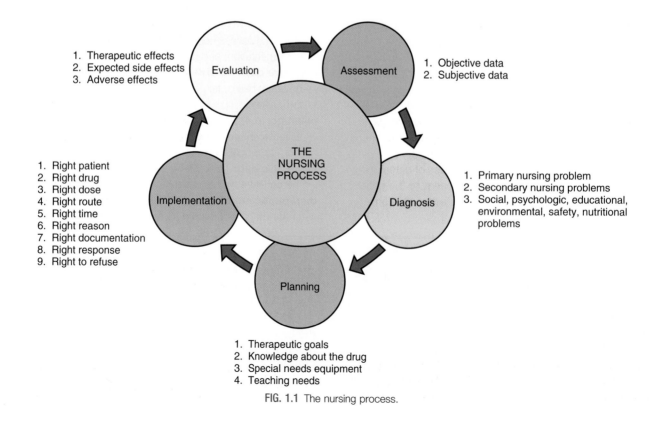

FIG. 1.1 The nursing process.

if the symptoms cannot be felt by anyone other than the patient. In such cases you would report, "The patient states that..." Other examples of subjective data that you may learn about from a patient interview are:

- the chief problem according to the patient (in the patient's own words)
- the patient's belief about what caused the problem
- the patient's description about what relieves the problem
- the patient's report of the severity of the problem

Objective data are data that can be seen, heard, felt, or measured by someone other than the patient. These include information obtained when the healthcare provider performs a physical examination or orders laboratory tests, x-rays, and other diagnostic tests. Typically the RN or physician will conduct a comprehensive physical assessment. As an LPN/VN, it will be important to assess vital signs (respiratory rate, pulse, blood pressure, weight, height, temperature), physical findings based on careful observation, auscultation (listening with the stethoscope), and light palpation as appropriate for your clinical setting and your state Nurse Practice Act. Other examples of objective data include:

- presence of edema
- quality of a cough
- percentage of foods eaten at a meal
- measures of intake and output

It is especially important to gather subjective and objective assessment data when the patient is first seen or on admission to the healthcare setting. This provides initial information that can be used as a baseline for comparison as care progresses. In addition to the physical examination, it is important to gather a good patient history. Thus asking questions and listening carefully to the patient may be just as important as the physical examination or the results of laboratory tests. Because the LPN/VN is often with the patient, he or she will play a very important role in continuing to listen to what the patient says and report new information to the other healthcare team members.

The nurse may not always be the one gathering the subjective and objective data; however, the nurse and everyone else on the healthcare team should learn whatever information they can from the chart, the physician, the family, and other team members, and use that information to plan the patient's care. Understanding the difference between subjective and objective information will help you in reporting, or charting, the information. Based on our previous example, if the patient reports nausea (subjective information), your charting should say, "The patient reports nausea," rather than "The patient is nauseated," because you do not objectively see nausea. On the other hand, if the patient vomits (objective information), you will record the time, color, and amount.

Much of your role in assessing can be reporting data you collect to the RN (or to other members of the healthcare team). The primary role you play in assessing

the patient is defined by your state Nurse Practice Act, which lists what actions LPN/VNs may and may not do. In addition, your role may vary according to your healthcare setting's policies and procedures.

Factors to Consider in Assessing the Patient

Certain information is very helpful in planning the care of the patient who is receiving drug therapy. As mentioned earlier, the baseline nursing assessment is conducted at the time of the patient's admission to the healthcare setting. One important part of the assessment is the patient's drug history. The patient is typically the best source; however, you may also include reports from caregivers (such as the spouse, close relatives, or friends) and past medical records (often in the electronic medical record [EMR]).

When asking about the patient's drug history, you will want to make assessments in the following areas:

1. Symptoms, signs, or diseases that explain the patient's need for a drug (such as high blood glucose levels, high blood pressure, or pain)
2. The names and, when possible, dosages of all the drugs the patient is taking, for example:
   - prescription drugs (patients often forget to mention birth control pills as well as implanted birth control measures in this category)
   - over-the-counter drugs such as aspirin, vitamins, laxatives, cold and sinus preparations, and antacids
   - alcohol or street drugs used for recreational purposes (such as marijuana or cocaine)
   - alternative therapies such as herbal agents or nutritional supplements
3. Any problems that the patient has had with drug therapy, for example:
   - allergies: include the name of the drug and the type of the reaction that the patient experienced (in other words, whether it was a mild or severe effect)
   - diseases that may prohibit or limit use of some drugs (such as sickle cell disease, glucose-6-phosphate dehydrogenase deficiency, history of drug addiction, or immune deficiencies)

Assessments for all of these areas are important because this information can help prevent drug interactions or complications of drug therapy. You will also use this information as you monitor your patient's response and any changes in patient condition or status that may influence drug therapy during the time the patient is in the healthcare setting. This will help you determine whether the drug is helping the patient.

Memory Jogger

Nursing assessment is using your observational, questioning, and listening skills to learn information about the patient that can be used to ensure you are safely giving drugs.

DIAGNOSIS

Once the assessment information has been collected, the nurse and other healthcare team members must make a diagnosis (a name [label] for the patient's disease or condition). The physician will decide the medical diagnoses. The RN will determine the nursing diagnoses. Although you will come to some decisions about how sick the patient is and how carefully you need to monitor him or her, your role does not include the development of formal diagnoses. Nevertheless, you will use knowledge about the diagnoses as you contribute to the plan of care. Examples of follow-up questions you will need to ask relating to giving drugs include:

- What are the major health-related problems of this patient?
- What drugs is the patient likely to require?
- What special knowledge or equipment is required in giving these drugs?
- What special concerns or cultural beliefs does the patient have?
- How much does this patient understand about the treatment and drugs prescribed?
- What factors affect the patient's ability to care for himself or herself?

The answers to these questions will (1) help you contribute to the goals of nursing care, (2) affect strategies you will use to care for the patient, and (3) tell you what type of patient teaching will be needed. Answering these questions may be more challenging with children, older adults, or people whose language or culture is different from yours. However, just as a physician must have the correct diagnosis to prescribe the right treatment, finding the correct answers to these questions helps you to plan the best care for the patient.

PLANNING

Based on the data you help collect, the medical and nursing diagnoses are made, goals are set, and nursing care plans are written. As a member of the healthcare team, the LPN/VN will be able to assist with the planning step. The nursing care plan involves a collaboration with nurses and the patients or caregivers. Using the information gathered in the assessment about the patient's history, medical and social problems, risk factors, and how ill the patient may be, goals will be set on either a short-term or a long-term basis. For example, short-term goals may be written that "the patient will describe pain at a level of 3 or below on a scale of 0 to 10, 30 minutes after receiving a drug for pain." An example of a long-term goal would be, "The patient will show how to rotate injection sites for using his or her insulin pen by the time of discharge."

> ### 💡 Memory Jogger
>
> When collecting the drug history, make sure to include the patient's use of over-the-counter drugs, such as herbal and nutritional supplements, because these may interfere with prescription drugs.

DRUG ORDERS AND THE NURSING CARE PLAN

Physicians, nurse practitioners, nurse midwives, nurse anesthetists, clinical nurse specialists, and physician assistants may write drug orders according to individual state laws. Large hospitals may have a staff *hospitalist*, a physician or nurse practitioner who practices in the hospital, to oversee care for all patients. Teaching hospitals may have resident doctors who are still in educational programs.

Once the drug is ordered, the nurse must verify that the order is accurate. This is usually done by checking the drug administration record or electronic medical record against the original order. You will need to learn and follow the procedures of the agency where you work when checking drugs and drug orders. In all care environments you must carefully check each time you give a drug. This is essential to maintaining patient safety and minimizing the risk for error or adverse effects.

The nurse must also apply knowledge about the drug to the specific drug order to determine whether the drug and the dose ordered seem to be correct. No part of the order or the reason for giving the drug should be unclear. (Chapter 2 lists what information is required for a clear and legal drug order.) Any questions about whether a drug is appropriate or safe for that patient *must* be answered before the drug is given. The electronic medical record may alert the nurse if there is a problem with the order. However, good clinical judgment in carrying out the drug order is very important. If you determine that (1) any part of the order is incorrect or unclear, (2) the patient's condition would be made worse by the drug, (3) the person ordering the drug may not have had all the information needed about the patient when drug therapy was planned, or (4) there has been a change in the patient's condition and a question has arisen about whether the drug should be given, then the drug should be *withheld* (that is, not given) until the question can be answered and the healthcare provider called. If you believe there is a problem with the drug order and the provider cannot be contacted or does not change the order under question, notify the charge nurse and the nursing supervisor as soon as possible. Most hospitals have clear policies about whom to contact, how to report this problem, and what to do next.

Once you have the drug order, and have decided to give the drug, include in your plan those patient problems that may increase the risk for issues relating to the drug's side effects. For example, a patient who has poor vision may have a risk for falling in an unfamiliar hospital or nursing home setting. This will be important if you are giving a diuretic and the patient needs to go to the bathroom frequently. You will need to plan ahead so that the patient can safely get to the bathroom. The importance of these problems may change over time as the patient's condition changes. Ongoing communication between nurses and the healthcare team is important to maintain safe, quality, and cost-effective patient care.

Factors to Consider in Planning to Give a Drug

Planning to give a drug involves four important steps:

1. Know the reason you are giving the patient the drug. (In other words, what is this drug supposed to do for the patient?)
2. Learn specific information about the drug including:
   - the major action of the drug;
   - negative side effects that may develop;
   - the usual dosage, route, and frequency;
   - situations in which the drug should not be given (contraindications); and
   - main drug interactions (in other words, the possible influence of another drug given at the same time).
3. Plan for special storage or procedures, techniques, or equipment needs.
   - Does the solution need to be shaken before giving?
   - Should the drug be refrigerated?
   - Do you need a specific syringe (such as an insulin syringe)?
   - What special techniques are necessary for giving the drug, such as using an inhaler or not applying pressure to the site after giving certain injectable drugs?
4. Develop a teaching plan for the patient, including:
   - what the patient needs to know about the drug's action and side effects,
   - what the patient needs to know to take the drug correctly, and
   - what the patient needs to report to the nurse or physician if there are any problems.

As you develop your plan, make sure to use the information you gathered in your assessment and your knowledge about the drug. You will use this information as you prepare to implement your plan. Whether to give the drug will be dependent on your assessment, your knowledge, and your professional judgment.

🔷 Top Tip for Safety

Drug Orders

Make certain that you understand each part of the drug order. Do not give the drug if you have a question about any part of the order.

The planning step of the nursing process is also the time to:

- Get any special equipment you need to give the drug (such as intravenous [IV] infusion pumps, alcohol wipes, or nebulizers).
- Review any special procedures you will need to give the drug (such as the Z-track injection technique or for giving a rectal suppository).

All of this information can be documented in the nursing care plan into the paper or electronic medical record so that other team members can see the plan.

IMPLEMENTATION

Implementation involves carrying out your plan of care as you safely give the drugs to the patient. In planning care, you learned why each drug was ordered, the drug's actions, and how to safely give the drug. For example, if you are giving an angiotensin-converting enzyme inhibitor (see Chapter 8) to a patient with high blood pressure, you will need to check the patient's blood pressure before giving the drug. On the other hand, if you are planning to give the ordered penicillin antibiotic (see Chapter 5) and you notice the patient has a red rash on his or her chest and arms, you would hold the next dose of the drug until you have reported the rash to the healthcare provider because it may indicate an allergic reaction. Then after you have carried out the plan, you will record in the patient's chart or electronic medical record that you have given the drug.

THE 9 RIGHTS OF DRUG ADMINISTRATION

A major strategy for giving drugs to patients is called the **9 Rights of Drug Administration**. There are nine commonly recognized rights of drug administration that the nurse must always keep in mind (Box 1.1).

You may have heard nurses in the clinical setting discuss the importance of the "five rights," "six rights," or "eight rights." Over time, nursing has continued to emphasize those essential components of safe drug administration and added more rights.

For our purposes the nine rights ensure that you identify the *right patient* and give the *right drug* with the *right dose* using the *right route* at the *right time* for the *right reason*. Then you use the *right documentation* to record that the dose has been given. You will then monitor the patient to assess the *right response*. The final right is that patients do have the *right to refuse* the drug. You might wonder: How can I remember nine things? A runner who really enjoyed racing in 15K races (9.3

Box 1.1   The 9 Rights of Drug Administration

- The right patient—use at least two identifiers.
- The right drug—check the drug label at least three times.
- The right dose—make sure that you use the right amount of the drug; double-check the dose.
- The right route—never change the route of administration without an order.
- The right time—make sure that the drug has not been given recently or should be given at a different time of day.
- The right reason—does this make sense for this patient? Know your patient and the drug.
- The right documentation—document after you have given the drug, never before.
- The right response—how is the patient responding to the drug? Does it work?
- The right to refuse—patients have the right to refuse; make sure to ask the patient to clarify his or her reason, provide good patient teaching, and document.

miles) said that he liked them the best because he could divide them into three 5Ks (3.1 miles) so it seemed easier. You can do the same with the nine rights.

We will review each right and explain the reason these are essential for safe, quality, and cost-effective care.

> **Memory Jogger**
>
> **The 9 Rights of Drug Administration (Three at a Time)**
> - Right patient, right drug, right dose
> - Right route, right time, right reason
> - Right documentation, right response, right to refuse

The Right Patient

Before you give any drug, you need to make sure that you identify the right patient. The National Patient Safety Goals claim that the purpose of this is to: (1) reliably identify the individual as the person for whom the treatment is intended, and (2) match the treatment to the person. To properly identify the patient, you will use at least two identifiers. **Identifiers** are information that is used to reliably prove an individual is the person for whom the drug treatment is intended. Identifiers may be the person's full name, his or her medical record identification number, birth date, or even telephone number. These may be compared with the patient's identification bracelet (wristband) if appropriate. Healthcare agencies may specify the main identifiers to be used in the setting and/or use a bar code system to scan the drug to the wristband.

For patients who are alert and oriented, asking them their full name and birthdate, and comparing with the medical record number is very clear. On the other hand, for those who are hard of hearing, confused, very young or very old, or are critically ill, make sure to compare the name, birthdate, or medical record against the patient's wristband (Fig. 1.2). Best practice is for you to directly ask the patient to "tell me your full name." This is much safer than asking the patient, "Are you Joe Jones?" A patient who is confused may not understand the question and say yes or no regardless of whether that is his correct name. In the hospital setting, never give a drug to a patient who is not wearing a wristband. Some long-term care settings use photographs of patients to assist the nurse in identifying patients who might be confused. Never identify the patient solely by the room or bed number.

▶ The Right Drug

Each drug that is prescribed for the patient has a particular intended action. You will need to make sure that you give the right drug. You will need to carefully compare the drug order with the drug label. Do not just assume that the correct drug has been sent by the pharmacy.

Be sure that the drug is in the correct form prescribed, because some drugs can come in multiple forms (e.g., tablets, capsules, or syrup). Also, many drugs have

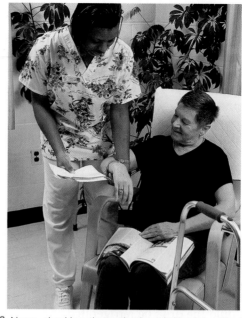

FIG. 1.2 Nurse checking the patient's wristband for identification. (From Hoffmann Wold G: *Basic geriatric nursing*, ed 5, St. Louis, 2012, Mosby.)

Table 1.1	Examples From Institute for Safe Medication Practices Common Confused Drug Names		
DRUG NAME	**CONFUSED DRUG NAME**	**DRUG NAME**	**CONFUSED DRUG NAME**
Aciphex	Accupril	Diprivan	Ditropan
Adderall	Inderal	Flonase	Flovent
Allegra	Viagra	Lantus	Lente
Benadryl	benazepril	Lexapro	Loxitane
Bextra	Zetia	Microzide	Micronase
captopril	carvedilol	Paxil	Plavix
Cozaar	Zocor	Pyridium	pyridoxine

Brand name drugs always start with a capital letter. Generic drug names always start with a lowercase letter.

names that sound or look nearly the same as the names of other drugs (sometimes called "look-alike, sound-alike drugs"). The Institute for Safe Medication Practices (ISMP) has a List of Confused Drug Names (Table 1.1). In addition, the US Food and Drug Administration and ISMP recommend the Tall Man lettering system to reduce confusion for look-alike drug names (Table 1.2). For example, Lamisil (a brand name for an antifungal) is written as LamISIL. This helps highlight the "ISIL" so the nurse does not confuse it with Lamictal (an anti-seizure drug), written as LaMICtal. The Tall Man lettering system has been embraced by healthcare agencies as one more strategy to reduce drug errors.

Drugs may come individually wrapped in a unit-dose system package, as a prescription filled for one person, or in rare cases taken from a unit's stock drugs.

Table 1.2   Examples From Institute for Safe Medication Practices List of Drug Names With Tall Man Letters

DRUG NAME WITH TALL MAN LETTERS	CONFUSED DRUG NAME	DRUG NAME WITH TALL MAN LETTERS	CONFUSED DRUG NAME
busPIRone	bupropion	SOLU-Medrol	Solu-CORTEF
chlorproMAZINE	chlorproPAMIDE	SandIMMUNE	SandoSTATIN
glipiZIPyDE	glyBURIDE	SEROquel	SINEquan
NIFEdipine*	niCARdipine	ZyPREXA	ZyrTEC
cefTRIAXone	ceFAZolin	FLUoxetine*	PARoxetine*
KlonoPIN	cloNIDine	HumaLOG	HumuLIN
PriLOSEC	PROzac	hydroOXYzine	hydrALAZINE

Brand name drugs always start with a capital letter. Generic drugs typically start with lowercase letters. NOTE: Some generic drug names incorporate tall man letters. Generic drugs that start with tall man letters are identified with an asterisk.

Sometimes the drug label has a bar code that is scanned by a computer. However it is packaged, you must read the drug label at least three times.

Top Tip for Safety

Read the drug label three times!
1. Before taking the drug from the unit-dose cart or storage area
2. Before preparing or measuring the prescribed dose of drug
3. Before opening the drug at the time you give it to the patient

The Right Time

The drug order should say when the drug and how often the drug is to be given. In many situations you will work with the RN (and/or pharmacist) to determine the right time. Most healthcare agencies have guidelines that specify what time drugs will be given when they are ordered (e.g., "drugs given once a day are given at 9:00 a.m."). You must be familiar with your agency guidelines for general times of administration. Nevertheless, it will be important for you to report if the drug information suggests timing of the drug that conflicts with the usual guideline. For example, some statin drugs (given once a day) should be given before bedtime for best effect rather than in the morning. If you have any questions, make sure to notify the RN or the healthcare provider. It is always better to ask the question than to risk the mistake.

To be effective, many drugs must be given exactly on schedule day and night to keep the level of drug constant in the body. For example, if a patient is taking warfarin, an anticoagulant, to decrease the risk for blood clots, the drug must be given at the same time every day. Patients with infections should follow a very regular schedule to maintain a consistent level of the drug and decrease the risk for antibiotic resistance.

You may need to plan around other patient activities when you give drugs. A patient with a newly diagnosed infection may need a blood culture drawn *before* starting antibiotic therapy. You may want to *hold* (wait until later) giving a diuretic in the early morning if the patient is scheduled for an ultrasound so that the patient does not experience urinary urgency while having the procedure. As you go through each chapter on drugs, you will learn more on this topic.

Drugs are usually given when there is the best chance for the body to absorb it and the least risk for side effects. This may mean that some drugs should be given when the patient's stomach is empty, and others should be given with food to prevent gastrointestinal side effects. Some drugs require that the patient not eat certain foods. Others do not mix well with alcohol. Antacids interfere with the absorption of a number of drugs; therefore antacids need to be given 2 hours before or 2 hours after taking these drugs. When a patient is taking several drugs, check to ensure that the drugs do not interfere or interact with each other. (For example, some antibiotics may interfere with the action of birth control pills, so a sexually active woman taking both could become pregnant if she does not use another form of contraception.) Whenever you are giving a new drug or one you have never seen before, use your drug references to ensure the timing is correct.

Finally, one-time-only, as needed (PRN), or emergency drugs are especially important to confirm regarding the timing. *The nurse must be certain that no one else has already given the drug and that it is the appropriate time to give the drug.* Narcotics (opioids) are often ordered as "stat" (given within a few minutes of the order) or PRN drugs. Note on the patient's record as soon as possible that you have given a narcotic so that it is clear the patient has been given the drug. (For more information, see Chapter 2.) Box 1.2 lists the main factors to remember in giving a drug at the right time.

Even though it may be tempting if you are on a busy unit, never leave a drug at the patient's bedside for him or her to take later. If the patient cannot take the drug when you bring it to him or her, you can return with the drug later. As a nurse, you must document the time the patient actually takes the drug. If you are not present when the patient takes the drug, you cannot document it.

Box **1.2** **Factors to Consider in Giving a Drug at the Right Time**

- Always make sure to confirm the last time the drug was given to avoid giving too much in too short of a time period.
- Understand and follow the rules of your hospital regarding the times to give scheduled drugs.
- Check drug references for best times to achieve the best drug absorption and to limit risks for drug interactions with other drugs.
- Give drugs at times ordered to help keep blood levels of the drug constant.
- Plan drug therapy while keeping in mind other diagnostic and laboratory testing that your patient may be experiencing.

The Right Dose

As an LPN/VN, you will want to make sure you are giving the right dose. The amount of drug to be given is typically ordered by the healthcare provider as a dose for the "average" patient. A patient who is older, who has experienced severe weight loss as a result of illness, or who is small or very obese may require changes in the usual dosages. Pediatric patients often have doses ordered based on how much they weigh. Geriatric or older adult patients may be very sensitive to many drugs and may require a change in dosage. Patients with poor liver or kidney function may require changes in dosage necessary for effect. Also, the healthcare provider may order a specific dosage of the drug when treatment begins, but adjust the dose according to changes in the patient's condition.

Giving the correct dose of a drug also requires that you use the proper equipment (e.g., insulin must be measured in an insulin syringe), the proper drug form (e.g., oral or rectal, water or oil base, scored tablets or coated capsules), and the proper concentration (e.g., 0.25% versus 0.5% solution for eye drops), and that you accurately calculate the right drug dose. For high-alert drugs (see Chapter 4), many healthcare settings have policies that require two nurses to check any drug dose that must be calculated, particularly for drugs such as narcotics, heparin, insulin, or IV drugs, to reduce risk for error.

The Right Route

Each drug must be given by the right route. The drug order must state how the drug is to be given (route of drug administration). The nurse must never change routes without obtaining a new order. Although many drugs may be given by different routes, the dose is often different for each route.

The oral route is the preferred route if the patient is oriented (awake and able to understand) and can swallow without choking. In some cases, faster delivery or a higher blood level of a drug is needed, so the drug

may be given parenterally (e.g., subcutaneously or intravenously; see Chapter 4). There may be special precautions for drugs given through these routes (such as how fast they can be given or in what dosage). Review your drug references to ensure that you are giving the drug correctly.

For patients with breathing problems such as asthma, drugs that previously were given orally can now be given via an inhaler. This has decreased the number of side effects by getting the drug right where it is needed: in the lungs. You will need to teach the patient the techniques to achieve the greatest benefit from the inhaler. Other routes that you will see in practice are drugs given as eye drops, eardrops, topical agents, and even as part of shampoos. The most important thing is that you give the right form of the drug for the right route.

Top Tip for Safety

Make Certain the Patient Takes the Drug

Never leave a drug at the patient's bedside for him or her to take later.

The Right Documentation

Increasingly, electronic health record and charting systems are being used in healthcare settings. Whether the nurse records giving the drug in a paper chart or using an electronic chart, the basics are the same: You will want to make the right documentation. Record the time, route, and site of administration (if parenteral drug) after you have given the drug. It is very important to record this right away (do not delay or "wait until later"). As a tool of communication, failure to record means you did not give the drug. In an emergency or when a drug is used only once or twice, this is very important.

The documentation must always list the drug given, the dose, and the time it was actually given (not the time it was supposed to be given). In some offices or clinics where immunizations are given, the policy may require that the lot number listed on the bottle be recorded in the patient's chart. Most charting systems include a place to record the patient's response to the drug. Any patient reports of problems or adverse effects must be noted in the chart and reported immediately to the head nurse and the physician.

It is vitally important that you *never record drugs that were not given or record them before they are given.* If a patient does not receive the drug for any reason, notify the nurse in charge or the healthcare provider according to your healthcare setting policies.

Following the rules of your healthcare setting and carefully following the rights of drug administration will reduce the risk for drug error. Should an error be made, talking about it honestly and taking quick action to correct any damage is vitally important to protect the patient from harm. Acknowledging error is an essential, and ethical, part of nursing practice.

The Right to Refuse

Patients do have the right to refuse the drugs based on the principle of autonomy (right to self-determination). Although we recognize that patients can refuse, it is really important to talk with the patient regarding his or her reasons for refusal. In many cases, the refusals are based on a lack of understanding about the purposes of the drug so that you have the opportunity to teach or clarify information about it. Another example is a patient who refuses a laxative because he or she has diarrhea (clearly a good reason!). Whatever the reason, if the patient refuses after you have answered all of his or her questions, make sure to document the refusal in the medical record.

Of note, there may be clinical areas (such as psychiatric units) where patients may be a danger to themselves or to others. In those situations make sure to know your state laws that allow emergency treatment orders. If there is any question, make sure to check with the RN or the healthcare provider.

EVALUATION

Evaluation is the process of determining the right response and looking at what happens to the patient when the nursing care plan is put into action. It is the appraisal of the treatment's effectiveness. Evaluation requires the nurse to watch for the patient's response to a drug, noting both expected and unexpected findings. For example, when *antipyretics* (drugs that reduce fever) are given, you will take the patient's temperature to determine whether the drug lowered the fever. When drugs are given to reduce blood pressure, you will want to do regular blood pressure checks. For drugs used to reduce pain, you will evaluate whether the drug reduced the patient's pain according to your agency pain scale.

Evaluation of what happens when you give a drug helps the healthcare team decide whether to continue the same drug or make a change. Gathering such information is also a part of the continuing assessment of a patient during care that the nurse will record in the patient's chart. Thus the nursing process may be seen as a circle (see Fig. 1.1). For example, the patient's temperature can be part of the evaluation step of the nursing process, but it may also be part of the assessment step when you notice that the patient's temperature remains elevated, indicating that the patient needs a different dose of the drug, a different drug altogether, or some additional treatment measures.

Factors to Consider in Evaluating Response to Drug

The nurse checks for three types of responses to drug therapy: therapeutic effects, expected side effects, and adverse effects.

Therapeutic effects are seen when the drug does what it was supposed to do. If you understand why the drug is being given (the therapeutic goal of the drug), you will be able to decide whether that goal is being met. For example, if the patient's blood glucose is high and regular insulin is given, you should see a lower blood glucose level when the next blood glucose is checked. If the patient is constipated and takes a laxative, the patient should have a bowel movement.

Expected side effects are those unintended but not unusual effects that occur in many people taking the drug; they are usually mild and do not require that the drug be stopped. One example of an expected side effect is the sleepiness that most patients feel when taking an opioid (narcotic) for pain. All drugs have side effects, but not all patients have every side effect listed for any single drug. Always document side effects. Sometimes side effects such as nausea or vomiting may be stopped by decreasing the dosage or by giving the drug with food. Telling the healthcare provider about the side effects helps him or her decide whether the patient should keep taking the drug or it should be stopped.

Adverse effects are seen when patients do not respond to their drugs in the way they should or they develop new signs or symptoms. For example, a patient with pneumonia may be given penicillin. Although this antibiotic may be working to control the infection, the patient may develop shortness of breath, which may be an allergic reaction to the drug; in this case the penicillin must be stopped. A patient taking an anticoagulant to prevent blood clots must be closely watched for signs of bleeding or bruising that would indicate that the patient has taken too large of a dose or has a larger-than-expected response to the drug. *If you suspect a patient is having an adverse effect, make sure to report to the RN or the healthcare provider immediately.* Usually when serious adverse effects occur in response to a drug, the healthcare provider *discontinues* (stops) the drug.

The nurse is the healthcare worker most often with the patient and is in an important position to notice the patient's response to drug therapy. Carefully and repeatedly evaluating the patient and documenting your findings in the patient's medical record is vitally important in the delivery of safe, quality, and cost-effective care.

🔲 Top Tip for Safety

Evaluate Response to Drug

It is important to watch the patient and look for any signs of improvement or if there are any side effects, adverse effects, or allergic responses.

🔲 Top Tip for Safety

Use the nine rights each and every time you give a drug to a patient!

Get Ready for the NCLEX® Examination!

Key Points

- Use the nine rights each and every time you give a drug to a patient.
- Nursing assessment is using your observational, questioning, and listening skills to learn information about the patient that can be used to ensure you are safely giving drugs.
- When assessing a patient, always ask carefully about any current health problems, history of illnesses, history of surgeries, and drugs (including OTC and herbals) taken both now and in the past.
- Always know why you are giving the patient the drug.
- Check the label of each drug you are giving three times to ensure it is the right drug.
- Do not give a drug that was made for one route by any other route.
- When giving a one-time-only drug, take extra precautions to make certain that it has not already been given by someone else.
- Never record drugs that were not given or record them before they are given.
- Always use two unique patient identifiers when giving a patient a drug
- If a patient refuses to take a drug, clarify the patient's reason and make sure to document the refusal.
- All drugs have side effects, but not all patients have every side effect listed for any single drug.
- Any questions about whether a drug is appropriate or safe for that patient *must* be answered before the drug is given.
- If you suspect a patient is having an adverse effect, make sure to report to the RN or the healthcare provider immediately.
- Never leave a drug at the patient's bedside for him or her to take later.
- In the hospital, never give a drug to a patient who is not wearing an identification band.

Review Questions for the NCLEX® Examination

1. What is the most appropriate measurement to determine the therapeutic response of an antipyretic drug?
   1. Blood pressure
   2. Respiratory rate
   3. Temperature
   4. Radial pulse

2. Which of the following examples would be considered objective data? (Select all that apply.)
   1. "I have pain in my abdomen."
   2. Blood pressure is 160/90.
   3. Skin is mottled.
   4. "I had a lab test last week at my doctor's office."
   5. Child's mother states, "His temperature was 102 degrees before we came to the hospital."
   6. Weight gain of 2 pounds in 4 days.
   7. Patient states she has trouble breathing or "catching" her breath.

3. Which of the following would be considered examples of the nine rights? (Select all that apply.)
   1. Right patient
   2. Right time
   3. Right room number
   4. Right to refuse
   5. Right documentation
   6. Right reason

4. Which of the following examples would be considered a contraindication?
   1. Giving a drug for nausea to a patient who has just vomited.
   2. Giving a drug that causes birth defects to a patient who is 12 weeks' pregnant.
   3. Giving a drug that may cause dizziness to a patient with high blood pressure.
   4. Giving a drug that may cause an increase in heart rate to a patient who has asthma.

5. The LPN/VN is giving a patient her morning drugs due at 9:00 a.m. After you have already prepared the drug, the patient states, "No, I don't want that pill today." What is your best first action?
   1. Tell the patient she has to take the drug because it was ordered by the doctor.
   2. Ask the patient to tell you her reason for not taking the drug.
   3. Teach the patient why she needs it and give the drug.
   4. Ask the patient if she has any questions about the drug.

6. What is considered the best resource for current use of drugs at admission to the healthcare setting?
   1. The patient
   2. The medical record
   3. The caregiver
   4. The prescriber

7. The LPN/VN is assessing a patient before giving a drug to manage his blood pressure and notes the blood pressure to be 90/50 mm Hg. What is the nurse's best action?
   1. Hold the drug and report to the RN in charge.
   2. Give the patient a cup of coffee and give the drug.
   3. Come back in 30 minutes and recheck the blood pressure.
   4. Tell the patient to walk in the hall and give the drug.

8. What is the best way to check that you are giving the drug to the right patient?
   1. Ask the patient's name.
   2. Compare the patient with the room number.
   3. Check the patient's wristband.
   4. Check two unique patient identifiers.

9. Which of the following nine rights should you apply immediately after you give a drug?
   1. Right drug
   2. Right patient
   3. Right documentation
   4. Right dose

10. Which priority assessment must you make before giving any patient a drug by mouth?
    1. Quiz the patient about the action of each drug.
    2. Make sure the patient can swallow.
    3. Find out whether the patient prefers cold or room temperature liquids.
    4. Ask the patient to repeat his or her name and birthdate.

Learning Outcomes

1. Describe the legal, regulatory, and ethical responsibilities of a nurse for drug administration.
2. Explain the meaning of controlled substances (scheduled drugs) and why drugs are placed in this category.
3. Describe the legal responsibilities for managing controlled substances.
4. List the information required for a legal drug order or prescription.
5. Describe the four different types of drug orders.
6. List what you need to do if you make a drug error.

Key Terms

as needed or "PRN" drug order (p. 16) An order for a drug to be given as needed based on a nurse's judgment of safety and patient need.

black box warning (p. 20) A special designation from the FDA that the drug has a higher-than-normal risk for causing serious and even life-threatening problems in addition to its positive benefits for some people.

controlled substances (kŏn-TRŌLD SŬB-stăn-sĕz, p. 12) Drugs that are highly regulated because they are commonly abused. Also known as "scheduled drugs."

emergency or "stat" drug order (p. 16) A a one-time drug order to be given immediately.

high-alert drugs (p. 19) Drugs that have the potential to cause significant harm to patients.

legal responsibility (LĒ-gŭl, p. 14) The nurse's authority as defined by the state Nurse Practice Act. It involves the nurse's judgment and actions while performing professional duties. All nurses must know what is legal in regard to drugs in the state they practice in.

Nurse Practice Act (p. 16) The state law that licenses LPN/VN, registered nurses, nurse anesthetists, nurse practitioners, and nurse midwives. It describes the minimal educational preparation and professional requirements needed to perform specific functions, including drug administration, to protect the public safety.

over-the-counter (OTC) drugs (p. 12) Category of drugs identified by federal legislation as having low risk to patients and may be purchased without a prescription; have low risk for abuse; and are safe when directions are followed.

physical dependence (FĬZ-ĭ-kăl, p. 12) The actual physical symptoms that occur with drug withdrawal (e.g., shaking, increased heart rate, pain, confusion, seizures).

prescription drugs (prĭ-SKRĬP-shŭn, p. 12) Category of drugs regulated by federal legislation because they are dangerous and their use must be controlled; may be purchased only when prescribed. Examples are antibiotics or oral birth control pills.

prescriptive authority (prĭ-SKRĬP-tĭv ă-THŌR-ĭ-tē, p. 16) The authority designated by an individual state that determines who is legally permitted to write an order or prescription for drugs.

professional responsibility (prō-FĒSH-năl rĭ-spŏn(t)-să-BĬ-lĭ-tē, p. 17) The obligation of nurses to act appropriately, ethically, and to the best of their ability as a healthcare provider.

psychologic dependence (sī-kō-LŎJ-ĭk, p. 12) Feeling of anxiety, stress, or tension when a patient does not have a medication.

single drug order (p. 16) A one-time order to be given at a specified time.

standing drug order (p. 16) A drug order that indicates that the drug is to be given until discontinued or for a certain number of doses.

INTRODUCTION

As a nurse, each time you give a drug (medication), you are faced with making decisions about the drug that can affect your patient's safety or that can have legal or ethical consequences. For example, in assisted living or nursing home facilities, it is a common practice to mix drugs with food or drink mainly to help patients swallow their prescribed drugs more easily. Before you decide to give drugs mixed in food or drink, there are several things you should consider. First, you have an ethical responsibility to inform the patient's care provider, the patient, and/or the family that you will be giving the drugs in this manner. Failure to inform the provider, patient, or family of this practice is considered covert drug administration, which, although not illegal, is not considered a best practice in drug administration.

The mixing of drugs with food or drink must be documented in the patient's care plan and on the drug administration chart to address the legal aspects of this practice. Certain foods or drinks, such as grapefruit juice, should not be taken with certain drugs because this practice may influence the effect of that drug. So, it would be important for you to check your drug handbook before mixing drugs with food or drink. Another common practice for easing drug administration is the crushing of pills or opening of capsules before mixing them with food or drink. It is important to know which types of drugs cannot be crushed or have the capsule opened. For example, a 325-mg enteric-coated aspirin pill may be difficult for some patients to swallow, but crushing the drug affects the speed at which the drug is absorbed and increases the chance of the patient developing a stomach ulcer. Some drugs have a coating that slows the release of the drug. Crushing capsules and tablets releases all of the drug at once, instead of slowly over time, and can result in accidental overdose. The Institute for Safe Medical Practice has published a "do not crush" list that can be used for reference: http://www.ismp.org/tools/donotcrush.pdf.

An important legal and ethical issue facing nurses is known as *drug diversion*. Drug diversion is defined as the illegal transfer of regulated drugs (like narcotics) from the patient for whom it was prescribed to another person, such as a nurse, for their own (or others') use. When a nurse diverts a prescribed drug, it can result in significant threats to patient safety and is a liability to the healthcare organization that employs the nurse. The American Nurses Association has defined an *impaired nurse* as one who cannot meet the professional Code of Ethics because of excessive use of alcohol or drugs. When drug diversion is suspected, the organization is required to launch a full-scale investigation. The nurse involved will most likely face disciplinary charges that will include treatment resources for the nurse with drug or alcohol addiction and may include suspension or permanent loss of the nurse's license.

Nurse leaders have a legal and ethical obligation to protect patients and the profession from impaired nurses. Some keys to behaviors that may signal a drug or alcohol dependency problem in the nurse include increased absences, lateness to work, unexplained "disappearance" from the assigned unit, and decreased alertness. Drug diversion should also be suspected if patients continually report pain despite appropriate drug treatment and if inaccurate narcotic counts are noted.

REGULATION OF DRUG ADMINISTRATION

Nurses who give drugs are required to follow these three levels of rules:
1. federal laws, which describe rules that control how certain drugs may be given;

2. state laws and regulations, or rules, which say who may prescribe, dispense (give a supply), and administer (or give) drugs and the process to be used; and
3. individual hospital or agency rules, which may use other guidelines or policies about how and when drugs are given and the records that must be kept to record drug treatment.

FEDERAL LAWS

Laws are passed by Congress to make drugs as safe as possible for patients to take and to ensure that the drug does what it claims to do (effectiveness). Congress created the US Food and Drug Administration (FDA) to monitor or watch the testing, approval, and marketing of new drugs. These regulations are very strict and so US drugs are some of the purest and most protected drugs in the world. Many laws have been passed to control drugs that might easily be abused and are dangerous. These laws define the three drug categories in the United States:
1. **controlled substances**, which include opioids (narcotics) and some sedatives or tranquilizers;
2. **prescription drugs** such as antibiotics and oral contraceptives; and
3. **over-the-counter (OTC) drugs** that are available without a prescription.

Controlled Substances

Most regulations are written for controlled substances, because these drugs are most often abused by both patients and the general public. The Controlled Substances Act of 1970 classified these drugs into five "schedules"; they became known as scheduled drugs, which rates the likelihood of the drugs in each category being abused, causing dependency or addiction.

For example, schedule I drugs, such as heroin, have no medical use and are considered highly addictive. Schedule V drugs, such as cough medicine with low-dose codeine, have a low potential for abuse. The degree of control, the recordkeeping required, the order forms, and other regulations are different for each of these five classes. Table 2.1 describes the five drug schedules, with examples of drugs in each category. Sometimes the drugs are moved from one class to another if it becomes clear they are being abused. More recently, many states have now approved the medical use of marijuana for the treatment of certain conditions, mostly in the case of terminal illness.

> ### 💡 Memory Jogger
>
> **Physical dependence** results in actual physical symptoms that occur with drug withdrawal. Symptoms such as shaking, increased heart rate, pain, confusion, seizures, and other troubling symptoms can occur.
>
> **Psychologic dependence**, or addiction, is a mental desire associated with taking certain substances, such as cocaine or alcohol. Symptoms of mental dependence such as anxiety, anger, or depression can occur with psychologic dependence.

Table 2.1   Classification of Controlled Substances (United States)

SCHEDULE	DESCRIPTION	EXAMPLES
I	High potential for abuse No accepted medical use in treatment in the United States Lack of accepted safety for use of the drug or other substance under medical supervision	More than 80 drugs or substances of which the following are the most well-known: alpha-acetylmethadol, gamma-hydroxybutyric acid (GHB), heroin, lysergic acid diethylamide (LSD), marijuana, mescaline, peyote, quaaludes
II	High potential for abuse Currently accepted use for treatment in the United States Abuse may lead to severe psychologic dependence or physical dependence	More than 30 drugs or substances of which the following are the most well-known: amphetamines, cocaine, codeine, fentanyl, hydromorphone (Dilaudid), meperidine (Demerol), methadone, methylphenidate (Ritalin), morphine, oxycodone (Percodan), pentobarbital, secobarbital
III	Potential for abuse is less than the drugs or substances in schedules I and II Currently accepted medical use for treatment in the United States Abuse may lead to moderate or low physical dependence or high psychologic dependence	Most drugs are compounds containing some small amounts of the drugs from schedule II along with acetaminophen or aspirin such as Tylenol # 3 or # 4 and Fiorinal Other drugs include anabolic steroids such as testosterone preparations and sodium oxybate (Xyrem), a drug that contains GHB for use with the sleep disorder narcolepsy
IV	Low potential for abuse relative to the drugs or substances in schedule III Currently accepted medical use for treatment in the United States Abuse may lead to limited physical dependence or psychologic dependence relative to the drugs or substances in schedule III	Include diet drugs with propionic acid Other well-known drugs include benzodiazepines (lorazepam [Ativan], flurazepam [Dalmane], diazepam [Valium], midazolam [Versed], alprazolam [Xanax]), chloral hydrate, paraldehyde, pentazocine (Talwin), phenobarbital
V	Low potential for abuse relative to the drugs or substances in schedule IV Currently accepted medical use in the United States Abuse may lead to limited physical dependence or psychologic dependence relative to the drugs or substances in schedule IV	Include cough preparations with small amounts of codeine and drugs for diarrhea that also contain small amounts of opioids such as diphenoxylate with atropine (Lomotil)

Source: US Drug Enforcement Administration (DEA), Title 21, Section 81.

Federal and state laws make it a crime for anyone to have controlled substances without a prescription. Each state has a practice act that lists which healthcare providers may dispense or write prescriptions for controlled substances. Almost all states have prescription monitoring programs that monitor for controlled substance prescriptions that may be received by patients from several different providers to prevent prescription drug abuse. Physicians, dentists, nurse practitioners, physician assistants, and sometimes nurse midwives may write prescriptions for controlled substances. Pharmacists dispense the drugs according to the provider's orders. Licensed practical nurses (LPNs) or licensed vocational nurses (LVNs) may give controlled substances to a patient only if the state board of nursing permits it in the scope of practice, and must be under the direction of a healthcare provider who is licensed to prescribe these drugs.

LPNs/VNs work in many different settings; some settings may have high levels of technology for securing controlled substances, while others may use a double-lock system. Each state and healthcare agency has laws and policies that cover the ordering, receiving, storing, and recordkeeping of controlled substances. Opioids (narcotics) are scheduled drugs and they must all be counted every shift. Records must be kept for every dose given. Agency policy determines which nurses will be held responsible for handing over the control of controlled substances from one shift to the next and for the counting and securing of controlled substances. All controlled substances ordered for a patient but not used during the hospital stay are sent back to the pharmacy when the patient is discharged.

Nurses may not borrow a drug ordered for one patient to use for another patient, and may never use these drugs for themselves. In a time when drug abuse is so common, the nurse who has responsibility for the controlled substances must remain alert. About 8% to 15% of healthcare professionals have a history of substance abuse, and there is a risk for drug diversion. A pattern of drugs frequently being "dropped" or "spilled" or records that show a patient received large or more frequent doses of drugs without pain relief can serve as clues to possible drug diversion. As a nurse, you must know the federal, state, and agency rules about giving any type of drug, including controlled substances. The rules that govern controlled substances are very clear and very strict. If you violate the controlled substance laws, you may be punished by a fine, a prison sentence, or both. Nurses with proven drug abuse problems lose their license to practice, at least temporarily, and may have a hard time getting it back. Nurses have both an ethical and a legal responsibility to report suspected drug diversion. In most states, the state board of nursing has a program to help nurses with substance abuse that affects their ability to carry out their nursing duties.

Distribution for controlled substances and drugs. Both federal and state laws, as well as agency policies, are clear about how controlled substances are handled in hospitals and other agencies. The goal of all regulations and policies is to verify and account for all controlled substances. When controlled substances, particularly opioids (narcotics), are ordered from the pharmacy, they come in single-dose unit or prefilled syringes and are attached to a special inventory sheet. The nurse receiving the order from the pharmacy must inspect the drug and return to the pharmacy a signed record stating that all of the drug ordered was received and that it was in acceptable condition. As each drug is used, it must be accounted for on the inventory sheet by the nurse giving the drug.

The use of opioids (narcotics) is carefully monitored on the hospital unit. Drugs are stored in a special locked cabinet. The key to this cabinet is carried by the charge nurse or by a drug nurse. This individual has the legal responsibility for overseeing the use and recording of all opioids during that shift, regardless of whether they personally give the drugs to the patients. There are also automated drug dispensing systems. These systems may include dispensing of opioids or some kinds of routinely stocked drugs that nurses withdraw by giving a password or fingerprint instead of using a key to open a locked cabinet.

When controlled substances are ordered for a patient, the nurse who will give the drug first checks the order, the dosage, and the last time the drug was given before obtaining the controlled drug. All nurses giving controlled substances must officially sign out all drugs given during the shift. The agency's inventory report form is completed before the drug is removed from the cabinet. This report may be in the form of a written document or a patient's bar code may be used instead. The report form should include the patient's name, date, drug, dosage, and the signature of the nurse giving the drug. A follow-up note about the patient's response to the drug may also be required. If a dose is ordered that is smaller than that provided (so that some of the drug must be discarded), or if the drug is accidentally dropped, contaminated, spilled, or otherwise made unusable and unreturnable, *two nurses* must sign the inventory report and describe the

situation. Institutional policy may require additional actions.

At the end of each shift, the responsibility for all controlled substances and the key to the controlled substances cabinet are transferred to another authorized nurse from the new shift. Keys to or electronic access to controlled substances are never given to physicians or any other unauthorized healthcare worker. The contents of the locked cabinet are counted together by one nurse from each shift. The numbers of each ampule, tablet, and prefilled syringe in the cabinet must match the numbers listed on the inventory report form. Sealed packages are kept sealed. Opened drug packages must each be inspected and counted. Prefilled syringes must be examined to make sure they all have the same color, the same fluid levels, and the same amounts of air within them. Both nurses must sign the inventory report, officially stating that the records and inventory are accurate at that time.

Occasionally the inventory and the written report do not agree. Any errors in the number of remaining doses and the number listed in the inventory report must be explained. All nurses who have access to the key must be asked about drugs they have given. Steps must be retraced to see if someone forgot to record any drug. Patient charts can also be checked to see if a drug was given that was not signed for on the inventory report. If errors in the report cannot be found, both the pharmacy and the nursing service office must be notified, and an investigation is opened to determine if drug diversion has occurred. Depending on the type and magnitude of the issue, the institution or agency administrator and security police may be contacted as well.

⬆ Top Tip for Safety

Controlled Substances

Always verify all orders for controlled substances. Only authorized nurses can be responsible for access to and delivery of controlled substances. Follow all regulatory policies and procedures for safety and security of controlled substances. Report any suspicious findings that may point to possible drug diversion.

Prescription Drugs

In the United States, the safety and effectiveness of prescription drugs are regulated by the Federal Prescription Drug Marketing Act (1987), and it is the responsibility of the Food and Drug Administration (FDA) to decide which drugs will require a prescription to be obtained. This regulation is in place to prevent both prescription drug misuse and abuse. Access to these drugs is provided by a few healthcare professionals (physicians, dentists, nurse practitioners, and physician assistants).

Misuse or abuse of prescription drugs can lead to adverse drug events, including those caused by dangerous drug interactions. The most commonly abused prescription drugs include narcotics (opioids) and drugs given for sleep or anxiety disorders.

The Omnibus Budget Reconciliation Acts of 1989, 1990, and 1991 placed further controls on drugs for Medicare or older adult patients. According to one study, as many as 15% of older adults are at risk for potential major drug–drug interactions. Older patients are at high risk for problems with prescription drugs because they may not take the drug properly because of poor eyesight, memory, or coordination; they may take many drugs that interact with each other; or they may have chronic diseases that interfere with how the drug works.

The most recent legislation, Medicare Plan D, provides coverage of some types of drugs for those who pay for this option. More and more, insurance or government groups who pay for drugs limit the types and numbers of drugs that may be ordered to those on a "preferred drug" list. The preferred drug list may require the use of cheaper generic drugs to control costs because new or brand name drugs usually are more expensive. Many drugs are not FDA approved as safe and effective for either children or pregnant women. Prescription drugs make up most of the drugs you give to patients in assisted living, nursing homes, or hospitals. Prescription drugs are carefully tested for safety and effectiveness before they are put on the market. However, even though much may be known about a particular drug, each patient is different and may have different reactions to the drug. You must know the expected and adverse effects of drugs given to your patients and watch for signs that the drug is working the way it should. Any adverse reactions that may develop must be reported to the ordering provider. Because the patient often gets several drugs at the same time, the interaction among the drugs may make it hard to tell how each drug affects the patient, making your nursing knowledge of these drugs a critical part of safe nursing practice.

Over-the-Counter Drugs

The FDA has also found that many drugs are safe enough not to need a prescription. These drugs are known as over-the-counter (OTC) drugs. They are used to treat many common minor problems such as colds, allergies, headaches, minor burns, constipation, or upset stomach. These drugs may easily be purchased at a drugstore or pharmacy. They are often the first thing patients try before they go to the doctor. Although OTC drugs are widely available, they are not without some risk. Like all drugs, some OTC drugs may produce adverse effects in some patients. There is also the possibility of drug or food interactions, or harm caused by excessive doses. Patients should be taught to read the Drug Facts label that is included with all OTC products and to consult with their pharmacist or other healthcare provider if they have additional questions concerning OTC drug use. Accidental overdoses of common cold drugs in children have occurred because of confusion by parents over the correct dosage to give, so these drugs are no longer recommended for use in pediatric patients. Studies have shown that 40% of parents give their children incorrect dosages of liquid drugs. Cold and allergy products that contain pseudoephedrine can be used to make illegal drugs, are now stored behind the pharmacy counter, and are sold in limited quantities. OTC drugs that are given in assisted living, nursing homes, and the hospital require a legal prescriber's order before they are given. In fact, without an order in these settings, patients cannot take even their own OTC drugs brought with them.

CANADIAN DRUG LEGISLATION

The Canadian Health Protection Branch of the Department of National Health and Welfare is like the FDA of the US Department of Health and Human Services. This branch is responsible for the administration and enforcement of federal legislation such as the Food and Drugs Act, the Proprietary or Patent Medicine Act, and the Controlled Drugs and Substances Act. These acts, together with provincial acts and regulations that cover the sale of drugs and those that cover the healthcare professions, are designed to protect the Canadian consumer from health hazards; misleading ads about drugs, cosmetics, and devices; and impure food and drugs. The Canadian Food and Drugs Act divides drugs into various categories. Regulations covering the various categories or schedules of drugs differ from those in the United States. There are three major classes of drugs under the Food and Drugs Act: nonprescription drugs, prescription drugs, and restricted drugs.

The Proprietary or Patent Medicine Act provides for a class of products that may be sold to the general public by anyone. The drug formula is not found in the official drug manuals or printed on the label. The formulas for all such proprietary (trade secret) non-pharmacologic drugs must be registered and have a license under the Proprietary or Patent Medicine Act. The nurse needs to be aware of patients taking such drugs in the case of possible drug interactions.

The Canadian Controlled Drugs and Substances Act covers the possession, sale, manufacture, production, and distribution of opioids (narcotics) in Canada. Only authorized people may have opioids in their possession. All people authorized to be in possession of an opioid must keep a record of the names and quantities of all opioids dispensed, and they must ensure their safekeeping. Nurses are in violation of this act if they are guilty of illegal possession of opioids.

OTC drugs are regulated in Canada by the Canadian Food and Drugs Act. These drugs can be purchased without a prescription, but there are rules about the packaging, labeling, and dispensing of the drug. The nurse needs to be aware of the risks these drugs have and watch for possible adverse effects and interactions with other drugs. OTC drugs available in Canada differ from those available in the United States.

THE DRUG ORDER

LEGAL PRESCRIPTIONS

Both state law and agency policy require that all drugs given in hospitals and long-term care facilities must be ordered by licensed healthcare providers acting within their scope of practice. This generally restricts **prescriptive authority** (the authority to write an order or prescription for drugs) to physicians, dentists, nurse practitioners, nurse midwives, nurse anesthetists, and physician assistants. Providers who write the prescriptions are also called prescribers. Prescriptions for a hospitalized patient are written in the specified area of a patient's chart, or recorded in the electronic record, and the pharmacy is notified. In some agencies, the order must be transcribed, or rewritten by an authorized individual onto a special pharmacy order form, which is then sent to the pharmacy. Assisted living facilities and long-term care facilities may have providers who evaluate the patients and order or issue recurring orders for patient drugs. Every time a patient has a prescription filled, the pharmacy is required to give information about the drug and how it is to be given.

A legal prescription order must contain:

- the patient's full name
- date
- name of drug
- route of administration
- dose
- frequency
- duration
- signature of prescriber

Additional details about how to give the drug may also be written: for example, "Take with meals," "Avoid milk products with this drug," "Do not refill," "May cause drowsiness," or "Please label." Pharmacies also require the patient's age and address on the prescription. This information may help the pharmacist ensure the right drug dosage for the patient (e.g., a child or older adult) and help verify the patient's identity.

In emergencies, or if the provider is not available on-site, a *verbal order*, usually over the telephone, may be given. All agencies that employ nurses have policies about verbal orders. The agency decides who is authorized to take, transcribe, and implement verbal orders. The nurse taking the order is responsible for writing the order on the order form in the medical record, including both the name of the nurse and the name of the prescriber. Many institutions also require that a note be written to indicate that the order was read back to the prescriber for validation. The prescriber must then cosign this order, usually within 24 hours, for the order to be valid. The receiving and transcribing of verbal telephone orders may be the responsibility of the registered nurse (RN). *It your responsibility as an LPN/VN to make sure you are very familiar with the verbal order policy of the institution where you are practicing.*

TYPES OF DRUG ORDERS

Drug orders are classified into one of four types of orders: the standing order, the emergency or "stat" order, the single order, and the as needed or "PRN" order.

A **standing drug order** indicates that the drug is to be given until discontinued or for a certain number of doses. Hospital or institutional policy usually dictates that most standing orders expire after a certain number of days. A renewal order must be written by the prescriber before the drug may be continued. Examples are:

- amoxicillin 500 mg orally every 8 hours for 10 days
- ibuprofen 600 mg orally every 6 hours

An **emergency or stat drug order** is a one-time order to be given immediately. An example is:

- diphenhydramine 50 mg IV stat

A **single drug order** is a one-time order to be given at specified time. An example of a single drug order is:

- cefazolin 1 g IV at 10:00 a.m. before surgery

An **as needed or "PRN" drug order** is an order for a drug to be given as needed based on a nurse's judgment of safety and patient need. An example of a PRN order is:

- docusate 100 mg orally at bedtime as needed for constipation

STATE LAW AND HEALTHCARE AGENCY POLICIES

Although many regulations about giving drugs come from Federal laws, details about who may prescribe and who may give drugs are set by each individual state. This authority is spelled out for nurses in the **Nurse Practice Act** of each state and can be found at the National Council of State Boards of Nursing website.

Bookmark This!

National Council of State Boards of Nursing: https://www.ncsbn.org/npa.htm

---

Differences in practice from state to state make it essential that nurses learn what is legal with regard to drug administration and make sure that they abide by the rules and regulations. Because nurses may move from state to state, nurses must know exactly what is in the Nurse Practice Act of the state where they are licensed to work. Today, nurses often move between jobs, and some states recognize the nursing license of another state through an agreement called the Nurse Licensure Compact. There is a growing list of states that participate in the compact (available at https://www.ncsbn.org).

State rules about nursing practice often list the basic or minimum standards of practice. Therefore agency or institutional policies and guidelines may be more specific or restrictive than state Nurse Practice Acts.

Agencies that employ nurses must provide written policy statements about the educational preparation for nurses permitted to give drugs and an orientation to particular policies, procedures, and recordkeeping rules of the agency. When you accept a nursing job, it is implied that you are willing to obey the policies or procedures of that institution. It may be an agency's policy to require employment for a certain period, completion of special orientation and training sessions, and passing a probation period before being permitted to give drugs. Even when you have the legal authority to give drugs, a valid drug order signed by an authorized prescriber is needed.

Giving drugs is a responsibility reserved for those nurses who are named by law to give drugs and who can document the appropriate educational preparation to do so. Nurses who give drugs to patients accept **professional responsibility** for giving drugs correctly, ethically, and legally. This means nurses must accept both *ethical and legal* responsibility for good judgment and actions in drug administration and monitoring the effects of drugs given. Agencies expect nurses to carry out the steps of the nursing process, and you are responsible for good assessment, planning, implementation, and evaluation of the patient when drugs are given. You, as the nurse, will be held responsible for failure to perform any of these steps well.

The nursing process is a helpful system to be used when giving drugs. There is a professional, and an implied ethical and legal, requirement that nurses use this process. You must learn information about the patient's medical diagnosis, past medical history, current symptoms, allergies, and current drugs taken. You are responsible for learning about all of the patient's prescribed drugs, the dosage, route of administration, expected response, adverse reactions, and the monitoring that may be needed to ensure the drug is working as it should and to observe for drug interactions. You are also responsible for following all laws and agency policies that are related to giving drugs, including the *9 Rights of Drug Administration* (Table 2.2). Finally, you teach the patient and the family the information they need to know for continued and safe administration of this drug.

DRUG ADMINISTRATION SYSTEMS

As a nurse, you are responsible for checking that the drug order is correct. This may mean you need to confirm the order you have (using a drug Kardex/other paper drug system or in the electronic medical record [EMR] in a computerized system) against the original order by the provider. Every agency has its own drug order, distribution, and recording system for the patient's health record. Agency policy will tell you what information is to be placed in each section. After you give the drug or drugs ordered, you must record all required drug administration information.

Table 2.2	The 9 Rights of Drug Administration
Right patient	Check the patient's name using two methods to identify the patient.
Right drug	Check drug order. Check drug label.
Right dose	Check drug order. Confirm drug dose is appropriate.
Right route	Confirm the drug can be given by the route ordered. Confirm the patient can take or receive the drug by the route ordered.
Right time	Confirm the times the drug is ordered are correct. Check for correct time before giving the drug. Check the last time the drug was given.
Right documentation	Document drug administration after the drug is given. Chart the time, route, and any other specific information as necessary.
Right reason	Confirm the reason or need for the drug.
Right response	Confirm the drug has had the desired effect. Document any monitoring needed or adverse effects as needed.
Right to refuse	The patient has a right to refuse any prescribed drug.

Integrated within an electronic health record, many facilities now use a bar-coded drug administration system to allow drug orders to be sent to the pharmacy when they are written; the drugs are then sent back to the patient's room or floor, and the drug is then taken to the patient's bedside. Both the patient's bar-coded wristband and the bar code on each drug are scanned by the nurse using a handheld device (Fig. 2.1). This ensures that the right patient is getting the right drug as noted in the drug order. As the patient is observed taking the drug, the nurse notes that the drug has been given and the chart is electronically updated with this information. An electronic health record and an integrated bar-coded drug system have several obvious advantages. The use of a computer to create the record prevents illegible clinician handwriting—a common cause of drug errors. In addition, these systems avoid having orders transcribed several times as they are sent to the pharmacy, given to the nurse, and so on. This also results in fewer errors. Many systems are designed to indicate whether the dose ordered by the clinician is out of the acceptable dosage range or would interact with another ordered drug, whether there are other dosing errors, or if the patient has a recorded allergy to a prescribed drug.

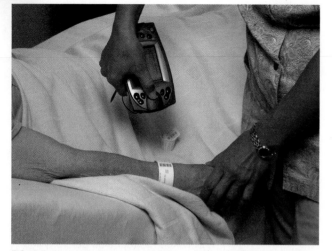

FIG. 2.1 Electronic scan of wristband. (From deWit SC, O'Neill P: *Fundamental concepts and skills for nursing,* ed 4, St. Louis, 2014, Saunders.)

KARDEX AND ELECTRONIC DRUG SYSTEMS

The Kardex is a pen and paper flip-file card system used for many years that has important patient information and the physician's orders. It is regularly updated and changed to reflect current orders. This format keeps important information about the patient easily available for all team members. When a unit-dose system is used, all drugs are listed in the Kardex or drug profile sheet (Fig. 2.2).

Memory Jogger

In every organization the patient will have either a paper or an electronic chart. The chart may differ in content and format depending on the type of healthcare organization. You are required to document all drug administration according to the agency policy and to record the patient's response to the drugs given and any adverse effects as needed.

DRUG ERRORS

Drug or medication errors are costly to patients who suffer adverse effects or even death as a result. In

---

MEDICATION KARDEX

PRN MEDICATIONS

Order date initials	Expir. date	Medication dose/frequency/route	Doses given											
			Date											
			Time											
			Initials											

IM Injection Site Code
1. Rt. posterior gluteal
2. Lt. posterior gluteal
3. Rt. anterior gluteal
4. Lt. anterior gluteal
5. Rt. anterolateral thigh
6. Lt. anterolateral thigh
7. Rt. deltoid
8. Lt. deltoid

Indicate the number of the site used with each IM dose given.

Record site with time.

Signatures/Initials
_____
_____
_____
_____
_____
_____
_____
_____
_____
_____
_____
_____

ALLERGIES _____   DIAGNOSIS _____

ROOM NO. _____   NAME _____   DOCTOR _____   AGE _____

FIG. 2.2 An example of a Kardex drug card.

addition, organizations pay a financial price for drug errors that occur. Every drug error that is prevented saves the agency approximately $7000. Drug errors can occur at any of three points in the drug administration process: (1) during drug preparation, (2) bringing the drug to the patient, and (3) giving the drug to the patient. Studies have pointed to the fast pace of current clinical practice, lower staffing levels, multitasking, and interruptions during the process of preparing and giving drugs as potential causes of drug errors. Efforts to minimize interruptions during all of the three points of drug administration can reduce errors.

? Did You Know?

The three most common points where drug errors are made are:
- during drug preparation
- bringing the drug to the patient
- giving the drug to the patient

Each agency has policies and procedures that cover what to do when a drug error is made. Agencies where drug errors are treated with blame and fear may have fewer nurses report errors when they are made. Nurses have an ethical responsibility to report drug errors because of possible harm to the patient. Regardless of whether the nurse believes the error may result in harm to the patient, all errors must be reported. If you suspect an error was made, immediately check the patient, notify the healthcare provider promptly, and follow any orders the provider gives to reduce the effect of the drug error. It is critical to watch the patient's condition through measuring vital signs, drawing blood for tests, or using any other method ordered by the provider. Also notify the nursing supervisor and fill out any other agency-required reports.

After the reports are made, an investigation into how and why the error occurred will be done. The investigation will include how it might be avoided in the future and will also consider any training of the nursing staff that may be needed. Consequences of drug errors vary and are often related to how severe the error was and if the patient was harmed. If the nurse was careless or negligent, she or he may be held professionally and/or legally liable. Although almost every nurse has made one drug error, repeated errors will not be ignored. Research in each institution helps determine whether the mistakes made in that institution are most commonly due to a "system error," a unique mistake, a failure to follow the *9 Rights of Drug Administration*, or a deliberate wrongdoing.

In a very important Institute of Medicine (IOM) report ("To Err Is Human," IOM, 2000) about the number of errors made in medical care, estimates suggest that adverse events, which include medical errors, occur in 3% to 4% of patients. The IOM report and other studies estimate that the costs of medical errors in the United States, including lost income, disability, and need for additional health care, may be between $17 billion and $136.8 billion or more annually. These costs come from a variety of drug-related problems, including patient compliance issues and medical or drug errors. Unfortunately, estimates suggest that more than half of the adverse medical events each year are because of medical errors that could be prevented. Because of this report, most agencies have tightened up ways to report and follow up on drug errors, and some improvement has been confirmed in the most recent studies. Nurses must make every effort to follow agency policies and work to minimize interruptions to prevent errors.

An independent, not-for-profit organization, The Joint Commission (TJC) accredits and certifies nearly 21,000 healthcare organizations and programs in the United States. The Joint Commission accreditation and certification is recognized nationwide as a symbol of quality that reflects an organization's commitment to meeting certain performance standards.

In an effort to cut down on drug errors, TJC has discouraged healthcare workers from using any abbreviations that might lead to confusion. That means that abbreviations that were used in the past (such as "hs" for nighttime, "cc" for cubic centimeter, and "QD" and "QOD" for daily and every other day) are no longer used in hospitals that wish to maintain their accreditation. Table 2.3 lists TJC's official "do not use" abbreviations.

🔖 Bookmark This!

Institute for Safe Medical Practices List of Abbreviations, Symbols, and Dose Designations

https://www.ismp.org/tools/errorproneabbreviations.pdf

In addition, a larger list of dangerous abbreviations can be found at: http://www.nccmerp.org/dangerous-abbreviations

High-Alert Drugs

A small category of drugs have a high risk for harm when associated with a drug error. We call these **high-alert drugs** because the consequences of the errors are very serious. Errors with these drugs can cause harm to the patient who receives it in error (i.e., was not prescribed to receive it), as well as to those who either receive too high a dose, too low a dose, or do not actually receive a prescribed dose. High-alert drugs are often packaged, stored differently, and given differently than others. Some agencies may require extra steps in the drug procedures before high-alert drugs are given.

Categories of common high-alert drugs can be remembered using the acronym PINCH. P is for potassium, I is for insulin, N is for narcotics (opioids), C is for cancer chemotherapy drugs, and H is for heparin or any drug type that interferes with blood clotting. Information about high-alert drugs in the hospital, community, and long-term care settings can be found online (https://www.ismp.org/Tools/highAlertMedicationLists.asp).

Table 2.3	The Joint Commission's Official "Do Not Use" List[a]	
DO NOT USE	**POTENTIAL PROBLEM**	**USE INSTEAD**
U, u (unit)	Mistaken for "0" (zero), the number "4" (four), or "cc"	Write "unit"
IU (International Unit)	Mistaken for IV (intravenous) or the number 10 (ten)	Write "International Unit"
Q.D., QD, q.d., qd (daily)	Mistaken for each other	Write "daily"
Q.O.D., QOD, q.o.d., qod (every other day)	Period after the Q mistaken for "I" and the "O" mistaken for "I"	Write "every other day"
Trailing zero (X.0 mg)[b]	Decimal point is missed	Write X mg
Lack of leading zero (.X mg)		Write 0.X mg
MS	Can mean morphine sulfate or magnesium sulfate	Write "morphine sulfate"
MSO$_4$ and MgSO$_4$	Confused for one another	Write "magnesium sulfate"

[a]Applies to all orders and all drug-related documentation that is handwritten (including free-text computer entry) or on preprinted forms.
[b]A trailing zero may not be used in drug orders or other drug-related documentation.
Adapted from the Joint Commission. *Facts about the Official "Do Not Use" List of Abbreviations.* Retrieved from https://www.jointcommission.org/PatientSafety/DoNotUseList. Updated June 9, 2017.

WARNING: RISK OF THYROID C-CELL TUMORS
See full prescribing information for complete boxed warning.
- Liraglutide causes thyroid C-cell tumors at clinically relevant exposures in rodents. It is unknown whether Victoza causes thyroid C-cell tumors, including medullary thyroid carcinoma (MTC), in humans, as human relevance could not be determined by clinical or nonclinical studies (5.1).
- Victoza is contraindicated in patients with a personal or family history of MTC or in patients with Multiple Endocrine Neoplasia syndrome type 2 (MEN 2) (5.1).

FIG. 2.3 An example of a "black box" warning; this warning was included in the Victoza package insert. (From Novo Nordisk: A black box warning. Retrieved from https://www.accessdata.fda.gov/drugsatfda_docs/label/2010/022341lbl.pdf.)

Memory Jogger

High-alert drug groups are *potassium*, *insulin*, *narcotics*, *cancer chemotherapy agents*, and *heparin*, and all other drugs that have interference with blood clotting as their main effect.

Black Box Designation

An additional way that some drugs are categorized is by their ability to harm the person taking it. Some drugs are assigned a black box warning by the FDA. When a drug has a **black box warning** it means that the drug has a higher-than-normal risk for causing serious and even life-threatening problems in addition to its positive benefits for some people. This black-bordered box is found on the drug insert sheet and may be included on the patient instruction sheet provided by some pharmacies. Fig. 2.3 shows an example of a black box warning. Prescribers must take extra care in deciding whether or not to prescribe a drug that has a black box warning. The patient is made aware of the potential problems the drug can cause. When you give a drug that carries a black box warning, you will need to monitor the patient even more closely than usual for possible problems.

MEDICATION RECONCILIATION

Medication (drug) reconciliation is the practice of comparing the patient's drug orders to all of the drugs that the patient has been taking. By doing so, drug errors caused by wrong dosages, duplication of drugs, and leaving out a drug can be avoided. The nurse compares the list of current drugs to the list of prescribed drugs to check for accuracy. This list includes all OTC drugs and any herbal supplements or vitamins, as well as prescription drugs the patient takes on a daily basis. Teach your patients to carry the most recent drug list with them to all healthcare provider appointments and to update this list as changes are made.

PROTECTION OF HEALTHCARE WORKERS

Patients with communicable diseases can place nurses and other healthcare workers at risk for infection. Many healthcare agencies require proof of vaccination to preventable diseases such as hepatitis B upon employment. Some unsafe clinical practices, such as the recapping of syringe needles, can result in needlestick injuries and exposure to bloodborne pathogens. Needlestick injuries expose nurses to serious infectious diseases such as hepatitis B, hepatitis C, and human immunodeficiency virus (HIV). Regulations require hospitals to have a written plan for reducing the risk for needlestick injuries among healthcare workers. Employers are required to provide the safest equipment available, regardless of cost. Such equipment includes needleless products, or those with engineering controls, which have built-in safety features to reduce risk. Also, sharps disposal units must be available in areas where needed in the unit. If a needlestick injury does occur, it is to be carefully recorded in the agency's needlestick injury documentation system. The exposure control plan, selection of safety products, and needlestick injury documentation system must be reviewed at least once every year.

> ⚠️ **Safety Alert!**
>
> Safe disposal of drugs is a primary concern for the health and safety of the population.
>
> The following tips are used for the safe disposal of prescription drugs:
> - Follow the disposal directions on the drug packaging or insert.
>
> - Unless directed, do not flush drugs down the toilet, because they can pollute the environment.
> - Bring unused or expired drugs to a local drug take-back program.
> - Consult with a pharmacist about drug disposal guidelines.

Get Ready for the NCLEX® Examination!

Key Points

- You are legally required to exercise judgment and responsibility in carrying out drug administration.
- Know the scope of your practice for drug administration as defined by your state's Nurse Practice Act.
- Always verify orders for all drugs to be given.
- Always account for all controlled substances prescribed and given to patients.
- Be aware of using unapproved abbreviations in transcribing drug orders for administration.
- Document all drugs given to a patient according to agency policy.
- Assess for and document the patient's response(s) to drugs you have given.
- Use extreme caution in preparing and giving high-alert drugs.
- Follow all clinical guidelines and agency policies to reduce drug errors and prevent injury to healthcare personnel.
- Do not dispose of unused drugs by flushing them down the toilet.

Review Questions for the NCLEX® Examination

1. According to the patient's record, a controlled substance has been ordered for pain relief. A review of the narcotics log and the patient's drug record indicates the drug has been given as ordered. However, the patient reports not receiving relief of pain. What may be a likely reason for the lack of pain relief?
   1. The patient may not be telling the truth.
   2. The drug is likely being diverted for illegal purposes.
   3. The patient has an allergy to opioids, and so they are not effective.
   4. The patient was offered the drug, but then refused the dose, and it was discarded.

2. Which patient is most likely to receive an incorrect dose of an over-the-counter (OTC) drug?
   1. A 2-year-old child given a liquid drug by his parents
   2. A 20-year-old woman who experiences frequent migraine headaches
   3. A 50-year-old man who is taking an anti-inflammatory drug for occasional arthritis pain
   4. A 13-year-old female student who was given acetaminophen for a headache by the school nurse

3. You have discovered that you made a potential drug administration error. What is the first step you should take?
   1. Fill out an incident report.
   2. Call the healthcare provider immediately.
   3. Check your patient and assess vital signs.
   4. Discuss your concerns with the nurse manager.

4. Which drug is classified as a schedule II controlled substance?
   1. Mescaline
   2. Morphine
   3. Pentazocine
   4. Tylenol #3

5. Which action is most likely to ensure you are giving the right drug to the right patient?
   1. Checking the patient's bed number
   2. Asking the patient if he is Mr. Jones
   3. Asking the patient if he has taken this drug before
   4. Checking the name on the patient's wristband

6. Which information is required for a prescription to be legal. (Select all that apply.)
   1. Patient's name
   2. The instruction "take with meals"
   3. Prescriber's signature
   4. How often the drug is to be taken
   5. When to notify the prescriber
   6. Drug dose
   7. Name of the pharmacist
   8. Route of administration
   9. How long to take the drug

7. What is the most important action to perform after giving a patient a drug that has a black box designation?
   1. Report the event as a drug error.
   2. Observe the patient closely for an adverse reaction.
   3. Be sure to sign out the drug according to agency policy.
   4. Remind the patient to stay in bed for 2 hours after receiving the drug.

3

Principles of Pharmacology

http://evolve.elsevier.com/Visovsky/LPNpharmacology/

Learning Outcomes

1. Define the keywords used in pharmacology and drug administration.
2. Explain the differences between the chemical, generic, and brand names of drugs.
3. Compare the drug actions of agonists, partial agonists, and antagonists.
4. Describe the four basic physiologic processes that affect drug actions in the body.
5. Explain the differences between side effects and adverse effects.
6. Discuss personal factors that influence drug therapy.
7. Describe how drugs affect persons at different lifespan changes.

Key Terms

absorption (ăb-SŎRP-shŭn, p. 24) Drugs enter the body and pass into the circulation to reach the part of the body it needs to affect through the processes of diffusion, osmosis, and filtration.

additive effect (ĂD-ĭ-tĭv, p. 28) When two drugs are given together and either make one drug stronger or make the action of the two drugs more powerful.

adverse reaction (ăd-VŬRS, p. 27) Severe symptoms or problems that can cause great harm.

agonist (ĂG-ō-nĭst, p. 24) Drugs that work by activating or unlocking cell receptors causing the same actions as the body's own chemicals.

allergy (ĂL-ĕr-jē, p. 27) An antigen-antibody response that can cause hives, rashes, itching, or swelling.

anaphylactic reaction (ăn-ă-fĭ-LĂK-tĭk, p. 27) A severe life-threatening form of an allergic reaction.

antagonist (ăn-TĂG-ŏ-nĭst, p. 24) Drugs that attach at a drug receptor site but do not activate or unlock the receptor.

bioequivalent (BĪ-ō-ĭ-KWĬV-ĭ-lent, p. 28) Drug products that are chemically the same or identical.

biotransformation (BĪ-ō-trăns-fŏr-MĀ-shŭn, p. 25) The transformation or altering of a drug into either active or inactive chemicals after it has been absorbed.

brand name (p. 23) The proprietary name that a manufacturer gives to a specific drug. Also known as a trade name.

buccal (BŬ-kĕl, p. 24) Drug placement against the cheek.

chemical name (KĔM—ĭ-kăl, p. 23) The names of the chemicals that actually form the drug.

desired action (ĂK-shŭn, p. 27) The drug does what it is supposed to do.

distribution (dĭs-trĭ-BŪ-shŭn, p. 25) Movement of a drug in the body to reach its site of action by way of the blood and lymph system.

drug interaction (ĭn-tĕr-ĂK-shŭn, p. 28) When one drug changes the action of another drug.

enteral (route) (ĔN-tĕr-ăl, p. 24) Giving a drug by way of the gastrointestinal system; oral, feeding tube, sublingual, and rectally.

first-pass (effect) (p. 26) After they are consumed, drugs are inactivated in the liver before being distributed to other parts of the body.

generic name (jĕn–ĔR-ĭk, p. 23) The most common drug name used by the manufacturer in all countries. Also known as the nonproprietary name.

half-life (p. 26) The time it takes the body to remove 50% of the drug from the body.

hepatotoxic (hĕp-ă-tō-TŎK-sĭk, p. 27) Adverse drug effects that can result in liver damage.

hypersensitivity (hĭ-pĕr-sĕn-sĭ-TĬV-ĭ-tē, p. 27) An exaggerated response to a drug. An allergy is an example of a hypersensitive response.

idiosyncratic response (ĭd-ē-ō-sĭn-KRĂ-tĭk, p. 27) Responses to a drug that are peculiar and unpredicted.

intramuscular (IM) (ĭn-trĕ-MŬ-skyĕ-lĕr, p. 24) Giving a drug by way of an injection deep into the muscle.

intravenous (IV) (in-tră-VĒ-nŭs, p. 24) Giving a drug by way of an injection into a vein or giving the drug into tubing that is connected to a catheter that is inserted into to a vein.

nephrotoxic (nĕf-rō-TŎK-sĭk, p. 27) Adverse drug effects that can result in kidney damage.

parenteral (route) (pĕ-RĔN-tĕr-ăl, p. 24) Giving a drug by way of an injection or an infusion underneath the skin.

partial agonist (PĂR-shăl ĂG-ō-nĭst, p. 24) Drugs that attach to the receptor site but produce only a partial effect rather than a full effect (agonist).

percutaneous (route) (pĕr-kū-TĀ-nē-ŭs, p. 24) Giving a drug by way of absorption through the skin. Topical creams, patches, or devices under the skin are common examples.

pharmacodynamics (FĂRM-ă-kō-dĭ-NĂM-ĭks, p. 23) The effects of a drug on body function (what a drug does to the body).

pharmacokinetics (FĂRM-ă-kō-kĭ-NĔT-ĭks, p. 23) The metabolism of a drug within the body (what the body does to a drug).

pharmacotherapeutics (FĂRM-ă-kō-thĕr-ă-PŪ-tĭks, p. 23) The use of drugs in the treatment of disease.

prodrug (p. 25) Drugs that must be metabolized before they are active.

receptor site (rē-SĔP-tŏr, p. 23) Small "lock-like" areas of cell membranes that control what substances either enter the cell or change its activity.

side effect (SĪD ĕf-FĔCT, p. 27) Mild but annoying responses to the drug. Nausea and headache are common and usual side effects to many drugs.

solubility (sŏl-ū-BĬL-ĭ-tē, p. 24) The ability of a drug to dissolve in body fluids.

subcutaneous (sŭb-kyū-TĀ-nē-ăs, p. 24) Drug placement into fatty tissue.

sublingual (sŭb-LĬNG-gwăl, p. 24) Drug placement under the tongue.

synergistic effect (sĭn-ĕr-JĬS-tĭk, p. 28) The effect of two drugs taken at the same time is greater than the sum of the effects of each drug given alone.

trade name (TRĀD), (p. 23) The proprietary name that a manufacturer gives to a specific drug. Also known as a brand name.

This chapter provides an overview of very basic information from chemistry, physics, anatomy, and physiology that explains the action of drugs in the body (**pharmacokinetics**, or what the body does to the drug). This involves the processes of absorption, distribution, metabolism/biotransformation, and excretion. It also covers basic information on the effects of drugs on body functions (**pharmacodynamics**, or what the drug does to the body). This information is vital in understanding **pharmacotherapeutics**, or the use of drugs in the treatment of disease.

DRUG NAMES

Drugs have several different names that may be confusing when you first learn to work with drugs. It is very important to know the different names of a drug so that the wrong drug is not given to a patient. Sometimes a drug is ordered by one name for the drug and the pharmacist labels it with another name for the same drug. For example, Valium (trade name) is also known as diazepam, its generic name. It is also common that one trade name drug is substituted for another trade name in the pharmacy. For example, Atarax (hydroxyzine) and Vistaril (hydroxyzine): hydroxyzine is the generic name, whereas Atarax and Vistaril are two different trade names (brand names) of hydroxyzine made by two different manufacturers. When one drug name is ordered and a drug with another name is supplied, it is important for you to know whether the drug is the same or a different drug.

The most common drug name used is the **generic name**. This is the name the drug manufacturer uses for a drug, and it is the same in all countries. It is also called the *nonproprietary name,* which is given to a drug before there is any specific trade name or when the drug has been available for many years and more than one company makes the drug. Examples would be ibuprofen and acetaminophen. The American Pharmaceutical Association, the American Medical Association,

and the US Adopted Names Council assign generic names. Generic names are not capitalized when written. It is becoming common in hospitals, extended care facilities, and other settings for drugs to be ordered by their generic names.

The **trade name**, or **brand name**, is the proprietary name or the name for the drug manufactured by one company. This name is often followed by the symbol ®, which indicates that the name is registered to a specific drug maker or owner and no one else can use that name for a drug. This is the drug name used in advertisements and is often descriptive, easy to spell, or catchy sounding so that prescribers will remember it easily and be more likely to use it. The first letters of the trade name are capitalized. Examples of trade names are Motrin, Tylenol, and Mylanta.

Chemical names are often difficult to remember because they include all of the chemicals that make up the drug. These names are usually long and hyphenated, and they describe the atomic or molecular structure. An example is ethyl 1-methyl-4-phenylisonipecotate hydrochloride, the chemical name for meperidine (Demerol). The chemical name is rarely, if ever, used by nurses or physicians and does not need to be remembered for safe drug administration.

DRUG ATTACHMENT

Drugs take part in chemical reactions that change the way the body acts. They do this most commonly when the drug forms a chemical bond at specific sites on body cells. **Receptor sites** are small, "lock-like" areas of cell membranes that control what substances either enter the cell or change their activity (Fig. 3.1). The chemical reactions between a drug and a receptor site are possible only when the receptor site and the drug can fit together like pieces of a jigsaw puzzle or a key fitting into a lock. The drug attaches to the receptor site and activates the receptor. The drug will have a similar effect to the body's own chemical effect. When drugs activate or unlock

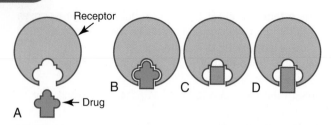

FIG. 3.1 (A) Possible drug receptor actions. (B) Complete attachment as in an agonist. (C) An attachment that does not give a response or blocks a response as in an antagonist. (D) A small response as in a partial agonist. (From Clayton BD, Stock YN, Cooper S: Basic pharmacology for nurses, ed 15, St Louis, 2010, Mosby.)

receptors and have the same actions as the body's own chemicals, they are known as receptor **agonists**. Here is an example: morphine (key) activates the opiate receptors (lock) and produces analgesia (pain relief). In the body, deep breathing (key) triggers the same opiate receptors (lock) to release the body's own endorphins to decrease pain. (You can teach patients to use this technique to decrease pain.)

Some drugs attach to the receptor site but produce only a partial effect. These drugs are called **partial agonists**. Buspirone (BuSpar) is an example of a partial agonist. When given, the drug partially locks into the serotonin receptors and helps relieve anxiety and depression. Although buspirone can be used alone, it is frequently used to boost the effects of other drugs for depression like Prozac, which are full serotonin agonists. When a drug attaches at a drug receptor site but does not activate or unlock it, there is no increase in cell activity and the drug is an **antagonist**. An important feature of an antagonist is that as long as the antagonist is attached to a receptor site, agonists cannot bind there. This antagonist effect blocks the action of agonists. Narcan (naloxone) is an example of an antagonist. In an opiate overdose, naloxone is given to completely reverse the effects of the opiate that is bound to the opioid receptor sites. The Memory Jogger box summarizes the various types of receptor site activity, and this is key information to memorize and understand.

> ### 💡 Memory Jogger
>
> *Agonist:* Drug attaches at receptor site and activates the receptor; the drug has an action similar to the body's own chemicals.
> *Antagonist:* Drug attaches at drug receptor site, but no chemical drug response is produced, and the drug prevents activation of the receptor.
> *Partial agonist:* Drug attaches at drug receptor site, but only a slight chemical action is produced.

BASIC DRUG PROCESSES

Drugs must be changed chemically in the body to become usable. Four basic processes are involved in

drug utilization in the body: absorption, distribution, metabolism, and excretion. Drugs have different characteristics, or pharmacokinetics, that determine to what extent these processes will be used. To safely give and monitor how a drug works in a patient's body, it is important for you to understand each of these processes for the specific drug or drugs prescribed.

ABSORPTION

Absorption is the way a drug enters the body and passes into the circulation to reach the part of the body it needs to affect. Absorption takes place through processes of diffusion, filtration, and osmosis. These mechanisms of absorption are more fully described in Box 3.1. How fast the drug is absorbed into the body through these processes depends on how easily the drug dissolves, how the drug is introduced into the body (by mouth or by injection), and whether there is good blood flow through the tissue where the drug is located.

All drugs must be dissolved in body fluid before they can enter body tissues. The ability of the drug to dissolve is called **solubility**. To achieve the best possible action, sometimes the drug must be dissolved quickly; at other times it should be dissolved slowly. Solubility is often controlled by the form of the drug. For example, liquids are more soluble than capsules or tablets because a liquid is absorbed faster than a tablet or capsule, which first must be dissolved. An injection with an oil base must be chemically changed before absorption can take place, and this delay in absorption holds the drug in the tissues longer, which may be the desired action, especially if it is an antibiotic. When your patient takes water with a tablet, it not only helps in swallowing but also helps dissolve the drug. That is why a full glass of water should be given with oral drugs unless the patient has a health problem that requires fluid restriction.

The route of administration also influences absorption. Drugs can be given in many different ways: the oral route (**enteral**) through the mouth, a nasogastric or feeding tube, or rectally; by injection (**parenteral**) underneath the skin; into the fat (**subcutaneous**); into the muscle (**intramuscular [IM]**); into the cerebrospinal fluid (epidural); into the bloodstream (**intravenous [IV]**); on top of the skin (topical or **percutaneous**); under the tongue (**sublingual**); against the cheek (**buccal**); or by way of breathing (inhalation).

In areas where the blood flow through tissues is very high, drugs are rapidly absorbed. The IV route delivers drugs directly into the bloodstream, and the drugs are immediately distributed to the tissues. The muscles (IM), the area under the tongue (sublingual), inside the nose (intranasal), and through the lungs (inhalation) have very high blood flow and so drugs given by these routes begin to work very quickly. Fig. 3.2 shows the action of drugs in the body from the fastest to the slowest onset.

Box **3.1**   Mechanisms Involved in Absorption

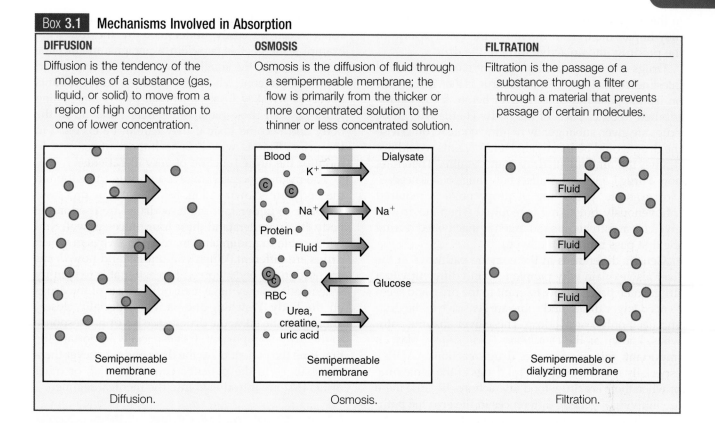

DIFFUSION	OSMOSIS	FILTRATION
Diffusion is the tendency of the molecules of a substance (gas, liquid, or solid) to move from a region of high concentration to one of lower concentration.	Osmosis is the diffusion of fluid through a semipermeable membrane; the flow is primarily from the thicker or more concentrated solution to the thinner or less concentrated solution.	Filtration is the passage of a substance through a filter or through a material that prevents passage of certain molecules.

Diffusion.   Osmosis.   Filtration.

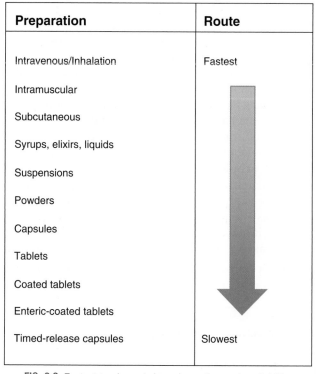

Preparation	Route
Intravenous/Inhalation	Fastest
Intramuscular	
Subcutaneous	
Syrups, elixirs, liquids	
Suspensions	
Powders	
Capsules	
Tablets	
Coated tablets	
Enteric-coated tablets	
Timed-release capsules	Slowest

FIG. 3.2 Fastest to slowest drug absorption and availability.

DISTRIBUTION

After a drug enters the body's circulation, it must reach the organ or tissues where it will have its action. Movement of a drug in the body is its **distribution**, which occurs by way of the blood and lymph system.

Distribution of the drug is usually uneven because of differences in how much blood is able to penetrate the tissue (perfusion), types of tissue (bone, fat, and muscle), and how easy it is for the drug to penetrate the cell membranes. For example, the tissue in the placenta and the brain make it difficult for the drug molecules to pass through. Some drugs will also bind together with many blood substances and proteins such as albumin. This binding allows only "free" drug (that which is not bound) to penetrate the tissues.

Some drugs are attracted to tissues other than the target receptor sites. For example, drugs that dissolve easily in lipids (fats) prefer adipose, or fat tissue, and stores of the drug may build up in these areas. Eventually this buildup of the drug in the fat cells will be released, making the effect of the drug last a long time. Diazepam (Valium), an antianxiety agent, is a highly lipophilic (fat-loving) drug, and the sedative effects last much longer than lorazepam (Ativan), a less lipophilic antianxiety agent.

METABOLISM

Once the drug is absorbed and distributed in the body, the body transforms or alters the drug into active or inactive chemicals. This process, known as **biotransformation**, happens mainly in the liver, where there are enzymes that break down the chemicals that make up the drug into its usable and unusable parts. Drugs that are known as **prodrugs** have to be transformed and activated by these enzymes before they can be used by the body. Biotransformation happens in various sites in the body, but mainly in the liver. Thus liver disease may impair the transformation of the inactive form of the prodrug into an active form of the drug.

Drugs move very quickly from the stomach or small intestines to the liver. A lot of the drug is then inactivated on its **first pass** through the liver before it can be distributed to other parts of the body. That is why some drugs are given sublingually or intravenously; otherwise the drug would be inactivated and patients would not receive the amount of drug they require. Therefore, how a drug is given may affect how much of it is needed. (For example, only 1 mg of propranolol is required intravenously, but 40 mg is required when the drug is given by mouth because so much is inactivated during the first pass through the liver.)

Genetic differences in the enzyme pathways in the liver also explain why people respond differently to a drug. Some people grow tolerant to the drug and seem to need larger doses, and some are sensitive to the drug and need only a small dose. These liver enzyme pathways, known as the *cytochrome P-450 system*, play an important role in adverse drug reactions (ADRs), especially when taking several drugs at the same time or when there are drug–food interactions. Because there are individual genetic differences in the enzyme pathways, different patients may respond differently to the same drug. For example, African American persons with hypertension require higher doses of some antihypertension drugs, and the drugs that they do respond to are different from that of white persons.

EXCRETION OR ELIMINATION

All inactive chemicals, chemical by-products, and waste (often referred to as *metabolites*) finally break down through metabolism and are removed from the body through the process of **excretion.** Fibrous or insoluble waste is usually passed through the gastrointestinal (GI) tract as feces. Chemicals that may be made water-soluble are dissolved and filtered out as they pass through the kidneys and then are lost in the urine. Some chemicals are exhaled from the lungs through breathing or lost through evaporation from the skin during sweating. Very small amounts of drug may also escape in

tears, saliva, or the milk of breast-feeding mothers. This concept can be easily understood by the following examples: the smell of penicillin, asparagus, and nicotine in the urine, or the smell of alcohol on the sweat and breath of someone who has consumed large amounts of beer or whiskey. If the patient has poorly functioning kidneys, then these metabolites may build up in the body and become toxic if they cannot be excreted in the urine. This is why it is so important for you to monitor the urine function of very ill patients.

The major processes involved in drug utilization in the body are shown in Fig. 3.3. These four processes are basic to understanding how drugs are used in the body. If you understand these four processes well, you will be able to understand many of the ways in which drugs are different. When you understand how drugs are used in the body, you will be better able to identify when patients may have toxic or ill effects of the drugs on the body. Watching the patient especially closely after he or she takes the drug to see his or her response to the drug is important. It is especially important the first time the patient takes the drug and whenever there are changes in the patient's condition, diet, or other drugs that are introduced into the medical regimen.

? Did You Know?

Grapefruit juice affects (usually reduces) the absorption of many drugs, such as antihistamines, cholesterol-lowering drugs, HIV drugs, and transplant drugs.

Some drugs enter and leave the body very quickly; other drugs remain for a long time. The standard method of describing how long it takes to metabolize and excrete a drug is the **half-life,** or the time it takes the body to remove 50% of the drug from the body. Because the rates of metabolism and excretion are usually the same for most people, the half-life helps explain the dose (how much drug should be taken), the frequency (how often it should be taken), and the duration (how long it will last) for different drugs. If a drug has a long half-life, it may need to be taken only once a day. If a person takes too much drug with a long half-life, an

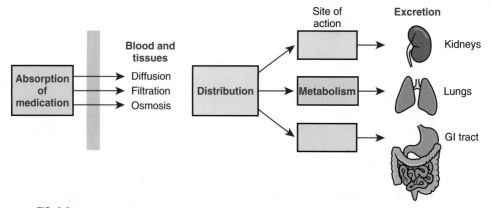

FIG. 3.3 Processes of absorption, distribution, metabolism, and excretion. *GI,* gastrointestinal.

adverse reaction may occur because the action of the drug lasts for such a long time. If the half-life of a drug is short, such as for many antibiotics, the person must take frequent doses to keep the correct level in the blood. If a person's liver or kidneys do not function correctly, drugs may not be properly metabolized or excreted, and this would mean that higher doses of the drug will circulate for a longer time and produce symptoms of overdosage. Drugs are often dosed based on kidney and liver function for this reason, which is why kidney and liver function blood work is drawn.

Some drugs such as narcotics and antihypertensive drugs come in an extended-release or long-acting form for ease of administration. Many of these drugs end in -contin, LA, or ER.

> ### Top Tip for Safety
>
> Long-acting or extended-release drugs *must never be crushed, chewed, opened (if it is a capsule), or cut* because this will result in an overdosage.

DRUG ACTIONS

When a drug is given to a patient, it is usually possible to predict the chemical reaction that will result and a change seen. However, because each patient is different, some unexpected chemical reactions are also possible. With each patient, giving a drug is somewhat of an experiment, so watching patients closely to monitor their reaction to the drug is an important role of the nurse. This is most important the first time a patient is given a newly prescribed drug.

The expected response of the drug is called the **desired action**. This is when the drug does what is desired, and the therapeutic goal is reached; for example, a fentanyl patch (Duragesic) relieves pain.

Because a drug may influence many body systems at the same time, the effect of the drug is often not restricted to the desired action. Other actions called *side effects* or *adverse reactions* may also take place. **Side effects** are usually seen as mild but annoying responses to the drug. Side effects are expected effects. For example, the drug used to relieve pain may make the patient very sleepy. Certain side effects, such as nausea, may be stopped if the dosage is reduced or the drug is given with food or a full glass of water. Some side effects are such a problem that the drug must be changed or stopped. An example of this is insomnia (inability to sleep) or making the patient pass out (syncope). Expected side effects that are very common are usually related to the GI system: nausea, constipation, and diarrhea.

Adverse reactions, or adverse effects, imply more severe symptoms or problems that develop because of the drug. Some adverse effects may require the patient to be hospitalized or may even be life-threatening. Examples include a necrotic skin condition called Steven-Johnsons syndrome or anaphylactic shock. If severe adverse effects such as damage to the kidney (**nephrotoxic** drug) or liver (**hepatotoxic** drug) or bleeding develop, the drug often must be stopped. You, as a nurse, are on the front line to notice whether and when an adverse reaction may occur and are responsible for the well-being of your patients.

Occasionally a patient may have a drug reaction that is a surprise. Strange, unique, peculiar, or unpredicted responses to drugs are called **idiosyncratic responses**. These reactions may be the result of missing or defective metabolic enzymes caused by a genetic or hormonal variation of that individual. They often produce either an unexpected result, such as pain or bleeding, or an over response to the drug. These types of reactions are usually rare. One type of idiosyncratic response is called a *paradoxical response*. In this situation, the patient's reaction may be just the opposite of what would be expected. For example, diphenhydramine (Benadryl) is an antihistamine with sedative (sleep-inducing) effects. It is in many over-the-counter sleep aids like Motrin PM. Instead of sedation, some people have a paradoxical response and remain awake and excited.

A second type of unexpected reaction is an increased reaction to a drug (**hypersensitivity**) or a sensitivity caused by antibody response to a drug (**allergy**). Some drugs (sulfa products, aspirin, penicillin) and some conditions (asthma) are more likely to produce allergic reactions than others. Allergic reactions usually occur when an individual has taken the drug and the body has developed antibodies to it. When the patient takes the drug again, the antigen–antibody reaction produces hives, rash, itching, or swelling of the skin. This type of allergic reaction is very common, so ask all patients about whether they have ever had a drug reaction. Patients with an allergy to one drug may be more likely to develop an allergy to another drug, but individuals may also develop a reaction to drugs they have taken before without problems or have been taking for a long time and only now show signs of an allergy.

> ### ? Did You Know?
>
> Allergic reactions to antibiotics can happen even after the first time a patient takes a drug because he or she may have been previously exposed to the antibiotics in milk or food that was fed to livestock.

Occasionally the allergic reaction is so severe the patient has trouble breathing, and the heart may stop. This life-threatening response is called an **anaphylactic reaction**. A patient who has a mild allergic reaction to a drug is much more likely to develop the more severe anaphylactic reaction if the drug is given again. An anaphylactic reaction is a true medical emergency because the patient may suffer severe breathing problems including swelling of their lips, throat, and trachea that prevent air from entering the lungs.

Patients often confuse an allergy with side effects, both of which may produce unpleasant symptoms. If a patient reports an "allergy" to a drug, make sure you ask the right questions to understand the exact past reaction to the drug. If the patient had nausea or stomach pain when taking aspirin, that is a side effect, but not an allergy. If the patient reported sedation when taking an antihypertensive drug, that is also not an allergy. Because patients often do not understand the difference between an allergy and a side effect, it is important for you to clarify the difference when patients say they have had an allergic reaction.

BIOEQUIVALENCE

After a new drug enters the market, an exclusive patent protects the financial interests of the drug company for some time, usually 17 years, by limiting other companies from producing that drug. After the patent ends, other companies may make the same drug under a generic name. Brand name drugs are usually more expensive than generic drugs because the maker of the brand name drug is attempting to recover the huge sums of money spent on research and drug development. Thus generic products are often less expensive because they do not face those costs.

Drug products seen as identical with respect to their active ingredients are known as *generic equivalents*. However, slight differences in processing or formulation may mean that the action of the generic drug in the body is slightly different from that of the brand name product. These differences most commonly cause variations in absorption, distribution, or metabolism. Thus the product a prescription is written for may vary according to what specific brand the pharmacist dispenses. Some products are chemically the same or identical and are thus **bioequivalent**. This may be particularly important for some cardiac or antiseizure drugs. An example is a prescription or an order written for Lanoxin, the brand name for digoxin. If the pharmacy dispenses a generic brand that is not considered bioequivalent, then the product may not have the same action on the body.

DRUG INTERACTIONS

When one drug changes the action of another drug, a **drug interaction** is present. These reactions often take place during the process of metabolism (or biotransformation) in the liver and are a result of the cytochrome P-450 enzyme pathways each person inherits genetically from his or her parents. The actions of a number of drugs may be altered when they are taken with other drugs; some examples include some antidepressants, respiratory drugs, anticlotting drugs, antibiotics, and opiates. Some drugs are given together on purpose because the combination produces an additive effect. The drugs work as a team so to speak. For example, probenecid is given with penicillin to increase the amount of penicillin that is absorbed. This is called an **additive effect**. Other drug interactions produce adverse effects. For example, many antibiotics make birth control tablets less effective, thus making it more likely a woman will get pregnant while taking both drugs if she is sexually active.

If one drug interferes with the action of another drug, it has an *antagonistic effect*. At times, one drug may replace another drug at a receptor site, decreasing the effect of the first drug (displacement). Flumazenil (Romazicon) is a drug that can be given to displace the effects of a sedative like diazepam (Valium). Sometimes *incompatibility* occurs when drugs do not mix well chemically. Attempts to mix them together, especially in a syringe or IV solution, may cause a chemical reaction, so neither of the drugs can be given. Heparin is an example of such a drug. If heparin is mixed together in a syringe or an IV line with many drugs, a white, hazy precipitate will occur. Finally, if the effect of two drugs taken at the same time is greater than the sum of the effects of each drug given alone, the drugs have a **synergistic effect**. For example, acetaminophen is given with codeine for added pain relief.

Food, Alcohol, and Drug Interactions

Food, alcohol, and most drugs taken by mouth must travel through the liver for chemical changes before they can be used by the body. Thus the risk for drug interaction with food or alcohol is high because these products also go through the liver. When taken together, food or alcohol and drugs may alter the body's ability to handle a particular food or drug. Part of these interactions may be caused by activation of the P-450 enzyme system or competition for receptor sites. The classification of antidepressant drugs called *monoamine oxidase inhibitors* are some of the drugs most noted for drug–food interactions. They cannot be taken with aged cheese, red wine, or many processed foods. Information every patient should know about possible drug interactions includes:

1. Cigarette smoking can decrease the effect of drugs or create other problems with some drugs by increasing metabolism.
2. Caffeine, which is found in coffee, tea, some soft drinks, chocolate, and some drugs, can also affect the action of some drugs.
3. Drugs should never be taken during pregnancy or by a patient trying to get pregnant without the advice of the healthcare provider.
4. If the patient has any problem related to drugs, the healthcare provider or a pharmacist should be contacted immediately.
5. Some drugs are blocked from being absorbed by the body by grapefruit juice, fatty meals, milk products, or other drugs.

Some drugs or foods increase or decrease the action of the anticlotting drug warfarin, by increasing or decreasing the blood clotting time, and thus can increase the risk for stroke or heart attacks. Other drugs might raise the blood pressure, increase vasoconstriction in tissues, or cause other vascular changes that might be harmful to the patient. Almost every drug has the potential to have an effect on other drugs that the patient is receiving, so you will need to be aware of potential drug interactions as you learn about different drug categories.

The amount of alcohol use is very high in the US population. It has been estimated that approximately 70% of adults consume alcohol at least occasionally. Many patients may not be aware that alcohol is one of the products that react most commonly with drugs. The extent to which a drug dose reaches its site of action is called *availability*. Alcohol can influence whether a drug is effective by changing its availability.

It is estimated that alcohol–drug interactions may be a factor in at least 25% of all emergency department admissions. "According to the National Institute on Alcohol Abuse and Alcoholism (NIAAA), more than 150 drugs have harmful additive or interactive effects when combined with alcohol." Narcotics, antianxiety agents, antidepressants, antihistamines, antihypertensive agents, and antibiotics are just a few of the drugs that will cause problems when combined with alcohol.

Older adults are more likely to suffer drug side effects compared with younger persons, and these effects tend to be more severe with advancing age.

Personal Factors That Influence Drug Therapy

Some personal factors affect how effective drugs are for any specific patient. All drug therapy requires adequate hydration and blood flow for drugs to be distributed to target tissues. So any problem that interferes with blood flow decreases drug effectiveness. Such problems include dehydration, overhydration, low blood pressure, shock, heart failure, or reduced blood flow to one or more body areas.

Use of other prescribed, over-the-counter, or illicit drugs, as well as alcohol intake often increase the activity of metabolic enzyme systems. This change increases the rate at which some drugs are deactivated and eliminated, often requiring that the doses be increased and/or given more frequently to be effective. For example, opioid drugs for pain are metabolized and eliminated much faster in the person who drinks alcohol on a daily basis. The dose then may need to be higher for the person to obtain pain relief.

Any person who has problems of the liver or the kidneys will retain a drug much longer, increasing the risk for adverse and toxic effects. For the patient who has either liver dysfunction or kidney problems, dosages usually need to be reduced and the drug given less frequently.

Body size and lean-to-fat ratios also affect drug therapy responses. For many drugs, bigger people (adults or children) require larger dosages of drugs. Drug dosages are based on kilogram of body weight or body surface area for children, as well as for drugs that are considered dangerous (e.g., heparin, chemotherapy drugs).

Ethnicity and genetic makeup change the expected drug response as well. For example, many people of Asian descent have a greater-than-usual response to the anticoagulant drug warfarin, which greatly increases their risk for excessive bleeding, hemorrhage, and stroke. As a result, the starting dosage of warfarin is lower for Asians and increased at a slower rate until the individual patient's response is known.

There is great variation in the activity of the P-450 system enzymes from one person to the next as a result of genetic differences. A person may be a rapid metabolizer of drugs and require higher-than-expected dosages to achieve the same desired effect. Another person may be a slow metabolizer and have more problems with side effects, adverse reactions, and toxic effects even from what are considered "normal" drug dosages.

These personal differences in drug therapy require all healthcare professionals to be aware of the possibility of unexpected patient responses. Thus one size does NOT fit all when it comes to drug therapy. This is especially true for drugs that have a narrow therapeutic range, which means that the dose that is effective is very close to the dose that causes adverse and toxic reactions. You are on the front line of drug therapy to prevent, as well as to recognize, unexpected patient responses.

DRUG THERAPY AND SPECIAL POPULATIONS

People respond to drugs differently at various lifespan stages. These differences are based on body size, water content, organ maturity, and general organ health.

PEDIATRIC DRUG THERAPY CONSIDERATIONS

Overview

Childhood extends from newborns to adolescents. During these years the processes of drug absorption, distribution, metabolism, and elimination continue to change. As children grow, total body water decreases (but is still greater than an adult's), body size increases, and body fat stores increase. Overall, body metabolism is highest in infants and slowly decreases as the child ages. However, healthy children have a higher metabolism than do adults. These normal changes alter a child's responses to drug therapy.

Drug Absorption

In neonates (less than 1 month of age), oral drugs are absorbed poorly from the GI tract because no gastric acid is present to help break down drugs, no intestinal bacteria or enzyme function is present to metabolize a drug, and the time it takes for a drug to move through the stomach and intestines is slow. Thus the effectiveness of oral drugs in this age group is not very predictable. In later infancy and childhood these factors change, making oral drugs more effective.

Absorption of IM injections is based on muscle mass and muscle blood flow. Neonates and infants have relatively small muscle mass and blood flow, which reduces IM absorption. In older children, muscle size and circulation in the muscles affect how rapidly a drug is absorbed. There is more rapid absorption from the deltoid muscle (shoulder and upper arm) than from the vastus lateralis muscle (thigh), and the slowest absorption is from the gluteal (buttock) muscles.

Drug Distribution

Distribution of water-soluble drugs is faster and more widespread in neonates, infants, and younger children because of their high percentages of total body water. For older children and adolescents, distribution is affected by the lean-to-fat body mass ratio in the same way that it is for adults.

Drug Metabolism

In neonates and young infants the systems that metabolize drugs in the liver are immature. As a result, prodrugs (drugs that must be metabolized before they are active) are slower to be activated and to become effective. For drugs that are active when absorbed, deactivation takes longer and drug levels can build up more quickly. This increases the risk for side effects, toxic effects, and overdosages in this age group.

Older infants and young children have higher metabolic rates and a rapid turnover of body water. This often results in greater drug dosage requirements per kilogram of body weight than those of the adolescent or adult. Often these young children require more frequent drug dosing to maintain blood drug levels.

For example, the dosing of digoxin, a heart drug that can become toxic very easily (narrow therapeutic index) is four times higher in the neonate than in the adult.

During adolescent growth spurts, metabolism increases along with body weight. Drug dosages often must be increased at this time, especially for drugs that control seizure disorders.

Drug Elimination

As with metabolism, the growth and maturity of the child's organs have important effects on the child's ability to excrete drugs, which changes expected drug responses. Preterm infants, neonates, and infants younger than 6 months have less mature kidneys that may not excrete drugs effectively. Careful monitoring of responses and blood drug levels are needed to determine the most effective dosages and scheduling of drug therapy.

OLDER ADULT DRUG THERAPY CONSIDERATIONS

Older adult patients also react differently to drugs. Drugs are absorbed, metabolized, and excreted more slowly and less completely in older adults. In adults older than 65 years, problems with drugs are often due to a lack of understanding of the way drugs are processed in the aging body and the body's changed response to drugs. To further complicate matters, people age differently, and their individual body systems may also age at different rates.

Many older adults with chronic illnesses take drugs daily. These drugs are helpful in controlling disease, but they also present a very real hazard to older adult patients. ADRs are common in older adults. Issues such as falls, hypotension, delirium, kidney failure, and bleeding are common clinical manifestations. Many of the issues can also be attributed to aging, which leads to ADRs being frequently overlooked in this population. You are the person most likely to notice these ADRs and alert the prescriber to the possibility of the problem.

Because many older adult patients take several drugs, interactions among these different drugs may also cause problems for them. These patients may see several specialists, each of whom may prescribe different drugs. This is called *polypharmacy*. If the specialists do not know about all the different drugs a patient may be taking at the same time, the patient is at risk for adverse interactions.

All drugs have some risk or hazard, but those most dangerous to older adults are tranquilizers, sedatives, and other drugs that alter the mind and change what the patient thinks he or she sees, or causes the patient to become dizzy or lose balance. Diuretics and cardiac drugs pose special dangers and must be given with caution and careful observation of how the patient responds. Older adult patients may become dehydrated easily, thus allowing the amount of drug in the blood to increase. This places them at greater risk for side effects and toxicity with normal dosages. Diuretics lead to an increase in urination, and this can lead to loss of electrolytes. Electrolytes are important for electrical energy of all body functions like muscle contraction and nerve impulses, but particularly for the proper electrical function of the heart. Electrolyte levels must be monitored by blood tests, and electrolytes may have to be replaced if they are low.

Drug Absorption

The overall importance of changes in the absorption of drugs with aging is not completely clear. There may be some delay in the absorption process. Physiologic changes that affect the GI tract include a reduction in acid output, so there is a more alkaline environment, which may affect drugs that require an acid medium for absorption. Reductions in blood flow, enzyme activity, gastric emptying, and bowel motility may delay the absorption of some drugs. Compounds such as iron, calcium, and some vitamins that depend on active transport mechanisms for absorption may be affected by the decreased blood flow in the aging patient's GI tract.

Drug Distribution

The distribution of drugs in the body may also be affected by the aging process and is linked to the chemical makeup of the agent. There is a decline in total body water and lean body mass with aging that may result in less movement or distribution of water-soluble drugs into some tissues. If the dose of these drugs is not decreased, the patient may develop higher serum concentrations, leading to an increased effect or toxicity. Thus the usual rule is to start drugs using a low dose and then increase the dose slowly in older adult patients. You should be mindful of the distribution of the drug you are giving so you can be alert to possible toxic effects.

The distribution of fat-soluble drugs may also be changed by the aging process. With aging, there is usually a decrease in lean body mass and an increase in total body fat. Thus lipid-soluble drugs may be stored in larger amounts in fat tissues and remain in the body for a longer time. This can cause problems with drug toxicity, as well as safety issues for a patient.

Another important concern for some older adults is a decrease in serum proteins. When serum proteins are low, greater amounts of unbound drug may circulate and cause adverse or toxic reactions.

Drug Metabolism

Overall, a decrease in liver mass occurs with age, along with a reduction in liver blood flow. When blood flow is reduced, as may occur with aging, less of the drug is metabolized, so increased amounts of the active form may remain in the blood.

In an aging liver, there may also be changes in the phases of metabolism during which certain chemical and molecular changes occur to prepare the drug for metabolism. The drug may stay in the body too long and/or not be eliminated.

Drugs that are metabolized by the liver may have less or reduced metabolism because of other changes in the liver and also because of the influence of other diseases. The aging liver often gets smaller, has less blood flow, is affected by changes in nutritional status, and may become overloaded with fluid from diseases such as chronic heart failure or chronic renal failure. These factors may result in a loss of the liver's ability to handle all the different chemicals it must process. In this situation, the patient may have more risk for adverse effects when drugs are added to the existing treatment plan.

Drug Elimination

Kidney (renal) function is an important factor that causes ADRs. Changes in the aging kidney include decreases in the number of nephrons; decreases in blood flow, glomerular filtration, and tubular secretion rate; and kidney damage. In addition, damage to the arterial walls of blood vessels and lowered cardiac output reduce the amount of blood that flows to the kidneys by 40% to 50%. The creatinine clearance rate is an estimated measure of how well the kidney functions. This rate decreases with age, which allows drugs to remain in an older adult's system longer, increasing the risk for adverse and toxic effects.

Important factors to remember when caring for older adults who are taking drugs that will be excreted by the kidneys is that each patient may respond a little differently to the drug. The dosage ordered is adjusted by the prescriber based on the best creatinine clearance estimates, and low doses or longer intervals between doses are used if kidney damage is present. Drugs that depend on the kidneys for elimination include many antibiotics, some antivirals, anticancer drugs, antifungals, analgesics, and many cardiac drugs.

PATIENT TEACHING CONSIDERATIONS

Many older adults require special teaching about how to take their prescription drugs and about the danger of taking nonprescription drugs at the same time. Failure of older adults to follow their drug therapy plan may be because of the cost of the drug, difficulty in getting it from a pharmacy, poor memory, lack of desire to take the drug regularly, depression, and feelings of being overwhelmed by the responsibility of taking care of themselves. In some cases, arthritis or another disease that causes physical disability may make it difficult to open bottle lids or use an inhaler. Poor eyesight may make it hard to draw up insulin or read labels accurately. Some older adults share drugs and may cut pills in half or skip doses without realizing this action may interfere with the effectiveness of the drug.

DRUG THERAPY CONSIDERATIONS DURING PREGNANCY AND LACTATION

Pregnant and breast-feeding women may have both chronic diseases and acute problems that require drug therapy. In pregnancy the drug is really going to two people, so how the drug may affect the growing fetus is a consideration. The benefit of any drug to a pregnant patient must be carefully weighed against the possible (or potential) risk to the fetus. It is important for pregnant women to avoid as many drugs as possible, especially those drugs with *teratogenic* potential (i.e., likely to cause malformations or damage in the embryo or fetus).

Many drugs have been confirmed as teratogenic in humans. The US Food and Drug Administration (FDA) has new guidelines for drug use during pregnancy. The pregnancy letter categories on prescription drugs will be removed by June of 2020. Instead, additional content will create awareness of the risks involved in taking drugs during pregnancy.

Factors such as what drug the mother takes, how much is taken, and the age of the fetus when the drug is taken are related to different types of malformations. Taking a drug during the first 2 weeks after conception (before implantation) results in an all-or-nothing effect. The ovum either dies of exposure to a lethal dose of a teratogen or recovers completely with no adverse effects. The critical period for teratogenic effects in humans lasts from about 2 to 10 weeks after the last menstrual period. This period is the time of organ development (14–56 days), during which any teratogenic drug taken by the mother may produce major abnormalities in the embryo. Taking a teratogen later in the pregnancy during the fetal period (57 days to term) may result in minor structural changes, but abnormalities are more likely to involve problems with growth, mental development, and reproductive organ abnormalities. Clearly it would be best if all women could stop taking any drugs before they got pregnant and not resume them until the baby is born. Always ask about the possibility of pregnancy when giving a drug to a woman of childbearing age.

As the fetus grows, the placenta allows most drugs and foods to cross from the mother to the baby. However, the reaction of a fetus to a drug is different from that of the mother. Because of an immature blood–brain barrier, many drugs are able to pass into the brain of the fetus. Because of the immaturity of the liver, the fetus does not metabolize drugs well.

Many drugs can pass into human breast milk, and this is also a major concern for the baby. Nicotine, cocaine, heroin, marijuana, and angel dust are examples of some illicit drugs that pass into the breast milk.

If a mother is given a prescription while she is nursing, she can lessen the infant's drug exposure by taking the drug just before the infant is due to have a lengthy sleep period or right after a feeding. A bottle can then be substituted for the next scheduled feeding, and the affected breast milk can be expressed and discarded. Nevertheless, the infant should be watched for emotional changes, altered feeding habits, sleepiness, or restlessness. If short-term drug therapy is required, the mother may need to consider stopping breast-feeding for a short time and instead pumping and discarding her milk to maintain lactation until drug therapy is finished.

DRUG CARDS

Approximately 9000 drugs are on the market, with new drugs becoming approved by the FDA every day. Of these, approximately 200 drugs are frequently prescribed. By now you have realized how important it is for you to understand everything you can about the patient and drug that you will be giving. A good way to learn and remember drugs is to write drug cards on the most popular drugs, as well as any and all drugs you will give to a patient. The golden rule of drug administration is to never give a patient a drug with which you are not fully familiar. A drug card should include both the trade and generic names of the drug, the dosage range, the desired action, expected side effects, adverse effects, how to give the drug, and lastly, important information that you will need to know before giving the drug.

As you progress through the text you will notice that many drugs belong to a classification, and part of the drug's generic name provides a hint. For example, what do you notice about the suffix (ending of a word) of each generic drug mentioned in the following list?

acebutolol (Sectral)
atenolol (Tenormin)
bisoprolol (Zebeta)
metoprolol (Lopressor, Toprol XL)
nadolol (Corgard)
nebivolol (Bystolic)
propranolol (Inderal)

All of these drugs are examples of a classification of antihypertensives known as beta blockers. They all have a suffix of "olol," and the way they work in the body is similar. They block the action of epinephrine in the body's beta receptor sites. Beta blockers are antagonist drugs. If epinephrine, a neurotransmitter in the body, cannot connect with a beta receptor, then the result will be a decreased heart rate and relaxation of the veins and arteries (vasodilation). The desired action then is to decrease the blood pressure. The dosage range and specific information of each of these drugs may differ, but they all work in the same way. The nurse may want to make one "classification" drug card with all of the drugs listed whenever possible to become acquainted with the drugs that belong in that classification. Table 3.1 provides a list of common suffixes and prefixes.

Table 3.1 Common Generic Drug Prefixes and Suffixes

SUFFIX OR PREFIX	DRUG CATEGORY	ACTION	EXAMPLES
cef-	Cephalosporins	Antibiotic	Cefadroxil, cefaclor
ceph-	Cephalosporins	Antibiotic	Cephalexin
sulf-	Sulfonamides	Antibiotic	Sulfadiazine
-actone	Diuretics	Spare potassium, increase urine production	Spironolactone (Aldactone)
-azoles	Antifungals	Antifungal	Fluconazole
-azosin	Alpha blocker	Relaxes blood vessels	Doxazosin, prazosin
-caine	Local anesthetics	Block pain	Lidocaine
-calci	Calcium vitamin D	Supplements	Calciferol
-cyclovir	Antivirals	Antiviral	Acyclovir, valacyclovir
-cycline	Tetracyclines	Antibiotics	Doxycycline, minocycline
-dipine	Calcium channel blockers	Relax blood vessels, decrease heart workload	Amlodipine, felodipine
-drodonate	Bisphosphonates	Prevent loss of bone mass	Alendronate, etidronate
-floxacin	Fluoroquinolone	Antibiotic	Ciprofloxacin, levofloxacin
-lam and -pam	Benzodiazepines	Decrease anxiety	Alprazolam, lorazepam
-olol	Beta blockers	Relax blood vessels, decrease heart workload	Atenolol, metoprolol
-lone	Corticosteroids	Anti-inflammatory	Methylprednisolone, triamcinolone
-mycin	Aminoglycoside/macrolides	Antibiotic	Erythromycin, vancomycin
-prazole	Proton pump inhibitors	Reduces gastric acid	Omeprazole, pantoprazole
-pril	Angiotensin-converting enzyme inhibitors	Prevents constriction of blood vessels and excess water in the body	Benazepril, captopril, lisinopril
-profen	Nonsteroidal anti-inflammatory drug	Nonsteroidal anti-inflammatory	Ibuprofen, ketoprofen
-sartan	Angiotensin II antagonists	Prevent constriction of blood vessels and excess water in the body	Losartan, valsartan
-sone	Corticosteroids	Anti-inflammatory	Prednisone, dexamethasone
-tidine	H2 receptor blockers	Decrease gastric acid	Cimetidine, famotidine
-statin	Anticholesterol, antilipemics	Decrease cholesterol and lipids	Atorvastatin, lovastatin
-zine	Phenothiazines	Antipsychotics, antiemetic	Chlorpromazine, prochlorperazine

Get Ready for the NCLEX® Examination!

Key Points

- An agonist drug increases a cell's or organ's activity, and an antagonist drug slows or stops the activity.
- Drug absorption and availability are fastest with the IV and other parenteral routes, and slowest for extended-release oral drugs.
- *Do not crush or let the patient chew, open (if it is a capsule), or cut* long-acting or extended-release drugs because this will result in an overdosage.
- Most drugs are metabolized by the liver and eliminated by the kidneys.
- Patients with liver or kidney impairment often require drug dosages to be lower to prevent adverse effects.
- Side effects are common and usually mild expected reactions to drugs, although they may be annoying.
- Adverse reactions or effects are serious and sometimes life-threatening patient responses to drug therapy that may require stopping the drug.
- Always warn patients who have anaphylactic reactions about their allergy so they will not take the drug again.
- Teach patients with a drug allergy to wear a medical alert bracelet or necklace, or carry identification about their allergy.

Get Ready for the NCLEX® Examination!—cont'd

- Special considerations are needed when giving drugs to pediatric patients, pregnant and breast-feeding women, and older adults.
- Distribution of water-soluble drugs is faster and more widespread in neonates, infants, and younger children because of their high percentages of total body water.
- The critical period for adverse drug effects during pregnancy is between conception and 57 days.
- Older adults taking many different drugs are at risk for serious drug interactions.
- Ethnicity and genetics can affect drug action in certain individuals.
- All drugs that belong to the same category work in the same way and often have similar side effects.
- Agonist drugs activate a receptor and antagonists prevent the receptor from affecting a response.
- Alcohol can make a drug either more or less effective.
- Ethnicity and genetic makeup can change the expected response of drugs.
- Consider barriers in older adults that require special teaching regarding their drugs.
- Never give a drug with which you are not fully familiar.

Review Questions for the NCLEX® Examination

1. Which drug route has the fastest action?
   1. Drugs given by way of a feeding tube.
   2. Drugs given by subcutaneous injection.
   3. Drugs given sublingually.
   4. Drugs given intravenously.

2. The patient is given a drug that will help him sleep. Instead he stays awake all night. What is this outcome known as?
   1. Paradoxical response
   2. Adverse reaction
   3. Side effect
   4. Anaphylactic reaction

3. The patient is prescribed a drug that leads to very difficult breathing. What is the reason for this response?
   1. Adverse reaction
   2. Anaphylactic reaction
   3. Side effect
   4. Idiosyncratic response

4. The nurse is giving a drug that blocks the effect of a receptor. What is this response known as?
   1. Displacement
   2. Additive effect
   3. Antagonistic effect
   4. Interference

5. The nurse is giving two drugs and finds that the effect of the two drugs taken together is greater than the sum of the effects of each drug were it given alone. What is this response known as?
   1. Interference
   2. Synergy
   3. Displacement
   4. Incompatibility

6. Which organ(s) is (are) mostly responsible for the elimination of drugs?
   1. Liver
   2. Intestines
   3. Kidney
   4. Gallbladder

7. The physician has changed an order from morphine 10 mg intravenously every 2 hours to morphine 30 mg by mouth every 4 hours. What does this nurse recognize about this order?
   1. The increased dosage is needed because of the "first-pass" effect.
   2. The prescriber has made a drug error.
   3. The dosage change is needed because the patient excretes oral drugs faster than IV drugs.
   4. The change is needed because the patient reports the IV dose is ineffective.

8. A patient on a diuretic (increases urine production) complains of leg cramping. Which is the priority action of the nurse?
   1. Encourage the patient to walk.
   2. Review the patient's current electrolyte levels for abnormalities.
   3. Offer the patient a bedpan so he/she doesn't need to walk to the bathroom.
   4. Ask the prescriber to order aspirin for pain.

9. Why are drug dosages sometimes reduced in the older patient?
   1. Older patients have a decrease in total body fat.
   2. Older patients have an increase in lean body mass.
   3. Older patients have a decrease in lean body mass.
   4. Older patients have a decrease in hydrochloric acid.

10. Ampicillin is ordered for a child: 100 mg/kg per day every 6 hours. The child weighs 10 kg. Ampicillin is supplied as 250 mg/5 mL. What is the correct dose at 6:00 a.m.?
    1. 20 mL
    2. 10 mL
    3. 5 mL
    4. 5 mg

Drug Calculation: Preparing and Giving Drugs

4

http://evolve.elsevier.com/Visovsky/LPNpharmacology/

Learning Outcomes

1. Apply the appropriate formula to accurately calculate drug dosages.
2. Select the correct equipment to prepare and give parenteral drugs, including insulin.
3. Explain the different types of parenteral drug delivery.
4. Identify anatomic landmarks used for giving parenteral drugs.
5. Apply the correct formula for calculating intravenous flow rates for infusions.
6. Correctly apply Clark's rule used to accurately calculate drug dosages for children.
7. Explain the principles and procedures to safely and accurately give drugs by the enteral, parenteral, and percutaneous routes.

Key Terms

ampules (ĂM-pūls, p. 46) Small, breakable glass containers that contain one dose of drug for intramuscular or intravenous injection.

aseptic technique (ā-SĔP-sĭs, p. 41) Manipulation that does not contaminate the sterility of the drug and drug delivery system.

body surface area (BSA) (p. 38) The total tissue area (including height and weight) of a patient's body.

buccal route (p. 57) A drug that is given by being applied to or held in the cheek. The drug diffuses through the oral mucosa directly into the bloodstream.

capsule (CĂP-sūl, p. 41) Gelatin container that holds powder or liquid drug.

Clark's rule (p. 38) A method for determining pediatric drug dosage calculated by ratio and proportion, based on the child's body weight.

drop factor (p. 39) The number of drops per milliliter of fluid.

flow rate (p. 39) The rate at which intravenous fluids are given.

intradermal injections (ĭn-tră-DĔR-măl ĭn-JĔK-shănz, p. 47) Injections that are given into the dermis, just below the epidermis, most often used for allergy testing and tuberculosis testing.

intramuscular (IM) route (ĭn-tră-MŬS-kū-lăr, p. 49) Injections that deposit drugs past the dermis and subcutaneous tissue, deep into the muscle mass.

intravenous (IV) route (ĭn-tră-VĒN-ĕs, p. 39) The administration of drugs directly into the bloodstream.

Mix-o-Vial (MĬKS Ō VĪ-ăl, p. 46) A two compartment vial that contains a sterile solution in one compartment and the powdered drug in the second compartment, separated by a rubber stopper. The solution and drug powder are mixed together immediately before use.

nasogastric (NG) tube (nā-zō-GĂS-trĭk, p. 42) An enteral route of drug administration and oral feeding that bypasses the mouth by use of a tube going through the nose and esophagus into the stomach.

nomogram (NŌM-Ō-grăm, p. 38) A chart that displays the relationships between two different types of data so that complex calculations are not necessary.

parenteral route (pĕ-RĔN-tĕr-ăl, p. 43) Administration of a drug by injection directly into the dermal, subcutaneous, or intramuscular tissue; epidurally into cerebral spinal fluid; or through intravenous injection into the bloodstream.

percutaneous route (pĕr-kū-TĀ-nē-ŭs, p. 56) Administration of a drug through topical (skin), sublingual (under the tongue), buccal (against the cheek), or inhalation (breathing) methods.

piggyback infusion (ĭn-FŪ-zhŭn, p. 52) A second or secondary intravenous fluid bag or bottle containing drugs or solution that is connected to the main IV line rather than directly to the patient.

subcutaneous injections (sŭb-kū-TĀ-nē-ĕs, p. 48) Injections that place no more than 2 mL of drug solution into the loose connective tissue between the dermis of the skin and muscle layer.

sublingual route (sŭb-LĬNG-wĕl, p. 57) Application of a drug to the mucous membranes under the tongue.

tablet (TĂB-lĕts, p. 41) Dried, powdered drugs compressed into small shapes.

topical route (TŎP-ĭ-kăl, p. 56) Drugs applied directly to the area of the skin requiring treatment; most common forms are creams, lotions, and ointments.

transdermal (trăn(t)s-DĔR-măl, p. 56) Drugs applied to the skin for absorption into the bloodstream.

vial (VĪ-ăl, p. 45) Small, single or multiple dose glass drug container.

Z-track technique (p. 51) A type of IM injection technique used to prevent tracking (leakage) of the medication into the subcutaneous tissue (underneath the skin).

In this chapter, we give an overview of basic principles of drug administration. Major sections are divided into dosage calculations, drugs given by the enteral route, drugs given parenterally, and drugs given percutaneously.

CALCULATING DRUG DOSAGES

Giving the correct dose of a drug is one of the most important responsibilities of the licensed practical or vocational nurse (LPN/VN) to ensure patient safety. Many drugs are now prepackaged with the correct dosage already prepared for the patient (known as "unit dose" drugs); however, you will need to understand how to accurately calculate the correct drug dosage using basic math formulas. Sometimes the drug dose the healthcare provider orders is not what is available. You then will need to use a mathematical formula to figure out how much to give to the patient. Even a small error in dosage can have severe consequences for the patient. These number relationships form important building blocks for accurate drug dosage. The metric system is used to convert from one unit of measure to another. For example, the metric system is used in the calculation of drug dosages, the conversion of Fahrenheit to Celsius while taking temperatures, and the conversion of pounds to kilograms when weighing patients. In the following section, we provide a brief review of essential information to master in calculating drug dosages. If you need a review of basic mathematics associated with drug calculations, read this section carefully and then use the *Student Study Guide* or *Evolve* resources to practice fractions, percentages, proportions, and ratios.

FRACTION METHOD

When you are using fractions to compute drug dosages, write an equation consisting of two fractions. First, set up a fraction showing the number of units to be given over *x*—the unknown number of tablets or milliliters using what you *want* to give over what you *have* on hand.

$$\frac{Want}{Have} = \text{number of tablets to give}$$

For example, if the healthcare provider's order states, "ibuprofen 600 mg," you would write $\frac{600\,mg}{X\,\text{tablets}}$.

On the other side of the equation, write a fraction showing the drug dosage as listed on the drug to be given over the number of tablets or milliliters to be given. The ibuprofen bottle label states, "200 mg per tablet," so the second fraction is $\frac{600\,mg}{X\,\text{tablets}}$. The equation then reads:

$$\frac{600\,mg}{x\,\text{tablets}} = \frac{200\,mg}{1\,\text{tablet}}$$

Note that the same units of measure are in both numerators and the same units of measure are in both denominators. Now solve for *x*:

$$\frac{600\,mg}{x\,\text{tablets}} = \frac{200\,mg}{1\,\text{tablet}}$$

$$\frac{600}{x} = \frac{200}{1}$$

$$200x = 600$$

$$x = 3\,\text{tablets}$$

RATIO AND PROPORTION METHOD

A fraction uses a division line to describe the mathematical relationship between *two numbers*; for example, $\frac{1}{4}$ or ¼.

Proportions describe the relationship between *two sets* of numbers. For example, $\frac{1}{2} = \frac{2}{4}$, so when you multiply across the diagonal, 1×4 equals 2×2. In using the ratio method, first write the amount of the drug to be given and the quantity of the dosage (*x*) as a ratio. Using the previous example, this is 600 mg: *x* tablets. Next, complete the equation by forming a second ratio consisting of the number of units of the drug in the dosage form and the quantity of that dosage form as taken from the bottle. Again, using the previous example, the second ratio is 200 mg: 1 tablet. Expressed as a proportion, this is:

$$600\,mg : x\,\text{tablets} :: 200\,mg : 1\,\text{tablet}$$

Solving for *x* determines the dosage:

$$600 \times 1 = 200 \times x$$

$$600 = 200x$$

$$x = 600/200$$

$$x = 3$$

Using this method provides the answer of a dosage of *3 tablets*, which is correct.

DIMENSIONAL ANALYSIS METHOD

Dimensional analysis is a technique used in a select number of LPN/VN programs instead of using ratio and proportion to solve dosage problems. Dimensional analysis is a method of comparing and equating different physical aspects and quantities by using simple algebraic rules together with known conversion factors (called *equivalency ratios*). However, it does require additional steps. Dimensional analysis is often used to convert from one set of measurement units to another set of units by using conversion factors in such a way that unwanted units are canceled out. A person comfortable with this method of calculation can always account for these units.

A simple example of this method is how many pounds (lb) are in 20 kilograms (kg) of a given substance? One kilogram is equivalent to 2.2 lb (in medical measurement), so the conversion factor from kilograms to pounds is 2.2 pounds per kilogram (2.2 lb/kg). So multiply the 20 kg by the conversion factor, 20 kg × 2.2 lb/kg, or expressed as the following equation:

$$\frac{20\,kg}{1}\times\frac{2.2\,lb}{1\,kg}$$

Now cancel out the kg because this unit is in both the numerator and the denominator.

$$\frac{20}{1}\times\frac{2.2\,lb}{1}=\frac{44\,lb}{1}=44\,lb$$

As you can see, the kilogram unit is canceled out through simple algebra.

What about going the other way? How many kilograms are in 315 lbs? Flip the conversion factor over, so 1 kg/2.2 lb, and multiply the weight in pounds by the new conversion factor, 315 lb × 1 kg/2.2 lb, which results in 143.2 kg. The equation would look like this:

$$\frac{315\,lb}{1}\times\frac{1\,kg}{2.2\,lb}\,\text{(cancel the pound units)}$$

$$=\frac{315}{1}\times\frac{1\,kg}{2.2}=\frac{315\,kg}{2.2}=143.2\,kg$$

Once again, the weight unit (this time the pounds unit) was factored out.

These two simple examples highlight how this method could be used for longer problems and how it allows the nurse using it to keep track of the units involved.

Here is a dosage example:

A patient who weighs 220 lb is prescribed a dose of drug at 12.5 mg/kg body weight. The concentration of the drug solution on hand is 125 mg/mL, and the patient wants to take the drug orally, by teaspoon. How many teaspoons of drug solution will the patient need to take per dose?

Use the following dimensional analysis steps for the conversions and accounting:

Step 1: 1 kg = 2.2 lb, so the weight conversion ratio is 1 kg/2.2 lb; the patient weighs 100 kg, so 220 lb × 1 kg/2.2 lb or

$$\frac{220\,lb}{1}\times\frac{1\,kg}{2.2\,lb}=\text{the patient weighs 100 kg}$$

Step 2: The weight (amount) of drug needed based on body mass is 12.5 mg/kg × 100 kg = 1250 mg or

$$\frac{12.5\,mg/kg}{1}\times\frac{100\,kg}{1}=\frac{1250\,mg}{1}=1250\,mg$$

Step 3: 1 tsp = 5 mL, so the volumetric conversion ratio is 5 mL/tsp.

The concentration in teaspoons is now 125 mg/mL × 5 mL/tsp = 625 mg/tsp or

$$\frac{125\,mg}{1\,mL}\times\frac{5\,mL}{1\,tsp}\,\text{(cancel out the mL)}=\frac{625\,mg}{1\,tsp}$$

$$=625\,mg/tsp$$

Step 4: The final dose in teaspoons is 1250 mg divided by 625 mg/tsp = 2 tsp, or

$$\frac{1250\,mg}{625\,mg/tsp}\,\text{(cancel out the mg)}=\frac{1250}{625/tsp}$$

$$=2\text{ teaspoons}$$

Steps 1 and 3 were conversions in which dimensional analysis was explicitly used. Steps 2 and 4 were simple calculations, but using dimensional analysis to solve for them allows for a higher degree of accountability and understanding of the units involved.

> ### Memory Jogger
>
> **Steps to Solving Drug Dosage Calculations**
>
> 1. Change dosages to the same unit of measurement if they are different.
> 2. Set up your equation as what dose is ordered (*want*) over what dose you have on hand (*have*).
> 3. Calculate the dosage, using fractions or ratios and proportions.
> 4. If preferred, use dimensional analysis to solve the problem.
> 5. Check your answer for correctness. Ask yourself, "Does this make sense knowing the dosage range for the drug?"

DRUG CALCULATION USING UNITS

Insulin is an example of a parenteral drug that is not given by milligrams (mg), but by units (u). Great accuracy is important in preparing and giving insulin, because the quantity given is very small, and even minor variations in dosage may result in severe consequences in the patient.

The preparation and calculation of insulin in insulin dosages is unique in the following three ways:

1. There are many kinds of insulin, available in short- and long-acting forms. All types of insulin come in a standardized measure called a *unit*. Insulin is available in 10-mL vials and in a specific strength (concentrations): U-100 (100 units per 1 mL of solution) (Fig. 4.1).
2. Insulin should be drawn up in a special insulin syringe that is marked or calibrated in units (Fig. 4.2).
3. The insulin order, the insulin bottle, and the insulin as drawn up should always be rechecked by another nurse for maximum accuracy.

To draw up a dose of U-100 insulin, use the corresponding 100-unit syringe. Next, draw up the number of units ordered. For example, the order reads: "48 units NPH insulin U-100 1 hour before breakfast." Using a U-100 syringe, you would draw up 48 units of NPH insulin.

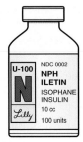

FIG. 4.1 U-100 vial.

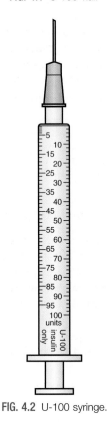

FIG. 4.2 U-100 syringe.

Occasionally an order will be written by the healthcare provider for two different types of insulin. In some cases, both types of insulin may be given at the same time in the same syringe. Usually, one type of insulin is cloudy and one type is clear. Some insulins cannot be mixed at all. For example, *never* mix Lantus or Levemir insulin with any other insulin preparation. Be sure to check with your healthcare provider, pharmacist, or diabetes educator before mixing. Chapter 17 has complete information on the processes used to give insulin. *Be certain that you are using the correct type of insulin.*

Top Tip for Safety

- Insulin is a *high-alert drug* that can cause serious harm to a patient if given at too high or too low a dose, or if it is not given to a patient for whom it was prescribed.
- You must be very accurate in these calculations. A small error makes a big change in insulin dosage. Use the correct syringe, the correct insulin, and the correct dose. Check your calculations, insulin type, and dose with another nurse or licensed healthcare professional.

CALCULATING DRUG DOSAGES FOR INFANTS AND CHILDREN

Recently, much attention has been given to drug administration errors that can lead to patient harm (see Chapter 2). This is especially true in the pediatric setting, where drug errors by both healthcare professionals and parents occur more frequently and have the potential for greater harm. Pharmaceutical companies list the recommended dosages of their drugs for a child or infant, and these dosages are much smaller than the recommended adult dosage. Although children's dosages were once frequently calculated, there remain only a few drugs that require the nurse to determine how much to give a child. In past years, several general rules were developed to calculate these special reduced dosages for infants and children. The Joint Commission, a nonprofit agency that credentials and certifies healthcare organizations, now recommends that all dosages for children be weight-based, usually in kilograms.

One of the most widely accepted methods for determining a child's dosage based on the child's body weight is **Clark's rule**. This rule is used to calculate drug doses for children aged 2 to 17 years. Just as for adult drug dosage calculations, ratios and proportions may be used to calculate the pediatric value. Assuming that an average adult weighs 150 lbs and we know the adult dosage, it follows that if we know the child's weight, we can calculate the child's dosage. The formula for calculating pediatric drug doses based on Clark's rule is as follows:

$$\text{Pediatric child dose} = (\text{weight of child}/150 \text{ lbs}) \times \text{adult dose}$$

Although you, as a nurse, should be familiar with the fact that there is a need to adjust adult drug dosages for use in children, the healthcare provider would be responsible for calculating the pediatric child dose using Clark's rule when ordering the drug.

Another way to calculate drug dosages in the pediatric patient uses **body surface area (BSA)**, or total tissue area (including height and weight), of the child. This is the most accurate method for determining pediatric dosages. The reason for using the BSA is that children have a greater surface area than adults in relation to their weight. For drugs that require careful dosage, charts known as **nomograms** are used to calculate the BSA in square meters. Nomograms (BSA charts) are constructed from height and weight data. Even with the use of standardized charts, the calculated dosages are more accurate for children than for very young infants. When giving drugs to infants or children, an important nursing responsibility is to *double-check* the original order and confirm the correct dose was calculated *before* giving the drug. Most healthcare organizations require any dose calculations for this population to be double-checked by two individual nurses to prevent drug errors that can have severe consequences to the pediatric patient. Your agency pharmacist is also an invaluable resource for any questions or concerns that arise regarding infant or child drug dosage and administration.

CALCULATIONS FOR IV INFUSIONS

Drugs can also be given through the **intravenous (IV) route**, which deposits the drug directly into the bloodstream. Drugs delivered in this manner are directly infused into the circulatory system though a vein. IV therapy can be used to correct dehydration in a patient or to give drugs directly and immediately into the bloodstream. Some drugs cannot be taken by mouth or by subcutaneous or intramuscular (IM) injection into the skin because of issues with drug absorption. However, because IV fluids and drugs enter the bloodstream directly, the potential for adverse events such as fluid overload or an adverse drug reaction is a concern. *Adverse drug reactions* are unintended responses associated with the use of a drug in a patient. These can range from mild allergic reactions to severe problems resulting in tissue damage or death.

An IV fluid administration order has several components:
- the specific IV fluid to be infused
- the amount (volume) of fluid to be infused
- the duration of the time the IV fluid should be infused
- the rate (how fast) the IV fluid should be infused

The **flow rate** of an IV fluid refers to how fast the IV fluid infuses. The flow rate tells how many milliliters are given to the patient in an hour. The diameter of the IV tubing determines the flow rate of the IV. IV tubing with a larger diameter will permit larger drops into the vein and more fluid into the body. The number of drops used to make a milliliter (mL) of IV fluid is called the **drop factor**.

Regulating the IV infusion rate is a common nursing responsibility. Some institutions have automatic infusion pumps that make flow rate calculations easy. Each nurse will learn to use the equipment available at their place of employment. However, all nurses must learn to calculate infusion rates without relying on equipment, in case of power or equipment failures or when working in agencies where no automatic pumps are available.

A complete IV infusion order specifies not only the type of solution and the volume to be infused (usually 500 or 1000 mL), but also the length of time over which the total volume of IV is to be infused. IV infusions that contain drugs need to have the flow rate calculated to determine how fast the drug will be infused. You can consult with the pharmacist or healthcare provider if the IV order is not clear, or not complete, or if you are infusing a high-alert drug, such as heparin, and wish to verify your calculations.

You must be familiar with two mathematical procedures regarding IV infusions:

- calculating the flow rates for IV fluid administration, and
- calculating total administration time for IV fluid.

To calculate the flow rate for IV fluid administration, you must understand two concepts: the flow rate and the drop factor. The rate at which IV fluids are given is the flow rate, and this is measured in drops per minute. The **drop factor** is the number of drops per milliliter of liquid and is determined by the size of the drops. The drop factor is different for different manufacturers of IV infusion equipment, and it must be checked by reading it on the infusion set itself. Regular infusion sets *(macrodrip)* generally range between 10 and 15 drops/mL. Other infusion sets are supplied in *microdrops* that are generally 60 drops/mL, which are most commonly used with pediatric patients or in skilled nursing or home care settings.

CALCULATING IV FLOW RATE

Once you know the drop factor for the equipment being used, you can calculate the flow rate by using the following formula:

$$\text{Drop factor} \times \text{mL/min} = \text{flow rate (drops/min)}$$

Occasionally, you may see an order for an IV fluid to "keep vein open" (KVO) or "to keep open" (TKO). This stand-alone order does not meet the criteria for safe drug administration. A flow rate must be specified, or the institution may have a specific policy that addresses the flow rate for a KVO order. For example, a KVO IV order may equal 20 drops/min in one institution, but 25 drops/min at another institution. Either way the flow rate must be clearly established by a healthcare provider order or institution policy.

CALCULATING IV ADMINISTRATION TIME

The order reads: "1000 mL normal saline (NS) to be given over 5 hours." The drop factor is 15. To calculate the flow rate, use:

$$\frac{\text{Total of fluid to give}}{\text{Total time (min)}} \times \frac{\text{Drop factor}}{\text{(drops/mL)}}$$

$$= \text{Flow rate (drops/minute)}$$

$$\frac{1000 \text{ mL}}{300 \text{ min}} \times 15 \text{ drops/mL} = \frac{15,000 \text{ drops}}{300 \text{ min}}$$

$$= 50 \text{ drops/min}$$

CALCULATING TOTAL INFUSION TIME

Calculating the total administration time for IV fluid depends on calculating the *total number of drops to be infused*. Using this information, plus the drop factor, you can easily determine the total infusion time by using the following formula:

$$\frac{\text{Total drops to be infused}}{\text{Flow rate (drops/min)}} \times 60 \text{ (drops/hr)}$$

$$= \text{Total infusion time (hr and min)}$$

To calculate the total infusion time:

1. *Determine the total number of drops ordered.* The total number of drops to be infused comes from the healthcare provider's order for the total amount of fluid to be infused. This amount of fluid to be infused is multiplied by the drop factor (read from the infusion set) to determine the total number of drops.

2. *Determine the number of minutes the IV is to flow.* The number of drops per minute is multiplied by the drop factor to give the number of drops infused in 1 hour. *This will give the number of hours and minutes for the total infusion.*

For example, the order reads: "1000 mL D5W to be given at 50 drops/min with a drop factor of 10 drops/mL." Thus:

$$1000 \text{ mL} \times 10 \text{ drops/mL} = 10,000 \text{ drops}$$

$$\frac{10,000 \text{ drops}}{3000 \text{ drops/hr}} = 3.33 \text{ hr or 3 hr, 20 min}$$

FACTORS THAT INFLUENCE IV FLOW RATES

Many other factors influence the flow rate of an infusion, such as the age, size, and condition of the patient, as well as the size of the patient's veins. Other factors may be changed or altered to assist in infusion of IV fluids, such as the size of the needle, the needle's position in the vein, the height of the IV pole or pump, and the positioning of the patient. If the fluid does not infuse at the calculated rate, the entire IV system should be carefully checked from the IV solution all the way down to the IV catheter insertion site for any of the following: level of fluid in the IV set drip chamber, air in the tubing that obstructs flow, patency of the IV, or signs of IV infiltration (e.g., redness or swelling of the area).

FLOW RATES FOR INFANTS AND CHILDREN

Infants and small children are very sensitive to extra amounts, or volumes, of fluids. Smaller total amounts of IV fluids are often ordered, and the infusions are given in very small drops to prevent accidental fluid overload and ensure patient safety. Usually 60 microdrops/mL is the drop factor for infants. As with adults, the drop factor must be determined from the infusion setup. For calculating the flow rates in infants, the same formula is used, but the *microdrop* drop factor must be used for the formula.

An example of a microdrip calculation formula is:

$$\frac{\text{Total of fluid to give}}{\text{Total time (min)}} \times \frac{\text{Drop factor}}{\text{(microdrops/mL)}}$$

$$= \text{Flow rate (drops/min)}$$

For example, if the IV infusion order reads: "Give 50 mL D5W [5% dextrose in water] IV in 4 hours." The drop factor is 60 microdrops/mL. Thus:

$$\frac{50 \text{ mL}}{240 \text{ min}} \times 60 \text{ microdrops/mL}$$

$$= 12.5 \text{ microdrops/min}$$

Modifications to the IV flow rate or IV drug dosage for an infant or child are strictly controlled and are ordered only by the healthcare provider.

Memory Jogger

- The *drop factor* for infusions depends on the type of equipment and must be read from the IV set label.
- The *flow rate* is calculated by using the following formula:

    Drop factor × mL/min = flow rate (drops/min)

- IV administration time is calculated using the following formula:

    $$\frac{\text{Total of fluid to give}}{\text{Total time (min)}} \times \text{drop factor (drops/mL)}$$

    $$= \text{flow rate (drops/min)}$$

- The *total infusion time* depends on the total number of drops to be infused, the amount of fluid to be infused, and the number of minutes the IV is to flow.

GENERAL PRINCIPLES OF DRUG ADMINISTRATION

The process of oral drug administration involves several steps and safety measures to ensure you have correctly adhered to the *9 Rights of Drug Administration* (see Chapter 1 for details on this topic), the nursing process, and your institution policy. In general, you are responsible for knowing the drug you are giving, the reason the drug is being given, side effects that can be expected, and the adverse effects for which the patient should be monitored. You must also know any specific allergies your patient may have, and how these may relate to drugs ordered. Some drugs have specific limits on when and if they can be safely given. For example, you would not give a drug for hypertension (high blood pressure) if the patient's blood pressure was below a certain point. The healthcare provider may include these types of limits in the original order, or you may use your nursing judgement to "hold" giving a certain drug until you clarify the order with the prescriber.

The following steps are a general guide for giving drugs to your patient:

- Follow the *9 Rights of Drug Administration.*
- Minimize interruptions and distractions while preparing drugs (see Chapter 2).
- Wash your hands to avoid contamination of the drugs.
- Assemble necessary equipment, such as medication cups, and water for swallowing drugs.
- Follow the written drug order. Compare drug order with the written order, medication administration record (MAR), and the drug label. Be careful of

look-alike and sound-alike drug names, as this is a significant source of drug error!
- Accurately identify the patient before giving any drugs by checking the patient's wristband and by asking the patient his or her name and date of birth. For bar-coded drug administration systems, scan the patient's wristband to confirm that the correct drug, dose, and route is given to the correct patient.
- Do not unwrap or remove the drug from the container until you are with the patient.
- Follow **aseptic technique** for oral drugs by not touching the drug or the inside of the drug container. Pour the oral liquid or pills into the appropriate medication cup. Hold liquid drugs at eye level to avoid errors.
- Follow sterile technique when handling needles and syringes for giving subcutaneous, IM, or IV drugs. Dispose of needles and syringes properly immediately after giving the drug.
- Follow the institution procedure for proper documentation (charting) after giving the drug, or if the patient refuses the drug.

ENTERAL DRUGS

Enteral drugs are given directly into the gastrointestinal (GI tract) extending from the mouth through the anus. Enteral drugs can be given by the oral (PO), nasogastric (NG), or rectal route.

GIVING ORAL DRUGS

The most common way of giving drugs is by the oral route. Oral drugs come in several different forms, and each form serves a specific purpose. For example, different forms of oral drugs can either increase absorption, delay absorption, or reduce irritation to the stomach. Some oral drugs can come in tablet or capsule form, but patients may still call this type of drug form a "pill," which is an outdated term for health professionals. Tablets may be covered with a special coating that resists the acidic pH of the stomach, but will dissolve in the alkaline pH of the intestine.

Advantages of oral preparations are:
- Oral drugs are convenient, economical, and noninvasive.
- There is a variety of short- or long-acting formulations, and some have enteric coating to protect the stomach.

The major disadvantages of oral preparations are:
- They cannot be given to patients who are nauseated, vomiting, or who are unconscious.
- Oral drugs cannot be given to patients who cannot swallow.
- Older adult patients may need additional time to swallow oral tablets or capsules.
- Some drugs become ineffective when mixed with the acid and enzymes in the stomach and intestines.
- The drug onset of action may vary because the drug absorption in the GI tract is unpredictable.

> **⚠ Safety Alert!**
>
> You are responsible for the following aspects of patient safety:
> - You have the responsibility to ensure that patients safely take the drug(s) given to them. Do not leave drugs at the bedside for patients to take later.
> - Never give a drug poured or prepared by another nurse or healthcare provider to a patient. *You may only give drugs that you have prepared.*

Giving Oral Tablets or Capsules

Tablets and capsules are different forms of oral drugs. A **tablet** is made up of dried, powdered drugs that have been compressed into small shapes, whereas a **capsule** is gelatin container that holds powder or liquid drug. Before you give oral drugs, you must make sure the patient can safely swallow any drug given. If the patient is unable to swallow the drug as ordered, notify the healthcare provider who ordered the drug. Be sure you have followed all the steps in the correct procedure for drug administration (see earlier) and have a glass of water ready for the patient. If the drug is in the form of a lozenge, it is meant to be sucked, not swallowed.

All oral drugs are brought to the patient's bedside unwrapped, or in the original container, and can be placed in a paper soufflé cup using aseptic technique before giving the drug.

Do not crush tablets or break capsules without checking with the pharmacist. Many drugs have special coatings that are essential for proper absorption. If they are broken, cut, crushed, or chewed, drug absorption can be so rapid that adverse effects are more likely.

If a patient has difficulty swallowing the drug, have him or her take a few sips of water before placing the drug in the back of the mouth, then follow with more water. Help patients keep their heads forward while swallowing, as they do when they eat. It is generally not helpful to tilt the head backward.

You are responsible for making sure the patient takes all drugs safely, and on schedule. Do not leave drugs at the patient's bedside to be taken later, or ask another person to give them for you.

Giving Liquid-Form Oral Drugs

Liquids or solutions often must be shaken before they are poured to ensure the drug is evenly distributed throughout the liquid. Check to make sure the lid on the bottle is tightly closed before shaking. Take the lid off the bottle and place the lid upside down (outer surface down) on a flat surface. This protects the inside of the lid from dirt or contamination. When pouring liquids from a bottle into a plastic medication cup, hold the bottle so the label is against the hand. This prevents the drug from running down onto the label so that it cannot be read. Hold the medication cup at eye level

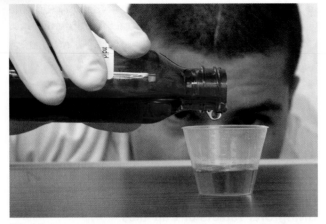

FIG. 4.3 Checking the drug dose in a medication cup. (From Potter AG, Perry P: *Clinical nursing skills and techniques*, ed 7, St. Louis, 2009, Mosby.)

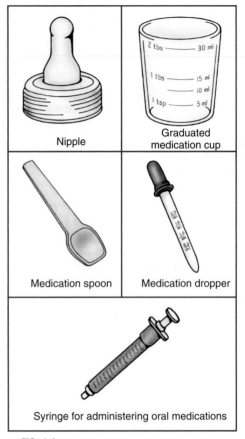

FIG. 4.4 Oral drug delivery for infant or child.

to read the proper dose (Fig. 4.3). Read the level at the lowest point in the medication cup. The drug could also be drawn up from the bottle or medication cup with a syringe or a medicine dropper (Fig. 4.4). These methods are useful in helping you to be accurate when a small dose is ordered or when giving drugs to infants or small children. The syringe or medicine dropper is placed halfway back in the baby's mouth, between the cheek and gums, and slowly emptied, giving the baby time to swallow it. The drug in the syringe or medicine dropper can be emptied into a nipple for an infant to suck the dose (see Fig. 4.4). Wipe any extra drug from the bottle top and replace the lid quickly to avoid contamination. Do not dilute a liquid drug unless ordered to do so by the prescriber.

Lifespan Considerations

Older Adults: Giving Drugs

Allow extra time when giving drugs to older adult patients. These individuals often are slower to take a drug, in swallowing drugs and water, and in understanding the answers provided to questions about their drugs.

GIVING DRUGS BY NASOGASTRIC OR PERCUTANEOUS ENDOSCOPIC GASTROSTOMY TUBE

Patients who cannot swallow, are nauseated, or who have bowel obstruction may be able to take drugs through an NG or percutaneous endoscopic gastrostomy (PEG) tube. A **nasogastric (NG) tube** is an enteral route of drug administration and oral feeding that bypasses the mouth by use of a tube going through the nose and esophagus into the stomach. The tubing and a clamp allow the nurse to easily give drugs in this way. The PEG tube is similar, but instead of going through the nose it is placed by surgical endoscopy directly through the abdomen wall and into the stomach. As with any other oral drug administration, check with the pharmacist before crushing tablets or opening capsules. Some tablets may be

crushed, mixed with 50 mL of water, and given through the NG or PEG tube. Others drugs cannot, and a liquid formulation must be ordered. It is important to know that some drugs are not compatible with feeding formulas (phenytoin [Dilantin]) or are degraded more quickly after crushing, making them less effective (enteric-coated pantoprazole). Sustained-release drugs are meant to be delivered over a period of time, so crushing this type of tablet can release the drug too quickly, resulting in increased drug blood levels and toxicity.

Top Tip for Safety

Do not open, cut, crush, or allow a patient to chew a sustained-release drug because these actions can release the drug too quickly and result in toxicity.

Follow the general procedure for preparing for drug administration. Double-check the prescriber's order to make sure you are giving the drug by the correct route, because all nonliquid drugs will need to be crushed or capsules opened to give drugs through NG or PEG tubes. Wash your hands and use gloves as needed following the agency's policy/procedure during this procedure. Place the patient in an upright position. For NG tube drug administration, check that the NG tube is in the stomach. Aspirate (remove) some stomach contents with a syringe and test the pH of the stomach contents. If the pH is 0 to 5, then the tube is most likely in the stomach. Auscultation over the area of the stomach and listening for a *whooshing* sound is no longer considered a reliable way to test NG tube placement.

The process for giving a drug through a PEG tube is very similar to that for the NG tube. In addition to the tubing, the PEG has a gastrostomy feeding button (a small, flexible silicone device that has a mushroom-shaped dome at one end and two small wings at the other end) that can be used to close the tube between uses. Irrigate this button with sterile water or normal saline after the drug has been given and clean the area according to institution policy.

In general, avoid crushing all tablets or capsules together; drugs should not be mixed together for administration through an NG or PEG tube. Each drug should be given separately because of possible incompatibilities, tube blockage, or changes in the pharmacodynamics of the drugs. Crushing enteric-coated drugs breaks them into small pieces that, when mixed with water, can result in clogging the tube. Always rinse the tube with sterile water or sodium chloride before and after giving the drug(s).

⬆ Top Tip for Safety

- Do not give sustained-release (long-acting), chewable, or enteric-coated capsules through an NG or PEG tube.
- If you are unsure if a drug can be given through an NG or PEG tube, ask the pharmacist.

Patients Who Are Receiving Enteral Feedings

For patients receiving enteral feedings, once tube placement is checked, the residual (amount) of stomach contents must also be checked. Drug administration may be held if the residual amount of feeding exceeds the standards set by the institution. Clamp the NG tube and attach a bulb syringe. Next, pour the drug mixed with water into the syringe, unclamp the NG tube, and let the drug run in by gravity. Add 50 mL of sterile water or normal saline according to the institution's policy to flush and clean out the tubing when all the drug has passed through the tube. Clamp the feeding tube for 30 minutes before and after drug administration to minimize interactions with the feeding formula, making sure to rinse the feeding tube well with sterile water or normal saline.

Patients With Nasogastric Tube to Suction

If suction is attached to the NG tube, disconnect it and clamp the suction tube shut for 30 minutes before drug administration. Attach a bulb syringe, pour the drug mixed with sterile water or normal saline into the syringe, unclamp the NG tube, and let the drug run in by gravity. Add 50 mL of sterile water or normal saline according to the institution's policy to flush and clean out the tubing when all of the drug has passed through

the tube, making sure to rinse the feeding tube well with sterile water or normal saline. Keep the feeding tube clamped for 30 minutes before and after drug administration to minimize interactions with the feeding formula.

The tube remains clamped for at least 30 minutes before the suction tube is reattached so that there is time for the drug to be absorbed. For additional information on this procedure, refer to your nursing fundamentals textbook.

PARENTERAL DRUGS

GENERAL PRINCIPLES

Giving drugs by the **parenteral route** refers to any drug given by intradermal, subcutaneous, IM, or IV route. Drugs are given parenterally for the following reasons:
- The patient cannot take an oral drug.
- The patient needs a drug that can act quickly.
- The drug needed may be destroyed by gastric enzymes.
- A steady blood level of the drug is needed.
- The drug is not available in an oral form.

For example, patients with severe, life-threatening infections may need IV antibiotics, or a patient may receive continuous IV heparin for anticoagulation.

IV drugs are injected directly into the bloodstream, and they act quickly, whereas drugs given by IM or subcutaneous injection require time for the drug to reach the bloodstream, so the onset of action is slower than for drugs given IV. Some IV drugs are effective for only a short time, requiring frequent doses. If an overdose of an IV drug is accidentally infused, the consequences to the patient can be very serious, because the effects are almost instantaneous. Once injected, the drug cannot be withdrawn, so accurate administration of the correct drug and dose is essential. When giving subcutaneous or IM drugs, you must accurately locate the appropriate injection site to avoid pain or tissue damage. Aseptic (sterile) technique must be followed to prevent infection.

Potential exposure to blood or body fluids can occur when giving parenteral drugs. Therefore the Centers for Disease Control and Prevention (CDC) issued standard precautions that include the wearing of gloves when there is risk to exposure to blood, body fluids, broken skin, or mucous membranes to prevent disease transmission. Therefore always wear gloves when giving any parenteral drugs.

When giving parenteral drugs, it is important that you do not recap needles and that you dispose of them properly in a designated "sharps" container to prevent needlestick injury. Usually these containers are present within a patient's room or in other patient care areas. Many hospitals and clinics now use needleless systems, retractable needles, or needles with a plastic safeguard to protect healthcare workers from needlestick injuries. Needle-free syringes dispense the drug using a high-pressurized air cartridge, although only a few drugs are available for delivery using this system. The needleless syringe is disposable anywhere because it does not come in contact with the skin and is a one-time use component of the device (Fig. 4.5).

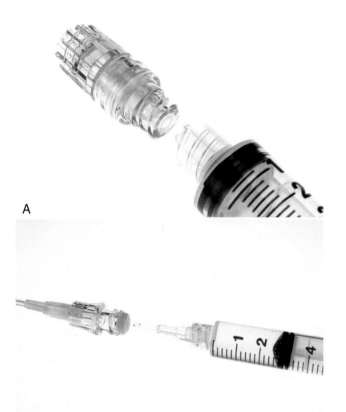

A

B

FIG. 4.5 Needleless syringe system. (© Baxter Healthcare Corp., Deerfield, IL.)

Syringes

Syringes come in a variety of sizes and are made up of three main parts. The tip is the portion that holds the needle. The needle screws onto the tip or fits tightly so it does not fall off. The barrel is the container for the drug. The calibrations are printed numbers on the barrel, and they indicate the amount or volume of drug in milliliters (mL), units, or cubic centimeters (cc) (Fig. 4.6).

The plunger is the inner portion that fits into the barrel of the syringe. When the plunger is pushed into the barrel, the drug is forced out through the needle.

Needles

The needle is made up of the hub, which attaches to the syringe; the shaft, which is the hollow part through which the drug passes; and the pointed or beveled tip, which pierces the skin (Fig. 4.7). The longer the pointed tip of the needle, the more easily the needle enters the skin. The diameter of the needle is called the *gauge*. The larger the number of the gauge, the smaller the hole (e.g., a 25-gauge needle is smaller than a 17-gauge needle). Thick solutions require larger diameters for injection. The needle gauge is written on the needle hub and on the package. Needles also come in varying lengths. Generally, the smaller the needle (larger the gauge), the shorter the needle. The smallest needles are used for intradermal or subcutaneous injections because they do not need to go very far into the skin and do not enter other tissues. Filter needles are also available for use when a drug is drawn from an ampule to prevent uptake of glass shards and risk of injection.

The sizes of the needle and syringe are determined by how viscous (thick) the drug is and by the amount to be injected. For example, blood is very thick and requires a 15- to 18-gauge needle. Sometimes when the

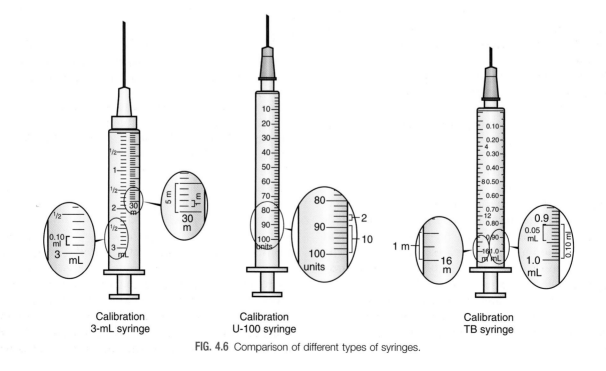

Calibration	Calibration	Calibration
3-mL syringe	U-100 syringe	TB syringe

FIG. 4.6 Comparison of different types of syringes.

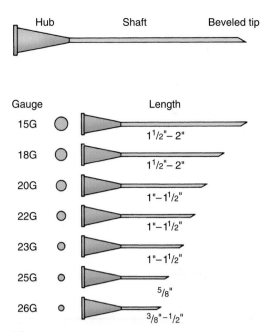

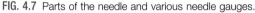

FIG. 4.7 Parts of the needle and various needle gauges.

| Table **4.1** | Suggested Guide for Selecting Syringe and Needles |

ROUTE	GAUGE (G)	LENGTH (INCHES)	VOLUME TO BE INJECTED (mL)
Intradermal	25–27	3/8–1/2	0.01–0.1
Subcutaneous	25–27	1/2–1	0.5–2
Intramuscular	20–22	1–2	0.5–2
Intravenous	15–22	1/2–2	Unlimited

volume is very small and the dosage must be very accurate (as with heparin or insulin), a small-gauge needle (such as a 27-gauge) is used so that no drug is lost. If more than 3 mL of drug is to be given IM, the drug must be divided and given in two injections so that a large pool of drug does not form in the tissue, which would irritate the tissue. A general guide for choosing the best syringe and needle size is presented in Table 4.1. Various needleless syringes are also used because it removes the risks associated with both reuse and disposal of needles.

PROCEDURE FOR PREPARING AND GIVING PARENTERAL DRUGS

The basic procedure for preparing and giving parenteral drugs is similar to that for oral drugs (Box 4.1). The type of parenteral injection and the specific drug to be given require the selection of the appropriate equipment and injection techniques. Inspect all syringe and needle packages to ensure they are sealed and the sterilization date has not expired. Any drug with a questionable seal that has changes in color or appearance or is expired is to be returned promptly to the pharmacy unused.

| Box **4.1** | Giving Parenteral Drugs |

STEP ONE: PREPARATION
Check the drug order as written for the patient, allergies, and the time to be given.
Wash hands well to avoid contaminating the drug and equipment.
Assemble all the necessary equipment (needles, syringes, alcohol swabs, and drug ordered).
Make certain the equipment is sterile and not expired.
Compare the drug order with the drug label. Check for the right patient, drug, route, dosage, and time to be given. Attach the needle to the syringe, keeping the needle covered with a cap.
Open the drug vial or ampule, cleansing the top of the drug container as appropriate.
Insert the needle into the drug container and fill the syringe with the proper amount of drug. Remove any air bubbles.
Do not mix more than one drug in a syringe unless they are compatible.
Replace the needle for a new sterile needle after the drug has been drawn up through a rubber stopper, multidose vial, or glass ampule.

STEP TWO: GIVING THE DRUG
Accurately identify the patient per institution policy.
Explain what drug is being given and answer any of the patient's questions.
Examine previous injection sites for signs of necrosis, infection, or swelling. Examine the site to be injected.
Put on gloves. Clean the skin with alcohol. Follow the specific procedure for intradermal, subcutaneous, or IM injection.
Dispose of the syringe per institution procedure and then wash your hands.
Document the drug was given as ordered per institution policy.
Check the patient, noting the response or adverse effects that must be recorded and reported.

Top Tip for Safety

- Check all equipment and drugs to ensure they are correct, sterile, and not expired before preparing the drug.
- *Always* wear gloves when giving parenteral drugs to avoid exposure to blood and body fluids.
- Clean the skin from the center outward, using a circular motion to minimize risk for infection.
- Do not recap needles! Recapping needles can result in needlestick injury and disease exposure.

Preparation of Parenteral Drugs

Parenteral drugs are supplied in a variety of different forms. A **vial** is a small, single- or multiple-dose glass or plastic container of a drug. The top of the glass container is fitted with a rubber diaphragm and a small aluminum lid. To draw up drugs from a vial, the metal lid is removed, and the rubber diaphragm is cleansed with alcohol. An amount of air equal to the amount of solution to be withdrawn is injected with

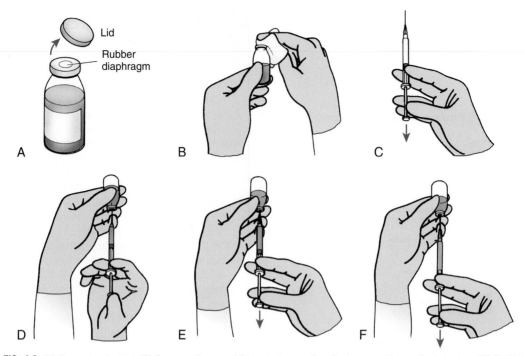

FIG. 4.8 (A) Example of a vial. (B) Remove the metal lid and cleanse the diaphragm with an alcohol wipe. (C) Pull into the syringe an amount of air equal to the amount of solution to be withdrawn. (D) Insert the needle with the bevel up and inject the air into the space above the solution. (E) Withdraw the drug. (F) Move the needle downward to allow the needle to continue to fill.

a syringe into the vial to assist the withdrawal of the drug (Fig. 4.8). Needles are always inserted into the vial bevel up so you can inspect the needle as it goes into the rubber stopper. The vial may contain a solution, or it may contain a powder to which a liquid diluent is added to make a solution. Read the label carefully to determine the type and amount of diluent that is required. Roll the vial carefully to make certain all of the powder is dissolved in the liquid. If the powder does not completely dissolve, do not give the drug and notify the pharmacy.

Ampules. **Ampules** contain one dose of a drug in a small, breakable glass container. The narrow neck of the base usually has a line (score) or ring around it, indicating a weakened area where the top can be broken off. All of the drug can be shifted to the bottom of the ampule by flicking the top lightly with a finger. Grasp the top above the scored or ringed area with a small gauze pad and pull down quickly on the glass top, breaking the ampule at the level of the line, or scored area, allowing insertion of the needle into the ampule to draw up the drug (Fig. 4.9). A filter needle is used to draw up the drug to prevent any glass shards from being drawn up into the syringe.

Mix-o-Vials. Parenteral drugs may come in a two-compartment vial called a **Mix-o-Vial.** The top compartment contains a sterile solution; the bottom compartment contains the drug powder. A rubber stopper separates the two areas. Pressure on the rubber plunger of the top compartment forces the stopper to fall below into the bottom compartment, letting in a solution that

dissolves the powder. Roll the vial gently between your palms to help dissolve the powder. When the powder is dissolved, insert the needle of the syringe to withdraw the solution (Fig. 4.10).

Multiple-dose vials. Any multiple-dose vial or newly mixed (reconstituted) powdered solution must be clearly labeled with the date, time, drug concentration and expiration time, and your initials. Once you withdraw a drug dose from a multiple-dose vial, change the needle before injecting the drug into the patient. Forcing the needle through the rubber stopper makes it dull and causes pain when injected into skin.

Mixing two parenteral drugs. Occasionally, two drugs are ordered that may be given in the same syringe. For example, two compatible drugs are often given together as preoperative sedation before surgery. Two types of insulin (regular and NPH) may be ordered to be given together. In contrast, many antibiotics must be given in separate syringes because they *precipitate* (form solid particles) or become inactive if mixed together.

Memory Jogger

It is important when *mixing two drugs in one syringe* to remember:
- The compatibility of the two drugs must be known; check with an up-to-date drug resource or your pharmacist.
- Air must be injected into both vials before any drug is withdrawn (to avoid accidental injection of a drug already in the syringe into the second vial).

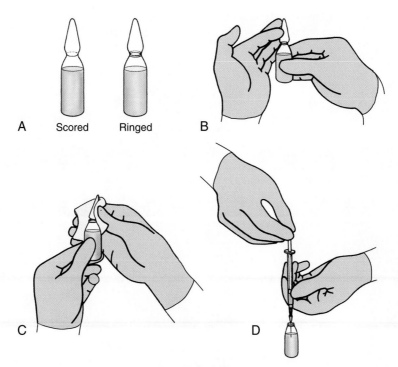

FIG. 4.9 (A) Examples of scored and ringed ampules. (B) Shift drug from the top to the bottom portion of the ampule by flicking the top lightly with a finger. (C) Wrap a gauze pad around the neck of the ampule and use a snapping motion to break off the top of the ampule along prescored line at the neck. Always break away from the body by bending the top toward you. (D) Insert the filter needle into the ampule and draw up the drug.

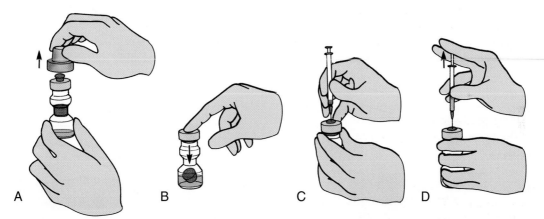

FIG. 4.10 Example of a Mix-o-Vial. (A) Remove the protective sterile cap from the Mix-o-Vial. (B) Push the rubber plunger on the top compartment; this will force the rubber stopper into the bottom compartment and let the solution dissolve the powder. The solution is mixed by gently rolling the container. (C) The needle is inserted through the top rubber diaphragm into the solution. (D) The required dose is withdrawn into the syringe.

Prefilled syringes or cartridges. Prefilled syringes and cartridges packaged this way are a convenient and reliable way of giving parenteral drugs. For patients, the advantages are ease of preparing and injecting drugs at home. Many opioids (narcotics) and emergency drugs (epinephrine) come in prefilled syringes and cartridges. These drug cartridges may be quickly slipped into a plastic holder and screwed into place (Fig. 4.11). The drug may then be quickly and accurately given.

Giving Intradermal Drugs

Intradermal injections are used for several purposes, such as for allergy sensitivity testing, tuberculosis exposure testing, and some vaccinations. Intradermal injections consist of a drug injection into the intradermal space between the upper two layers of the skin—the epidermis and the dermis (Fig. 4.12). Injections are made into the inner aspect of the forearm, the scapular area of the back, and the upper chest, if these areas are reasonably hairless. The blood supply to this area of the skin is less than that in other areas, so there is very slow absorption from the intradermal layer. Usually just a small volume is injected, producing a small bump like a mosquito bite, called a *bleb*. Once the drug has been injected, instruct the patient not to wear tight clothing over the area.

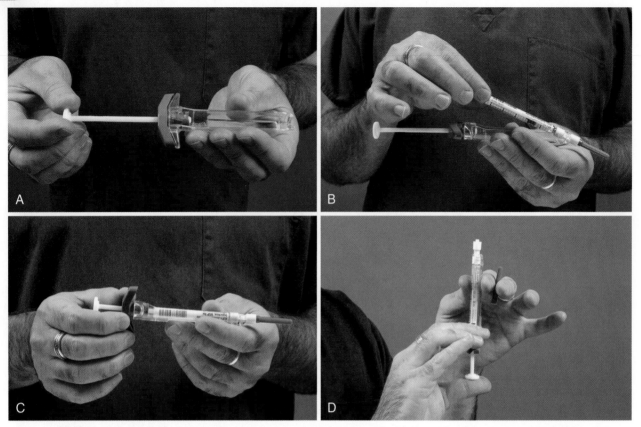

FIG. 4.11 (A) Example of a syringe and prefilled sterile cartridge with needle. (B) Assembling the syringe-needle system. (C) The cartridge slides into the syringe barrel, turns, and locks at the needle end. The plunger then screws into the cartridge end. (D) Expel excess drug to obtain accurate dose. (From Potter PA, Perry AG: *Fundamentals of nursing*, ed 7, St. Louis, 2008, Elsevier.)

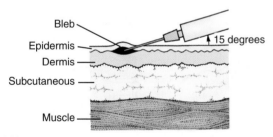

FIG. 4.12 Anatomy of skin showing placement for intradermal injections.

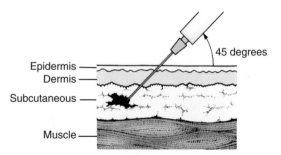

FIG. 4.13 Anatomy of skin showing placement for subcutaneous injections.

For intradermal injections, choose a needle that is both small (25-gauge) and short (3/8 inch). Wash your hands and don gloves. Cleanse the skin before giving the injection. Once you draw up the drug, insert the needle firmly at a 15-degree angle, with the bevel of the needle pointing upward. Do not aspirate (pull back) the syringe plunger before giving the drug. Inject the drug and then quickly remove the needle. The small bleb should be seen on the skin at the point where the drug was injected into the intradermal space. After giving the injection, check the patient's skin for sensitivity or an allergic reaction to the injection. You may see an immediate reaction, or reactions may take hours to several days to develop. Tuberculin tests are given

intradermally and are checked for reactivity in 48 to 72 hours after the injection. Making a circle mark around the injection site with a pen as soon as the drug is given can help you identify the site of the injection and the size of the reaction. Document any reaction noted and notify the healthcare provider.

Giving Subcutaneous Drugs

Subcutaneous injections are given into the tissue between the dermis of the skin and the muscle layer (Fig. 4.13). There will be a slow but long duration of drug action because less blood is normally supplied to this area. Heparin and insulin are the drugs most frequently given by subcutaneous injection. See Chapters 14 and 17 for

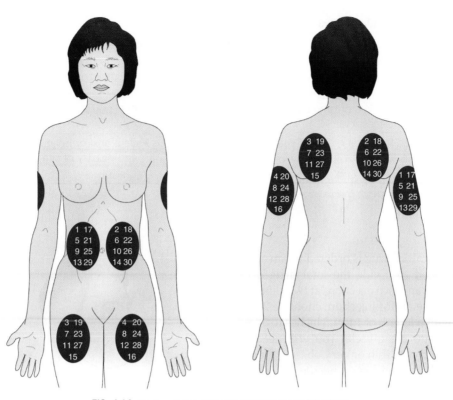

FIG. 4.14 Body rotation sites for subcutaneous injections.

detailed information on these drugs. The drug volume given in a subcutaneous injection is usually between 0.5 and 1 mL per injection. When giving subcutaneous drugs daily over a long time period, you will need to rotate the injection sites to avoid irritating the tissue or causing changes in the tissue with repeated injections in the same area.

Subcutaneous injections require a small syringe and needle. Usually a 25- or 27-gauge needle with a 3/8-inch needle length is used. Subcutaneous injections may be given in the upper arms, upper back, scapular region, anterior thighs, and abdomen. Before giving the injection, wash your hands and don gloves, then cleanse the appropriate skin area with alcohol. To give a subcutaneous injection, insert the needle bevel up into the skin at a 45-degree angle. Do not aspirate before giving the drug to prevent bruising and other tissue damage. Inject the drug and remove the needle. Once the needle is removed, apply slight pressure to prevent bleeding. Apply additional or pressure of longer duration if the patient is at risk for bleeding. Document the injection site (location) and any skin or other reactions to the injection.

⌂ **Top Tip for Safety**

Do not aspirate before giving a drug subcutaneously to prevent bruising and other tissue damage.

If a patient is to continue subcutaneous drug administration for any length of time at home, teach the patient

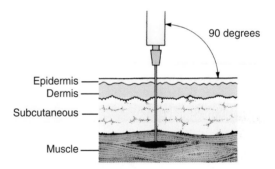

FIG. 4.15 Anatomy of skin showing placement for IM injections.

about the drug, expected effects and adverse effects to report, and proper techniques for drug administration. Teach the patient and family to develop a plan for rotating injection sites. The front view in Fig. 4.14 shows areas usually used for subcutaneous self-injection. The back view shows less commonly used areas that may be accessed for injection by the family.

Giving IM Drugs

Drugs given by the **intramuscular (IM) route** are deposited deep into the muscle mass (Fig. 4.15), where the rich blood supply allows for a more rapid drug absorption as compared with the subcutaneous route. The muscles also contain large blood vessels and nerves, so it is important to place the needle correctly to avoid damage to these structures.

IM injections for adults typically range from 1 to 3 mL, and infants and children rarely receive more than

Table **4.2**	IM Injection-Site Advantages and Disadvantages	
INJECTION SITE	**ADVANTAGES**	**DISADVANTAGES**
Deltoid (upper arm)	Easily accessible Useful for vaccinations in adolescents and adults	Poorly developed in young children Only small amounts (0.5–1 mL) can be injected
Vastus lateralis (thigh)	Preferred site for infant injections Relatively free of large blood vessels and nerves Easily accessible	Intake of drug is slower than the arm but faster than buttocks
Ventrogluteal (hips)	Used for children aged 7 years or older and adults Less likely to be inadvertently injected subcutaneously	Patient anxiety because of unfamiliarity with site and visibility of site during injection

From Workman ML, LaCharity L: *Understanding pharmacology*, ed 2, St. Louis, 2016, Elsevier.

1 mL. If more than 3 mL of drug is ordered for an adult patient, you will need to divide the total drug dose between two syringes, and two injections at two different sites are given. To give an IM injection, choose a 20- to 22-gauge needle with a length of 1 to 1.5 inches to allow deeper placement into the muscle. You will need to make adjustments for very thin or very obese patients, who will require a shorter or longer needle for proper drug placement.

The sites for IM injections include the deltoid, vastus lateralis, and ventrogluteal muscles. Each site has advantages and disadvantages, and you must be able to correctly identify each site for giving IM drugs safely. Table 4.2 describes the advantages and disadvantages of each IM injection site. The dorsogluteal site is *not* recommended because the presence of nerves and blood vessels in the area increase the risk for tissue damage.

> ### Top Tip for Safety
>
> The dorsogluteal site is *not* recommended for IM injections because the presence of nerves and blood vessels in the area increase the risk for tissue damage.

Before preparing the IM drug for injection, carefully select the site and identify the landmarks. Figs. 4.16 through 4.18 show how to identify sites for IM injections. Position the patient properly to be able to access the injection site. Wash your hands and put on gloves. Clean the injection area with alcohol. Insert the needle firmly, at a 90-degree angle, and inject the drug. *Aspiration is not recommended for IM injection of vaccines or immunizations.* If aspiration is required for a certain drug, pull back the plunger after inserting the needle and check for the presence of blood being drawn up into the syringe. If this occurs, remove the needle and discard the drug and syringe properly. You will then need to prepare a new dose of the drug and inject into a different site. After withdrawing the needle, apply gentle pressure to the site with a dry cotton ball. Avoid massaging the area of injection. Rotate the site of injection when repeated injections are needed. Note the time and site of the injection, and be sure to check

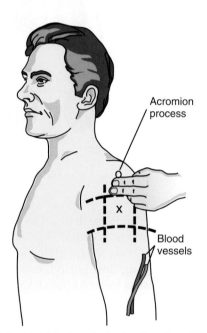

FIG. 4.16 Deltoid IM injection-site landmarks. (From Workman ML, LaCharity L: *Understanding pharmacology*, ed 2, St. Louis, 2016, Elsevier.)

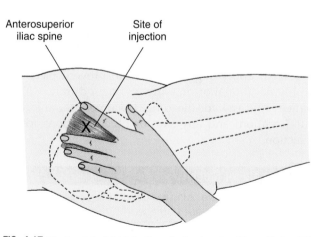

FIG. 4.17 Ventrogluteal IM injection-site landmarks. (From Potter PA, Perry AG: *Fundamentals of nursing: Concepts, process, and practice*, ed 8, St. Louis, 2013, Mosby.)

the patient for both expected and adverse effects of the drug; document your findings.

The **Z-track technique** may be used for IM injections of drugs that can stain the skin or are known to be irritating to the tissues (Fig. 4.19). To give drugs using the Z-track technique, draw up the drug as usual, plus 0.1 to 0.2 mL of air. The injection of the air seals the injection site, preventing leakage of the drug. Drugs of the type that require the Z-track technique are injected into the ventrogluteal site. Once the injection site is prepared, pull the tissue downward and away from the injection site. Inject the drug and allow the skin to move back into place before you remove the needle. This action allows the tissue to make a seal over the injection site, sealing the drug in place. *Do not massage the injection site.*

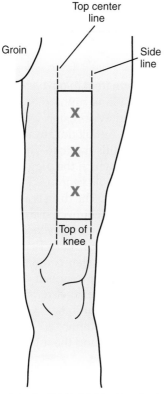

FIG. 4.18 Vastus lateralis (thigh) IM injection-site landmarks. (From Workman ML, LaCharity L: *Understanding pharmacology*, ed 2, St. Louis, 2016, Elsevier.)

Giving IV Drugs

Intravenous drugs are delivered by IV "push" or bolus route, IV "piggyback" or intermittent infusion, or continuous IV infusion. The IV route injects a drug directly into the vein, where it enters the bloodstream immediately. The rate of absorption and the onset of action are faster for the IV route than for the oral and IM routes because IV drugs have not been exposed to other enzymes or tissues before reaching the bloodstream. In addition, some drugs cannot be given orally, and may be very painful or irritating if given IM. In emergencies, a drug may be injected directly into a vein, but usually the IV drug is given on a scheduled basis or infused slowly through IV tubing or an infusion line that is already in the vein.

Greater skill and knowledge are needed to give IV drugs, and care is needed to prevent infection at the needle site. In addition, because the effect of the drug is immediate, drug overdosages, errors in dosage calculation, or failure to control the rate of administration may produce serious or fatal consequences for the patient. Thus you have an increased responsibility for implementing and evaluating the drug given. Registered nurses are usually the nurses who will give these types of drugs, but an LPN/VN often assists in this procedure. In some states the LPN/VN may give IV drugs into an already existing IV set up either by piggyback or as an IV push dose. Initiating the actual IV system is not within the LPN/VN scope of practice in many states. Be sure to check your state's Nurse Practice Act to determine your legal role in IV drug administration.

Top Tip for Safety

- You are responsible for checking the provider's IV drug order to ensure it is both complete and clear.
- The drug, dose, timing, and type of IV administration (IV push, intermittent, or continuous infusion) must be specified, along with the rate of infusion.
- A drug order that states to give an IV drug "slowly" is not acceptable because it leaves the timing open to interpretation and may prove harmful to the patient if done improperly.

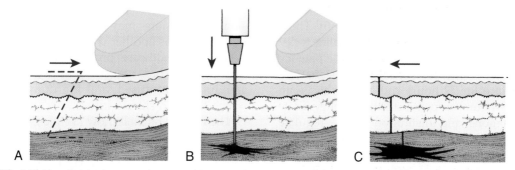

FIG. 4.19 Z-track injection technique. (A) Pull the tissue laterally. (B) Insert the needle straight down into the muscle and inject the drug. (C) Release the tissue as the needle is withdrawn; this allows the skin to slide over the injection track and seal the drug inside.

All IV drugs that are prepared directly in advance of administration must be clearly labeled and given only by the person who drew it up. All IV drugs that need to be reconstituted (powders to be mixed with liquid) must be mixed using the recommended liquid in the reconstitution process to prevent crystals or other harmful precipitates from forming. Before giving drugs into an existing IV connected to an IV pump, make sure you have been oriented to the proper use of the pump to prevent infusion errors.

Always use aseptic technique, which is manipulation that does not contaminate the sterility of the drug and drug delivery system when giving IV drugs. You must wash your hands and don gloves in preparation for giving IV drugs. Make sure you disinfect the diaphragm of the drug vial and the injection portal before giving the IV drug or injecting it into a piggyback or IV solution. Make sure you use the proper personal protection equipment if you will be exposed to blood or body fluids. Use a filter syringe to withdraw a drug from a glass vial, changing the needle (or use a needless syringe) before injecting the drug.

Giving IV push drugs. Many IV drugs are commonly given by syringe through an IV infusion that is already running as a direct "push" or "bolus" dose. In this way the drug most directly enters the patient, rather than the IV bottle or bag. In addition to the directions presented here, review your nursing fundamentals textbook for more information about this procedure.

Wash your hands and don a pair of gloves. Clean the drug injection portal with alcohol, then slowly inject the drug into the IV line, using the portal closest to the patient and according to the prescribed rate of IV push infusion for that drug. There are specific guidelines for the length of time of IV push injection for all drugs able to be given in this manner. Once all the drug is injected, the needle is withdrawn. The main IV solution is restarted at the specified infusion rate. Document the IV injection, note if the effects of the drug have been achieved (e.g., pain relief), and monitor the patient for any adverse effects.

Giving drugs by peripheral IV locks. A patient may have a butterfly or scalp vein needle inserted and left in place without being attached to a primary IV solution, to serve as a means for giving drugs intermittently. These units may be referred to as peripheral IV or saline locks, because normal saline is used to maintain the patency of these devices. Peripheral IV or saline locks are typically left in place for 72 hours and are flushed with saline every 8 hours or per institution policy. State practice regulations and institution policy regulate whether an LPN/VN may give drugs through these systems. Follow institutional policy if you, as an LPN/VN, are permitted to give drugs in this manner.

To begin, wash your hands and don gloves. Use an alcohol wipe to cleanse the top of the rubber diaphragm at the end of the tubing. Follow the institution's policy

and procedures for flushing the tubing before and after giving the drug. Refer to your nursing fundamentals textbook to review this procedure. Be sure to inject the drug over the specified length of time recommended for that drug and observe for expected and adverse effects.

Adding drugs to an IV solution container. Make certain that the drug is compatible with the solution into which it will be injected. Wash your hands and don a pair of gloves. Identify the proper portal and cleanse it with an alcohol wipe. Fill the syringe with the drug and inject it slowly with a small needle through the portal into the IV container. Label the IV bottle or bag with the date, time, dosage, and drugs added and sign your initials. Monitor the patient for the desired drug effects or any adverse effects (e.g., allergic reaction) that may occur. Document drug administration in accordance with your institution's policy. Review your nursing fundamentals textbook for more information on this procedure.

Giving drugs by intermittent (piggyback) infusion. While an existing IV infusion is running, it may be clamped off to allow a second IV infusion for giving drugs by intermittent infusion. Antibiotics are an example of drug types often given in this manner. The drug order will specify the time over which the piggyback IV solution containing the drug should be infused. Wash your hands and don a pair of gloves. The drug is added to a second, small IV bottle or bag connected to the drug portal. This second IV container, or **piggyback infusion**, is hung slightly higher than the primary IV solution with the tubing to the primary IV clamped off to allow the piggyback IV containing the prescribed drug to be infused. The piggyback IV is to be labeled with the time, date, drug, and dosage, and your initials. Once the piggyback is infused, the setup is removed, the clamp on the primary IV is reopened, and the infusion is reset to the prescribed drops/minute.

IV infusions. Giving IV fluids is considered another IV drug delivery system. Remember that whenever you infuse fluids or drugs directly into the vein, they immediately enter the bloodstream. When IV fluids are given, this is known as a continuous intravenous infusion. IV infusions may be given for the purpose of hydration or as another way to give parenteral drugs. When the healthcare provider orders IV fluids for hydration, the order must include the type of fluid, the amount to be infused, and the duration (time) over which the fluid should infuse.

The IV flow rate tells how fast the IV infusion should run. The healthcare provider's order must state the amount (in milliliters) over time. For example, the order may instruct you to give 250 mL of a solution over 1 hour. The size of the tubing influences the rate of the infusion. Thicker tubing will give more drops per minute as compared with smaller, thinner tubing. Each tubing has what is known as a drop factor, which is the number of drops needed to make a milliliter of fluid. Each manufacturer places the drop factor on each IV administration tubing set.

IV tubing is divided into two types: *macrodrip* and *microdrip* tubing. The actual *drip chamber* (the clear plastic cylinder attached to the IV tubing) of the IV tubing differs considerably. Fig. 4.20 shows the differences between the macrodrip and microdrip chambers.

When the IV tubing is *primed* to be ready for IV fluid administration, the drip chamber is filled only halfway so you can see the fluid dripping and count the number of drops per minute, if needed. Depending on the manufacturer, the drop factor for a macrodrip IV set is 10, 15, or 20 drops/mL. However, all microdrip tubing delivers 60 drops/mL. This information is important, because you need to know the drip factor for every IV calculation. Fig. 4.21 shows the different parts of the IV infusion set.

IV fluid regulation. To regulate the flow of IV fluids, you will need to calculate the drip rate, as described in the Calculations for IV Infusions section earlier in this chapter. Recall that the drip rate is the number of drops per minute needed to have the IV infused in the amount of time ordered by the prescriber. There are essentially two ways to regulate IV fluids: You can use the roller clamp on the tubing to regulate the flow of the IV solution, or more commonly, an IV pump is used. An IV pump is an electronic device that infuses the IV solution into the vein by pressure. The IV pump has buttons for specific settings that are involved in infusion of IV fluid that can be manually programmed. Fig. 4.22 shows an example of an IV pump.

The IV pump settings are:
On/Off
Start/Enter
Stop

Silence
IV Lock (prevent tampering)
Primary (controls the main or primary IV solution infusion)
IVPB (controls piggyback or secondary infusion)

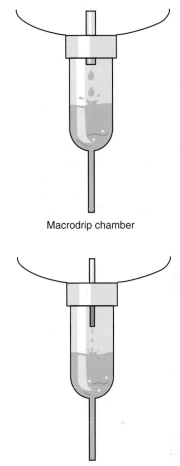

Macrodrip chamber

Microdrip chamber

FIG. 4.20 Macrodrip chamber and microdrip chamber. (From Workman ML, LaCharity L: *Understanding pharmacology*, ed 2, St. Louis, 2016, Elsevier.)

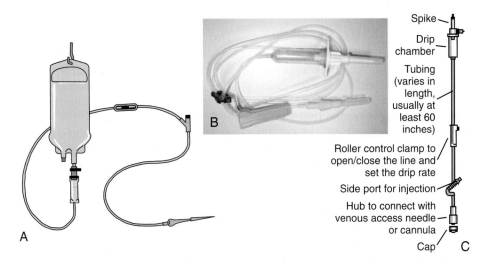

Spike
Drip chamber
Tubing (varies in length, usually at least 60 inches)
Roller control clamp to open/close the line and set the drip rate
Side port for injection
Hub to connect with venous access needle or cannula
Cap

FIG. 4.21 IV tubing administration sets. (A) Administration set connected to an IV solution bag. (B) Photo of IV tubing administration set. (C) Details of IV tubing administration set. (From Workman ML, LaCharity L: *Understanding pharmacology*, ed 2, St. Louis, 2016, Elsevier.)

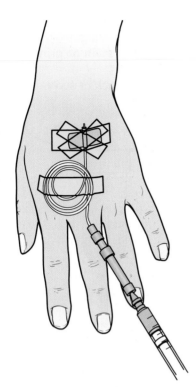

FIG. 4.22 Example of an IV pump. SIGMA Spectrum infusion system. (© Baxter Healthcare Corp., Deerfield, IL.)

IV pumps are made by different companies, so you will need to be oriented to the IV pumps used in your facility and follow the manufacturer's directions. Some IV pumps are set to deliver the IV solution in milliliters per hour and others in drops per minute.

Memory Jogger

To infuse IV fluids properly, you will need to know these four items:
- the correct type of fluid ordered,
- the volume (how much) to be infused,
- the duration (how long) of the infusion, and
- the rate (how fast) the IV solution is to be infused.

The healthcare provider's order must address the type of fluid to be infused, the amount (volume) to be infused, and the duration (length of time) the fluid should be infused over. You will need to calculate the rate of the infusion. For example, the order may read: "Infuse 1000 mL of 0.9% normal saline over 12 hours." You can use this information to program the IV pump. You will need to note the start and stop times of the infusion. Many factors influence the gravity flow, so a solution may not necessarily continue to flow at the rate originally set. Therefore IV infusions must be monitored to verify that the fluid is flowing at the intended rate. Mark the IV bag or bottle with tape with the start time of the infusion. The flow is calculated when the solution is originally hung and

then rechecked at least hourly to ensure it is infusing on time.

Calculating the IV flow rate. As discussed earlier in this chapter, the IV flow rate is the rate at which IV fluids are given. Recall that you will need to know the IV tubing drop factor plus the duration of time (in minutes) the IV solution is to run over to perform this calculation.

The basic formula is:

$$\frac{\text{drop factor}}{\text{minutes}}$$

Macrodrip calculation. Using our previous example, 1000 mL of normal saline is to be infused over 12 hours. The first step is to find out the number of milliliters to be run over 1 hour (flow rate).

$$\text{Divide 1000 by 12: } \frac{1000}{12} = 83 \text{ mL/h}$$

Now calculate the number of drops per minute needed to have the IV infuse at 83 mL/h.

$$\frac{\text{Volume (in milliliters)}}{\text{Time}} \times \text{drop factor (drops/mL)}$$
$$= \text{drops/min}$$

A check of the IV administration set shows a drip factor of 10.

$$\frac{83}{60} \times 10 = 1.38 \times 10 = 13.8 \text{ drops/min. You may round}$$

up to 14 drops per minute.

Microdrip calculation. Recall the drop factor for microdrip tubing is 60 drops/mL, the same as the number of minutes in 1 hour. Use the same formula as for the macrodrip set.

$$\frac{83}{60} \times \frac{60}{1} \text{ (drop factor)}$$
$$= \frac{83}{1} \text{ (the 60 and 60 cancel each other out)}$$
$$= 83 \text{ microdrops/min}$$

You can see that the flow rate always equals the drop rate when using a microdrip set. Calculation of the milliliters per hour provides the drops per minute.

Completing IV therapy. When IV therapy is to be discontinued, clamp the tubing, loosen the adhesive tape, and put on gloves. Holding a gauze pad in the non-dominant hand, apply gentle pressure on the venipuncture site with the gauze pad and carefully withdraw the needle with the dominant hand. The area is then cleaned with an alcohol wipe and elevated, if possible, and direct pressure is applied to stop any bleeding at the site. Check for bleeding after 1 to 2 minutes. Follow institutional procedure for any additional steps regarding

Table 4.3 Complications of Intravenous Infusions

PROBLEM	APPROPRIATE NURSING ACTION
Failure to infuse properly	Check for bent tubing, needle against vein wall, or small clot at needle end; the intravenous (IV) pole may be too low, or the needle may be out of the vein. Check for damage done from tissue infusion. Stop infusion and report problem to the registered nurse.
IV infiltration	Check to see whether any tissue was damaged. Notify healthcare provider of any necrosis or sloughing. Apply wet compresses to the area to reduce pain. Stop infusion and report problem to the registered nurse.
Signs of infection	Check for local and systemic symptoms. Stop infusion and notify healthcare provider. Treat symptomatically. Save the solution for testing.
Allergic reactions	Stop infusion and notify the healthcare provider.
Circulatory problems	Watch for symptoms of pulmonary edema: shortness of breath, poor color, weight gain, restlessness, and edema. Notify the healthcare provider.
Other	Watch for symptoms of pulmonary embolus: poor color, shortness of breath, chest pain, and coughing up blood. Notify the healthcare provider.

ointments or pressure dressings as needed. Dispose of all contaminated equipment per institution policy.

Evaluation for complications of IV therapy. There are six primary areas for evaluation of patients receiving IV therapy. Table 4.3 summarizes the problems and complications that may occur with an IV infusion and the appropriate nursing actions to take.

The first step for evaluating the situation if an IV fails to infuse properly is to check the patient for bending of the IV tubing or lying on tubing, obstructing flow. If the rate of infusion is very slow, a small clot may form at the end of the needle, blocking the flow. The IV container may have to be elevated to keep adequate pressure for infusion. Check every part of the infusion setup for any problems that can block infusion, including lack of blood return to the tubing, leading you to suspect that the needle is out of place or blocked.

Infiltration. When the needle becomes dislodged from the vein, allowing infusion of fluid into the tissues, this is known as *infiltration*. This produces pain, swelling of the area, and redness. When the infiltrating fluid irritates or damages the surrounding tissue, it is known as *extravasation*. When an IV infiltration is discovered, inspect the infusion site carefully for signs of infection or injury. Discontinue the infusion and contact the healthcare provider who ordered the IV. Report any swelling, redness, tissue loss, or necrosis. Warm, moist compresses may be ordered to be applied to the area. In the case of necrosis, more intensive treatment would be needed; promptly notify the pharmacist as well as the healthcare provider.

Infection. Signs of infection from an existing IV or inflammation of the vein (*phlebitis*) include redness, swelling, warmth, and burning along the course of the vein. Inflammation and infection can be associated with irritating solutions or certain drugs such as potassium, antibiotics, or anticancer drugs. In these cases, stop the IV and notify the healthcare provider. Warm, moist compresses may be applied to the area.

Allergic reactions. Because IV infusions directly enter the vein and bloodstream, there is potential for an allergic reaction to drugs. Monitor the patient receiving IV drugs for shortness of breath, temperature elevation, or rash. Reactions to blood or blood products are not common, but they can be harmful to the lungs and kidneys and can cause itching, shaking chills, temperature elevations, back pain, dark urine, and shortness of breath. Stop the drug infusion or blood transfusion immediately, obtain vital signs, and remain with the patient while another colleague notifies the healthcare provider.

Fluid overload. The potential for fluid overload is a concern for older adult patients, infants, and children because they are more sensitive to the amount of fluid infused. These individuals may have heart, lung, or kidney problems that decrease their ability to handle extra fluid. Fluid overload may develop when fluids are infused too rapidly or when the volume to be infused is too great. Signs of fluid overload include dyspnea, weakness, lethargy, reduced urine output, edema of the extremities, sacral edema weak, rapid pulse, and shallow, rapid respirations. If the excess fluid accumulates primarily in the lungs, producing coughing, difficulty breathing, crackles in the lung sounds, and frothy sputum, slow the infusion immediately, monitor the patient's vital signs, and notify the healthcare provider.

Top Tip for Safety

- Check IV patency flow rates hourly.
- Observe the patient for signs of fluid overload (shortness of breath, edema).
- Monitor the patient's urinary output. Urinary output should be at least 30 cc/h.
- Observe the IV site for redness or swelling that may indicate infiltration.
- Monitor the patient for signs of allergic reactions to any IV drug.

PERCUTANEOUS DRUGS

The **percutaneous route** is the delivery of drugs by application to the skin or mucous membranes. Using this route makes it difficult to predict how well the drug will be absorbed. The amount of drug absorbed through the skin or mucous membranes depends on several factors:

- the size of the area covered by the drug;
- the concentration or strength of the drug;
- the length of time the drug stays in contact with the skin; and
- the general condition of the skin, including any areas of skin irritation or breakdown, skin thickness, and the general hydration, nutrition, and tone of the skin.

Methods of percutaneous administration include:

- giving drugs into the mucous membranes of the ear, eye, nose, mouth, or vagina;
- applying topical creams, powders, ointments, or lotions;
- inhaling aerosolized liquids or gases to carry drugs to the nasal passages, sinuses, and lungs; and
- application of transdermal patches or topical gel systems.

Follow the same general procedures and patient safety considerations outlined for other routes of administration when applying drugs to the skin or mucous membranes. The general method for giving percutaneous drugs is outlined in Box 4.2.

GIVING TOPICAL AND TRANSDERMAL DRUGS

Drugs given by the **topical route** are applied directly to the area of skin that requires treatment. The most common forms of topical drugs include creams, lotions, and ointments, although there are many others. Each form of topical application has specific advantages and characteristics. **Transdermal** drugs are semipermeable membranes and adhesive patches that are applied to the skin, where the drug is absorbed into the bloodstream. Drugs using a transdermal delivery system include fentanyl, nitroglycerin, birth control pills, scopolamine, testosterone, and clonidine. Various antismoking programs also use nicotine patches.

Topical Drugs

1. Choose the skin site carefully. Avoid skin that has been tattooed, skin that has lesions, or broken skin, all of which can affect absorption.
2. Clean the skin before applying topical drugs to reduce the risk for infection, and remove remaining drug from the previous application to prevent drug buildup.
3. Wear gloves for protection, because the drug you are giving can also be absorbed through your skin.

Apply a thin layer of the topical drug with a tongue depressor, a cotton-tipped applicator, or a gloved finger. The topical drug may also be applied directly onto a gauze pad and placed on the skin if the site requires a dressing, as shown in Fig. 4.23. Anchor the dressing as ordered by the healthcare provider.

Transdermal Patches

1. Follow steps 1 through 3 in the previous section as for giving topical drugs.
2. To apply transdermal patches, carefully pick up the patch and remove the clear plastic backing as shown in Fig. 4.24.
3. Firmly press the patch drug side down onto the skin. The adhesive on the edges will hold the patch tightly to the skin.
4. Transdermal patches are changed on a regular schedule, as indicated by the provider's order. Transderm-Nitro, fentanyl patches, Nitro-Dur, and birth control patches may be worn while showering; all other drug patches are to be applied after bathing.

Many topical or transdermal drugs are continued after the patient leaves the hospital. Teach the patient how to clean the area, apply the drug, and dress the area, as needed. Note the site where ointments (nitroglycerine) or patches (fentanyl, nitroglycerine) are placed, along with the date and time.

Box **4.2**   Giving Percutaneous Drugs

STEP ONE: PREPARATION

Check the drug order as written for the patient, allergies, and time to be given.

Wash your hands well to avoid contaminating the drug or equipment used.

Assemble all the necessary equipment (drug, gloves, and plastic wrap).

Compare the drug order with the label on the container. First check for the right patient, drug, route, dosage, and time to be given.

STEP TWO: GIVING THE DRUG

Accurately identify the patient per institution policy.

Explain what drug is being given, and answer any of the patient's questions.

Apply the drug as ordered to the appropriate area.

When complete, discard all used dressings and gloves. Wash hands.

Document the drug was given as ordered per institution policy.

Check the patient, noting the response or adverse effects that must be recorded and reported.

⬆ Top Tip for Safety

Avoid touching topical or transdermal drugs with your bare hands or fingers to prevent absorbing the drug through the skin into your system.

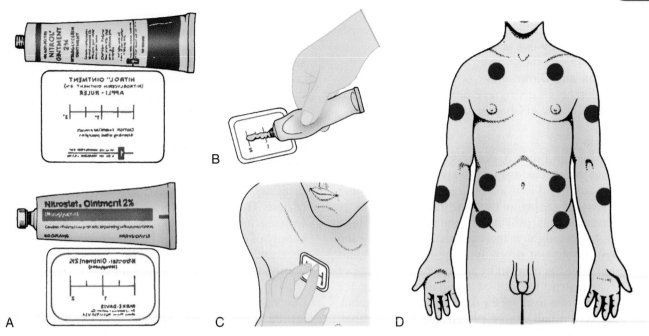

FIG. 4.23 (A) Nitroglycerin ointment and special application papers. Note that the papers are printed backward. (B) The correct amount of ointment is squeezed onto the paper. (C) The paper is applied to the patient's skin in one of the sites shown in (D). Clear plastic wrap may be applied over the paper to increase absorption and protect clothing from staining.

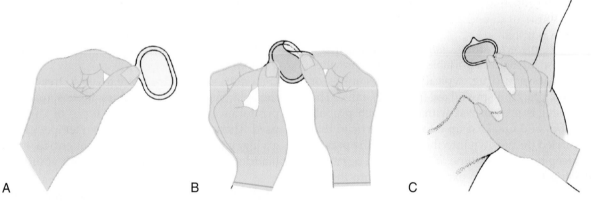

FIG. 4.24 (A) Nitroglycerin patch. (B) Remove the plastic backing, being careful not to touch the drug inside. (C) Place the side with drug on the patient's skin and press the adhesive edges into place.

GIVING DRUGS THROUGH MUCOUS MEMBRANES

The mucous membranes are the other major route of percutaneous drug administration. Different mucous membranes throughout the body can be used for giving drugs. Drugs can be given by the **sublingual route** (under the tongue); **buccal route** (against the cheek); in the mucous membranes of the eye, nose, or ear; or inhaled into the lung through an aerosol. Vaginal suppositories or creams and drugs given rectally also represent treatment through mucosal membranes. Drugs for mucous membranes might come as small tablets, drops, ointments, creams, suppositories, or metered-dose inhalers.

Before giving drugs through the mucous membranes, follow all the general steps noted earlier in this chapter for safe drug administration, wash your hands, and don a pair of gloves.

Sublingual and Buccal Drugs

Place sublingual drugs, such as nitroglycerine tablets or spray, under the tongue. There is a rich blood supply in this area, so the drug is absorbed quickly. Teach the patient not to chew or swallow the drug, because drugs meant for the sublingual route are less effective if absorbed by the GI tract. Teach the patient to avoid food or drink until the drug is completely dissolved.

To give drugs by the buccal route, place the drug between the cheek and teeth of the upper jaw. Lozenges are often given by this route.

Eye Drops and Ointments
Information about giving eye drops and ointments is provided in detail in Chapter 18.

Ear Drops
As described in Box 4.3, position the patient on one side, with the affected ear up. You will need to pull the ear lobe (pinna) down in children who are younger than 3 years of age before instilling the drops. For older children and adults, pull the ear lobe up and out. These actions help straighten the ear canal. Now place the required amount of drops into the ear canal. Avoid contaminating the dropper by not touching the dropper to the ear. Instruct the patient to remain in position for at least 5 minutes to allow the drug to coat the ear canal. A small cotton ball can be placed into the ear canal. Repeat on the opposite ear if both ears are affected.

Respiratory Mucosa
Drugs can be given and inhaled through the respiratory mucosa. Common types of aerosols used for inhaled drug delivery are the pressurized metered-dose inhaler, the dry-powder inhaler, and continuous aerosol therapy. Table 4.4 lists the advantages and disadvantages for inhaled drugs.

Pressurized metered-dose inhaler. A pressurized metered-dose inhaler is a portable device that provides multiple doses of a drug, typically corticosteroids or bronchodilators, by a specialized (metered) valve. The drug canister is pressurized with gas, which propels the drug out and breaks it up into small particles that can be carried deep down into the lungs as the patient takes a deep breath. This type of device must be *primed* by pressing the device to expel the drug into the air before the first use and periodically thereafter. Otherwise the drug and propellant fail to combine, and the correct dose may not be delivered.

Dry-powder inhaler. A dry-powder inhaler is an aerosol device that delivers the drug in a powdered form when the patient takes a deep breath. For both types of inhalers, place the patient in an upright position. Shake the container before use. Instruct the patient to exhale and then on the next inhalation (following the specific directions for the inhaler) to release the drug. Ask the patient to hold his or her breath as long as possible before exhaling. This action allows the drug to settle before taking another puff as ordered. You will need to teach the patient the proper technique to avoid the drug simply being delivered into the back of the throat or nose. The nebulizer must be cleaned with water after each use. It is important that the patient keep an adequate supply of drug on hand. Many metered-dose canisters click and count each spray (Fig. 4.25). For those that do not, teach the patient to count every spray.

Continuous aerosol therapy. Continuous aerosol therapy is used to treat an acute asthma attack. The drug typically comes ready as a small, disposable container that is then opened and placed in the nebulizer chamber. Oxygen is used to deliver the drug while the patient uses the mouthpiece to inhale in and out slowly and deeply, while in a upright position. The nebulizer treatment is continued in this way until the drug is completely gone from the nebulizer chamber, about 10 to 20 minutes. The equipment is then cleaned after use. Each patient has his or her own nebulizer equipment, and these are not shared between patients to avoid contamination.

Vaginal Drugs
Generally, vaginal drugs are given to treat infection in the area. Vaginal creams, jellies, tablets, foams, or suppositories are examples of the types of vaginal drugs used. These drugs are kept at room temperature. Before giving vaginal drugs, ask the patient to empty her bladder. As described in Box 4.4, wash your hands and

Table 4.4	Advantages and Disadvantages of Inhaled Drug Delivery
Advantages	
Drug dose is reproducible when used correctly	
Able to deliver a smaller drug dose with fewer side effects	
Faster effect of the drug when delivered directly to the respiratory mucosa	
Disadvantages	
It may be difficult for patients to coordinate the hand and breath action needed to dispense the drug.	
The equipment/mouthpiece may become contaminated, providing a source for infection if not cleaned properly.	

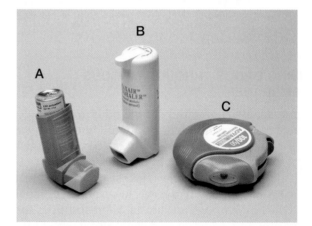

FIG. 4.25 Types of inhalers. (A) Metered-dose inhaler (MDI). (B) Breath-activated inhaler. (C) Dry-powder inhaler (DPI). (From Lilley LL, Collins SR, Snyder JS: *Pharmacology and the nursing process*, ed 6, St. Louis, 2011, Mosby.)

Box **4.3**   **Instructions for Giving Buccal, Sublingual, Ear, and Eye Drugs**

STEP 1: PREPARATION
Always follow the *9 Rights of Drug Administration*.
Check the drug label.
Gather the necessary equipment, including gloves, cotton ball, if needed, and the correct drug. Wash your hands before giving any drug.
Correctly identify the patient. Explain the procedure to the patient.
For optic or otic drugs, identify the correct eye or ear to be treated.

STEP 2: GIVING BUCCAL AREA DRUGS
Place the drug into the patient's mouth using a gloved hand.
Instruct the patient to hold the drug between the cheek and molar teeth.

Dispose of gloves and then wash your hands.
Drugs given here are rapidly absorbed into the bloodstream, reaching the systemic circulation without metabolism by the liver.

Giving Sublingual Drugs
Using a gloved hand, instruct the patient to lift the tongue. Place the tablet under the tongue, where it dissolves. Dispose of gloves and then wash your hands.

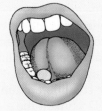

The drug is then rapidly absorbed through the blood vessels. This site is used for nitroglycerin tablets to relieve chest pain.

Giving Drugs for the Ear
Localized infection or inflammation of the ear is treated by dropping a small amount of a sterile drug solution into the ear. Be sure the drug label indicates it is for otic (ear) usage.
Instruct the patient to lie on his or her side with the affected ear up. Shake the drug well and then draw it up into the dropper. Instill the ear drops, being sure not touch the dropper to the ear.
For children younger than 3 years, gently pull the earlobe down and back.

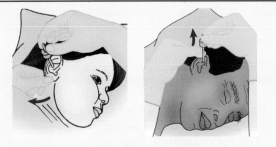

For adults, gently pull the earlobe up and out. This will straighten the external canal for proper drug placement.
Keep the patient in the same position for 5 minutes to allow the drug to coat the inner canal.
A cotton ball may be ordered for insertion to keep the drug in place.
Repeat in the other ear if indicated.
Dispose of gloves and then wash your hands.

Giving Drugs for the Eye
Sterile drops or ointments may be used to treat inflammation or infection of the eye.
Be sure that the drug is specifically labeled for ophthalmic (eye) use.
Any discharge from the eye may be removed with a cotton ball saturated with normal saline, wiping from the inner canthus out to prevent contamination of the eye. Use one cotton ball per stroke.
Instruct the patient to look up, then pull out the lower lid to show the conjunctival sac. Instill the prescribed drops or ointment into the eye.

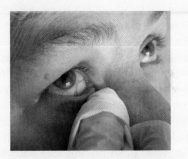

Do not touch the eye with the dropper or the ointment tip. Drop the drug or squeeze the ointment into the conjunctival sac, not onto the eye itself.
Apply gentle external pressure with a tissue to the inner corner of the eyelid on the bone for 1 to 2 minutes to ensure adequate concentration of drug and prevent drug from draining rapidly into the nose.
Apply sterile dressing, if ordered.
Dispose of gloves and then wash your hands.
Instruct the patient to move his or her eyes around with eyelids closed to spread the ointment over the surface of the eye.
Sterile dressings may be ordered to cover the eye at the conclusion of treatment.
For All of the Above:
Document drug administration in accordance with institution policy.
Assess the patient's response to the drug.

Photo from Workman ML, LaCharity L: *Understanding pharmacology,* ed 2, St. Louis, 2016, Elsevier.

Box 4.4 Giving Vaginal Drugs

Drugs to treat local vaginal infections or irritation include creams, jellies, tablets, foams, suppositories, or irrigations (douches).

STEP 1: PREPARATION

Always follow the *9 Rights of Drug Administration*.
Check the drug label.
Gather the necessary equipment, including gloves, lubricant (if needed), and the correct drug. Wash your hands before giving any drug.
Correctly identify the patient. Explain the procedure to the patient.

STEP TWO: GIVING VAGINAL DRUGS

Room-temperature suppositories are inserted into the vagina with a gloved hand, much like a rectal suppository is inserted.
Creams, jellies, tablets, and foams are inserted with a special applicator that comes with the drug.

With the patient lying down, the filled vaginal applicator is inserted as far into the vaginal canal as possible and the plunger is pushed, depositing the drug.
Instruct the patient to remain lying down for 10 to 15 minutes so that all of the drug can melt and coat the vaginal walls.
Offer the patient a perineal pad to catch any drainage or prevent staining.

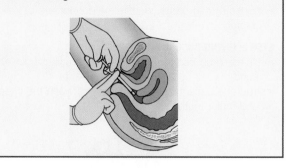

---

don a pair of gloves. Instruct the patient to lie down. Suppositories may be lubricated before insertion into the vagina. Creams, jellies, and foams typically have their own specialized applicators and are placed into the vagina as far as possible. There is a plunger-type applicator that is used to give the drug. Instruct the patient to lie down for 15 minutes after inserting a vaginal drug to prevent drug loss.

Rectal Drugs

Drugs may need to be put into the rectum for either local (within the GI system) or systemic effects. The rectal route is preferred in nausea or vomiting, for reducing fever in children, for pain relief, or for promoting a bowel movement for patients who are constipated. Rectal suppositories should be refrigerated to keep them from melting. As described in Box 4.5, prepare for rectal drug administration by first washing your hands. Place the patient in Sims' position. Put on a pair of nonsterile

gloves and use a water-soluble lubricate on the tip of the suppository for easy insertion. Insert the drug past the internal anal sphincter. If the suppository is inserted improperly, the patient might expel it before the drug can dissolve and be absorbed. Have the patient remain in a supine position for about 5 minutes afterward to ensure drug absorption.

The procedure for giving drugs by rectal enema is similar: insert the lubricated tip of the enema into the rectum and squeeze the enema liquid into the rectum. Instruct the patient to use the anal sphincter muscles to "hold" the enema as long as possible. Remain near, but provide the patient privacy. Offer a bedpan or escort the patient to the toilet when needed. Record the results of the enema. Finally, document all drugs given; note the site for any drug (patches) that requires the site to be rotated and the condition of the skin where topical drugs are placed. Document the expected actions and any adverse effects experienced.

Box 4.5 Giving Rectal Drugs

STEP ONE: PREPARATION

Always follow the *9 Rights of Drug Administration*.
Check the drug label.
Gather the necessary equipment, including gloves, lubricant (if needed), and the correct drug. Wash your hands before giving any drug.
Correctly identify the patient. Explain the procedure to the patient.
Assemble the drug and the necessary equipment (lubricant and rubber gloves).

STEP TWO: GIVING THE DRUG

Accurately identify the patient per institution policy.
Explain what drug is being given and answer any of the patient's questions.

Turn the patient over on his or her side with one leg bent over the other in a Sim's position.
Protect the patient's modesty as much as possible.
Put on gloves. Remove the *suppository* from the foil packet and place a small amount of water-soluble lubricant on the tip of the suppository and on the inserting finger. Instruct the patient to take a deep breath and to bear down slightly. This will relax the sphincter so the suppository may be pushed into the rectum about 1 inch.
Instruct the patient to remain on his or her side for about 20 minutes. With children, it may be necessary to hold the buttocks together to prevent release of the suppository.

Box 4.5   Giving Rectal Drugs—cont'd

If the drug is being given by *disposable enema*, follow the same procedure with the lubricated tip inserted into the rectum and the 50 to 150 mL of drug is slowly squeezed from the disposable container.
Dispose of equipment and gloves.

Wash your hands.
Document your actions per institution policy.
Check the patient, and note any response or adverse effects that should be documented and/or reported.

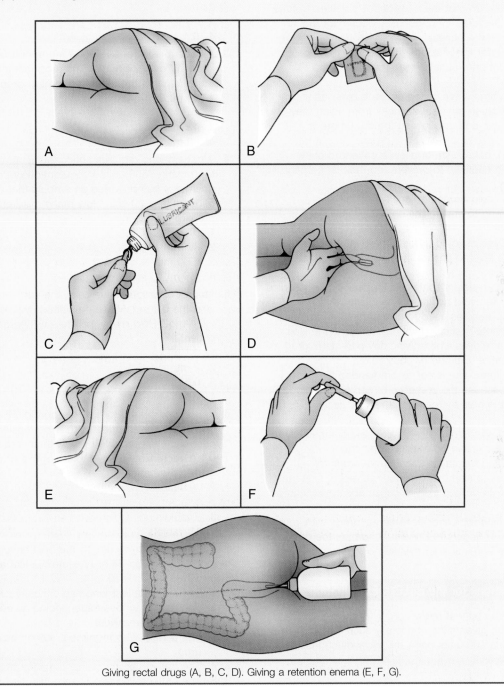

Giving rectal drugs (A, B, C, D). Giving a retention enema (E, F, G).

Get Ready for the NCLEX® Examination!

Key Points

- Always wash your hands before preparing to give a drug regardless of route.
- Never leave a drug at the bedside for a patient to take later because you cannot honestly document that it was taken by the patient.
- The drop factor for infusions depends on the type of equipment and must be read from the setup label.
- Allow extra time when giving drugs to older adult patients because physical changes from aging may make handling and swallowing the drug more difficult.
- Never open, cut, crush, or allow a patient to chew an oral drug capsule, to prevent too rapid absorption of the drug.
- Shake oral liquid drugs and solutions well before pouring to ensure the drug is evenly distributed.
- Read the dose of liquid drugs poured into medicine cups at eye level to ensure the correct amount is present.
- Use puncture-resistant containers for disposing all needles and sharps to avoid accidental needlestick injuries.
- Never recap needles used to give parenteral drugs, to avoid accidentally sticking yourself or someone else.
- Always wear gloves when giving any parenteral drug to avoid exposure to blood or body fluids.
- The dorsogluteal site is *not* recommended for IM injections because the presence of nerves and blood vessels in the area increases the risk for tissue damage.
- Do not aspirate before giving a drug subcutaneously to prevent bruising and other tissue damage.
- Avoid applying topical or transdermal drugs for systemic use to skin that has been tattooed, skin that has lesions, or broken skin, because absorption can be affected.
- Avoid touching topical or transdermal drugs with your bare hands or fingers to prevent absorbing the drug through the skin into your system.

Review Questions for the NCLEX® Examination

1. Your diabetic patient has an order for 30 units of NPH insulin to be given subcutaneously each morning. The vial contains 100 units per 1 mL. How much insulin must be given?
   1. 0.3 mL
   2. 30 mL
   3. 1 mL
   4. 0.5 mL

2. A patient preparing for surgery has an order for cefazolin sulfate (Ancef) 500 mg IV. The drug is available in a vial of powder and is labeled with the following instructions: "Add 2.0 mL of sterile water for injection. This will provide 250 mg/mL." How many milliliters of solution should you prepare?
   1. 2 mL
   2. 0.2 mL
   3. 4 mL
   4. 0.4 mL

3. A patient is to receive 1000 mL of normal saline to infuse IV over 24 hours. The drop factor is 10 drops = 1 mL. What is the flow rate in mL/h of this infusion?
   1. 84 mL/h
   2. 24 mL/h
   3. 42 mL/h
   4. 60 mL/h

4. A patient who requires anticoagulation has an order for heparin 7500 units subcutaneously daily. The pharmacy has provided an ampule that contains 5000 units per 1 mL. How many milliliters should you prepare for this injection?
   1. 0.15 mL
   2. 0.75 mL
   3. 0.50 mL
   4. 1.5 mL

5. As part of preoperative care, the surgeon has ordered atropine 0.2 mg IM. The multidose vial reads: "1 mL = 0.1 mg." How many milliliters will be given to this patient?
   1. 0.1 mL
   2. 2 mL
   3. 0.2 mL
   4. 1 mL

6. You are preparing to give metoprolol 50 mg orally twice daily for a patient with hypertension. The pharmacy has provided you with scored tablets of 0.1 g each. How many tablets of this drug should you give to the patient?
   1. ½ tablet
   2. 1 tablet
   3. 2 tablets
   4. 1½ tablets

7. Which patient(s) would be the best candidate to receive drugs by IM or IV route? Select all that apply.
   1. The older patient who has difficulty swallowing
   2. The patient who is experiencing an episode of prolonged weakness
   3. The patient who requires a steady blood level of the drug
   4. The patient experiencing vomiting after surgery
   5. The patient who needs an antibiotic for bronchitis
   6. The patient who is a child younger than 1 year

Get Ready for the NCLEX® Examination!—cont'd

8. You are preparing to give an intradermal injection for allergy testing to your patient. Which of the following reactions should you expect to see from this injection?
   1. Blister
   2. Bleb
   3. Bruise
   4. Contusion

9. You are preparing to give an IM injection of penicillin. What would be the correct angle at which to give this injection?
   1. 90 degrees
   2. 45 degrees
   3. 30 degrees
   4. 15 degrees

10. You have just entered the medication room, where a fellow nurse has just finished pouring capsules for a patient when he is called away in an emergency. The nurse requests that you give the patient the drugs that have been poured into a medication cup and left at the bedside. What would be your best course of action?
    1. Give the patient the drugs due at this time that the other nurse prepared.
    2. Ask the charge nurse to give the patient the drugs that the other nurse prepared.
    3. Tell the other nurse that he or she cannot leave until the prepared drugs are given.
    4. Remove the drugs from the bedside and discard them. Pour the drugs yourself to give.

5 Anti-Infective Drugs: Antibacterial, Antitubercular, and Antifungal Agents

http://evolve.elsevier.com/Visovsky/LPNpharmacology/

Learning Outcomes

1. Explain how infections, pathogens, drug spectrum, drug resistance, and drug generation affect antibiotic drug therapy.
2. List the names, actions, possible side effects, and adverse effects of the penicillins and cephalosporins.
3. Explain what to teach patients and families about penicillins and cephalosporins.
4. List the names, actions, possible side effects, and adverse effects of the common tetracyclines, macrolides, and aminoglycosides.
5. Explain what to teach patients and families about tetracyclines, macrolides, and aminoglycosides.
6. List the names, actions, possible side effects, and adverse effects of the common sulfonamides and fluoroquinolones.
7. Explain what to teach patients and families about sulfonamides and fluoroquinolones.
8. List the names, actions, possible side effects, and adverse effects of first-line antitubercular drugs.
9. List the names, actions, possible side effects, and adverse effects of antifungal drugs.
10. List the names, actions, possible side effects, and adverse effects of antiparasitic drugs.

Key Terms

antibacterial (ăn-tē-băk-TĬR-ē-ăl, p. 66) Antimicrobial drugs that kill or slow the reproduction of bacteria only. Often used interchangeably with antibiotics.

antibiotic (ăn-tĭ-bī-ŎT-ĭk, p. 66) Any drug that has the ability to destroy or interfere with the development of a living organism. Often used interchangeably with antibacterials.

antimicrobial drug (ăn-tĭ-mī-KRŌ-bē-ăl, p. 66) A general term for any drug that has the purpose of killing or inhibiting the growth of pathogenic microorganisms.

antimicrobial resistance (ăn-tĭ-mī-KRŌ-bē-ăl rĭ-ZĬS-tăn(t)s, p. 66) The ability of an organism to resist the killing or growth suppressing effects of anti-infective drugs.

antifungal drug (ăn-tĭ-FŬN-găl, p. 84) Any drug used to treat a fungal infection, also called a fungicide or fungistatic.

bacteria (băk-tēr-ē-ă, p. 65) Microscopic living organisms that exist everywhere and are both beneficial and dangerous. They are capable of both preventing and causing infection.

bactericidal (băk-tēr-ĭ-SĪD-ăl, p. 66) Drugs with mechanisms of action that kill bacteria.

bacteriostatic (băk-tēr-ē-ō-STĂT-ĭk, p. 66) Drugs with mechanisms of action that only suppress or slow bacterial growth.

fungus (FŬN-gŭs, p. 65) A group of microorganisms that are everywhere and exist by absorbing nutrients from a host organism. Includes yeasts and molds. A fungal infection is called a mycosis.

generation (JĔN-ĕr-Ā-shun, p. 67) A new group of drugs developed from other similar drugs is called a drug generation. Each new generation of antibiotics manufactured from the original generation has significantly greater antimicrobial properties than the preceding generation.

normal flora (p. 65) Organisms of many different types that are usually present on the skin, the mouth, the intestinal tract, and the vagina of a healthy individual and do not cause infection unless the person has reduced immunity or the organisms are located in the wrong body area.

parasite (PĂR-ă-sīt, p. 65) An organism that lives on or in a human and relies on the human for its food and other functions.

pathogen (PĂTH-ō-jĕn, p. 65) An organism that that is expected to cause infection even among people with a strong immune system.

pseudomembranous colitis (sū-dō-MĔM-bră-nŭs kō-LĪ-tĭs, p. 67) An abnormal intestinal reaction to a strong antibiotic that causes excessive watery, bloody diarrhea, abdominal cramps, and low-grade fever and can lead to dehydration, as well as damage the walls of the intestinal tract.

spectrum (SPĔK-trŭm, p. 67) The number of different specific organisms the drug is effective against.

virus (p. 65) A small infectious agent that can replicate (reproduce itself) only inside the living cells of organisms.

INFECTION

An infection is an invasion of body tissue by disease-producing pathogens that multiply and produce toxins that react in a dangerous way and produce illness in a host organism. Infections can be caused by bacteria, viruses, parasites, fungi, and insects. Anti-infective drugs are some of the most commonly given drugs because of the many different types of infections that these drugs have been developed to treat. These drugs are most effective and have fewer side effects when taken correctly. Thus it is important for you to learn as much as possible about these drugs and what to teach patients who are taking them.

NORMAL FLORA

Organisms of many different types are always on the skin, the mouth, the intestinal tract, and the vagina of a healthy person. These organisms are known as **normal floras** and are considered *nonpathogens* because they usually do not cause infection. Conditions in which normal floras can cause infection include when a person has very low immunity, if the organisms are present in excessive amounts and overwhelm the body, or if they are located in the wrong place. For example, if *Escherichia coli*, which are normal floras in the bowel, are present in the bladder or other parts of the renal/urinary system, they can cause an infection in the urinary tract. If skin floras enter a surgical incision, a wound infection can develop. Infants, young children, people with AIDS, anyone receiving cancer chemotherapy, anyone who is taking a drug that suppresses the immune system, and older adults have the greatest risk for infection. Other factors that increase the risk for infection include poor circulation, poor nutritional status, or chronic diseases.

Antibiotic use can upset the normal flora balance in the body and cause yeast or fungal infections to occur. Candida is a common body yeast and often overgrows to cause a fungal infection. When a person is given antibiotics to kill infectious bacteria, the normal flora is killed off as well. The gut, mouth, and vaginal mucosa have bacterial flora that acts as a barrier against fungal infections. When the barrier weakens, yeast infections can occur. If a yeast infection occurs after antibiotic therapy, it is known as a secondary infection or a superinfection. There is evidence to support using probiotic bacteria with an antibiotic as a strategy to prevent yeast infections. Probiotic (beneficial) bacteria can be found in many foods, as well as in capsule form. Yogurt, dark chocolate, miso soup, pickles, and sauerkraut are some foods that can easily be added to a diet. The healthcare provider can prescribe probiotics in capsule form and recommend any necessary dietary changes.

PATHOGENS

An organism that is expected to cause infection even among people with a strong immune system is a pathogen. A variety of pathogenic organisms exist and may cause disease in different ways. For example, they may be able to divide rapidly and overwhelm the immune system or produce toxins. **Bacteria** are a large domain of single-celled microorganisms that exist everywhere. Bacteria are both beneficial and dangerous. For example, *E. coli* bacteria in the intestines benefit digestion but become infective if overgrowth occurs. Bacteria have different shapes and characteristics. They are shaped as rods, spheres, or spirals; they can survive with oxygen (*aerobic*) or without oxygen (*anaerobic*). When stained with a Gram solution, they can stain either violet (*gram-positive*) or red (*gram-negative*). Gram-positive bacteria have a thick cell wall and outer capsule. The cell wall of gram-negative bacteria is much more complex, with an outer capsule and two cell wall membranes. This complex cell wall makes gram-negative bacterial infections more difficult to treat. It is harder for the antibiotic to penetrate the gram-negative bacterial wall.

A **fungus** is a member of a large group of microorganisms that include yeasts and molds, which have cell features that are similar to those of human cells. Fungi are everywhere and exist by absorbing nutrients from a host organism. A fungal infection is called a *mycosis*. A **virus** is a small infectious agent that can replicate (reproduce itself) only inside the living cells of organisms. Viral infection and antiviral drugs are discussed in Chapter 6. A **parasite** is an organism that lives on or in a human and relies on the human for its food and other functions. Common human parasites include worms (helminthes), amoebas, and protozoa, to name only a few examples.

> **Memory Jogger**
>
> Gram-negative bacteria have cells walls that antibiotics have a difficult time penetrating, which makes infections caused by gram-negative bacteria more difficult to treat.

DETERMINATION OF INFECTION

Some infections are diagnosed by the healthcare provider based on the patient's symptoms and the type of organism that commonly causes a specific infection type in that community. In this situation the healthcare provider usually knows what the most likely organism is and which drug or drugs are effective against it. Prescribing a drug without identification of the specific organism is called *empiric treatment* or *empirical therapy* and is based on experience and clinical expertise.

However, at other times the cause of the infection is not known, and the infection must be evaluated to identify the specific pathogenic organism and the drug that will be most effective against it. Bacteria are often stained, cultured, and tested to determine which drugs are effective against them (*antimicrobial* sensitivity). A specimen of the infective material is taken for culture and sensitivity testing that is performed before anti-infective therapy is begun. Learning what organism is present allows the healthcare provider to order the correct drugs that will kill or stop the reproduction of that organism before the illness worsens.

ANTI-INFECTIVES

Anti-infective agents are drugs that can either kill or inhibit the spread of an infectious agent such as bacteria, viruses, fungi, or protozoans. It is a general term used synonymously with the term *antimicrobial*. A few **antimicrobial drug** classification examples are antibacterials, antivirals, antifungals, and anthelminthics (also called *anthelminthics*). These drugs are classified by their chemical structures, mechanisms of action, and type of organism they effectively combat. For example, antimicrobials that kill or slow the reproduction of bacteria are called **antibacterials**. An **antibiotic** is any drug that has the ability to destroy or interfere with the development of a living organism. In anti-infective therapy the term *antibiotic* is used interchangeably with *antibacterial*.

DRUG SUSCEPTIBILITY AND RESISTANCE

Overuse or unnecessary use of antibiotics has led to several current problems for infection management. When antibacterials are overused, prescribed for conditions not responsive to these drugs, or taken improperly, drug-resistant strains of bacteria develop. **Antimicrobial resistance** is the ability of an organism to resist the killing or growth-suppressing effects of anti-infective drugs. Organisms that either can be killed or have their reproduction suppressed by anti-infective drugs are *susceptible*. Those that are neither killed nor suppressed by anti-infective drugs are *resistant* organisms. Many organisms, especially bacteria, that were once susceptible to a variety of anti-infective drugs are now resistant to most types. When an organism is resistant to three or more different types of drugs to which it was once susceptible, it is a *superbug* or a *multidrug-resistant (MDR) organism*.

Each year more organisms have become resistant to standard anti-infective drugs. Infections caused by resistant organisms cost more to treat, increase the length of hospital stays, and lead to higher mortality rates. Often the drugs used against MDR organisms are more powerful and have more side effects than standard anti-infective drugs. Drug resistance has developed in many disease-causing bacteria, viruses, retroviruses, fungi, and some parasites. The Centers for Disease Control and Prevention (CDC) has identified 18 drug-resistant threats in the United States. Of those threats, three are considered urgent: *Clostridium difficile (C. diff.)*, carbapenem-resistant Enterobacteriaceae (CRE), and Neisseria gonorrhoeae.

> ### 📑 Bookmark This!
> Bacterial resistance to antibiotics is a constant threat. To keep current on bacterial resistance and treatment options, check out the CDC at: https://www.cdc.gov/drugresistance/index.html.

Beta-lactamases (or penicillinase) are enzymes that some bacteria produce that give them resistance against beta-lactam antibiotics, which include penicillins, cephalosporins, monobactams, and carbapenems. Inhibitor agents are added to the primary antibiotic (e.g., amoxicillin/clavulanate potassium) to make the antibiotics less resistant to β-lactamases.

GENERAL CONSIDERATIONS FOR ANTI-INFECTIVE (ANTIMICROBIAL) DRUG THERAPY

Drug management for infection is very common and usually short-term. Even though there are many different types of antimicrobial drugs, some nursing interventions are the same for all of them. In addition, many of the points to teach patients and families about these drugs are the same. Box 5.1 describes these common nursing interventions, and Box 5.2 describes general patient teaching points. Specific interventions and patient teaching issues are listed in the individual drug categories.

> ### 🍂 Lifespan Considerations
> **Breast-feeding**
>
> Breast-feeding should be avoided during antimicrobial therapy because most of these drugs are excreted into breast milk and the infant (who may not have an infection) will be exposed to the actions, side effects, and adverse effects.

ANTIBIOTICS

Antibiotics work in different ways to affect pathogenic bacteria (Fig. 5.1). They may attack a bacterium's internal cellular processes, which are vital to its existence, or they may destroy the external cell wall, making it weaker or unable to reproduce; in some cases, they actually kill the organism. Drugs that are **bactericidal** kill the bacteria; those that are **bacteriostatic** limit or slow the growth of the bacteria, weakening or eventually leading to the death of the bacteria.

> ### 💡 Memory Jogger
> The *cidal* or *static* part of the word describing the antibiotic gives a hint about its activity.
>   Bactericidal drugs kill the bacteria (think about the word *homicide*).
>   Bacteriostatic drugs only limit or slow the growth of bacteria, relying on the patient's immune system to kill the organism.

Box 5.1   General Nursing Implications for Antimicrobial Drug Therapy

ASSESSMENT

- Take a complete drug history from the patient to prevent possible drug interactions.
- If ordered, obtain specimens for culture and sensitivity before starting antibiotic therapy to ensure drug sensitivity.
- Do a focused assessment to include the current condition of the infectious site, vital signs, WBC count, and other baseline laboratory data like liver enzymes, kidney function, and drug levels that may be ordered before therapy to establish a baseline.
- A patient can have an allergy to any anti-infective drug. Always ask patients about specific drug allergies and what specific type of problem occurred as part of the allergy before starting any new antimicrobial drug.
- Have emergency drugs and equipment available to treat allergic and/or anaphylaxis (diphenhydramine, epinephrine, crash cart).
- If a female patient is on oral contraceptives and does not wish to be pregnant, an alternative or additional method of contraception should be recommended while taking antibiotic therapy.

PLANNING AND INTERVENTION

- If the patient develops a rash or itching while on the drug, immediately report the problem to the healthcare provider. If the patient has difficulty breathing, a lump in the throat, or a sudden, severe drop in blood pressure, call the emergency team.
- A common and expected side effect of anti-infective therapy, especially the antibacterial drugs, is diarrhea. This response is caused by the drug reducing the numbers of normal floras in the intestinal tract that have the job of helping digestion. With less intestinal floras, diarrhea results. This is *not* an allergy.
- Some very strong antibiotics can cause severe and damaging inflammation of the colon when there is overgrowth of the organism *C. diff*. This serious and abnormal complication is **pseudomembranous colitis** with symptoms that include excessive watery, bloody diarrhea, abdominal cramps, and low-grade fever.
- Many antibiotics allow yeast to overgrow when normal flora are reduced in the mouth and vagina. In the mouth, white patches (thrush) appear especially on the tongue and roof. In the vagina, an itchy discharge may occur. Both problems may need antifungal therapy.
- Antimicrobials work best against infection when blood drug levels remain consistent, so it is best to give them on an even schedule around-the-clock. If an antibiotic is ordered to be given four times a day, the schedule

should be every 6 hours. For example, remind the prescriber or the person making the schedule to use 6:00 a.m., noon, 6:00 p.m., and midnight instead of 9:00 a.m., 1:00 p.m., 5:00 p.m., and 9:00 p.m. If the drugs were given on the 9, 1, 5, and 9 schedule, during the 12 hours the drugs were not given, the blood level would be so low that the organisms would start growing again.
- Many antimicrobials given parenterally have interactions with other drugs. Be sure to consult a pharmacist or drug reference to determine whether a specific drug can be given in the same IV line used for other drugs.
- Most parenteral antimicrobial drugs must be given slowly, over 30 to 60 minutes. Consult a pharmacist or drug reference to determine the time needed to give a specific drug intravenously.
- Some antimicrobial drugs have toxic side effects and their use has a time limit. For example, the aminoglycoside antibiotics can damage the nerves of the ear and cause hearing loss. Usually these drugs are used for only 5 days. It is important for you to know the start and stop dates of antimicrobial drugs to prevent accidental excessive exposure to the drug.
- Duration of antimicrobial therapy varies for different types of infections. For example, some uncomplicated bladder infections (*cystitis*) may require only 3 days of a specific antibacterial drug for complete therapy. In contrast, tuberculosis (TB) usually requires at least 6 months of four different types of drugs to suppress the infection. Most often the duration of antibiotic therapy is 10–14 days.

EVALUATION

- A major nursing responsibility with antimicrobial therapy is evaluating the effectiveness of the drug prescribed for the infection. Therefore it is important to know the patient's infection symptoms and monitor them daily to assess whether the drug therapy is reducing them.
- If symptoms continue at the same intensity beyond 72 hours or become worse, notify the prescriber.
- Whatever duration is prescribed, it is important for the patient to receive all of the therapy. Stopping antimicrobial therapy after infection symptoms are no longer present but before the prescribed duration is completed leads to increased risk for infection recurrence and for the development of drug-resistant organisms.
- Reevaluate any laboratory work that has been ordered so that adverse effects like liver and kidney damage or altered drug levels can be prevented.

Bacteria are often classified as gram-positive or gram-negative. The number of different specific organisms the drug is effective against is described as its **spectrum**. Some antibiotics are effective against only a few types of bacteria and are called *narrow-spectrum drugs*. Other drugs that are effective against more types of bacteria, including both gram-negative and

gram-positive bacteria, are known as *broad-spectrum drugs*.

Some drugs have become more refined, purified, and sensitive as a result of long-term testing. Each new group of these drugs developed from other, similar drugs is called a drug **generation**. The original drugs are referred to as first-generation drugs, and later groups are called

| Box **5.2** | General Teaching Points for Patients and Families During Antimicrobial Drug Therapy |

- Explain to patients that ordinary diarrhea is an expected side effect and not an allergic response to antimicrobial drugs. It is not generally a reason to stop the drug. However, excessive watery and bloody diarrhea with severe abdominal pain and fever is a complication and needs to be reported to the prescriber immediately.
- Stress to patients that if they develop a lump in the throat, difficulty breathing, or swelling of the lips, tongue, or throat to call 911 immediately.
- Instruct patients to take their prescribed antimicrobial drugs exactly as prescribed and for as long as prescribed to prevent infection recurrence and drug resistance.
- Instruct patients to stop taking the drug and notify the healthcare provider if a rash or hives develop while

taking an antimicrobial drug. A drug allergy can develop at any time after the patient begins treatment.
- Remind patients to report to the healthcare provider any new symptoms that occur while taking antimicrobial therapy because they may represent an adverse reaction.
- Tell patients that even though it may be inconvenient to take a drug in the middle of the night, it is important to space the drugs out evenly during the 24 hours for best results.
- Instruct patients not to save antimicrobial drugs because many expired drugs deteriorate and become less effective.

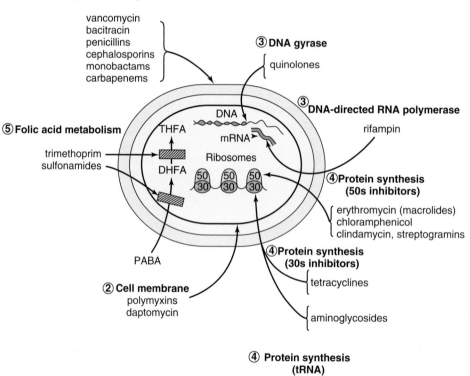

FIG. 5.1 Sites of antimicrobial bactericidal or bacteriostatic action on bacterial pathogens. Five general actions include: (*1*) inhibition of synthesis or building of cell wall; (*2*) damage to cell membrane; (*3*) modification of nucleic acid synthesis; (*4*) modification of protein synthesis (at ribosomes); and (*5*) modification of energy metabolism within the cytoplasm (at the folate cycle). *DHFA*, Dihydrofolic acid; *mRNA*, messenger RNA; *PABA*, para-aminobenzoic acid; *THFA*, tetrahydrofolic acid; *tRNA*, transfer RNA. (From Wecker L: *Brody's human pharmacology*, ed 5, Philadelphia, 2009, Elsevier.)

second-generation drugs, third-generation drugs, and so on.

Usually each new generation of drugs has certain advantages over the older-generation drugs. For example, the newer drugs may have improved effectiveness, fewer side effects, or a faster onset of action. Some of the newer generation of drugs have a narrower spectrum of bacteria that are susceptible to them but

are more powerful than previous generations against the susceptible bacteria.

PENICILLINS

All bacteria have plasma membranes just like human cells do (see number 2 in Fig. 5.1). In addition to a plasma membrane, some bacteria also have the extra protection of cell walls that surround the bacterium outside of the plasma membrane (see number 1 in Fig. 5.1). The cell walls are much tougher than plasma membranes and are built like a brick wall. Just like a brick wall, the cell wall needs to be continuously maintained and repaired to prevent holes and wall crumbling, which would make the rest of the bacterium inside the cell wall less protected. A variety of substances work like bricks and mortar to hold the wall together. Different enzymes help make the mortar, replace old or crumbling bricks, and keep the cell wall intact.

Action

Penicillins are one type of a class of drugs known as *cell wall synthesis inhibitors*. They interfere with the creation and repair of bacterial cell walls. They also bind or stick to specific enzymes that the bacteria need so the bacteria cannot use them. This process makes the bacterial cell weak and allows it to break down more easily. This action is bactericidal for bacteria susceptible to penicillin actions. Pure penicillin may be combined with other ingredients to make the drug stay in the body longer or to prevent the drug from being destroyed by bacterial enzymes. Penicillin and other cell wall synthesis inhibitors are effective only against bacteria that have cells walls, and they have no action against bacteria without cells walls. Although penicillin can be very effective, over time many organisms have become resistant to its killing effects.

Uses

Penicillin was created in 1929 from a fungus by Alexander Fleming. It was used as an antibiotic throughout World War II. Since that time five generations of synthetic penicillins have been developed. Sadly, bacterial resistance to many penicillin drugs have developed as well. Regardless of the increased resistance, penicillin G remains the drug of choice for many infections, including syphilis and certain types of endocarditis. Penicillins are used for infections that occur in the mouth, throat, skin, soft tissue, heart, lungs, and ears. Penicillin is also used for *prophylactic* (preventive) treatment against bacterial endocarditis in patients with rheumatic or heart disease before they have dental procedures or surgery of the upper respiratory tract, genitourinary tract, or GI tract. Some penicillins may be used for treating exposure to agents of biological warfare. Penicillins are still considered the safest antibiotics and are the broad-spectrum drugs of choice for susceptible gram-negative and gram-positive organisms.

Many penicillin products are available in a variety of forms, ranging from oral drugs to parenteral drugs. There are five generations of penicillins.

1. *Natural penicillins* (e.g., penicillin G and penicillin V) combat non-beta-lactamase–producing gram-positive cocci, including *Streptococcus viridans*, group A Streptococci, *Streptococcus pneumoniae*, and *Anaerobic streptococcus*.

2. *Penicillinase-resistant penicillins* (e.g., dicloxacillin, nafcillin, and oxacillin) combat *Staphylococcus* but are not effective against methicillin-resistant *Staphylococcus aureus* (MRSA) or methicillin-resistant *Staphylococcus epidermidis* (MRSE). Methicillin is no longer manufactured.

3. *Aminopenicillins* (e.g., ampicillin and amoxicillin) combat the same bacteria as the natural penicillins but have improved activity against some gram-negative bacteria. Combining an aminopenicillin with a beta-lactamase inhibitor (clavulanic acid or sulbactam) treats infections caused by beta-lactamase–producing organisms.

4. *Carboxypenicillins* (e.g., carbenicillin and ticarcillin) have increased activity to penetrate the cell wall, so they are used for gram-negative bacteria such as *Pseudomonas aeruginosa* and *Proteus*.

5. *Ureidopenicillins* and *piperazine penicillin* (e.g., piperacillin) are the latest class of penicillin antibiotics that combat gram-negative bacteria such as *Klebsiella*. When a beta-lactamase inhibitor is added (piperacillin and tazobactam), it becomes a very powerful broad-spectrum antibiotic against many gram-positive and gram-negative bacteria, and it is used only in cases where other antibiotics have been ineffective to prevent resistance. These penicillins and the carboxypenicillins are only used intravenously.

Table 5.1 lists examples of common penicillins, their dosages, and nursing implications. Be sure to consult a drug reference book or a pharmacist for information about a specific penicillin.

Expected Side Effects

Penicillin overall has fewer side effects and fewer drug interactions than other antibiotics. The most common side effect of penicillin (and many other antibiotics) is simple diarrhea of two to four loose stools daily. This is not an allergy but is caused by the drug killing off some of the normal floras of the GI tract that help digest food. If the diarrhea is severe, the healthcare provider needs to be notified for any additions or changes that need to occur with therapy. Other common and expected side effects include nausea, vomiting, and epigastric distress.

C. diff. is an infectious form of diarrhea caused by antibiotic use, particularly with amoxicillin/clavulanate potassium. If *C. diff.* is suspected, notify the healthcare provider and obtain a stool culture before treatment with another antibiotic.

Adverse Reactions

Allergy to penicillin occurs in 2% to 5% of the population, producing rash, *erythema* (redness or inflammation), *urticaria* (hives), *angioedema* (swelling of the skin and mucous membranes), *laryngeal edema* (swelling of the larynx), and *anaphylaxis* (shock). These allergic reactions may occur suddenly or after the patient has been taking

Table 5.1   Examples of Common Penicillins and Cephalosporins

Penicillins and cephalosporins are cell wall synthesis inhibitors that kill susceptible bacteria within cell walls by preventing cells walls from being made and maintained.

PENICILLINS	
DRUG/ADULT DOSAGE RANGE	**NURSING IMPLICATIONS**
amoxicillin (Moxatag) 500 mg orally every 12 hours *or* 775 mg to 1 g orally once daily amoxicillin/clavulanic acid (Augmentin) 875/125 mg combination orally every 12 hours (immediate-release formula) penicillin G benzathine (Bicillin L-A) 1.2 million units IM as a single injection penicillin G procaine 600,000 to 1.2 million units IM once daily for 10 days penicillin VK (Veetids) 250–500 mg orally every 6 hours	• Shake the liquid suspension drugs thoroughly before giving because this drug form separates. • Give Moxatag within 1 hour of the patient completing a meal for best absorption and fewer GI side effects. • Remind patients not to chew the extended-release forms to avoid counteracting the slow-release feature. • Penicillin G procaine is ***never*** injected into a blood vessel because the procaine it contains can cause severe neurovascular complications. • With penicillin G, use the Z-track method of IM injection deep into the muscle to prevent drug from leaking out through the tissues and causing pain or damage. • Aspirate before injecting the IM dose to ensure the drug is not injected into the bloodstream. • Do not interchange the various suspensions of amoxicillin clavulanic acid because they contain different amounts of clavulanic acid. • Concentrations of Penicillin V are higher when taken on an empty stomach, but if GI upset occurs, it can be taken with food.
CEPHALOSPORINS	
DRUG/ADULT DOSAGE RANGE	**NURSING IMPLICATIONS**
First Generation cefazolin 250–1000 mg IM or IV every 8 hours cephalexin (Keflex) 500 mg orally every 12 hours **Second Generation** cefaclor 250–500 mg orally every 8 hours cefuroxime (Ceftin) 250–500 mg orally every 12 hours *or* 750 mg IM or IV every 8 hours **Third Generation** cefdinir (Omnicef) 300 mg orally every 12 hours *or* 600 mg orally once daily ceftriaxone 1–2 g IM or IV every 12–24 hours **Fourth Generation** cefepime (Maxipime) 0.5–2 g IM or IV every 8–12 hours	• Make sure to check for a penicillin allergy before giving a cephalosporin because patients may have a cross-sensitivity to the drug. • Do not give oral cephalosporins within 1 hour of taking antacids because they interfere with absorption of cephalosporins. • Give IM cefazolin, cefuroxime, ceftriaxone, and cefepime using the Z-track method of IM injection deep into the muscle to prevent drug from leaking out through the tissues and causing pain or damage. • Aspirate before injecting the IM dose to ensure the drug is not injected into the bloodstream. • Reconstitute parenteral cephalosporins only according to manufacturer's direction to ensure the greatest potency of the drug. • Cefaclor extended-release tablets must be taken whole with food and never crushed to avoid getting too much of the drug at one time. • Cefuroxime tablets and suspension cannot be substituted milligram to milligram because they are not bioequivalent. • Cefuroxime suspension must be given with food to ensure a consistent blood drug level. • IV ceftriaxone cannot be given with Ringer lactate because Ringer lactate contains calcium and will precipitate the drug. • IV ceftriaxone and cefepime cannot be given by IV push and must be infused over 30 minutes to reduce the risk for immediate cardiac side effects. • Warn patients not to drink alcohol while taking cephalosporins to reduce the side effects of copious vomiting, hypotension, dyspnea, and chest pain.

Table 5.1   Examples of Common Penicillins and Cephalosporins—cont'd

VANCOMYCIN	
DRUG/ADULT DOSAGE RANGE	**NURSING IMPLICATIONS**
vancomycin (Vancocin) 500 mg IV every 6 hours *or* 1 g IV every 12 hours; 125 mg orally every 6 hours for pseudomembranous colitis caused by *Clostridium difficile*	• Ask patients who are prescribed vancomycin whether they have a corn allergy because they may also be allergic to this drug. • Vancomycin tablets must be swallowed whole, not crushed, to avoid altered dosing. • Regularly assess hearing and monitor urine, BUN/creatinine intermittently; notify the healthcare provider for outlying values because this drug is toxic to the ears and kidneys, and accumulates in the body. • IV vancomycin must be infused over *at least* 60 minutes or no more than 10 mg/min to avoid red man syndrome, a histamine response. Stopping or slowing the infusion will decrease the response. • Parenteral doses of vancomycin must be monitored using serum vancomycin concentrations peak and trough levels because the drug can accumulate to toxic levels quickly. Make sure that the trough is drawn within 30 minutes before the next dose is to be given (so it accurately reflects the drug's lowest level) and that the peak is drawn 1–2 hours after the dose is infused to accurately reflect the drug's highest level. • Monitor urine output and renal blood tests very closely when vancomycin is given with other renal-toxic drugs (such as aminoglycosides) because renal toxicity occurs even faster. • Administration of vancomycin with cidofovir is contraindicated because these drugs together cause severe renal toxicity.
CARBAPENEMS	
DRUG/ADULT DOSAGE RANGE	**NURSING IMPLICATIONS**
imipenem (Primaxin) 500–1000 mg IV every 6–8 hours *or* 500–750 mg IM every 12 hours meropenem (Merrem) 1–2 g IV every 6–8 hours ertapenem (Invanz) 1 g IM or IV once daily	• Do not use the IM formulation of imipenem or ertapenem for IV use because it contains lidocaine, which can cause severe cardiac side effects. • Give IM injections of the carbapenems using the Z-track method of IM injection deep into the muscle to prevent the drug from leaking out through the tissues and causing pain or damage. • Aspirate before injecting the IM dose to ensure the drug is not injected into the bloodstream. • Monitor patients receiving carbapenems closely for confusion and seizure activity because these drugs can cause central nervous system (CNS) changes. • Carbapenem use with ganciclovir or valproic acid can cause seizures because simultaneous use increases the risk for seizure activity. • Monitor patients receiving carbapenems with warfarin for bleeding abnormalities and changes in the international normalized ratio (INR) levels because carbapenems increase warfarin action, which increases the risk for bleeding. • When carbapenems are used along with other antibiotics, monitor urine and laboratory tests closely and report abnormal results to the healthcare provider because the combination greatly increases the risk for kidney damage.

the drug for some time and may cause life-threatening anaphylactic shock. Some patients with penicillin allergy may also have an allergy to the cephalosporins because of a cross-sensitivity.

Drug Interactions

Other bacteriostatic antibiotics such as tetracycline and erythromycin may decrease the bactericidal effect of penicillin. Probenecid blocks the excretion of penicillin, prolonging blood levels and making the antibiotic more effective. Ampicillin reduces the effectiveness of oral contraceptives, which can lead to an unplanned pregnancy. Indomethacin, phenylbutazone, or aspirin may increase serum penicillin levels. Antacids may decrease the absorption of penicillin. Penicillin may change the results of some laboratory tests.

> ### Top Tip for Safety
> Teach women who are taking oral birth control pills to use another reliable method of pregnancy protection while taking penicillin and for 1 month after completing penicillin therapy to prevent an unplanned pregnancy.

❖ Nursing Implications and Patient Teaching

In addition to the general nursing implications and teaching points for all antimicrobial drugs, specific ones for the penicillins are listed in Table 5.1.

> ### Top Tip for Safety
> With all IM injections, including penicillin, use the Z-track method and aspirate before injecting the drug. If blood appears in the syringe, remove the syringe, dispose of the drug, and prepare another dose.

Take the patient's vital signs before giving IM penicillin injections to have baseline information. In an office or clinic setting, keep the patient for 30 minutes after giving the first dose orally or IM to observe him or her for signs of adverse or allergic reactions.

CEPHALOSPORINS

Action

Cephalosporins are cell wall synthesis inhibitors that are chemically similar to penicillin and work in the same way to kill bacteria. Over the years, five generations of cephalosporins have been developed, all of which have broad-spectrum activity (see Table 5.1).

Uses

The first generation of cephalosporins have mostly gram-positive coverage and limited coverage against gram-negative bacteria (e.g., cefazolin and cephalexin). The second-generation drugs have the same gram-positive coverage as the first generation and are more effective against gram-negative and anaerobic organisms (e.g., cefoxitin and cefotetan). Third-generation drugs are more potent against gram-negative bacteria than

the earlier generations but are less active against gram-positive bacteria (e.g., ceftriaxone and ceftazidime). The fourth-generation cephalosporin (cefepime) has increased activity against both gram-negative and gram-positive bacteria and is only available intravenously. The fifth generation (e.g., ceftaroline) is also only available in IV form and has the broadest spectrum against both gram-negative and gram-positive bacteria. It is the only cephalosporin that can treat MRSA.

> ### Memory Jogger
> Most cephalosporin drugs have *ceph*, *cef*, or *kef* in their names.

Cephalosporins are used for uncomplicated skin and soft tissue infections; infections of the lower respiratory tract, central nervous system (CNS), genitourinary system, joints, and bones; and for serious infections, such as bacteremia and septicemia (infections of the blood).

Expected Side Effects

Common side effects of cephalosporins are similar to those of penicillin. Nausea, vomiting, and diarrhea are frequent but usually mild.

Adverse Reactions

The most common adverse effect is acute *hypersensitivity* (allergy). Although some patients may have only a minor rash and itching, a major event with anaphylaxis is possible. Patients who are allergic to penicillins have a risk of also being allergic to cephalosporins because cephalosporins are so similar to penicillins. This is known as a *cross-sensitivity*, and if a cephalosporin must be used, it is used with caution. If a patient had an anaphylactic reaction to penicillin, then cephalosporins should not be used at all.

Nephrotoxicity (kidney toxic effects) has been reported with some cephalosporins, and the incidence is greater in older adult patients and in patients with poor renal function. There may also be severe pain at the injection site.

Drug Interactions

Alcohol taken with cephalosporins may produce a disulfiram reaction (a drug used to prevent alcohol use by producing a severe sensitivity to alcohol). The effects result in severe flushing, copious vomiting, throbbing headache, dyspnea, tachycardia, hypotension, and chest pain.

Antacids and iron can cause decreased absorption of some cephalosporins, and probenecid can decrease elimination of the drug.

❖ Nursing Implications and Patient Teaching

In addition to the general nursing implications and teaching points for all antimicrobial drugs, those specific for the cephalosporins are listed in Table 5.1.

Many cephalosporins are given by the IV or IM route because some formulations are not absorbed from the GI tract. Table 5.1 presents a summary of the names, dosages, and nursing implications of common cephalosporins. Be sure to consult a drug reference book or a pharmacist for information about a specific cephalosporin.

OTHER CELL WALL SYNTHESIS INHIBITORS

Two other very powerful cell wall synthesis inhibitors are vancomycin and a group known as carbapenems (see Table 5.1). The carbapenems (imipenem/cilastatin, meropenem, ertapenem, and doripenem) have the broadest spectrum of antibacterial activity against gram-positive and gram-negative bacteria. These drugs generally are used for infections caused by MDR bacteria in hospitalized patients. Side effects and adverse effects are severe, so the use of these drugs is generally limited to severe and life-threatening bacterial infections. Vancomycin is used to treat MRSA and other drug-resistant infections. Vancomycin-resistant enterococci (VRE) and CRE now exist. Enterococci are bacteria present in the intestines and in the female genital tract, and Enterobacteriaceae such as *E. coli* and *Klebsiella* are normal floras in the intestines. Usually only hospitalized or nursing home patients who are critically ill and on numerous antibiotics are susceptible to these resistant bacteria.

These drugs are given intravenously by IV push or by infusion over an hour or more in an acute care setting. Dosages and schedules are based on the patient's weight, organ health, and the severity of the infection. Vancomycin has an oral form that is used to combat the pseudomembranous colitis caused by *C. diff.* Imipenem/cilastin comes in an IM form that contains lidocaine.

Expected Side Effects and Adverse Reactions

Nausea, vomiting, diarrhea, headache, rash, fever, and chills can occur with these powerful drugs. Vancomycin often causes flushing and hypotension. An unusual response is a deep red rash on the upper body known as red man syndrome that is produced by a histamine-released reaction. Slowing the infusion rate and pretreating the patient with antihistamines and an H2 receptor blocker offers protection against red man syndrome.

Carbapenems can cause adverse CNS effects such as confusion and seizures. Vancomycin and carbapenems in high doses can produce nephrotoxicity and ototoxicity.

Drug Interactions

Carbapenem drugs compete with probenecid, so these drugs should not be given at the same time. The drug may reduce the activity of valproic acid, which is given to prevent seizures. Simultaneous use of carbapenems with ganciclovir increases the risk for seizures.

Vancomycin adds to the toxicity of other antibiotics such as the aminoglycosides and other drugs that are ototoxic or nephrotoxic. Cholestyramine and colestipol decrease the absorption of the oral form of the drug.

Memory Jogger

When a drug is nephrotoxic (toxic to the kidneys), it is ototoxic (toxic to the ears) as well because ear and kidney tissue are immunologically and biologically related.

TETRACYCLINES

Action

Tetracyclines are one type of a group of antibacterial drugs classified as *protein synthesis inhibitors* (tetracyclines, macrolides, and aminoglycosides). All protein synthesis inhibitors (not to be confused with cell wall synthesis inhibitors) enter the bacterium and interfere with the processes used by the bacterium to make important proteins needed for growth. If the bacteria cannot make protein, it will either not be able to reproduce or it will die. Usually tetracyclines only have bacteriostatic action against susceptible organisms. This means that bacterial reproduction is reduced and that the patient's immune system must rid the body of the organism.

Uses

The tetracyclines are broad-spectrum drugs that are similar to penicillins in that they are effective against many gram-negative and gram-positive organisms. Many other drugs are more effective against those organisms, so tetracyclines are the first choice drugs in only a few diseases, such as acne, urinary tract infections, infections of the skin and respiratory tract, Lyme disease, stomach ulcers caused by *Helicobacter pylori*, *Chlamydia*, Rocky Mountain spotted fever, typhoid fever, sexually transmitted diseases (chlamydia, syphilis, and gonorrhea), and inhalation anthrax exposure.

Expected Side Effects

The tetracyclines commonly produce mild episodes of nausea, vomiting, and diarrhea that may require stopping the drug. These effects are often dose related, and they result from irritation of the GI tract, changes in the normal bacteria in the bowel, and overgrowth of yeast. The tetracyclines increase the sensitivity of the skin to the sun and severe sunburns are possible, even among people with dark complexions. Yeast infections of the mouth (thrush) and the vagina are common when tetracycline therapy lasts longer than 10 days or in patients who are immunosuppressed or have diabetes. Yeast infections can be treated either topically or orally with antifungal drugs.

Adverse Effects

Use of tetracycline is contraindicated in women who are pregnant or breast-feeding, as well as in children younger than 8 years. These drugs may cause inadequate bone or tooth development, produce permanent yellow-brown tooth discoloration, and/or cause permanent damage (skeletal retardation) to a developing fetus.

Tetracycline should be used with caution in patients with poor liver function, because the drug may cause liver toxicity. In high doses, tetracyclines can decrease kidney function. Persistent dizziness, blurred vision, ringing in the ears, confusion, and headache can occur and may indicate increased pressure inside the brain.

> ### 🍃 Lifespan Considerations
>
> Unless an infection is life-threatening and the organism is sensitive only to tetracycline, this drug is not given to pregnant women or young children. Tetracycline interferes with bone development and the development of tooth enamel. Exposure can cause permanent tooth staining.

Drug Interactions

Food, dairy products, aluminum, magnesium and calcium interfere with the intestinal absorption of tetracyclines. For this reason tetracycline is best taken with water on an empty stomach 1 hour before eating or 2 hours after eating. In addition to the general nursing implications and teaching points for all antimicrobial drugs, those specific for the tetracyclines are listed in Table 5.2.

MACROLIDES

Actions

Macrolides are protein synthesis inhibitors that work in the same way as tetracyclines do. Macrolides are either bactericidal or bacteriostatic depending on the organisms and the dose used. Azithromycin and clarithromycin are considered advanced-generation macrolides compared with erythromycin, which was the first macrolide antibiotic. The later macrolides have a longer duration of action than erythromycin, fewer side effects, and can penetrate the tissues better, making them more effective at destroying bacteria. Their blood levels remain higher longer, so fewer doses are needed daily and therapy is often of shorter duration.

Uses

The macrolides are effective against many of the same infectious organisms that are sensitive to penicillin. Macrolides are used as alternatives to penicillin for patients who have a penicillin allergy and for infections caused by organisms that are resistant to penicillin. These drugs are effective against aerobic and anaerobic gram-positive cocci. They are not effective against MRSA or some other staphylococcus bacteria, as well as some types of streptococci.

Additional uses of macrolides include *Mycoplasma pneumoniae* and *Chlamydia* infections. They are also used in Legionnaires' disease and in the treatment of pertussis ("whooping cough").

Expected Side Effects

The most common side effects of macrolides are associated with the GI tract and include mild abdominal pain, nausea, flatulence, and diarrhea. In addition, these drugs increase the sensitivity of the skin to sunlight. Severe sunburns are possible even among people with darker skin.

Adverse Effects

Macrolides can impair the liver and cause jaundice. When macrolides are given intravenously, phlebitis and other types of vein irritation are common.

Drug Interactions

Macrolides are protein bound and metabolized by the liver, making them capable of having numerous drug interactions. Macrolides enhance the action of digoxin, theophylline, warfarin, cyclosporine, and carbamazepine. Toxic effects of these drugs can occur if levels are not followed closely. The combination of a macrolide with other drugs, such as ergotamine for migraines or pimozide for Tourette syndrome, can precipitate life-threatening cardiac dysrhythmias. Anesthetic agents and anticonvulsant drugs may interact to cause high serum drug levels and toxicity. Consult a drug reference book or a pharmacist for information when other drugs are prescribed during macrolide therapy.

❖ Nursing Implications and Patient Teaching

The major differences between erythromycin and the newer macrolides include better GI tolerability, a broader spectrum of activity, and less dosing frequency for the newer products. The strength of erythromycin varies by product. Stomach acid inactivates erythromycin. This is the reason erythromycin is prepared as an enteric-coated drug combined with other products to form different drugs such as erythromycin base, erythromycin estolate, erythromycin ethylsuccinate, or erythromycin stearate. There are differences in dosages among these different erythromycin preparations. Thus one type of erythromycin tablet should never be substituted for another type unless advised to do so by the pharmacist or healthcare provider.

Many macrolides may be given orally or parenterally. Topical application should be avoided to prevent sensitization. Keep the patient well hydrated (supplied with fluids). Drinking extra fluids to ensure a minimum urine output of 1500 mL decreases the odds of renal toxicity. In addition to the general nursing implications and teaching points for all antimicrobial drugs, those specific for the macrolides are listed in Table 5.2.

Table 5.2   Examples of Common Tetracyclines, Macrolides, and Aminoglycosides

Tetracyclines, macrolides, and aminoglycosides are all protein synthesis inhibitors that are able to get inside the bacterium and prevent it from making important life-cycle proteins. Most are bacteriostatic rather than bactericidal and depend on the patient's immune system to fully rid the body of the infectious organisms.

TETRACYCLINES

DRUG/ADULT DOSAGE RANGE	NURSING IMPLICATIONS
doxycycline 100 mg orally every 12 hours minocycline hydrochloride (Minocin) 100–200 mg orally or intravenously every 12 hours tetracycline 250–500 mg orally every 6–12 hours	• Remind patients taking tetracyclines to wear sun-protective clothing and sunscreen when going outdoors because these drugs increase skin sun sensitivity and can cause severe sunburns. • Instruct patients to take these drugs 1 hour before a meal or drinking milk or 2 hours after eating a meal or drinking milk because food and milk inhibit intestinal absorption. • Ask patients if they are using retinoids (isotretinoin, acitretin) for acne because using these drugs with tetracycline can cause a severe rise in intracranial pressure and is contraindicated.

MACROLIDES

DRUG/ADULT DOSAGE RANGE	NURSING IMPLICATIONS
azithromycin (Zithromax) 500 mg orally for one dose then 250 mg orally once daily for 4 days clarithromycin (Biaxin) 250–500 mg orally every 12 hours clarithromycin extended release (Biaxin XL) 1000 mg orally once daily erythromycin (E.E.S.) 250–500 mg by mouth every 6–12 hours	• Consult with the healthcare provider and the pharmacist for patients taking other drugs with macrolides because they interact with many drugs. • Clarithromycin and erythromycin should not be used with moxifloxacin, pimozide, thioridazine, or other drugs that may prolong the QT interval because life-threatening dysrhythmias can occur. • Tell patients that if palpitations and chest pain occur while taking clarithromycin or erythromycin to seek emergency help immediately because these drugs can cause cardiac dysrhythmias. • Instruct patients to take erythromycin with food or milk because the drug is not absorbed as well if taken on an empty stomach. • Monitor liver enzymes and assess for jaundice in patients taking a macrolide because this drug can cause liver damage, especially in older people.

AMINOGLYCOSIDES

DRUG/ADULT DOSAGE RANGE	NURSING IMPLICATIONS
amikacin 15–30 mg/kg IV every 8–12 hours gentamicin 3–5 mg/kg per day IV or IM streptomycin 1–2 g IM every 6 or 12 hours	• Be sure to give these drugs only for as long as prescribed because they can cause kidney damage and hearing loss. • When giving these drugs intravenously, be sure to dilute them well and give over 30–60 minutes to reduce vein irritation and prevent cardiac side effects. • Assess patients for confusion, weakness, sleep disorders, or eye disorders because these drugs, especially streptomycin, can induce nervous system toxicities. If these appear, notify the healthcare provider immediately to prevent severe complications.

MISCELLANEOUS PROTEIN SYNTHESIS INHIBITORS

DRUG/ADULT DOSAGE RANGE	NURSING IMPLICATIONS
clindamycin (Cleocin) 150–450 mg orally every 6 hours	• Give with food or a full glass of water to minimize GI irritation.
linezolid (Zyvox) 600 mg orally or IV every 12 hours	• If patients are on an selective serotonin reuptake inhibitor antidepressant, monitor their blood pressure and heart rate because the risk for serotonin syndrome is increased. • Ask patients if they are on monoamine oxidase inhibitor antidepressants because use with linezolid could cause severe cardiac problems and is contraindicated. • Tell patients that if unusual bruising or bleeding occurs to notify their healthcare provider because these may be symptoms of a low platelet count. • Tell patients to avoid alcohol and tyramine-containing foods to avoid severe hypertension.
dalfopristin/quinupristin (Synercid) 7.5 mg/kg IV every 12 hours	• Mix the drug according to manufacturer's instructions and give the infusion over 60 minutes to reduce vein irritation and injection-site reactions. • Consult with the pharmacist for patients taking other IV drugs with macrolides because this drug is not compatible with some other IV drugs. • Consult with the healthcare provider and the pharmacist for patients taking other drugs with dalfopristin/quinupristin because it interacts with many drugs.

AMINOGLYCOSIDES

Action

Like other protein synthesis inhibitors, aminoglycosides weaken the bacteria by limiting the production of protein, which is essential to the life of the bacteria.

Uses

Aminoglycosides, such as gentamicin and amikacin, are used in the treatment of serious aerobic gram-negative infections, including those caused by *E. coli*, *Serratia*, *Proteus*, *Klebsiella*, and *Pseudomonas*; aerobic gram-negative bacteria; mycobacteria; and some protozoans. Some drugs are used to sterilize the bowel before intestinal surgery and to treat hepatic encephalopathy.

Expected Side Effects

When given intravenously, aminoglycosides are irritating to the veins. Additional common side effects include nausea, vomiting, rash, lethargy, and fever.

Adverse Reactions

Aminoglycosides can cause serious adverse effects including damage to the kidney (*nephrotoxicity*) that is usually reversible if the drug is stopped quickly. They can also produce permanent damage to the inner ear (*ototoxicity*), or hearing impairment, dizziness, loss of balance, ringing in the ears, and persistent headache or other types of neurotoxicity, particularly with drugs such as gentamicin.

Aminoglycosides have a narrow therapeutic range (when the lowest and highest acceptable drug levels are not far apart). This requires that the sample for the antibiotic blood level be drawn just before the next scheduled dose is given. This sample will show the lowest blood level of the antibiotic (*trough*), rather than a blood level at a higher range (*peak*). The lowest blood level will determine whether the dosage needs to be adjusted to stay within the therapeutic range and not reach the toxic level or go below the effective level. Aminoglycoside dosage is calculated on the basis of the patient's weight. Dosage is adjusted based on creatinine clearance that is based on creatinine blood levels so that a therapeutic level is maintained without nephrotoxicity. Blood urea nitrogen (BUN) and glomerular filtration rates are also closely monitored.

Drug Interactions

Using aminoglycosides with many other drugs, particularly vancomycin, increases the risk for nephrotoxicity. Ototoxicity is also increased with aspirin, furosemide, ethacrynic acid, and many other drugs. Consult a drug reference book or a pharmacist for information when other drugs are prescribed during aminoglycoside therapy.

❖ Nursing Implications and Patient Teaching

In addition to the general nursing implications and teaching points for all antimicrobial drugs, those specific for the aminoglycosides are listed in Table 5.2. Aminoglycosides are given parenterally for systemic bacterial infections because they are poorly absorbed from the GI tract.

Patients should have frequent hearing and urine tests to monitor for ototoxicity and nephrotoxicity, respectively.

For patients taking these aminoglycosides, particularly in the hospital, the nurses will be involved in monitoring the blood levels of these drugs. The drug levels peak and trough (go up and down) and thus close monitoring is important.

MISCELLANEOUS PROTEIN SYNTHESIS INHIBITORS

Three other classifications of protein synthesis inhibitors do not fit into other categories and are not used commonly: lincosamides, oxazolidinones, and streptogramins. They are usually given intravenously to treat bacterial infections that have not responded to other antibiotics, and their use is limited to life-threatening infections such as MRSA and VRSA. Clindamycin is a lincosamide that can be given orally for skin infections such as impetigo, cellulitis, and complicated skin and soft tissue infections such as diabetic foot ulcers. It is used intravenously for bone infections, intra-abdominal abscess, peritonitis, cellulitis, septicemia, bacteremia, and anaerobic pneumonia. Clindamycin is an older drug, and more organisms are resistant to it. In addition, it is more likely to cause antibiotic-associated diarrhea, including *C. diff.* colitis, than other antibiotics.

Linezolid (Zyvox) is an oxazolidinone that can be given orally or intravenously. It is used for MRSA, VRE, and sepsis after treatment with vancomycin has failed. Dalfopristin/quinupristin can only be given intravenously and is reserved for patients with bacteremia or sepsis. See Table 5.2 for specific implications when giving these drugs.

> **⚠ Safety Alert!**
>
> Do not confuse Zyvox with Zovirax or Zyban.
> Zyvox is an antibiotic, Zovirax is an antiviral, and Zyban is a drug used for smoking cessation.

> **🔖 Bookmark This!**
>
> For a full list of sound-alike drugs, you can download a pdf file from the Institute of Safe Medical Practices at https://www.ismp.org/Tools/confuseddrugnames.pdf.

SULFONAMIDES

Action

Sulfonamides are antibacterial drugs from a class known as metabolism inhibitors. They enter the bacteria and prevent them from making the final form of folic acid, which is needed for bacterial growth and function.

Sulfonamides are bacteriostatic rather than bactericidal because they do not actually kill the bacteria.

Uses

Sulfonamides have a broad spectrum of activity. They are eliminated by the kidneys, so they have a high concentration of activity in the kidneys. This makes sulfonamides a good choice for treating acute and chronic urinary tract infections, particularly cystitis, pyelitis, and pyelonephritis. The drug sulfamethoxazole is combined with trimethoprim (Bactrim or Septra) and is the most commonly used sulfonamide. It is effective for infections caused by *E. coli*, *Klebsiella*, *Proteus mirabilis*, and *S. aureus*. However, resistant strains of these bacteria are developing because sulfonamides have been used for many years.

Other indications for sulfonamide use include respiratory infections from susceptible organisms, and prevention and treatment of pneumocystis pneumonia in patients with HIV. Additional uses include treatment of otitis media from *Haemophilus influenza*, community-acquired MRSA in children, toxoplasmosis, CNS infections, and MRSA infections of the skin and joints.

Expected Side Effects

Common side effects of sulfonamides include many minor but irritating problems such as headache, drowsiness, fatigue, dizziness, *insomnia* (inability to sleep), *anorexia* (lack of appetite), nausea, vomiting, and abdominal pain. More problematic effects include *vertigo* (feeling of dizziness or spinning), *tinnitus* (ringing in the ears), hearing loss, and *stomatitis* (inflammation of the mouth).

Adverse Reactions

Sulfonamides can crystalize in the kidney and cause kidney damage. Allergic reactions to sulfonamides are relatively common, including anaphylaxis. Typically, sulfonamides cause skin reactions, such as a rash that begins with a fever. Increased sun sensitivity (photosensitivity) reactions are common and can result in a severe sunburn. These drugs can suppress bone marrow function, increasing the risk for anemia, bleeding, and reduced immunity during and for several weeks after therapy is completed.

Drug Interactions

Sulfonamides may increase the effect of sulfonylureas that are used to treat diabetes type 2 and cause hypoglycemia. They may increase the neurologic toxic effects of phenytoin and increase warfarin drug levels, which leads to excess bleeding. If other drugs eliminated by the kidneys are taken at the same time, sulfonamides can increase the risk for nephrotoxicity. The effect of sulfonamides may be decreased by local anesthetics. Use of sulfonamides with some phenothiazine antipsychotic drugs can cause lethal cardiac dysrhythmias. Patients with an allergy or sensitivity to thiazide diuretics, oral sulfonylureas, or carbonic anhydrase inhibitors may exhibit the same allergy or sensitivity to sulfonamides. Consult a drug reference book or a pharmacist for information when other drugs are prescribed during sulfonamide therapy.

❖ Nursing Implications and Patient Teaching

In addition to the general nursing implications and teaching points for all antimicrobial drugs, those specific for the sulfonamides are listed in Table 5.3. Warn the patient to stay out of the sun, because severe photosensitivity (abnormal response to exposure to sunlight) can occur if the patient's skin is exposed to excessive amounts of sunlight or ultraviolet light.

Sulfonamide dosage depends on the severity of the infection being treated, the drug used, and the patient's response to and tolerance of the drug. Short-acting sulfonamides usually require a special first dose (initial loading dose) that is larger than the dose that will then be taken regularly.

Sulfonamides should be taken with food, milk, or a full glass of water to minimize stomach irritation. To prevent formation of crystals in the urine, the patient must drink at least 1.5 L/day unless this is contraindicated.

FLUOROQUINOLONES

Action

Fluoroquinolones destroy bacteria by inhibiting two enzymes needed for DNA synthesis and reproduction. They are a type of bactericidal DNA synthesis inhibitor.

Uses

All four generations of fluoroquinolones are effective against gram-negative pathogens. The newer ones are significantly more effective against gram-positive microbes. They are primarily excreted by the kidneys, making them a good choice for treating complicated urinary tract infections. These drugs are also used in the treatment of respiratory, GI, gynecologic, skin, and soft tissue, bone, and joint infections. Ciprofloxacin (Cipro) is the drug of choice for anthrax exposure in a bioterrorist attack.

Expected Side Effects

Nausea, vomiting, diarrhea, abdominal pain, and headache are the most common side effects of fluoroquinolones. These drugs concentrate in the urine, making it more irritating. For patients who dribble urine or who are incontinent, the skin in the genital area can become red and sore. This problem is reduced by having the patient increase his or her fluid intake to dilute the urine.

Adverse Reactions

Arthropathy (joint pain and disease) can occur especially in children who are receiving fluoroquinolones.

Table 5.3 Examples of Common Sulfonamides and Fluoroquinolones

Sulfonamides: drugs known as metabolism inhibitors that work by entering the bacteria and preventing them from making the final form of folic acid, which is needed for bacterial growth and function

DRUG/ADULT DOSAGE RANGE	NURSING IMPLICATIONS
sulfamethoxazole/trimethoprim (Bactrim, Septra) 400 mg/80 mg orally every 12 hours sulfamethoxazole/trimethoprim (Bactrim DS, Septra DS) 800 mg/160 mg orally once daily	• Have the patient drink a full glass of water whenever he or she takes the drug and increase fluids to 1.5 L/day if there are no fluid restrictions to prevent crystals from forming in the kidney and causing kidney damage. • Remind patients to stay out of the sun while taking sulfonamide drugs to prevent severe sunburns. • Warn patients who are on sulfonylureas (drugs for diabetes type 2) that fatigue, shakiness, anxiety, and irritability (hypoglycemia) may occur.

Fluoroquinolones: drugs known as DNA synthesis inhibitors that prevent bacterial reproduction and induce bacterial death by suppressing enzymes needed for DNA synthesis and important life-cycle activities

DRUG/ADULT DOSAGE RANGE	NURSING IMPLICATIONS
ciprofloxacin (Cipro, Cipro XR) 250–750 mg orally every 12 hours or 1 g orally once daily or 200–400 mg IV every 12 hours levofloxacin (Levaquin) 250–750 mg orally or IV once daily	• Give with food (no dairy) to ensure absorption. • These drugs are not used for children younger than 18 years because they interfere with the growth of bones, muscles, and tendons. • Teach patients to stop the drug and call their healthcare provider if they develop joint pain or inflammation because these drugs can cause tendon rupture. • IV dosages should be mixed according to manufacturer's directions and given over 60–90 minutes to reduce vein irritation and injection-site reactions. • Teach patients to drink increased fluids to dilute urine to prevent crystallization of urine. • Teach patients to avoid sunlight to prevent severe sunburn. • Teach patients with diabetes to check blood glucose levels frequently because fluctuations in glucose levels can occur and cause hyperglycemia or hypoglycemia. • Teach patients to notify the healthcare provider if numbness, tingling, or pain occurs in hands or feet to avoid complications from peripheral neuropathy. • Teach patients to notify the healthcare provider for tendonitis symptoms that might occur (ache, pain, redness, and swelling in a joint or area where a tendon attaches to a bone).

Life-threatening heart rhythm changes can occur if fluoroquinolones are used with antidysrhythmic drugs such as quinidine, sotalol, or amiodarone. Fluoroquinolones are generally contraindicated in patients on antidysrhythmics. Tingling, burning, and numbness in the feet and hands (*peripheral neuropathy*) can occur. Rupture of a tendon in the shoulder, hand, arm, wrist, legs, or heel can occur, especially in patients with decreased renal function, older age, and those taking prednisone.

Drug Interactions

Fluoroquinolones should be taken 2 hours before or 4 hours after multivitamins, minerals, antacids, and iron because these agents reduce the absorption of the antibiotic by as much as 90%. When taken with warfarin, fluoroquinolones increase the anticoagulant effects of warfarin. Dairy products and enteral tube feedings reduce the absorption of fluoroquinolones. In patients taking antidiabetic drugs, hyperglycemia or hypoglycemia may occur. Consult a drug reference book or a pharmacist for information when other drugs are prescribed during fluoroquinolone therapy.

❖ **Nursing Implications and Patient Teaching**

In addition to the general nursing implications and teaching points for all antimicrobial drugs, those specific for the fluoroquinolones are listed in Table 5.3. Fluoroquinolones are to be taken with food, but not dairy products, to decrease adverse GI effects. Keep older patients well hydrated to prevent decreased renal function.

ANTITUBERCULAR DRUGS

Tuberculosis (TB) is a common lung infection caused by a slow-growing aerobic bacterium, *Mycobacterium tuberculosis*. It is primarily a disease of the lungs but may also be seen in bones, bladder, kidneys, and other parts of the body. TB is transmitted by infected humans, cows (bovine), and birds (avian). Droplets ejected during coughing or sneezing are inhaled by an uninfected host. Once the bacterium is inhaled, it rapidly multiplies in the oxygen-rich lung tissue. The lesion that is formed is inflamed and filled with bacteria. If the person's immune system is intact, the bacillus is encased in a *granuloma*, which is a collection of macrophages that

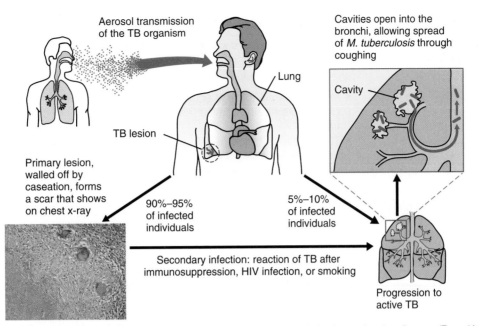

FIG. 5.2 Primary tuberculosis (TB) infection with progression to secondary infection and active disease. (From Kumar V, Abbas A, Fausto N, Aster J: *Robbins and Cotran pathologic basis of disease*, ed 8, Philadelphia, 2009, Saunders. Photo courtesy Dominick Cavuoti, DO, Dallas, Texas.)

walls off the bacteria to stop its growth. The person will not become sick, but the TB test will remain positive because the immune system continues to recognize the exposure. A person who is exposed to the TB infection but who has no disease symptoms is said to have latent or inactive TB. Patients with latent TB can still develop active TB (called *secondary TB*) at a later time if he or she becomes immunocompromised (Fig. 5.2). Depending on the patient, often the healthcare provider will decide that treatment is warranted to kill the encased bacterium.

The immune process takes between 2 and 10 weeks after exposure and is confirmed by an intradermal TB skin test that shows a 10-mm or larger *induration* (hardened red area). If the person does not have resistance to the disease because of reduced immunity from advanced age, disease, or repeated exposure, the bacteria will multiply, grow, and spread into more places in the lungs. The bacterium can also enter into the bloodstream, which is how other organs become infected.

Memory Jogger

Symptoms of Active TB infection

Symptoms of active TB infection include productive cough, bloody sputum, poor appetite, weight loss, night sweats, fever, and chills.

Far more adults are infected by this airborne infection than actually experience development of active TB. Even when a person is heavily exposed to the organism and inhales it deeply and often, if the immune system is functioning well, no actual disease will develop. Active TB is more commonly seen in underdeveloped nations,

where living conditions are crowded and unsanitary. However, it is also increasingly found in the United States among immigrants (particularly Asian and Hispanic individuals), drug users, alcoholics, homeless people, malnourished people with HIV/AIDS, prisoners, and people on immunosuppressive drugs.

The TB organism is slow-growing, so standard antibacterial drugs are not effective in controlling it. Four special drugs taken as a combination are used as first-line treatment to control uncomplicated active TB and prevent its transmission. Therapy continues until the disease is under control. The combination multiple-drug regimen controls the TB organisms as quickly as possible and reduces the development of drug-resistant organisms. Treatment usually last 6 months or longer. People with TB are generally thought to no longer be infectious to others after they have been receiving drug therapy for several weeks, are feeling better, and are symptom free.

The first-line TB drug therapy recommended by the CDC is the use of isoniazid (INH), rifampin (Rifadin), pyrazinamide, and ethambutol (Myambutol) for the first 8 weeks, which is the *initial* phase of treatment. The *continuation* phase lasts another 18 weeks, and the patient takes INH and rifampin either daily or 5 days a week. There are three more treatment regimens in the CDC guidelines that should be used for patients with HIV/AIDS or when treatment is difficult. The same drugs are used to prevent TB in people who have been living with TB patients before diagnosis was made and treatment was started (Table 5.4).

Many patients with TB are infected with MDR organisms that require susceptibility tests and alternate methods of treatment to control infection. Most

Table 5.4 First-Line Drug Therapy for Tuberculosis

Isoniazid: kills actively growing mycobacteria outside the cell and inhibits the growth of dormant bacteria inside macrophages and granulomas.

DRUG/ADULT DOSAGE RANGE	NURSING IMPLICATIONS
For Uncomplicated TB: isoniazid (INH) 300 mg orally for 2 months, followed by 300 mg orally three times per week for 2–4 months **For Prophylaxis:** isoniazid (INH) 300 mg orally daily for 9 months *or* 900 mg orally twice weekly for 9 months isoniazid (INH) 5 mg/kg (maximum dose 300 mg) IM once daily	• Instruct patients to avoid antacids and to take the drug on an empty stomach (1 hour before or 2 hours after meals) to prevent slowing of drug absorption in the GI tract. • Teach patients to take a daily multivitamin that contains the B-complex vitamins or vitamin B_6 while taking this drug because the drug can deplete the body of this vitamin and cause numbness and tingling in feet and hands (peripheral neuropathy). • Remind patients to avoid drinking alcoholic beverages while on this drug because the liver-damaging effects of this drug are potentiated by drinking alcohol. Acetaminophen should also be avoided for the same reason. • Tell patients to report darkening of the urine, a yellow appearance to the skin or whites of the eyes, and an increased tendency to bruise or bleed, which are signs and symptoms of liver toxicity or failure. • Ask patients about all drugs they are taking because many drugs can interact with INH. • The IM route can be used only if oral therapy is not practical.

Rifampin (Rifadin): kills slower-growing organisms, even those that reside inside macrophages and granulomas.

DRUG/ADULT DOSAGE RANGE	NURSING IMPLICATIONS
For Uncomplicated TB: rifampin 150–300 mg orally daily for 6 months **For Prophylaxis:** rifampin 150–300 mg orally daily for 4 months, usually with isoniazid rifampin 10 mg/kg (maximum dose 600 mg) IV	• Instruct patients to avoid antacids and to take the drug on an empty stomach (1 hour before or 2 hours after meals) to prevent slowing of drug absorption in the GI tract. • Warn patients to expect a reddish orange staining of the skin, urine, and all other secretions. • Tell patients not to wear soft contact lenses while on therapy with this drug because they will become permanently stained. • Remind patients to avoid drinking alcoholic beverages and taking acetaminophen while on this drug because the liver-damaging effects of this drug are potentiated by alcohol and acetaminophen use. • Tell patients to report darkening of the urine, a yellow appearance to the skin or whites of the eyes, and an increased tendency to bruise or bleed, which are signs and symptoms of liver toxicity or failure. • Teach patients with diabetes to check blood glucose levels frequently because fluctuations in glucose levels can occur and cause hyperglycemia or hypoglycemia. • Ask the patient about all other drugs in use because this drug interacts with many other drugs. • The IV route can be used only if oral therapy is not practical. • Mix IV doses according to manufacturer's instructions and give over 30 minutes to 3 hours to reduce the chances for shocklike reactions and CNS symptoms.

Pyrazinamide: can effectively kill organisms residing within the very acidic environment of macrophages (which is where the tubercle bacillus isolates itself). This drug is used in combination with other anti-TB drugs.

DRUG/ADULT DOSAGE RANGE	NURSING IMPLICATIONS
For Uncomplicated TB: pyrazinamide 1.5–2 g orally once daily for 6 months *or* 3 g orally once daily three times per week	• Ask whether the patient has ever had gout because the drug increases uric acid formation and will make gout symptoms worse. • Instruct patients to drink at least 8 ounces of water when taking this tablet and to increase fluid intake to prevent uric acid from precipitating, making gout or kidney problems worse. • Teach the patient to wear protective clothing, a hat, and sunscreen when going outdoors in the sunlight because the drug causes photosensitivity and greatly increases the risk for sunburn. • Remind the patient to avoid drinking alcoholic beverages while on this drug because the liver-damaging effects of this drug are potentiated by drinking alcohol. • Tell the patient to report darkening of the urine, a yellow appearance to the skin or whites of the eyes, and an increased tendency to bruise or bleed, which are signs and symptoms of liver toxicity or failure.

Table 5.4   First-Line Drug Therapy for Tuberculosis—cont'd

Ethambutol: inhibits bacterial RNA synthesis, thus suppressing bacterial growth. It is slow-acting and is bacteriostatic, rather than bactericidal. Thus it must be used in combination with other anti-TB drugs.

DRUG/ADULT DOSAGE RANGE	NURSING IMPLICATIONS
For Uncomplicated TB: ethambutol (Myambutol) 15 mg/kg per dose (maximum 1.5 g) orally once daily for 6 months	• Teach patients to take the drug with food to prevent or minimize stomach irritation. • Instruct patients to immediately report any changes in vision, such as reduced color vision, blurred vision, or reduced visual fields, to the primary healthcare provider because the drug can cause optic neuritis, especially at high doses, and can lead to blindness. Minor eye problems are usually reversed when the drug is stopped. • Remind the patient to avoid drinking alcoholic beverages while on this drug because the drug induces severe nausea and vomiting when alcohol is ingested. • Ask whether the patient has ever had gout because the drug increases uric acid formation and will make gout worse. • Instruct patients to drink at least 8 ounces of water when taking this drug and to increase fluid intake to prevent uric acid from precipitating, making gout or kidney problems worse.

TB, Tuberculosis.

commonly the drugs are given orally and some are combined to reduce the number of separate drugs the patient has to take every day. When patients are hospitalized and are unable to take the oral form of the drugs, parenteral forms are available. There is an extensively drug-resistant tuberculosis (XDR-TB) that is rare but resistant to almost all drugs currently used to treat TB. Patients who have XDR-TB have a poor prognosis.

Action and Uses

The main action of first-line antitubercular drugs takes place within and outside the cell walls of the bacteria that slow down the reproduction of *M. tuberculosis* bacteria. The drugs used to treat TB are both bactericidal and bacteriostatic. Antitubercular drugs are used to control the active disease and prevent its spread to various organ systems in the infected patient or to other people. The drug therapy is used for direct treatment of TB infection and for prophylaxis in people who have been heavily exposed to the organism but have no symptoms of the disease.

Isoniazid (INH) inhibits the enzymes of the TB organisms needed for reproduction and growth. It is a bactericidal drug. INH can inhibit the enzymes of the TB bacteria that are in an infectious as well as a dormant state. It is metabolized by the liver and is available in oral and IM form.

Rifampin inhibits a TB enzyme needed for making its DNA and proteins. This drug is effective in preventing the reproduction of the TB organism both in infected tissues and in the macrophages and TB granulomas. Rifampin can be bactericidal if the concentration of the drug is high enough in infected tissues.

Pyrazinamide appears to work by making the pH of infected cells lower (more acidic) than the TB organism needs to reproduce and grow. It is especially effective at slowing the growth of TB organisms that are inside macrophages and in granulomas.

Ethambutol appears to interfere with the RNA and protein synthesis of the TB organism, which reduces bacterial reproduction. It is bacteriostatic and is always used in combination with other drugs. See Fig. 5.3 for sites of drug activity on the TB organism.

Lifespan Considerations
Pediatric
Children who either have active TB or who are heavily exposed and require prophylaxis are prescribed isoniazid, rifampin, and pyrazinamide as first-line therapy. Ethambutol is not prescribed for infants or young children because they are unable to report visual changes that may indicate a complication that can lead to permanent blindness.

Bedaquiline (Sirturo) is a new drug that has been approved for use in confirmed pulmonary MDR TB or if INH and Rifampin therapy is unsuccessful. It has a half-life of 4 to 5 months and is used for 24 weeks in combination with INH, rifampin, pyrazinamide, and ethambutol. Bedaquiline is liver toxic and can cause life-threatening dysrhythmias. Baseline ECGs and serum electrolyte values are obtained and then monitored periodically throughout treatment to assess for cardiotoxicity. The dose is 400 mg orally every day for 2 weeks, then 200 mg three times a week for the next 24 weeks. The drug has not been studied in children, persons with HIV/AIDS, or women who are pregnant; therefore it is not used in these populations.

Expected Side Effects

Most of the first-line drugs against TB cause nausea, vomiting, diarrhea, headache, and sleeplessness. INH causes pyridoxine (vitamin B₆) deficiency, so

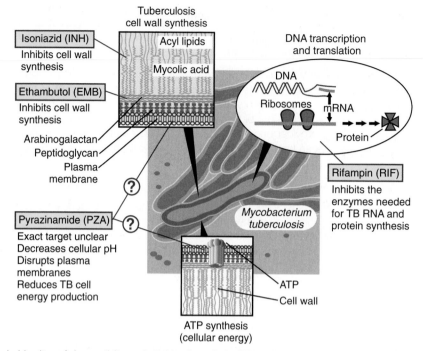

FIG. 5.3 Probable sites of drug activity against the tuberculosis (TB) organism. *ATP*, Adenosine triphosphate; *mRNA*, messenger RNA. (From Workman ML, LaCharity LA: *Understanding pharmacology*, ed 2, St. Louis, 2016, Elsevier.)

supplements of vitamin B$_6$ are generally given during treatment. Rifampin discolors urine and other body fluids a reddish orange color. It may even stain soft contact lenses. Pyrazinamide increases sun sensitivity and causes muscle aches and acne. Both pyrazinamide and ethambutol increase the formation of uric acid, which causes gout or makes the symptoms worse.

Adverse Reactions

All first-line drugs for TB treatment are toxic to the liver. The toxicity is worsened if patients drink alcohol or use other liver-toxic drugs such as acetaminophen during TB therapy. INH, because it causes a deficiency in vitamin B$_6$, causes peripheral neuropathy with loss of sensation in the hands and feet. Ethambutol may cause confusion and optic neuritis that can lead to vision loss if the drug is not stopped. Pyrazinamide may interfere with blood clotting time and cause anemia. INH and ethambutol may cause psychological changes in some patients.

Contraindications for the use of TB drugs are severe drug allergy and major renal or liver dysfunction. However, because of the fatal nature of TB, the risks may outweigh the benefits in these patients and the contraindications may be lifted. Patients with allergies can be given supportive therapy such as antihistamines and steroids during treatment if drug allergies exist.

Drug Interactions

The drug treatment plan for TB is often complicated. No other drugs should be taken at the same time as or right after antitubercular drugs are swallowed. Even topical agents on the skin are avoided while the patient is receiving anti-TB therapy. This is because other drugs may increase the significant risk for neurotoxicity and nephrotoxicity. All drugs taken by the patient should be checked closely for drug interactions, which are common among the antitubercular drugs. Consult a drug reference book or a pharmacist for information when other drugs are prescribed during antitubercular therapy.

❖ Nursing Implications and Patient Teaching

◆ *Assessment.* Assess the patient for signs and symptoms of active TB (productive cough with thick and often bloody sputum, low-grade fever, night sweats, anorexia, unplanned weight loss, and fatigue). It is important that the patient be a full partner in TB treatment because the drug therapy lasts for many months and is critical in controlling the disease. Assess whether the patient understands the importance of correctly taking the drugs every day. Also check whether he or she understands how to prevent infection spread.

Laboratory values are obtained before therapy begins to establish baseline levels and also to prevent adverse effects from starting the drugs. These usually include a complete blood count (CBC) to assess for anemia, BUN and creatinine to assess kidney function, liver enzymes to assess liver function, and a uric acid level to assess for gout.

Drug resistance is likely to develop if only one drug is used for active TB or if the patient does not take the drugs as prescribed. If patients are homeless, homeless clinics and outreach services can be enlisted to ensure treatment success. If the patient cannot be relied on to take the drugs exactly as prescribed, he or she may need to be enrolled in a program of *directly observed therapy (DOT)* in which the drugs are given by an authorized person who watches to ensure the patient actually swallows the drugs. Your local or state public health department, hospital, or pharmacy can provide more information on DOT programs.

◆ *Planning and implementation.* Drug toxicity is a special problem because of the long-term nature of the required treatment. Ask patients on TB therapy about symptoms of adverse reactions. If toxic effects, adverse reactions, or allergic reactions occur, drugs are stopped, and the healthcare provider immediately begins further evaluation to determine which drug or drugs are responsible.

Check for yellowing of the skin and eyes, light-colored stools, and darkening of the urine, which would indicate liver toxicity. Ask about any numbness or tingling or pain in hands and feet that could indicate peripheral neuropathy from vitamin B_6 deficiency. Symptoms of urinary retention such as low abdominal discomfort, inability to urinate, painful urination, and bladder distention may indicate urinary retention. Ask patients about joint pain and swelling that may indicate gout. Assess vision frequently, especially for patients taking ethambutol. Ask whether the patients have noticed any changes in reading or driving, and whether they have any pain or blurring of vision. These symptoms can indicate optic neuritis. Look for any changes in personality such as anxiety, withdrawal, or depression. Report all changes and unusual symptoms to the healthcare provider because all of these changes indicate possible adverse reactions to the drugs.

All drugs, unless stated otherwise, should be taken at the same time each day, preferably in the morning. If parenteral administration is required, the injection sites should be rotated and each site inspected for signs of tenderness, swelling, or redness.

Rifampin and isoniazid are best absorbed on an empty stomach. They should be taken either 1 hour before or 2 hours after a meal.

◆ *Evaluation.* The positive skin test for TB does not change during therapy. Patients are assessed on a monthly basis for improvement of TB symptoms and the presence of active organisms in sputum cultures. Vital signs and new symptoms should be monitored for recurrence of acute infection. Weigh patients at each visit to monitor their general health status. Report weight loss to the healthcare provider because it may indicate worsening of the disease. Diet changes and nutritional supplements may be indicated.

◆ *Patient and family teaching.* In addition to the general nursing implications and teaching points for all anti-microbial drugs, those specific for first-line antitubercular therapy are listed in Table 5.4. Patients must take their drugs for a long time, so it is important to give clear instructions at the scheduled visits about the importance of continuing to take the drugs as ordered and the problems that should be reported to the healthcare provider. Stress the following important instructions:

- Do not drink alcohol for the entire duration of your TB treatment because all of these drugs can damage your liver and the damage is worse when alcohol is consumed.
- Set a regular time each day to take your anti-TB drugs to help you remember to take them.
- Take these drugs exactly as directed. If a dose is missed, take it as soon as you remember it unless it is almost time for the next dose. Then do not take the missed dose, just follow the regular dosing schedule.
- Report any new symptoms promptly to your healthcare provider. Symptoms to report include any episodes of easy bruising, fever, sore throat, unusual bleeding, skin rashes, mental confusion, headache, tremors, severe nausea, vomiting, diarrhea, malaise, yellowish discoloration of the skin, visual changes, excessive drowsiness, severe pain in knees, feet, or wrists, or changes in personality or affect (seem not to respond to things).
- Remember that while taking rifampin, your urine will be reddish orange. Although it can stain your clothing and toilet, this is normal.
- Do not wear soft contact lenses while taking the combination drugs for TB because rifampin can permanently stain contact lenses.
- Do not take other drugs without the knowledge and permission of your healthcare provider.
- Take rifampin and isoniazid 1 hour before or 2 hours after eating or taking an antacid because food and antacids delay absorption of the drugs and may reduce their effects.
- Take ethambutol with food to reduce stomach irritation.
- Keep all appointments with your healthcare provider and laboratory tests so that progress can be measured.

ANTIFUNGAL DRUGS

Fungi are microorganisms that include yeasts and molds. Fungi are found everywhere in the environment and they thrive in dark, moist places. Most of the time fungi exist in harmony with humans; however, fungi can become pathogens and cause an infection. A fungal infection is called a *mycosis* or a *mycotic infection*. Fungi can be ingested or inhaled, and they easily grow on skin and nails. Some fungal infections are *localized* (kept to a specific area), such as athlete's foot, whereas others may become *systemic* (spread throughout the patient's whole body), such as an invasive candidiasis.

When fungi come into contact with a person who has reduced immunity, they take advantage of the weakened immune system and cause infection. For this reason they are called *opportunistic infections*. Patients at increased risk for developing a fungal infection are patients with diabetes, pregnant women, women on birth control, patients taking corticosteroids, persons who are taking antibiotics (particularly women), and newborns. Transplant patients who are taking immunosuppressive drugs, cancer patients on chemotherapy, and patients with AIDS are at risk for developing severe systemic fungal infections.

Fungi are more complex organisms than bacteria and more closely resemble human cells. Thus they require drugs that act in a different way than antibacterials. In addition, because antifungal drugs often work on the same structures that human cells have, they usually have more side effects and reactions when taken systemically.

Action and Uses

Antifungal drugs are used orally, intravenously, topically, and vaginally to treat a variety of fungal or mycotic infections. Antifungal drugs have six classifications: the azoles, the polyenes, the allylamines, antifungal antibiotics, antimetabolites, and echinocandins. Azoles, polyenes, and allylamines all prevent the production of a lipid-like substance from forming the fungal cell membrane. Without the cell membrane, the fungus becomes damaged and either cannot reproduce (*fungistatic*) or dies (*fungicidal*). The antifungal drug griseofulvin stops the fungus from reproducing. Antimetabolites (flucytosine) disrupt the metabolic pathway of the fungal cell and interfere with both reproduction and growth of the fungus. Echinocandins damage the cell wall of the fungus, killing it. They are the newest class of antifungals and are given only by the IV route for the treatment of invasive candidiasis, especially in critically ill patients.

The actions and specific uses of common systemic antifungal drugs are described in Table 5.5. Instructions for patients using topical antifungal agents for superficial fungal infections are presented in Box 5.3.

> ### Memory Jogger
> Fluconazole, ketoconazole, itraconazole, posaconazole, and voriconazole all have the suffix of -azole and are fungistatic and fungicidal at higher doses.

Expected Side Effects and Adverse Reactions

Nausea, vomiting, and diarrhea are the most common expected side effects of antifungal drugs. Adverse reactions are associated with more severe problems such as toxicity to the neurologic, cardiac, hematologic, liver, and renal systems. Skin reactions, rashes, and a rare serious rash such as *Stevens-Johnson syndrome* can occur. Stevens-Johnson syndrome begins with a painful red or purple rash, blisters, and flu symptoms. It is a medical emergency.

Amphotericin B in particular, which is given intravenously, is associated with numerous adverse reactions, and patients are premedicated with antihistamines, antipyretics, corticosteroids, and opiates to prevent adverse effects. Amphotericin B is associated with serious adverse effects, and these patients must be closely monitored. Increased sun sensitivity (photosensitivity) can cause severe sunburn when taking ketoconazole, voriconazole, or griseofulvin. Griseofulvin can cause liver toxicity and numbness and tingling of hands and feet (paresthesia). Terbinafine (Lamisil) and flucytosine (Ancobon) can increase the risk for infection because they can reduce the white blood cell (WBC) count. Terbinafine is also associated with hair loss in some individuals. Azoles at high doses given intravenously can cause life-threatening cardiac dysrhythmias.

> ### Top Tip for Safety
> Adverse reactions to systemic antifungals, such as peeling, blistering, itching, burning, and redness of the skin, are similar to the symptoms of the diseases they are intended to cure. Therefore it is sometimes difficult to determine whether the patient needs more or less drug.

Drug Interactions

Superinfections can result when antifungals are given together with corticosteroid therapy because corticosteroids reduce the immunity response, making the person more vulnerable to a fungal infection. Oral anticoagulant activity is decreased when used at the same time as griseofulvin. Fluconazole and itraconazole increase the effects of anticoagulants, causing patients to bleed, and can cause hypoglycemia when used with an oral hypoglycemic. Voriconazole interferes with many antidysrhythmic drugs and can cause life-threatening dysrhythmias. Antacids, anticholinergics, and H2 blockers (e.g., Pepcid, Zantac) change GI pH and interfere with drug absorption.

Toxicity can result when flucytosine is used together with other drugs that depress bone marrow or when used during radiation therapy. Use of flucytosine with hepatotoxic or nephrotoxic drugs should be avoided. The use of flucytosine also decreases leukocyte and platelet counts and hemoglobin levels. Consult a drug reference book or a pharmacist for information when other drugs are prescribed during antifungal therapy.

❖ Nursing Implications and Patient Teaching

◆ *Assessment.* Ask about any allergy, bone marrow depression, use of alcohol or other drugs that may produce drug interactions (particularly corticosteroids), and the possibility of pregnancy. Some antifungal drugs may be *teratogenic* (cause birth defects).

The patient may have a history of fever and chills at the onset of infection. Many patients report itching if they have a fungal infection. A history of recent antibiotic therapy is common. Inspect the mouth for the classic signs of thick, white nonmovable plaques that coat the tongue and *erythema* (redness or irritation) associated with *thrush* (*Candida* infection). The patient may also have a history of multiple scaly or blistered red patches on the skin, itching and soreness of infected areas, or brittle nails with yellow discoloration and separation from the nail bed. Check current laboratory

Table 5.5   Examples of Common Antifungal Drugs

Azoles: work by altering the cellular membrane of the fungus by depleting a lipid-like substance (ergosterol), which damages the fungus and will not allow it to reproduce. At higher doses azoles will kill the fungus. They are used to provide prophylaxis in high-risk patients and to treat topical and systemic infections caused by *Candida* and other fungi that are susceptible to their action.

DRUG/ADULT DOSAGE RANGE	NURSING IMPLICATIONS

fluconazole (Diflucan)
    200 mg–400 mg orally daily *or*
    200–800 mg IV daily *or* 150 mg
    orally one time for treatment of
    vaginal candidiasis
 ketoconazole (Nizoral, Extina)
    200 mg–400 mg orally once a
    day (ketoconazole can also be
    applied topically)
	• Length of treatment depends on the nature of the infection, so tell patients to take the drugs as prescribed for as long as they are prescribed to ensure adequate protection against infection or adequate treatment of infection.
	 • Instruct patients to monitor for rash, redness, or blistering because this could indicate a serious medical emergency. If these symptoms occur, they must notify the healthcare provider immediately.
	 • Instruct patients on oral antidiabetic drugs to monitor glucose levels closely because these drugs can cause fluctuations in glucose control.
	 • Monitor blood urea nitrogen (BUN), serum creatinine, and liver function studies because these drugs can cause kidney and liver damage.
	 • Tell patients to report yellow skin, light-colored stools, dark urine, and yellowing of the eye sclera to the healthcare provider because these are indications of adverse liver reactions.
	 • Mix IV doses of fluconazole according to manufacturer's direction and give no faster than 200 mg/h to reduce the risk for cardiac dysrhythmias.
	 • Teach patients how to take their pulse daily and report a pulse greater than 100 beats per minute or lower than 60 beats per minute, or a newly irregular heart rate to the healthcare provider because these drugs can cause cardiac rhythm problems.
	 • Instruct patients to take ketoconazole with an acidic beverage such as cola to increase its absorption.
	 • Teach sexually active women to use effective birth control while taking azoles because these drugs may cause birth defects.

Griseofulvin: stops fungal reproduction interfering with cell division. It is effective in the treatment of superficial dermatophyte infections such as tinea infections (ringworm, jock itch, athlete's foot, and toenail fungus).

DRUG/ADULT DOSAGE RANGE	NURSING IMPLICATIONS

griseofulvin (Gris-PEG, Grifulvin)
    300–750 mg orally once
    daily (ultramicrosize) *or*
    750–1000 mg orally once
    daily (microsize)
	• Teach patients to take the drug with a fatty meal to increase absorption.
	 • Teach patients to check for numbness and/or tingling of the feet and report these to their healthcare provider because these drugs can cause peripheral neuropathy.
	 • Tell patients to wear sunscreen and protective clothing when outdoors to prevent a severe sunburn because this drug increases sun sensitivity.
	 • Teach patients to alert their healthcare provider if symptoms such as rash or hives develop because these may indicate an allergy (hypersensitivity) to the drug.
	 • Tell patients to report yellow skin, light-colored stools, dark urine, and yellowing of the eye sclera to the healthcare provider because these drugs can damage the liver.
	 • Advise patients to avoid alcoholic beverages while taking griseofulvin because they may experience a rapid heart rate, sweating, and flushing.
	 • Teach sexually active women to use effective birth control because these drugs can cause birth defects.

Nystatin: alters fungal cell membranes by depleting a lipid-like substance (ergosterol), which damages the fungus and will not allow it to reproduce. At higher doses azoles will kill the fungus. It is used to treat candidiasis infections such as thrush and diaper dermatitis and skin infections.

DRUG/ADULT DOSAGE RANGE	NURSING IMPLICATIONS

nystatin (Bio-Statin, Nyata)
    400,000–600,000 units oral
    suspension in oral cavity four
    times a day *or* 200,000–
    400,000 units orally by
    troche dissolved in mouth
    four to five times daily *or*
    500,000–1,000,000 units by
    tablet orally three times a day
    (can also be applied as a
    powder, cream, or solution)
	• Teach patients to prepare only a single dose of the nystatin powder for suspension because it does not contain preservatives and will not stay fresh.
	 • Teach patients to shake the suspension liquid well before taking it because the drug separates quickly.
	 • Teach patients to take half of the dose in each side of the mouth to completely cover the oral tissues.
	 • Teach patients to retain the suspension in the mouth for several minutes before swallowing to ensure the drug comes into contact with any oral fungus.
	 • Warn patients who have diabetes and are taking nystatin suspension that it may increase their blood glucose levels because it contains sucrose.

Box **5.3** **Teaching Points for Patients Using Topical Antifungal Drugs**

GENERAL

- Report any indication of an allergic reaction (new redness, swelling, blisters, or drainage) to the prescriber.
- Wash your hands to remove all traces of the drug from your hands immediately after applying it.
- Avoid getting any antifungal drug in your eye. If the drug does get into your eye, wash the eye with large amounts of warm, running tap water and notify the prescriber.
- Use the drug exactly as prescribed and for as long as prescribed to ensure the infection is cured.

POWDERS

- Ensure skin area is clean and completely dry before applying the powder to prevent the powder from caking together.
- Hold your breath while applying to avoid inhaling the drug.
- For the foot area, be sure to get the powder between and under your toes. Wear clean cotton socks (night and day). Change the socks at least twice daily.
- For the groin area, wear clean, close-fitting (but not tight) cotton underwear (briefs or panties) to keep the drug in contact with the areas that are infected.

LOTIONS, CREAMS, AND OINTMENTS APPLIED TO THE SKIN

- Ensure the skin area is clean and dry before applying the drug to ensure best contact with the affected area.
- Be careful to apply it only to the skin that has the infection. Keep it off of the surrounding skin to prevent healthy skin from reacting to the drug.
- Apply a thin coating as often as prescribed.
- Wash the area and dry it right before reapplying the next dose to ensure the fresh drug is able to come into contact with the affected area.
- Loosely cover the area to prevent spreading the drug to other body areas, clothing, or furniture.

ORAL LOZENGES

- Brush your teeth and tongue before using the tablet or troche to remove as much of the organism as possible so that the drug can come into direct contact with the affected area.
- Let the tablet or troche completely dissolve in your mouth for maximum release of the drug.
- Clean your toothbrush daily by running it through the dishwasher or soaking it in a solution of 1 part household bleach with 9 parts water. After using bleach, rinse the toothbrush thoroughly. Cleaning keeps the infection from recurring.

VAGINAL CREAMS/SUPPOSITORIES

- Vaginal creams or suppositories should be placed just before going to bed to help keep them within the vagina longer.
- Wash your hands before inserting the drug to avoid getting other organisms into the vagina.
- Insert the suppository (rounded end first) into the vagina as far as you can reach with your finger so that the drug reaches all affected areas.
- Insert an applicator full of the cream as far into the vagina as is comfortable for you so that the drug reaches all affected areas.
- Wash the applicator and your hands with warm, soapy water, rinse well, and dry to prevent reinfecting yourself with organisms left on the applicator.
- A sanitary napkin can be worn to protect your clothing and the bed from drug leakage.
- Avoid sexual intercourse during the treatment period. If you do have intercourse, the drug can make holes in a condom or damage a diaphragm and increase your risk for an unplanned pregnancy. In addition, you could spread the infection or get reinfected with the yeast.

Adapted from Workman ML, LaCharity LA: *Understanding pharmacology,* ed 2, St. Louis, 2016, Elsevier.

work for CBC, platelet count, BUN, creatinine, and liver enzymes to establish a baseline and to prevent kidney, liver, or hematologic damage. Check and document vital signs, an accurate height and weight, as well as culture and sensitivity reports.

Top Tip for Safety

Closely monitor renal and hepatic functioning when giving ketoconazole and fluconazole.

Closely monitor hematologic, renal, and hepatic status when giving flucytosine.

◆ *Planning and implementation.* Observe the patient for any signs of allergic reactions, such as hives, swelling of the lips and face, rapid pulse, and lower blood pressure. Alert the rapid response team immediately for any of these symptoms because they indicate an anaphylactic reaction.

Check the skin for rashes, blisters, or increased itching that may indicate an adverse reaction or worsening of the fungal infection.

Assess the site of infection daily for any changes and document your findings. Assess vital signs as ordered daily and alert the healthcare provider for changes, particularly changes in temperature and pulse rate.

Check the patient daily for signs of jaundice that may indicate hepatotoxicity: yellow skin, yellowing of the eye sclera, dark urine, clay-colored stool, and abdominal pain.

Check the ongoing ordered laboratory work for any abnormalities that can indicate an adverse reaction or worsening of disease symptoms. Alert the healthcare provider as soon as possible for any changes from baseline levels.

◆ *Evaluation.* Observe the patient for therapeutic effects: chills or fever associated with some infections should disappear, and signs and symptoms should improve.

Also watch for development of adverse effects and signs of GI distress. Remind the patient to continue to take the drug for the length that the dose is prescribed and/or until the laboratory tests show that normal function has returned.

Top Tip for Safety

If you are monitoring a patient receiving amphotericin B, give prescribed drugs to prevent adverse effects before the start of the infusion and avoid giving any other drugs during the infusion. Monitor vital signs closely and watch for reactions such as fever, chills, abdominal pain, cramping, diarrhea, nausea, vomiting, headache, flushing, and decreased blood pressure. Monitor for pain and inflammation at the infusion site.

◆ *Patient and family teaching.* Stress the following important instructions to the patient and family:
- Do not take any over-the-counter drugs and let your healthcare provider know of all drugs you are currently taking or any drugs that another practitioner may prescribe for you during treatment because antifungals have many possible drug interactions.
- Take griseofulvin with high-fat foods or meals like cheeseburgers, whole milk, or ice cream. This causes more of the drug to be absorbed and reduces possible stomach upset.
- Avoid direct sunlight and wear sunscreen and protective clothing while outside to prevent severe sunburn when taking ketoconazole, voriconazole, and griseofulvin.
- Notify your healthcare provider if you have dark urine, light-colored stool, or yellowing of the whites of the eyes because these are signs of liver problems.
- Notify your healthcare provider if you have increased fatigue and shortness of breath, which may indicate an anemia.
- Be alert to flu symptoms, rash, or blisters and notify your healthcare provider immediately because these symptoms can indicate a severe adverse reaction to the drug and require hospitalization.
- Notify your healthcare provider about any skin rash or worsening nausea, vomiting, or diarrhea.
- When taking more than one capsule per dose, taking one capsule every 15 minutes or more can reduce the likelihood of GI upset.
- If symptoms do not resolve within 2 to 3 days, notify your healthcare provider.
- Finish all of the drugs you were given even if your symptoms improve so that the infection does not return and resistance to the antifungal does not develop.
- If you take an "azole," do not take the drug with grapefruit juice and limit the amount of grapefruit juice you drink daily because it increases the potency of the drug, thus increasing the risk for adverse effects.

ANTIPARASITIC DRUGS

A parasite is an organism that can survive only by living in or on a host organism. Billions of people worldwide and millions of people in the United States are affected by parasites that cause serious illnesses and can even cause death, especially in immunocompromised individuals. Parasites can be picked up from food, water, or insects and can be transmitted from person to person. Three main classes of parasites can cause disease in humans: protozoa, helminthes, and ectoparasites (fleas and lice).

PROTOZOA

Amoebiasis and *giardiasis* are usually contracted from food and water contaminated by feces or by unwashed hands after using the bathroom or changing a diaper. These infections reside in the intestinal tract, and common symptoms are diarrhea, abdominal pain, vomiting, and foul-smelling stools. Amoebiasis is able to invade other parts of the body if it reaches the bloodstream and it can cause liver abscesses.

Toxoplasmosis is usually asymptomatic in a healthy individual but can cause serious illness in people with chronic disease. It is contracted from contaminated raw food and water or by handling contaminated soil, cat litter, and raw meat and then touching the mouth, nose, or eyes.

Trichomoniasis is transmitted through sexual exposure. Symptoms of trichomoniasis include burning, itching, redness, and vaginal or penile discharge.

Malaria is common in southeast Asia and Africa. It is spread through the bites of mosquitoes that have been infected by malaria-causing parasites (*Plasmodium*). The parasite migrates to the liver, where it matures and then enters the bloodstream. It lives and reproduces in the blood, using the hemoglobin and nutrients inside the red blood cell (RBC) until the blood cell ruptures and causes anemia. Treatment for malaria is guided by the CDC and depends on where the person contracted the disease. The CDC also has a prophylaxis treatment guide for persons traveling to areas where malaria is prevalent. Malaria signs and symptoms include fever, chills, sweating, headaches, extreme fatigue, body aches, and nausea and vomiting. Even after treatment the disease is able to relapse.

Bookmark This!

For information on the malarial disease process and up-to-date prophylaxis and treatment options, visit the CDC at www.cdc.gov/malaria.

ANTIPROTOZOAL DRUGS
Action and Uses

Antiprotozoal drugs work in several different ways inside the cell, affecting the function of DNA and/or RNA to kill the protozoan parasites. Antiprotozoals used to treat amebiasis, giardiasis, toxoplasmosis, and trichomoniasis are metronidazole (Flagyl) and iodoquinol (Yodoxin). Metronidazole is also used to treat bacterial vaginitis in conjunction with antibiotics used for the treatment of pelvic inflammatory disease.

Drugs used to either prevent or treat malaria include quinine, chloroquine (Aralen), hydroxychloroquine (Plaquenil), mefloquine (Lariam), and primaquine. Chloroquine, hydroxychloroquine, quinine, and mefloquine inhibit the DNA and RNA enzymes necessary for the parasite to reproduce and live. They also raise the pH inside the parasite so it is unable to use the hemoglobin in the human RBC to live and reproduce. All of these actions cause damage to the parasite. Pyrimethamine inhibits enzymes necessary for the parasite to produce substances necessary for its survival. The combination of malarial drugs together kill the malarial parasite in different life cycles. Antimalarial drugs are sometimes used to treat other parasitic diseases as well. Table 5.6 provides a summary of antiprotozoal and antimalarial drugs.

Expected Side Effects and Adverse Reactions

All drugs used to treat parasitic infections may cause nausea, vomiting, headache, anorexia, diarrhea, or GI distress. Additional drugs to support minimizing these side effects may be warranted. Iodoquinol (Yodoxin) is an iodine-based drug, so patients may experience hypothyroidism or hyperthyroidism, and thyroid function tests may be altered. Iodoquinol may also cause a yellow-brown nail, hair and skin discoloration, as well as discolored sweat. Optic neuritis can occur with symptoms of eye pain or vision changes. Permanent vision loss can occur if the drug is not stopped quickly. Peripheral neuropathy symptoms such as numbness and tingling of the fingers can occur with prolonged therapy. Metronidazole (Flagyl) can cause peripheral neuropathy as well as confusion. Fungal superinfections may occur with the use of metronidazole.

Common side effects of drugs used to treat malaria are similar to those used to treat other parasitic conditions: diarrhea, nausea, vomiting, headache, and GI distress. Primaquine can cause hemolytic anemia, leukopenia, and life-threatening dysrhythmias. Hydroxychloroquine can cause visual defects and possible loss of vision. Chloroquine and hydroxychloroquine can cause CNS changes such as personality changes, anxiety, and depression.

Drug Interactions

There are no significant drug interactions with the use of iodoquinol. Metronidazole increases the effects of warfarin, and serious bleeding can occur when the two drugs are taken together. Alcohol-containing drinks, food, or mouthwash taken with or used during metronidazole can result in severe nausea, vomiting, headache, shortness of breath, and hypotension (disulfiram-like reaction). Chloroquine can decrease

levels of valproic acid and increase levels of digoxin. Mefloquine and primaquine interact with many antidysrhythmic drugs like quinidine, beta blockers, and calcium channel blockers and can increase the risk for life-threatening dysrhythmias. Consult a drug reference book or a pharmacist for information when other drugs are prescribed during drug therapy for parasitic infestations.

❖ Nursing Implications and Patient Teaching

◆ *Assessment.* Ask the patient about any allergy to drugs, current use of alcohol or disulfiram, the possibility of pregnancy, or the existence of chronic renal, hematologic, cardiac, thyroid, or liver disease. These conditions are contraindications or precautions to the use of antiparasitics and drugs used to treat malaria. Baseline laboratory tests should be completed before therapy begins.

◆ *Planning and implementation.* Observe the patient for any signs of allergic reactions such as hives, swelling of the lips and face, rapid pulse, and lower blood pressure. Alert the rapid response team immediately for any of these symptoms because they indicate an anaphylactic reaction.

Monitor nutritional status and encourage adequate food and fluid intake to help fight infection.

Monitor for superinfections and notify the healthcare provider for any changes. Assess vital signs as ordered daily and alert the healthcare provider for any changes, particularly in temperature.

Check the patient daily for signs of jaundice that may indicate hepatotoxicity: yellow skin, yellowing of the eye sclera, dark urine, clay-colored stool, and abdominal pain.

Check the ongoing laboratory work as it is ordered for any abnormalities that can indicate an adverse reaction or worsening of disease symptoms. Alert the healthcare provider as soon as possible for any changes from baseline levels.

◆ *Evaluation.* After drug therapy, periodic laboratory blood and stool tests are required to make certain that the disease has been controlled or eliminated. These tests may be needed monthly for up to 1 year after therapy. Be alert to signs of drug toxicity. If severe symptoms appear, the drug may have to be stopped.

◆ *Patient and family teaching.* Stress the following important instructions to the patient and family:

- Take antiparasitics with or after meals to decrease the chances of stomach upset.
- Take antiparasitics with a full glass of water to prevent stomach upset.
- Report worsening symptoms of infection such as increased fever, increasing fatigue, or anorexia.
- Take the entire course of drug, even if symptoms improve, to prevent relapse or worsening infection.
- If taking metronidazole, avoid all forms of alcohol so that severe adverse effects do not occur.
- When traveling to areas where malaria is common, take prophylactic doses as prescribed.

Table 5.6   Examples of Common Antiparasitic Drugs

Antiparasitics (not used for malaria): work in several different ways inside cell DNA and/or RNA to kill the protozoal parasites.

DRUG/ADULT DOSAGE RANGE	NURSING IMPLICATIONS
metronidazole (Flagyl) 500–750 mg orally three times daily iodoquinol (Yodoxin) 650 mg orally three times daily	• Teach patients to swallow metronidazole extended-release tablets whole; do not crush, break, or chew to prevent the release of drug too rapidly, which can lead to adverse effects. • Give metronidazole at least 1 hour before or 2 hours after meals to ensure best absorption. • Give iodoquinol with a meal or directly after a meal to minimize stomach upset. • Advise patients to take metronidazole and iodoquinol with a full glass of water to support excretion by the kidney. • Check patient's baseline liver and kidney function laboratory tests and alert the healthcare provider if there are abnormalities, because these drugs are metabolized by the liver and excreted by the kidney and could cause damage in compromised individuals. • Remind patients taking metronidazole to avoid alcohol or products that contain alcohol because severe side effects can occur with the use of metronidazole. • Consult with the healthcare provider and the pharmacist for patients taking other drugs with metronidazole because it interacts with many drugs, leading to life-threatening dysrhythmias. • Tell patients taking iodoquinol to contact their healthcare provider for any visual changes because the drug can cause optic neuritis and permanent vision loss. • Advise patients taking iodoquinol to contact their healthcare provider for any worsening symptoms of thyroid problems because the drug can interfere with drugs used for thyroid disorders.

Antimalarials: inhibit the DNA and RNA enzymes necessary for the parasite *Plasmodium* to reproduce and live.

DRUG/ADULT DOSAGE RANGE	NURSING IMPLICATIONS
Chloroquine (Aralen) **For Malaria Treatment:** 1000 mg orally, then 500 mg orally in 6–8 hours, then 500 mg orally once daily for 2 days **For Malaria Prophylaxis:** 500 mg orally weekly on the same day of each week, starting 2 weeks before entering the endemic area and continuing for 8 weeks after leaving the area. **Primaquine** **For Treatment of Malaria:** 52.6 mg orally daily for 14 days in combination with chloroquine **For Prophylaxis of Malaria:** 52.6 mg orally once daily for 1–2 days before travel to the malaria-risk area; continue once daily while in the malaria-risk area and once daily for 7 days after leaving the malaria-risk area	• Give chloroquine and primaquine with meals to minimize stomach upset. • Observe patients for corneal opacities and changes in vision because chloroquine can cause retinopathy especially in older adults. If visual changes occur, contact the healthcare provider immediately because retinal changes can be permanent if the drug is not stopped. • Warn patients with psoriasis that chloroquine may worsen psoriasis symptoms of red, scaly skin patches. • Teach family members to watch for any changes in personality and to notify the healthcare provider should they occur because these drugs can affect the CNS. • Tell patients taking chloroquine who also take either valproic acid or digoxin that they may need more frequent drug levels drawn. Chloroquine decreases valproic acid levels, increasing the risk for seizures, and increases digoxin levels, increasing the risk for digoxin toxicity. • Teach patients taking primaquine to observe for increased fatigue, darkening of the urine, and a feeling of fullness in the stomach area that may indicate an enlarged liver because the drug may impair liver function. If these symptoms occur, the healthcare provider should be notified immediately. • Consult with the healthcare provider and the pharmacist for patients taking other drugs with primaquine because it interacts with many drugs, increasing the risk for life-threatening dysrhythmias.

Anthelmintics: destroy worms by paralyzing the parasite, killing it, and dislocating its adherence to the host site.

DRUG/ADULT DOSAGE RANGE	NURSING IMPLICATIONS
praziquantel (Biltricide) 20–25 mg/kg orally three times daily for 1 or 2 days	• Tell patients to take tablets with food and a full glass of water to minimize stomach upset. • Warn patients to check for yellowing of the eyes, darkening of the urine, or light-colored stools and report these symptoms to their healthcare provider because this drug can damage the liver. • Tell patients with a history of cardiac dysrhythmia to contact their healthcare provider if dizziness or irregular heart rate occur and to call 911 if chest pain occurs, because this drug can cause cardiac dysrhythmias.

- Notify your healthcare provider if expected side effects of nausea, vomiting, diarrhea, or abdominal pain cannot be controlled or worsen.
- When taking metronidazole for trichomoniasis or other sexually transmitted disease, refrain from sexual intercourse until told to do so by your healthcare provider to prevent spreading the infection to others.

ANTHELMINTICS
Action
When a patient has *helminthes* (worms), the infestation is called *helminthiasis*. The condition is usually caused by flatworms, roundworms, tapeworms, and flukes. The worm gains entrance to the body through unclean food or water, unwashed hands, or the skin. Anthelmintic drugs are specific for the worms they can kill, so accurate identification of the worm is necessary. Identification is done by analyzing the stool, urine, blood, sputum, or tissue from the host to look for the larvae or eggs of the parasitic worm.

Uses
Albendazole (Albenza), ivermectin (Stromectol), pyrantel (Reese's pinworm medicine, Walgreen's pinworm medicine), and praziquantel (Biltricide) are examples of anthelmintic drugs that are currently being used. Albendazole (Albenza) is used to treat certain types of tapeworms, flatworms, and roundworms. Albendazole kills the larvae by destroying the cytoplasm of the worm (not the host cells). This disrupts the cellular function necessary for the survival of the worm. Ivermectin (Stromectol) paralyzes certain kinds of roundworms. Praziquantel (Biltricide) kills certain types of flukes and tapeworms by moving calcium into the cell membrane, which causes contraction and paralysis of the worm, dislodging it from the host site and killing it. Pyrantel also causes paralysis of the worm, which dislodges it from the intestines and allows it to be expelled through the stool. It is used for certain types of roundworm infestations (pinworms being a type of roundworm) and is available without a prescription. Table 5.6 provides a summary of anthelmintics.

Expected Side Effects and Adverse Reactions
Nausea, vomiting, headache, abdominal pain, and drowsiness are common with anthelmintic drugs. Praziquantel can worsen symptoms of asthma. The number of side effects increases with higher dosages and longer length of treatment.

Drug Interactions
Anthelmintic drugs work against each other (antagonistic) if they are given together. The drugs also may interfere with a number of specific drugs and a variety of laboratory tests. Consult a drug reference book or a pharmacist for information when other drugs are prescribed during drug therapy for helminthic infestations.

❖ Nursing Implications and Patient Teaching
◆ *Assessment.* Obtain a history and physical examination from the patient, including any history of liver disease or drug allergies. Ask about a history of any foods eaten and how they were prepared that may indicate the source of the infection. Obtain a diet history, height, weight, appetite, and energy level. Other family members may also be infected and require assessment and treatment.

◆ *Planning and implementation.* Severe pruritus (itching) may occur in the treatment of a type of hookworm (cutaneous larva migrans), and the patient may need an anti-inflammatory agent for comfort.

Patients with a recent history of malaria should be treated with an antimalarial agent *before* giving them anthelmintics to prevent a relapse.

Patients may develop allergic reactions to the dead microfilaria and may need treatment for symptoms. Antihistamines or corticosteroids may be necessary to reduce allergic effects.

◆ *Evaluation.* Determine whether the patient is taking prescribed drug as ordered and performing other actions that are prescribed parts of the therapy. Reevaluate weight, energy level, and appetite to evaluate therapeutic results. Collect laboratory specimens after treatment and as ordered to make sure the worms are gone.

◆ *Patient and family teaching.* Stress the following important instructions to the patient and family:
- Take this drug as prescribed. Therapy usually involves an initial treatment that should kill all worms, but in some cases a second course must be taken.
- Report any symptoms that do not disappear after treatment.
- Worms passed in bowel movements are still alive and capable of infecting others. Use good hand washing and cleanliness to avoid transmission to others.
- Some people have diarrhea and abdominal discomfort while taking the drug.
- You may need iron supplements and an iron-rich diet to counteract anemia during hookworm treatment.

Get Ready for the NCLEX® Examination!

Key Points

- Before giving a patient the first dose of a prescribed anti-infective drug, ask the patient about previous allergic reactions to these drugs.
- Give antibiotics on an even schedule around-the-clock to maintain blood drug levels for best effect.
- Stopping antimicrobial therapy after infection symptoms are no longer present but before the prescribed duration is completed leads to increased risk for infection recurrence and for the development of drug-resistant organisms.
- Bactericidal drugs kill the bacteria (think about the word *homicide*).
- Bacteriostatic drugs only limit or slow the growth of bacteria, relying on the patient's immune system to kill the organism.
- Breast-feeding should be avoided during antimicrobial therapy because most of these drugs are excreted into breast milk and the infant (who may not have an infection) will be exposed to the actions, side effects, and adverse effects.
- Patients who are allergic to penicillin are often allergic to the cephalosporins because the chemical structures are similar. Inform the prescriber about a penicillin allergy.
- Instruct patients taking drug therapy for TB not to drink alcohol for the entire duration of the treatment because these drugs are all toxic to the liver and alcohol increases the risk for liver damage.
- Antifungal drugs have many adverse effects; the most common is anemia.
- Azoles should not be given with grapefruit juice, and grapefruit juice should be limited to less than 24 ounces a day because this food increases the blood level of the drugs, which can lead to adverse reactions.
- Amphotericin B has numerous expected side effects, and patients must be premedicated with antihistamines, antipyretics, corticosteroids, and opiates to maintain comfort and prevent adverse effects.
- Superinfections can result from giving antifungals and corticosteroids together.
- Rash, flu symptoms, and blisters can indicate severe reactions to antifungals and are considered a medical emergency.
- Advise patient to take antiparasitics with or after meals and with a full glass of water to decrease the chances of stomach upset.
- Patients who are taking metronidazole for trichomoniasis or other sexually transmitted disease need to refrain from sexual intercourse until told to do so by the healthcare provider to prevent transmitting the infection to others.
- Worms passed in bowel movements are still alive and capable of infecting others. Teach the patient the importance of good hand washing and cleanliness to avoid transmission.

Review Questions for the NCLEX® Examination

1. How are bactericidal drugs different from bacteriostatic drugs?
   1. Bacteriostatic drugs are more likely to cause an allergic response than bactericidal drugs.
   2. Bacteriostatic drugs work only against bacteria, whereas bactericidal drugs are effective against other types of organisms.
   3. Bactericidal drug actions actually result in the killing of the bacteria, whereas bacteriostatic drugs only slow bacterial growth.
   4. Bactericidal drugs require assistance from the patient's immune system to be effective, whereas bacteriostatic drugs are effective even when function is poor.

2. The patient receiving antibiotics for 3 days reports a skin rash over the chest, back, and arms. What is the nurse's first action?
   1. Ask the patient whether he or she has ever developed a rash while taking another drug.
   2. Reassure the patient that many people have this expected reaction to antibiotic therapy.
   3. Ask the patient whether the rash itches, burns, or causes other types of discomfort.
   4. Document the report as the only action.

3. Which drug categories work by interfering with bacterial cell wall synthesis and maintenance? (Select all that apply.)
   1. Aminoglycosides
   2. Carbapenems
   3. Cephalosporins
   4. Macrolides
   5. Penicillins
   6. Sulfonamides
   7. Tetracyclines
   8. Vancomycin

4. Which administration technique does the nurse teach the family of a patient with memory problems for best adherence to first-line drug therapy for tuberculosis?
   1. Having one family member responsible for giving the drugs and watching the patient swallow them
   2. Setting up the patient's drugs using a daily pill dispenser that has separate slots for each individual drug
   3. Asking the patient every night whether he or she has remembered to take all the drug doses that day
   4. Crushing all the drugs together and placing them in the patient's coffee so that he or she is unaware of taking them

Get Ready for the NCLEX® Examination!—cont'd

5. Which precautions are important to teach a woman using a vaginal cream form of an antifungal drug? (Select all that apply.)
   1. Wear gloves to insert the cream.
   2. Wash the applicator with soap and water.
   3. Do not take baths until treatment is completed.
   4. Avoid sexual intercourse during the treatment period.
   5. The cream can make holes in a condom or diaphragm.
   6. Stop the drug immediately if you think you are pregnant.
   7. Stop the drug when symptoms have disappeared to avoid unnecessary exposure to it.

6. A patient has been given a prescription for doxycycline (Vibramycin). Which patient teaching points are important to tell the patient about doxycycline? (Select all that apply.)
   1. This drug should be taken 1 hour before or 2 hours after a meal.
   2. Doxycycline should not be taken with dairy products to avoid absorption issues.
   3. Wear protective clothing and sunscreen while on doxycycline or a severe sunburn can result.
   4. Numbness and tingling of the hands and feet can be prevented by taking a B-complex vitamin pill every day.
   5. Orange-colored urine is common when taking this drug and is not an important problem.

7. A patient calls the clinic and states that her right arm below the elbow is reddened and painful since being prescribed ciprofloxacin (Cipro) for a urinary tract infection. What is your best action?
   1. Tell the patient to stop taking the drug for now and that you will notify the healthcare provider for further instructions.
   2. Tell the patient that this is an expected side effect and to take acetaminophen for discomfort.
   3. Tell the patient to take the drug with a full glass of water to alleviate this expected side effect.
   4. Tell the patient to limit the use of her right arm and to wear a wrist splint.

8. Which drugs are used for first-line treatment of tuberculosis? (Select all that apply.)
   1. Vancomycin (Vancocin)
   2. Linezolid (Zyvox)
   3. Isoniazid (INH)
   4. Metronidazole (Flagyl)
   5. Rifampin
   6. Fluconazole (Diflucan)
   7. Pyrazinamide
   8. Ethambutol (Myambutol)

9. The patient has been prescribed vancomycin and is also receiving gentamycin. Which assessment status is most important when monitoring this patient?
   1. Mental status
   2. Visual acuity
   3. Urine output
   4. Energy level

10. The order reads: "Kefzol 400 mg IM every 6 hours."
    Reconstitution directions: Add 2 mL of 0.9% normal saline to a vial of Kefzol 500 mg to yield a total volume of 2.2 mL.
    How many mL should be given with each dose? (Round to the nearest tenth.)

Case Study

Bill Ellington, 64 years old, comes into the clinic with a temperature of 104°F. He is sweating profusely, feels nauseated, and says that he feels "horrible." He reports he has never felt this way before. He sits in the chair but twists and turns, rubbing his lower back as he talks. A urine specimen is positive for RBCs and protein, and a microscopic specimen shows bacteria and urinary casts. The nurse practitioner confirms that he has a urinary tract infection.

1. What antibiotics are used primarily for urinary tract infections and why?
2. What instructions would you give the patient if the nurse practitioner started the patient on Bactrim?
3. How would your nursing interventions and precautions need to change if Mr. Ellington has diabetes?
4. What other laboratory work besides a urinalysis might the healthcare provider order?
5. What other problems might Mr. Ellington experience?

Antivirals and Antiretrovirals

http://evolve.elsevier.com/Visovsky/LPNpharmacology/

Learning Outcomes

1. Describe the pathophysiology of viruses and retroviruses, and how they cause infections.
2. List the names, actions, possible side effects, and adverse effects of common antiviral drugs for herpes simplex viral infections and influenza infections.
3. Explain what to teach patients and families about the common antiviral drugs for herpes simplex viral infections and influenza.
4. List the names, actions, possible side effects, and adverse effects of antiviral drugs for cytomegalovirus and respiratory syncytial virus.
5. Explain what to teach patients and families about antiviral drugs for cytomegalovirus and respiratory syncytial virus.
6. List the names, actions, possible side effects, and adverse effects of antiviral drugs for hepatitis B and C.
7. Explain what to teach patients and families about antiviral drugs for hepatitis B and C.
8. List the names, actions, possible side effects, and adverse effects of the common reverse transcriptase inhibitors and protease inhibitors.
9. Explain what to teach patients and families about reverse transcriptase inhibitors and protease inhibitors.
10. List the names, actions, possible side effects, and adverse effects of the common entry inhibitors, fusion inhibitors, and integrase inhibitors.
11. Explain what to teach patients and families about entry inhibitors, fusion inhibitors, and integrase inhibitors.

Key Terms

AIDS (p. 98) The later stage of HIV disease that causes a breakdown in the immune system, leaving the patient unable to fight infection.

antiretroviral (ăn-tī-RĚT-rō-vī-răls, p. 99) Drugs that are a subset of antiviral drugs and specifically suppress the reproduction of retroviruses.

antiviral (ăn-tē-VĪ-răl, p. 94) Drugs capable of interfering with the ability of the virus to carry out its reproductive functions.

cART (p. 99) A combination of antiretroviral drugs that must be taken every day to combat the progression of HIV disease from becoming AIDS or to prevent HIV infection after exposure.

entry inhibitor (ĚN-trē ĭn-HĬ-bă-těr, p. 102) Antiretroviral drugs that *prevent* cellular infection with HIV by blocking the *CCR5* receptor on CD4+ T cells.

fusion inhibitor (FYŪ-zhŏn ĭn-HĬ-bă-těr, p. 102) Antiretroviral drugs that prevent cellular infection with HIV by blocking the ability of HIV's surface protein *gp41* to fuse with the host cell's CD4 receptor.

HIV (p. 98) The specific retrovirus responsible for the immune system problems associated with desruction of helper T cells (CD4 cells) when the infection results in HIV disease and progresses to AIDS.

integrase inhibitor (ĭn-TĚ-grās ĭn-HĬ-bă-těr, p. 102) Antiretroviral drugs that inhibit the HIV enzyme *integrase*, which the virus uses to insert the viral DNA into the host cell's human DNA.

non-nucleoside reverse transcriptase inhibitor (NNRTI) (nŏn-NŪ-klē-ă-sīd rĭ-VĚRS trăn-SKRĬP-ˌtās ĭn-HĬ-bă-těr, p. 99) Antiretroviral drugs that work by binding directly to the HIV-1 enzyme *reverse transcriptase,* preventing viral cell DNA replication, RNA replication, and protein synthesis.

nucleoside reverse transcriptase inhibitor (NRTI) (NŪ-klē-ă-tīd rĭ-VĚRS trăn-SKRĬP-ˌtās ĭn-HĬ-bă-těr, p. 96) Antiretroviral drugs that have a similar structure to the four nucleoside bases of DNA, making them "counterfeit" bases. When these counterfeit bases are used by the HIV enzyme *reverse transcriptase*, viral DNA synthesis and reproduction are suppressed.

opportunistic infection (p. 98) A virus, bacteria, protozoa, or fungi that takes the "opportunity" to cause an infection in an immunocompromised host.

protease inhibitor (PI) (PRŌ-tē-āz ĭn-HĬ-bă-těr, p. 99) Antiretroviral drugs that suppress the formation of infectious virions by inhibiting the retroviral protease enzyme.

retrovirus (RĚT-rō-vī-rŭs, p. 98) Viral organisms that carry special enzymes (reverse transcriptase, integrase, and protease) with them and use RNA (ribonucleic acid) instead of DNA as their genes to reproduce.

virion (VĪ-rē-ŭnz, p. 94) New viral particles reproduced in cells infected with retroviruses that can leave the cell and infect more human body cells.

virus (VĪ-rŭs, p. 94) A small infectious agent that can reproduce only inside other living cells, including human cells.

VIRUS

A **virus** is a small infectious agent that can reproduce only inside other living cells of a host organism, including human cells. Viruses consist of RNA or DNA genetic material and are surrounded by a protein or fatty (or combination) coating, known as a *capsid*. The virus inserts its own genetic information into the host cell's nucleus and hijacks the cell's function. This causes the host cell to produce and release more virus particles (**virions**), so the infection spreads. Damage, breakdown, and eventual death of the infected cell itself also occur with a viral infection. Viruses cannot survive or reproduce without the host. Viral infections are not killed or suppressed by antibiotics. Drugs that are capable of interfering with the ability of the virus to carry out its reproductive functions are called **antivirals**.

ANTIVIRALS

Antiviral drugs are used to treat a variety of common conditions caused by different viruses. These include viruses that cause herpes zoster, herpes simplex, genital herpes, varicella, some influenza infections, and hepatitis B and C.

Antiviral drugs must enter the infected cell and act at the site of infection to be effective. Antivirals do not kill the virus but rather stop viral reproduction. This action means that all antivirals are only virustatic, not virucidal. The antiviral drugs work in a variety of ways: by blocking the virus from entering the host cell, by targeting the enzymes and proteins inside the host cell that allow the viruses to replicate and leave the infected cell to then find new cells to infect, or by helping the host's immune system fight the viral infection.

ANTIVIRAL DRUGS FOR HERPES SIMPLEX VIRUS INFECTIONS

Herpes simplex virus type 1 (HSV-1) is the virus responsible for common "cold sores" of the mouth. This infection can become widespread in newborns and in anyone whose immune system is not functioning well. Herpes simplex virus type 2 (HSV-2) is the virus responsible for genital herpes infections and lesions. Just like all other viruses, once a person is infected, the viruses are always present in some tissues. However, actual symptoms come and go in patterns called *outbreaks*. An infected person is more likely to spread the virus to other people just before symptoms are present and during actual outbreaks. Outbreaks are uncomfortable and have other consequences; therefore the goal of HSV antiviral therapy is to prevent outbreaks (or at least reduce the frequency and intensity of symptoms), which also helps reduce spread of the disease.

Actions

The common antiviral drugs for HSV are acyclovir (Zovirax), famciclovir (Famvir), and valacyclovir (Valtrex) (Table 6.1). They are viral DNA polymerase inhibitors that work to reduce viral reproduction by forming "counterfeit" molecules that block the virus and its enzymes from making more genetic material and virions in an infected host cell. Without the genetic material, the virus cannot reproduce.

Uses

Drugs in this class are most often used to prevent and control HSV infections. However, although chicken pox and shingles are caused by a different virus (the varicella zoster virus [VZV]), these drugs can help to control the symptoms of VZV infections. This is because VZV and HSV are very similar and have similar enzymes.

ANTIVIRAL DRUGS FOR INFLUENZA

Actions

For influenza viruses to infect cells, they must first open their outer coats to be able to fuse with the host's cell membranes. In addition most viruses that cause common influenza (flu) use a special viral enzyme on their surfaces known as neuraminidase to help cause the infection. This enzyme helps the virus burrow its way into cells that line the respiratory tract. The enzyme also helps new viral particles (virions) made in the infected cells leave the infected cell to spread throughout the respiratory system and infect more cells. So the two types of drugs to treat for influenza are the neuraminidase inhibitors oseltamivir (Tamiflu) and zanamivir (Relenza), and drugs that prevent the virus from opening the outer coat are amantadine (Symmetrel) and rimantadine (Flumadine) (see Table 6.1).

Uses

All of the antiviral drugs for influenza are used either to prevent an infection in a patient who has been exposed to the virus or to reduce the symptoms of an existing influenza infection. They work best when given after exposure and before symptoms start or within 48 hours of the onset of symptoms. Those that prevent viral uncoating are most effective against influenza A, and the neuraminidase inhibitors are most effective against influenza B. They are used for short-term therapy, usually 2 to 4 days. Unfortunately many strains of influenza are becoming resistant to these drugs.

ANTIVIRAL DRUGS FOR CYTOMEGALOVIRUS AND RESPIRATORY SYNCYTIAL VIRUS

Cytomegalovirus (CMV) is a virus from the herpes family that can infect human cells. In people who have a fully functioning immune system, CMV infection causes few problems and may even go unnoticed. However, in the person whose immune system is not functioning well, such as people with AIDS, newborns, and people who are immunosuppressed from chemotherapy, CMV infection can cause serious problems such as brain infection (encephalitis), which can lead to brain

📋 Table 6.1 **Antiviral Drugs for Influenza and Herpes Simplex Virus**

Neuraminidase inhibitors: prevent influenza spread and reduce the symptoms of influenza by suppressing the viral neuraminidase enzyme. As a result, the influenza virus cannot enter uninfected cells and the virions in infected cells are not released for further spread.

DRUG/ADULT DOSAGE RANGE	NURSING IMPLICATIONS
oseltamivir (Tamiflu) 75 mg orally twice daily for 5 days zanamivir (Relenza): 2 oral inhalations of a 5 mg blister Diskhaler (total of 10 mg) twice daily for 5 days with an active influenza infection or for 10 days for uninfected adults in the same household with an infected person	• Before giving zanamivir, ask patients whether they have asthma because this orally inhaled drug can cause bronchospasms. • Before giving zanamivir, ask patients whether they have a true milk allergy because this is a contraindication to zanamivir therapy because there is cross-reactivity of the antibodies. • Observe patients for confusion, hallucinations, nightmares, and depression because these drugs cross the blood–brain barrier and can cause central nervous system (CNS) side effects.

Uncoating inhibitors: prevent initial influenza infection and spread of influenza infection by interfering with viral uncoating, which is needed for viral fusion with host cells, the first step of cellular infection.

DRUG/ADULT DOSAGE RANGE	NURSING IMPLICATIONS
amantadine (Symmetrel) 200 mg orally once daily or 100 mg orally twice daily within 24–48 hours of the onset of symptoms until symptoms are gone rimantadine (Flumadine) 100 mg orally once daily within 24–48 hours of symptom onset for 5–7 days	• Before giving either of these drugs, ask the patient about all other drugs he or she takes and check with a pharmacist because of the numerous possible drug interactions. • Observe patients for confusion, hallucinations, nightmares, and depression because these drugs cross the blood–brain barrier and can cause CNS side effects. • Warn patients to change positions slowly because these drugs can cause orthostatic hypotension.

Viral DNA polymerase inhibitors: work to reduce viral reproduction by forming "counterfeit" molecules that block the virus and its enzymes from making more genetic material and virions in an infected host cell.

DRUG/ADULT DOSAGE RANGE	NURSING IMPLICATIONS
acyclovir (Zovirax) 5 mg/kg intravenously for 7 days initially; 400 mg orally twice daily to decrease frequency of outbreaks famciclovir (Famvir) 1 g orally twice daily for the first day of an outbreak, followed by 500 mg orally twice daily for 7 days (HSV-2) penciclovir (Denavir): apply 1% cream every 2 hours while awake for 4 days when lesions appear valacyclovir (Valtrex) 1 g orally twice daily for 10 days at first sign of outbreak; 500 mg orally once daily continually to prevent a person with herpes from spreading it to an uninfected sexual partner	• Before giving any of these drugs, ask the patient about all other drugs he or she takes and check with a pharmacist because of the numerous possible drug interactions. • Assess urine output and teach patients to stay hydrated because these drugs can damage the kidneys. • Assess patients for fatigue and excessive bruising because these drugs decrease bone marrow production of red blood cells and platelets. • For patients taking acyclovir or famciclovir, assess for yellowing of the skin and sclera, and elevated liver enzymes because these drugs are liver toxic. • Tell families to watch for confusion or behavior changes because the systemic drugs can affect the CNS. • Warn patients that the skin may become red where the topical cream is applied to reduce their anxiety when the symptom appears. • Warn patients that excessive use of the topical cream can cause systemic side effects and adverse effects because of skin absorption of the drug. • Before giving acyclovir, ask patients whether they have a true milk allergy because this is a contraindication to acyclovir therapy because there is cross-reactivity of the antibodies.

damage and death, and serious eye infections (retinitis) that can lead to blindness.

Respiratory syncytial virus (RSV) is a common respiratory virus that infects the lungs and the bronchial tubes. It is a very common cause of chest colds, croup, and even pneumonia in children. For healthy people who have good immune function, the diseases it causes are mild, and most people recover in 5 to 7 days without treatment. However, in premature infants, newborns, small children who have chronic illnesses, and older adults with weakened immune systems, the respiratory infection can be severe and lead to death.

Actions and Uses

Drugs to treat CMV come from the viral DNA polymerase inhibitor class. These drugs inhibit the viral enzyme's need to make more DNA for viral reproduction. As a result, fewer virions are made and the infection

Table 6.2   Antiviral Drugs for Cytomegalovirus and Respiratory Syncytial Virus

Anticytomegalovirus drugs/DNA polymerase inhibitors: These drugs inhibit the viral form of the enzyme needed to make DNA for viral replication. As a result, fewer virions are made and the symptoms of the acute infection are stopped.

DRUG/ADULT DOSAGE RANGE	NURSING IMPLICATIONS
cidofovir (Vistide) 5 mg/kg intravenously once weekly for 2 weeks foscarnet (Foscavir) 40 mg/kg intravenously every 8–12 hours for 14–21 days	• Do not mix these drugs with other drugs because they are incompatible with most other drugs. • Be sure the patient receives adequate hydration during therapy because these drugs are very toxic to the kidneys. • Should not be used in women who are pregnant unless the infection is life-threatening because the risk for birth defects is high. • Ask patients whether they have a seizure disorder because these drugs increase the likelihood for seizures. • Assess patients frequently for signs of infection because bone marrow production of white blood cells is suppressed, increasing the risk for infections. • Give drugs by slow infusion to reduce the risk for immediate adverse reactions. • Frequently assess the patient's red blood cell counts because these drugs suppress the bone marrow and can cause severe anemia. • Assess the patient's heart rate, rhythm, and respiratory system frequently because these drugs can cause heart and respiratory adverse events. • Use gloves and masks when giving these drugs because they are both classified as "hazardous drugs" and precautions are needed to avoid exposure of these drugs to anyone except the patient. • For patients receiving foscarnet, check their serum electrolytes whenever they are drawn because this drug causes many electrolyte imbalances. • Before giving cidofovir, ask about allergies to sulfonamides or probenecid because cross-reactivity can result in a similar cidofovir allergic reaction.

Drugs for RSV: The only drug in this class is ribavirin, which directly damages genetic material, both RNA and DNA, and causes cell mutations. The mutated virions are unable to reproduce.

DRUG/ADULT DOSAGE RANGE	NURSING IMPLICATIONS

ribavirin (Virazole) aerosol or nasal inhalant of 190 mcg/L air or oxygen (for children and adults) 600 mg orally twice daily for adults receiving therapy for hepatitis C	• Avoid all contact with this drug because it is very hazardous. Use these precautions when giving the aerosol form:
	  • Wear gloves, a mask, and a gown during administration.
	  • Close the door to the patient's room to prevent the drug from entering the hallway and endangering others.
	  • If you are pregnant, ***do not give*** this drug because it can cause severe birth defects or fetal death.
	• Assess the patient's red blood cell counts frequently because these drugs suppress the bone marrow and can cause severe anemia.
	• Assess patients frequently for signs of infection because bone marrow production of white blood cells is suppressed, increasing the risk for infections.

symptoms subside. The drugs used for this purpose are cidofovir (Vistide) and foscarnet (Foscavir) (Table 6.2). They are both extremely toxic, are given intravenously, and are used on a short-term basis to reduce infection symptoms.

The only drug approved for RSV treatment is ribavirin (Virazole). It is also very toxic, even when given in aerosol form, and requires careful handling (see Table 6.2). It also has some efficacy for treating hepatitis C virus (HCV). For treating RSV, it is used only short-term as an aerosol. For hepatitis C, it is taken orally along with other drugs for years.

ANTIVIRAL DRUGS FOR HEPATITIS B AND HEPATITIS C VIRUSES

Hepatitis B virus (HBV) and HCV are both hardy viruses that can live in a variety of environments. In the United States and Canada the most common ways these viruses cause infection are by the blood-borne route and by sexual transmission. Both have a long incubation period (2–26 weeks) after infection followed by first an acute illness and then often a chronic illness. The acute phase of HBV may result in a noticeable illness in about 30% of infected people. For others the acute phase is so mild that there may be no obvious symptoms. For HCV, few infected individuals have any symptoms during the acute phase. With both HBV and HCV, active virus remains in the blood forever. Some people with HBV have chronic recurrence of symptoms from time to time. With HCV, the disease remains dormant for years (although it can be transmitted) and then causes profound liver damage with cirrhosis.

The major drugs used to treat HBV fall into three classes: the **nucleoside reverse transcriptase inhibitors**

Table 6.3 Drugs for Hepatitis B and Hepatitis C

DNA polymerase inhibitors: These drugs inhibit the viral form of the enzyme needed to make DNA for viral replication. As a result, fewer virions are made and blood levels of the virus decline.

DRUG/ADULT DOSAGE RANGE	NURSING IMPLICATIONS
adefovir (Hepsera) 10 mg orally once daily entecavir (Baraclude) 1 mg orally once daily telbivudine (Tyzeka) 600 mg orally once daily	• Assess patients for yellowing of the skin and sclera, and elevated liver enzymes because these drugs are toxic to the liver. • Assess patients for nausea, vomiting, and severe epigastric pain because these drugs increase the risk for pancreatitis. • Ask patients taking adefovir about bone pain because it can cause bone thinning and increased risk for fractures. • Give entecavir on an empty stomach because stomach contents interfere with its absorption.

Protease inhibitors: These drugs competitively block the viral protease enzyme, preventing viral replication and release of viral particles.

DRUG/ADULT DOSAGE RANGE	NURSING IMPLICATIONS
simeprevir (Olysio) 150 mg orally daily along with other antiviral drugs	• Assess patients for yellowing of the skin and sclera, and elevated liver enzymes because this drug is toxic to the liver. • Teach patients to protect themselves from the sun with clothing, hats, and sunscreen because this drug increases sun sensitivity and can result in severe sunburn. • Teach patients to take this drug with food to prevent GI side effects.

Combination agent: This drug, now reported to "cure" hepatitis C, is a combination antiviral agent containing the viral protein inhibitor ledipasvir and the viral DNA polymerase inhibitor sofosbuvir.

DRUG/ADULT DOSAGE RANGE	NURSING IMPLICATIONS
ledipasvir 90 mg/sofosbuvir 400 mg (HARVONI): 1 tablet orally daily for 8–12 weeks	• Assess patients for yellowing of the skin and sclera, and elevated liver enzymes because this drug is toxic to the liver. • Ask the patient and family about any changes in mood or increase in depression because a higher incidence of suicide ideation has been seen with this drug.

(NRTIs), the DNA polymerase inhibitors, and interferon. The NRTI drug is lamivudine. This is the same class of drugs used as part of treatment for HIV infection and AIDS (see the Antiretrovirals section later in this chapter for the actions and nursing implications of this drug). This oral drug works in the same way against HBV (although it is not a true retrovirus), at a lower dosage than what is needed for HIV infection. The DNA polymerase inhibitors are adefovir (Hepsera), entecavir (Baraclude), lamivudine (Epivir), and telbivudine (Tyzeka). This is the same class of drugs used to treat CMV infection, but these are oral drugs given once daily long term (Table 6.3). Interferon, specifically interferon alfa-2b (Intron A), is a synthetic injected drug similar to the interferon the human body makes to fight viral infections. Chapter 14 describes the mechanism of action, drug dosages, and nursing implications for interferon therapy.

General antiviral drugs used to treat HCV include ribavirin (Virazole) (discussed earlier in this chapter) and interferon alfa-2b (discussed in Chapter 14). Additional drugs are listed in Table 6.3. Of note is a new drug, Harvoni, which suppressed HCV replication and presence in the blood to such an extent that it is thought to result in a "cure." However, the extreme cost of this drug for 12 weeks of treatment (about $96,000 in 2016 prohibits many patients from using it and thus they continue with more standard therapy.

General Antiviral Expected Side Effects, Adverse Reactions, and Drug Interactions

Expected side effects to antivirals include vomiting, nausea, diarrhea, and headache. Adverse reactions are reported for some antivirals, and you should read current information before giving these drugs. Tables 6.1 through 6.3 provide specific adverse reactions and nursing implications for antiviral drugs. All drugs can cause hypersensitivity and/or anaphylactic shock. Always be aware of rashes, hives, difficulty breathing, and facial swelling. If hypersensitivity reactions occur, then the drug should be discontinued and the prescriber made aware. If an anaphylactic event occurs as indicated by difficulty breathing, swelling of the mouth and tongue, and unstable vital signs, emergency measures must be taken immediately.

Many antivirals also have drug interactions. As antivirals become more widely used these interactions may increase. Again, to be prudent, always look up current information. Some antivirals can be applied topically and as such do not have systemic interactions as they would if they were taken orally or by injection.

❖ Nursing Implications and Patient Teaching

Table 6.1 gives an overview of antivirals currently used to treat herpes infections and influenza infection or influenza prophylaxis. You may also notice that the antivirals have a common suffix of either -vir or -dine.

Table 6.2 gives an overview of some very toxic intravenous antivirals used for the more serious problems of CMV retinitis and RSV. You may not be giving these drugs, but you may be responsible for caring for these patients. All of these drugs carry serious warnings for patients and black box warnings for healthcare providers, so caution should be taken.

Top Tip For Safety

Only two antivirals are used in treating or preventing influenza in children: oseltamivir phosphate (Tamiflu) and zanamivir (Relenza).

◆ *Patient and family teaching.* Tell the patient and family the following:

- When using topical drugs for treatment of HSV-1 (cold sores) or HSV-2 (genital herpes), use gloves and wash your hands thoroughly so the infection does not spread.
- There is no cure for herpes. Antivirals can only treat herpes prophylactically or symptomatically.
- To be effective, oral drugs should be started at the first sign of infection or reinfection.
- The drugs must be used daily for suppression of the herpes virus.
- When using antivirals for flu, it is best to begin usage within 2 days of being sick; however, starting them later may still be helpful in preventing serious flu symptoms.
- Antivirals will not cure the flu, so there is still a need to reduce symptoms such as fever, cough, and pain.
- Check yourself daily for worsening symptoms that may indicate pneumonia or bacterial infection. If these are present, notify your healthcare provider immediately so that antibiotics can be started instead of antivirals.
- Antivirals can also be used for prevention or prophylaxis of the flu in unvaccinated persons who have been exposed to the disease. Prevention works best if these drugs are taken before flu symptoms are present or within the first 24 to 48 hours after they appear.
- Follow the specific storage instructions listed on the package for the drug.

RETROVIRUS

Retroviruses are organisms that differ from viruses in that instead of merely hijacking a cell's DNA or RNA to reproduce, they transmit their own information into the cell's DNA. Normally, cellular DNA is unzipped by an enzyme called *transcriptionase* and then transmitted by RNA to the ribosome, where protein synthesis takes place. Protein is the building block of all tissue and needs the DNA information to form. **Retroviruses** carry special enzymes (reverse transcriptase, integrase, and protease) with them and use RNA instead of DNA as their genes. The retrovirus inserts its own genetic material into the host cell DNA from its RNA. In this way the retrovirus can expand and multiply all the while using the host cell's metabolic systems to make *virions* (new viral particles) that can leave the cell and infect more cells.

HIV is the retrovirus responsible for the immune system problems when infection with this organism results in HIV disease and progresses to **AIDS.** Once a person has become infected with HIV, he or she will have the virus for life. HIV attacks the body's CD4 or helper T cells that are responsible for helping the immune system fight infections. If HIV is left untreated, the decreased number of CD4 cells in the body makes the person highly susceptible to infections such as tuberculosis, viruses such as CMV, and cancers such as non-Hodgkin lymphoma. These **opportunistic infections** signal that AIDS has developed in the person. AIDS is the later stage of HIV disease that causes a breakdown in the immune system, leaving the patient unable to fight any infection.

In the United States the groups at highest risk for development of AIDS include homosexual and bisexual men, although the fastest growing group to develop AIDS is minority heterosexual women. When compared with other racial and ethnic groups, HIV mostly affects African American and Hispanic individuals. Transgender women who have sex with men are among the groups at highest risk for HIV infection. Intravenous drug users remain at significant risk for acquiring HIV. Other groups at high risk are children born to HIV-positive women and individuals whose sexual partners have HIV/AIDS. According to the Centers for Disease Control and Prevention, in 2013 people 55 years and older accounted for 26% of all Americans living with diagnosed or undiagnosed HIV infection. Appropriate treatment with combined antiretroviral drugs has prolonged the lives of patients with HIV/AIDS for as much as 35 years.

The HIV life cycle occurs in seven steps, and the HIV drugs are designed to attack the virus at different steps. The steps in the HIV life cycle and where each category of HIV drug works are presented in the following list and shown in Fig. 6.1.

1. Attachment: The HIV binds or attaches to the outside of the CD4 (T helper) cell. Entry inhibitors work here to prevent the attachment.
2. Fusion: The HIV and the CD4 cell become locked or fused together and the HIV enters the cell. Fusion inhibitors work here to prevent the fusion.
3. Reverse transcriptionase: Inside the cell the reverse transcriptionase enzyme made by the HIV converts the HIV RNA into the DNA of the cell nucleus. This is where NRTIs and NNRTs work to prevent the transfer from occurring.
4. Integration: Inside the nucleus of the CD4 cell the HIV releases another enzyme integrase that places the viral DNA into the CD4 cell DNA. This is where

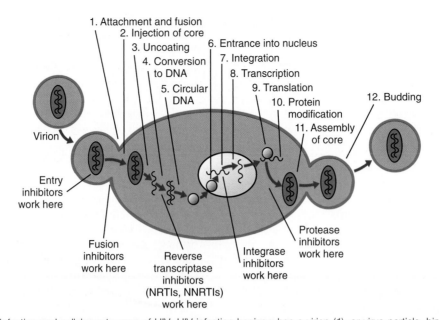

FIG. 6.1 Infection and cellular outcomes of HIV. HIV infection begins when a virion (*1*), or virus particle, binds to the outside of a susceptible cell and fuses with it (*2*), injecting the core proteins and two strands of viral RNA (*3*). Uncoating occurs, during which the core proteins are removed and the viral RNA is released into the infected cell's cytoplasm. The double-stranded DNA (*4*), or provirus, migrates to the nucleus, uncoats itself (*5*), and is integrated into the cell's own DNA (*6*). The provirus then can do a couple of things: remain latent (*7A*) or activate cellular mechanisms to copy its genes into RNA (*7B*), some of which is translated into virus proteins or ribosomes. The proteins and additional RNA are then assembled into new virions that bud from the cell. The process can take place slowly, sparing the host cell (*7B*), or so rapidly that the cell is lysed or ruptured (*7C*). (From Workman ML, LaCharity LA: *Understanding pharmacology*, ed 2, St. Louis, 2016, Elsevier.)

integrase inhibitors work to prevent the release of the enzyme integrase.

5. Replication: The HIV has completely changed the CD4 cell DNA and the RNA messenger. Now the CD4 cell starts to make long HIV protein chains that will later break up into smaller chains and begin to infect other cells.

6. Assembly: All of the new long HIV chains move under the surface of the CD4 cell and assemble. They are not infective yet.

7. Budding: The HIV chains burst out of the cell and release an enzyme protease, which breaks up the long chain into small buds of protein particles that are now free to infect more CD4 cells. This is where the **protease inhibitors (PIs)** work to prevent the release of protease.

ANTIRETROVIRALS

Antiretrovirals are an important group of drugs that slow the growth or prevent the duplication of retroviruses. They are used to limit or slow the advance of HIV and its progression to AIDS. Antiretroviral drugs are used in treating the patient infected with HIV or for adults and children at risk for acquiring HIV and AIDS. They do not cure HIV or AIDS, but they do help patients live healthier, longer lives by acting to interfere with the ability of the retrovirus to replicate (reproduce) and slowing the production of new retroviruses. All

antiretroviral drugs are virustatic rather than virucidal. *None of these drugs kill the virus.*

Drug therapy for HIV infection and AIDS works best when several different types of antiretroviral drugs are used together daily. This therapy is known as combination antiretroviral therapy (**cART**). The six categories of antiretroviral therapy drugs are NRTIs, **non-nucleoside reverse transcriptase inhibitors (NNRTIs)**, PIs, integrase inhibitors, fusion inhibitors, and entry inhibitors. They are all called *inhibitors* because, rather than killing the virus, they suppress retroviral reproduction either by preventing HIV from infecting host cells or by inhibiting different steps in the HIV life cycle. None of these drugs are useful or effective against HIV when used alone. Table 6.4 lists the common drugs in each category and their nursing implications. Fig. 6.1 shows where in the HIV infection process and life cycle different categories of antiretroviral drugs inhibit retroviral reproduction. These drugs are used only for the management of HIV disease.

Although cART is usually started and managed by healthcare providers in special settings and clinics for immune disorders, this drug therapy must continue for the rest of the patient's life. Therapy is effective only if the patient takes the prescribed drugs correctly and on time at least 90% of the time. So people who are HIV-positive and taking cART may be a patient or resident in any healthcare setting. Regardless of the setting, they must continue the prescribed therapy.

Table 6.4 **Examples of Antiretroviral Drug Therapy for HIV Infection**

Nucleoside reverse transcriptase inhibitors (NRTIs): These drugs have a similar structure to the four nucleoside bases of DNA, making them "counterfeit" bases. They fool the HIV enzyme *reverse transcriptase* into using these counterfeit bases so that viral DNA synthesis and replication are suppressed. All NRTIs are oral drugs.

DRUG/ADULT DOSAGES RANGE	NURSING IMPLICATIONS
abacavir (Ziagen) 300 mg orally twice daily *or* 600 mg orally once daily didanosine (Videx EC) 125–200 mg orally twice daily emtricitabine (Emtriva) 200 mg orally once daily lamivudine (Epivir) 300 mg orally once daily stavudine (Zerit) 40 mg orally twice daily tenofovir (Viread) 300 mg orally once daily zidovudine (Retrovir) 300 mg orally twice daily	• Remind patients to avoid fatty and fried foods with these drugs because they cause digestive upsets and may lead to pancreatitis when combined with NRTIs. • Teach patients to use precautions to prevent injury because these drugs induce peripheral neuropathy. • Teach patients taking abacavir to report flu-like symptoms to the provider immediately because these symptoms may indicate a hypersensitivity reaction that requires discontinuing the drug. • Instruct patients to avoid or severely limit alcoholic beverages to reduce the risk for liver damage while on these drugs. • Do not give abacavir to patients who test positive for the HLA-B 5701 tissue type because fatal allergic responses are likely. • Tell patients that the solution form and capsule form of emtricitabine (Emtriva) are not interchangeable on a mg per mg basis

Non-nucleoside reverse transcriptase inhibitors (NNRTIs): These drugs work by binding directly to the HIV-1 enzyme *reverse transcriptase*, preventing viral cell DNA replication, RNA replication, and protein synthesis. This action suppresses viral replication of the HIV-1 virus but does not affect HIV-2 viral replication. All NNRTIs are oral drugs.

DRUG/ADULT DOSAGE RANGE	NURSING IMPLICATIONS
delavirdine (Rescriptor) 400 mg orally three times daily efavirenz (Sustiva) 600 mg orally once daily at bedtime etravirine (Intelence) 200 mg orally twice daily rilpivirine (EDURANT) 25 mg once daily with a meal	• Check laboratory values for increases in liver enzymes and decreased red blood cells because the most common side effects are anemia and liver toxicity. • Teach patients to take these drugs at least 1 hour before or 2 hours after taking an antacid to avoid inhibiting GI absorption. • Instruct patients to notify the prescriber if a sore throat, fever, different types of rashes, blisters, or multiple bruises develop because these are indications of a serious adverse drug effect. • Do not give delavirdine or efavirenz to pregnant women because these two drugs have the potential to cause birth defects and developmental problems.

Protease inhibitors (PIs): These drugs competitively block the HIV protease enzyme, preventing viral replication and release of viral particles. The HIV initially produces all of its proteins in one long strand, which must be broken down into separate smaller proteins by HIV protease to be active. Thus, when inhibited, viral proteins are not functional and viral particles cannot leave the cell to infect other cells. All PIs are oral drugs.

DRUG/ADULT DOSAGE RANGE	NURSING IMPLICATIONS
atazanavir (Reyataz) 300 mg orally daily darunavir (Prezista) 800 mg orally twice daily fosamprenavir (Lexiva) 700 mg orally twice daily indinavir (Chemet, Crixivan) 800 mg orally every 8 hours lopinavir/ritonavir (Kaletra) 400 mg/100 mg orally twice daily nelfinavir (Viracept) 1250 mg orally twice daily with a meal saquinavir (Fortovase, Invirase) 500 mg orally twice daily tipranavir (Aptivus) 500 mg orally twice daily	• Instruct patients not to chew or crush these drugs because this action may cause the drug to be absorbed too rapidly and increase the risk for side effects. • Teach patients to report jaundice, nausea and vomiting, or severe abdominal pain because these drugs can induce liver toxicity. • Instruct patients to keep all appointments for laboratory work because these drugs increase blood lipid levels and increase the risk for atherosclerosis and pancreatitis. • Remind patients to avoid St. John's wort while taking these drugs because the supplement reduces the effectiveness of all PIs. • Teach patients taking atazanavir and ritonavir to check their pulse daily and report low heart rate to the prescriber because these two drugs can impair electrical conduction and lead to heart block. • Do not give darunavir or fosamprenavir to patients who have a known sulfa allergy because these two drugs contain sulfa.

Table 6.4   Examples of Antiretroviral Drug Therapy for HIV Infection—cont'd

Entry inhibitors/CCR5 antagonists: These drugs prevent cellular infection with HIV by blocking the *CCR5* receptor on CD4$^+$ T cells. (The virus's *gp120* must bind to the CD4 receptor and its *gp41* must bind to the *CCR5* receptor or to the *CXCR4* receptor for entry into host cells). These are all oral drugs.

DRUG/ADULT DOSAGE RANGE	NURSING IMPLICATIONS
maraviroc (Selzentry) 150–600 mg orally twice daily	• Instruct patients not to chew or crush this drug because this action may cause the drug to be absorbed too rapidly and increase the risk for side effects. • Teach patients to change positions slowly because hypotension is a common side effect, especially orthostatic hypotension. • Teach patients to report jaundice, nausea and vomiting, or severe abdominal pain because these drugs can induce liver toxicity. • Instruct patients to report pain or numbness in the hands or feet because this drug can induce peripheral neuropathy.

Fusion inhibitors: These drugs block the fusion of HIV with a host cell by blocking the ability of *gp41* to fuse with the host cell's CD4 receptor. Without fusion, infection of new cells does not occur.

DRUG/ADULT DOSAGE RANGE	NURSING IMPLICATIONS
enfuvirtide (Fuzeon) 90 mg subcutaneously twice daily	• Teach patients how to prepare and inject the drug subcutaneously to ensure correct dosage and effectiveness. • Assess injection sites for warmth, swelling, redness, skin hardening, or bump formation because these are indications of injection-site reactions. • Instruct patients to report pain or numbness in the hands or feet because this drug can induce peripheral neuropathy. • Teach patients to report jaundice, nausea and vomiting, or severe abdominal pain because this drug can induce liver toxicity. • Teach patients to observe for and report cough, shortness of breath, fever, and purulent mucus because this drug increases the risk for severe respiratory infections, including pneumonia.

Integrase inhibitors: These drugs inhibit the HIV enzyme *integrase*, which the virus uses to insert the viral DNA into the host cell's human DNA. Without this action, viral proteins are not made and viral replication is inhibited.

DRUG/ADULT DOSAGE RANGE	NURSING IMPLICATIONS
dolutegravir (Tivicay) 50 mg orally once or twice daily elvitegravir (Vitekta) 85–150 mg orally once daily raltegravir (Isentress) 400 mg orally twice daily	• Warn patients that diarrhea, nausea, rash, insomnia, and abdominal pain are common side effects of these drugs, because knowing the expected side effects decreases anxiety when they appear. • Suggest that patients take the drug with food to reduce the GI side effects. • Instruct patients not to chew or crush these drugs because this action may cause the drug to be absorbed too rapidly and increase the risk for side effects. • Instruct patients to report new-onset muscle pain or weakness because these drugs can cause muscle breakdown (rhabdomyolysis), especially in adults taking a "statin" type of lipid-lowering drug. • Teach patients with diabetes to closely monitor blood glucose levels because these drugs increase hyperglycemia. • Do not give raltegravir to pregnant women because it is associated with an increased risk for birth defects.

Combination products: Each ingredient has the same mechanism of action and nursing implications as the parent drug class.

Atripla (emtricitabine, tenofovir, and efavirenz)
Combivir (lamivudine and zidovudine)
Complera (emtricitabine, rilpivirine, and tenofovir)
Epzicom (lamivudine and abacavir)
Genvoya (elvitegravir, cobicistat,[a] emtricitabine, and tenofovir)
Stribild (elvitegravir, cobicistat,[a] emtricitabine, and tenofovir)
Triumeq (dolutegravir, abacavir, and lamivudine)
Truvada (emtricitabine and tenofovir)

[a]Cobicistat is a metabolizing enzyme inhibitor that allows other drugs in the combination to remain active longer, boosting their antiretroviral action.

ACTIONS OF DRUGS USED FOR ANTIRETROVIRAL THERAPY

Nucleoside Reverse Transcriptase Inhibitors

NRTIs are antiretroviral drugs that have a similar structure to the molecules that comprise DNA, making them "counterfeit" molecules. The NRTIs work by blocking the function of reverse transcriptionase and preventing the complete synthesis of the viral DNA. Without reverse transcriptase, HIV cannot make new virus copies of itself. These drugs work early in the life cycle of the HIV (see Fig. 6.1).

Non-nucleoside Reverse Transcriptase Inhibitors

NNRTIs bind directly to the HIV-1 enzyme *reverse transcriptase*, preventing viral cell DNA replication, RNA replication, and protein synthesis. With these actions interrupted, HIV reproduction is slowed or stopped. These drugs work fairly early in the HIV life cycle (see Fig. 6.1).

Protease Inhibitors

PIs are antiretroviral drugs that suppress the formation of infectious virions by inhibiting the viral protease enzyme. They act later in the life cycle of the virus (see Fig. 6.1). One of the final stages of the HIV life cycle is the production of HIV proteins, which are first produced as one large protein strand. This single, large protein must be separated by the HIV enzyme protease (which acts like "chemical scissors") into smaller activated proteins needed for the production of more infectious virions. PIs block the HIV enzyme protease and prevent these important proteins from being activated. As a result, infectious HIV virions are not produced and released.

Entry Inhibitors

Entry inhibitors, also known as CCR5 antagonists, are antiretroviral drugs that prevent cellular infection with HIV by blocking the HIV from attaching to special receptors on CD4$^+$ T cells. Each HIV must bind to both of two specific receptors on the CD4 T cell for entry into this host cells. Thus this class of drugs protects uninfected cells from HIV infection. (see Fig. 6.1).

Fusion Inhibitors

Fusion inhibitors are antiretroviral drugs that prevent cellular infection with HIV by blocking the ability of HIV's surface protein to fuse or lock with the host cell's CD4 receptor. Without fusion, infection of new cells does not occur. Just like the entry inhibitors, fusion inhibitors protect uninfected host cells from becoming HIV-infected. (see Fig. 6.1).

Integrase Inhibitors

Integrase inhibitors are antiretroviral drugs that inhibit the HIV enzyme *integrase,* which the virus uses to insert the viral DNA into the host cell's human DNA. Without this action, viral proteins are not made and viral replication is inhibited. Integrase inhibitors work early in the life cycle of HIV infection (see Fig. 6.1).

EXPECTED SIDE EFFECTS OF ANTIRETROVIRAL DRUGS

Most antiretroviral drugs are taken in combination; therefore determining which drug is causing side effects can be difficult. In addition some of the same problems are caused by the HIV disease as by the drugs used to treat it. Common expected side effects for all antiretroviral drugs include mouth ulcers, nausea, and diarrhea. Skin rashes and headaches are also common. Many patients report vivid dreams or nightmares while taking these drugs. Table 6.4 lists many of the common side effects of the drugs.

ADVERSE REACTIONS OF ANTIRETROVIRAL DRUGS

Antiretrovirals often cause severe toxic reactions. Most of these drugs can also cause damage to the liver (hepatotoxic) or kidneys (nephrotoxic). Many also cause inflammation of the pancreas known as pancreatitis. Other possible adverse effects include lactic acidosis, peripheral neuropathy (loss of nerve function, especially in the hands and feet), and diseases that affect the blood.

PRE-EXPOSURE PROPHYLAXIS

There is a new drug therapy to prevent HIV transmission to the uninfected sex partners of people who are HIV-positive and are using cART. The drug approved for this purpose is tenofovir 300 mg/emtricitabine 300 mg (Truvada), which is an oral tablet taken once daily for as long as the person remains at risk for infection. It can only be taken by people who are HIV-negative but are at high risk for becoming infected. After starting Truvada, the person must have his or her HIV status checked every 3 months. The person must take the drug as prescribed for at least 4 days before Truvada can begin to effectively protect against HIV infection.

❖ Nursing Implications and Patient Teaching

> ### 🍂 Lifespan Considerations
> #### Older Adults
>
> - Immunocompromised older adult patients may have other chronic diseases. This may mean that they are taking 8 or 10 drugs at a time. These patients often need encouragement to continue taking all of their drugs.
> - Monitoring for adverse effects from some of the drugs used to treat patients with HIV is more difficult in older adult patients. It is sometimes difficult to know which drugs are causing the adverse reactions because older adults have other health problems and take other drugs.

> ### ⚠ Safety Alert!
> #### Signs or Symptoms of Pancreatitis
>
> Upper abdominal pain and/or pain that radiates to the back, pain that worsens after eating, fever, rapid pulse, increased nausea, and vomiting may indicate pancreatitis, which is a medical emergency.

> ### ⚠ Safety Alert!
> #### Symptoms of Lactic Acidosis
>
> Weakness, fatigue, unexplained muscle pain, nausea, vomiting, dizziness, cold arms and legs, irregular heart rate, and difficulty breathing are symptoms of lactic acidosis.

◆ *Patient and family teaching.* The patient taking cART has probably been doing so for some time and may know more about these drugs than you do. However, it is important to remind the patient and his or her family about the following:

- Take the drugs exactly as ordered every day to ensure the drugs work properly and your disease does not become resistant to the drugs.
- Taking too little of the drugs or skipping doses leads to drug resistance and disease advancement. It is imperative not to skip doses or decrease the dosage.
- Use pillboxes, pill reminders, and/or diaries to maintain strict compliance.
- Take the drugs at the same time every day and use a cell phone reminder for time alerts. This way drug levels remain steady and viral suppression is ideal.
- Alert your healthcare provider immediately to specific symptoms that may indicate adverse reactions.
- Do not cut down or stop the drugs until told to do so by your healthcare provider.
- Safer sexual practice and standard precautions must be taken to prevent disease transmission.
- Impaired immunity makes it more likely to contract diseases. Avoid eating raw meats and fish, and fruits and vegetables that cannot be peeled or scrubbed.
- If you are lactating, stop breast-feeding your baby because there is a high risk for HIV transmission in breast milk.
- Report any new over-the-counter herbs, vitamins, illegal drugs, and nutritional supplements to your prescriber because they could cause increased adverse reactions.
- Do not miss clinic or laboratory appointments. CD4 counts guide treatment. These drugs are highly liver toxic, so liver enzymes must be measured frequently. Complete blood counts monitor infections and adverse effects. Amylase and lipase levels monitor pancreatitis, and lactic acid levels monitor lactic acidosis because symptoms of lactic acidosis are rather nonspecific.
- Avoid alcohol and recreational drugs because of the increased risk for liver damage associated with these drugs.
- Report signs of neuropathy: numbness; tingling in feet or hands, which spread to legs and arms; sharp, jabbing, throbbing, or burning pain in arms and legs; and decreased coordination and falling.
- If you have symptoms of pancreatitis (upper abdominal pain that may radiate to your back, pain that worsens after eating, increased nausea and vomiting), notify your healthcare provider immediately so treatment can begin early.

Get Ready for the NCLEX® Examination!

Key Points

- Viruses are organisms that cannot self-produce, so they "hijack" a cell to reproduce.
- Retroviruses do not just hijack a cell, they actually become a part of the cell and therefore are highly efficient at spreading their infection.
- All antiviral drugs are virustatic; they only suppress viral reproduction and do not kill the virus.
- Antiretroviral drugs are most effective when combinations of drugs from several antiretroviral categories are given daily. This type of therapy is known as cART (combination antiretroviral therapy).
- Teach patients to take antiviral drugs exactly as prescribed and not to stop unless ordered to do so by the prescriber.
- To be most effective in preventing HIV infection and slowing HIV reproduction, cART drugs must be taken correctly and on time at least 90% of the time.
- Except for the fusion inhibitor, enfuvirtide (Fuzeon), antiretroviral drugs are given orally.
- Antivirals used for CMV retinitis and RSV (ribavirin and cidofovir) carry a black box warning and are never to be used or *touched* by anyone who is pregnant or breast-feeding.
- Antivirals have many interactions with other drugs. Always check for interactions with a drug handbook before giving them.
- Antiretroviral drugs are highly toxic to the liver, kidney, and pancreas. Teach patients to be alert for signs and symptoms of toxicity.
- Some antiretroviral drugs need to be taken together on an empty stomach or with food. Teach patients the importance of taking the drugs exactly as they were prescribed.

Review Questions for the NCLEX® Examination

1. The patient has been started on an antiretroviral drug. He tells the nurse he has mouth ulcers. What does this finding suggest?
   1. It is indicative of an anaphylactic reaction.
   2. It is an expected side effect of the drug.
   3. It is an unexpected toxic reaction of the drug.
   4. It is indicative of liver or kidney damage.
2. Which classes of antiretroviral drugs are approved for use during pregnancy in HIV-positive women? (Select all that apply.)
   1. Entry inhibitors
   2. Fusion inhibitors
   3. Integrase inhibitors
   4. Non-nucleoside reverse transcriptase inhibitors
   5. Nucleoside reverse transcriptase inhibitors
   6. Protease inhibitors
3. Which antiretroviral drug belongs to the protease inhibitor class?
   1. darunavir (Prezista)
   2. dolutegravir (Tivicay)
   3. etravirine (Viramune)
   4. tenofovir (Viread)
4. For which antiretroviral drug does the nurse need to assess the patient's subcutaneous injection site for irritation, warmth, or bump formation?
   1. abacavir (Ziagen)
   2. indinavir (Crixivan)
   3. enfuvirtide (Fuzeon)
   4. raltegravir (Isentress)
5. Which antiviral is given by inhalation?
   1. famciclovir
   2. oseltamivir phosphate
   3. zanamivir (Relenza)
   4. acyclovir
6. Which drugs should not be used in persons with an allergy to milk products? (Select all that apply.)
   1. acyclovir
   2. famciclovir
   3. amantadine hydrochloride
   4. oseltamivir phosphate
   5. zanamivir
   6. penciclovir
7. Which antiviral can be given by mouth, by injection, or applied topically?
   1. famciclovir
   2. acyclovir
   3. zanamivir
   4. penciclovir
8. What is the action of a virustatic drug?
   1. The drug kills the virus.
   2. The drug stops the virus from producing.
   3. The drug increases the effectiveness of white blood cells.
   4. The drug blocks reverse transcriptase.
9. Which of the following foods should be avoided in persons taking cART?
   1. Oranges
   2. Bananas
   3. Sushi
   4. Kale
10. Which drug can be taken only by people who are HIV negative but are at high risk for becoming infected?
    1. tenofovir 300 mg/emtricitabine 300 mg
    2. delavirdine 200 mg
    3. lamivudine 300 mg/zidovudine 300 mg
    4. abacavir 600 mg
11. Order: "acyclovir 5 mg/kg intravenous every 8 hours." The patient weighs 165 lb.
    1. How many kilograms does the patient weigh?
    2. How many milligrams of acyclovir should be given with the first dose?
12. Order: "delavirdine 400 mg three times a day." The patient has HIV. Supplied: delavirdine 200-mg tablets. How many tablets will the patient need for a 10-day supply?

Get Ready for the NCLEX® Examination!—cont'd

Case Study

Mary Taft is a patient who has AIDS. She states that her symptoms include sharp, burning pains in her feet with numbness and sensitivity to touch. She has been receiving cART.

1. What disease process or syndrome does Mary's symptoms suggest?
2. If the symptoms are ignored, what might happen?
3. What is the treatment?
4. What drug changes would need to take place if Mary became pregnant?
5. What are the adverse effects of taking cART? How would you monitor for them?
6. Mary has developed a sensitivity and multiple blisters around her mouth. What disease process do these symptoms suggest?
7. Why are infections of this type common in immunocompromised individuals?
8. Mary is started on acyclovir. What are some ramifications of taking acyclovir?
9. What other opportunistic infections might Mary endure, and how can she best prevent them?

7 Drugs for Allergy and Respiratory Problems

Learning Outcomes

1. Describe the causes and symptoms of allergy, asthma, and chronic obstructive pulmonary disease.
2. List the names, actions, possible side effects, and adverse effects of antihistamines, leukotriene inhibitors, and decongestant drugs.
3. Explain what to teach patients and families about antihistamines, leukotriene inhibitors, and decongestant drugs.
4. List the names, actions, possible side effects, and adverse effects of beta-adrenergic agonists and anticholinergic antagonists for asthma and chronic obstructive pulmonary disease.
5. Explain what to teach patients and families about beta-adrenergic agonists and anticholinergic antagonists for asthma and chronic obstructive pulmonary disease.
6. Explain what to teach patients for correct use of drugs delivered by aerosol inhalers and dry-powder inhalers.
7. Explain how asthma controller (preventive) drugs are different from asthma reliever (rescue) drugs.
8. List the names, actions, possible side effects, and adverse effects of mucolytic and antitussive drugs.
9. Explain what to teach patients and families about mucolytic and antitussive drugs.

Key Terms

allergy (Ă-lĕr-jē, p. 107) An excessive reaction that leads to an inflammatory response when a person comes into contact with a substance (allergen) to which he or she is sensitive. It is a common immune response to substances such as pollen, animal dander, food, or dust. Also known as hypersensitivity.

antihistamine (ĂN-tī-HĬS-tă-mēn, p. 107) Drugs that stop histamines from attaching to histamine receptors in the tissues and producing inflammatory and allergic symptoms. This action counteracts the response of histamine in causing smooth muscle contraction and dilation and leakage of capillaries.

antitussive (ĂN-tī-TŬ-sĭv, p. 121) Drugs that work to prevent and/or relieve coughing.

asthma controller drug (p. 115) Drugs that have the main purpose of preventing an asthma attack. Also known as asthma prevention drugs. These drugs must be taken daily even when no asthma symptoms are present. Also known as *prevention* drugs.

asthma reliever drug (p. 115) Drugs that have the main purpose of stopping an asthma attack once it has started. Also known as asthma *rescue* drugs.

bronchodilator (brn-k-D-I-trz, p. 115) Drugs that relax the airway smooth muscles allowing the lumen of the airways to widen.

cholinergic antagonist (p. 116) Drugs that block the action of acetylcholine thereby inhibiting the parasympathetic nervous system response. Also known as cholinergic blockers, parasympatholytics, or anticholinergic drugs.

corticosteroid (kōr-tĭ-kō-'STĚR-oid, p. 112) Drugs built on the structure of cholesterol that are able to prevent or limit inflammation and allergy by slowing or stopping production of the mediators histamine and leukotriene.

decongestant (dē-kăn-JĚS-tănt, p. 112) Drugs that reduce the swelling of nasal passages by shrinking the small blood vessels in the nose, throat, and sinuses so breathing is easier.

leukotriene inhibitor (lū-kō-TRĪ-ēn ĭn-HĬ-bă-tĕr, p. 111) Drugs that block the leukotriene response and lessen or prevent the symptoms of allergy and asthma.

long-acting beta-adrenergic agonist (LABA) (ă-dră-NĚR-jĭk Ă-gă-nĭst, p. 116) Orally inhaled drugs that bind over time to beta$_2$-adrenergic receptors and are used as asthma controller drugs that must be taken on a daily schedule to prevent bronchospasms and asthma attacks even when symptoms are not present.

mast cell stabilizer (cromone) (p. 112) Drugs that work on the surface of mast cells and prevent them from opening to release the inflammatory mediators.

mucolytics (myū-kă-LĬ-tĭks, p. 119) Drugs that decrease the thickness of respiratory secretions and aid in their removal. Also called expectorants.

short-acting beta-adrenergic agonist (SABA) (ă-dră-NĚR-jĭk Ă-gă-nĭst, p. 116) Orally inhaled drugs that bind rapidly to beta$_2$-adrenergic receptors and can start smooth muscle relaxation within seconds to minutes. Also known as asthma reliever or rescue drugs.

sympathomimetics (SĬM-pă-thō-mă-MĚ-tĭks, p. 112) Drugs that mimic the sympathetic nervous system and have the same actions as the body's own adrenalin. Also called beta- and/or alpha-adrenergic agonists.

ALLERGY

An **allergy** is an excessive reaction that leads to an inflammatory response when a person comes into contact with a substance or allergen to which he or she is sensitive. It is estimated that one in five people in the United States suffer from allergies. Allergens are usually harmless substances and include things people are surrounded with every day such as dust mites, plant pollen, pet dander, food, and insect bites. These substances only cause allergic reactions in people who are overly sensitive to them. Allergies are also known as *hypersensitivities* and occur when the immune system overacts and develops a response to substances in the environment. When the immune system overreacts to an allergen, symptoms appear where the allergen entered or touched the body, usually in the nose, lungs, throat, or on the skin.

The purpose of the immune system is to protect the body from living substances that cause infections such as bacteria, viruses, and fungi. The immune system also protects the body from nonliving substances it views as dangerous, such as drugs, toxins, and chemicals. These "invaders" are known as *antigens* because they are not part of the body and can trigger the immune system to take protective actions. These protective actions occur when the immune system produces an antibody directed against the offending antigen. The antibodies are produced by specific immune system cells known as *lymphocytes* in the bloodstream. The action of an antibody is to either neutralize the offending antigen or cause it to be destroyed and eliminated from the body. The lymphocytes make five different antibodies or immunoglobulins (Igs) for protection: IgA, IgD, IgE, IgG, and IgM. The IgE class of antibody is the body's defense against allergens.

Once the antibodies are released in response to the allergen, they trigger other immune system cells and mast cells to produce internal chemicals, known as *mediators*, to start and continue inflammation. The important mediators released by WBCs when antibodies react with allergens are *histamine* and *leukotriene*. Histamine starts the inflammation and leukotriene works with histamine to keep the inflammatory response going once it has started. These mediators start actions in tissues and blood vessels resulting in inflammation and its symptoms. As described more completely in Chapter 11, these mediators, especially histamine, cause contraction of smooth muscle and dilation and leakage of capillaries, which explains the symptoms of swelling, redness, tissue irritation, and mucous production. Think about the person who has an allergy to pollens and develops hay fever. The symptoms include red, itchy eyes that produce tears to flush out the invader. The nasal passages swell, the nose is stuffed up to prevent entrance of more antigens, and the sinuses drain to get rid of the offender. Sneezing rids the invader from the airway passages. Contraction of the smooth muscle

of the bronchioles or bronchoconstriction caused by histamine and by leukotriene release prevents entry into the lungs and causes breathing difficulties. Unfortunately, in an attempt to protect the body from the invaders, oxygen is also prevented from entering the body.

Air must be able to move from the upper respiratory system (the oral and nasal cavities, sinuses, pharynx, larynx, and trachea) to the lower respiratory system (the bronchi and lungs) for gas exchange to take place. The alveoli in the base of the lungs exchange life-giving oxygen on inspiration for the waste product of carbon dioxide on expiration. Anything that interrupts this passage of air from the airway to the alveoli can cause death (Fig. 7.1). Disruptions that create problems can be a narrow or constricted opening (a bronchospasm), or a blockage from mucus, infection, or edema in the bases of the lungs (pulmonary edema) or collapse of the bronchioles and the alveoli themselves.

DRUG THERAPY FOR ALLERGY

Drugs used to treat allergies are those that interfere with inflammation. These include antihistamines, leukotriene blockers, and corticosteroids. Leukotrienes are also used to treat asthma because allergies often trigger asthma attacks. Decongestants are other drugs that can help lessen the symptoms of allergy but do not interfere with inflammation. Drugs used for allergies may be taken orally, used as a nasal spray, or inhaled into the lungs when inflammation triggers asthma. They can also be applied topically to the skin when allergic reactions are present in the skin. Table 7.1 lists the common drugs for allergy together with the nursing implications.

> **Bookmark This!**
>
> Research is always expanding treatment and drugs. For more patient and healthcare professional education regarding allergens and asthma, check out the American Academy of Allergy, Asthma, & Immunology at https://www.aaaai.org.

ANTIHISTAMINES

Actions

Antihistamines are drugs that stop histamines from attaching to histamine receptors in the tissues and producing inflammatory and allergic symptoms. Allergens activate mast cells that are the chief controllers of the immune system. They are manufactured in the bone marrow and are present in all tissues of the body. When the mast cells are activated, they release histamine. There are two types of histamine: H_1 and H_2. Antihistamines do not prevent histamine from being released. They block the receptors on the tissues. Blocking H_1 receptors limits the blood vessel vasodilation, capillary leak, swelling, and bronchoconstriction. Blocking H_2 receptors decreases stomach acid production, which is discussed

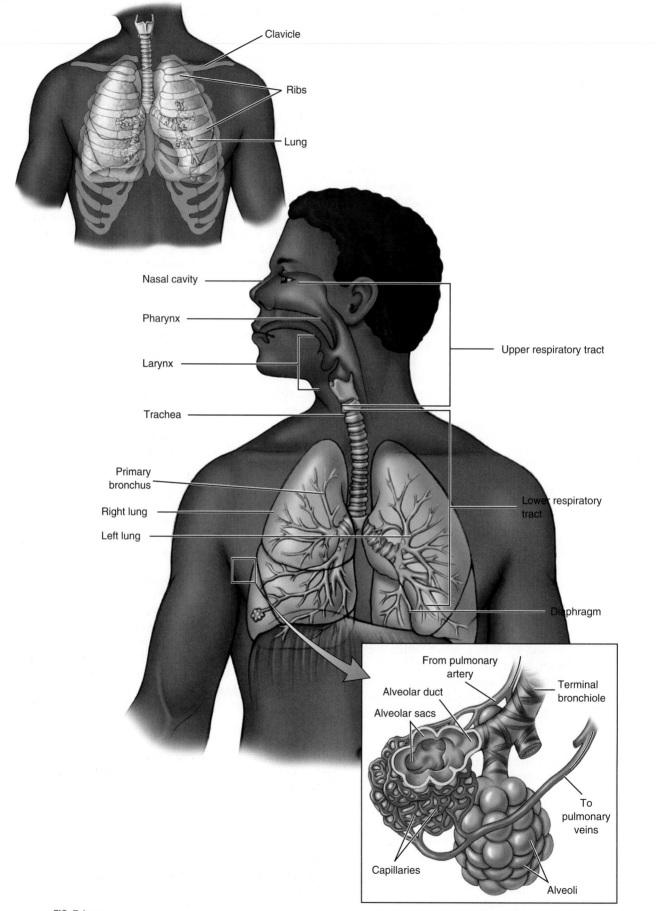

FIG. 7.1 The respiratory system. (From Herlihy B: *The human body in health and illness*, ed 5, St. Louis, 2014, Elsevier.)

Table 7.1 **Examples of Common Antihistamines, Leukotriene Inhibitors, and Mast Cell Stabilizers**

First-generation antihistamines: work by preventing histamine from attaching to the tissue receptor sites, thus decreasing allergic symptoms. These drugs have safety concerns because they cause CNS depression.

DRUG/ADULT DOSAGE RANGE	NURSING IMPLICATIONS
diphenhydramine (Benadryl) 25–50 mg orally three to four times a day *or* 10–50 mg slow IM or slow IV over 10 minutes every 4–6 hours PRN diphenhydramine cream (topical agent) brompheniramine (Dimetapp) 12–24 mg orally once daily (oral) *or* 10 mg IV slowly, IM, or subcutaneously every 6–12 hours PRN	• Warn patients not to drive or operate hazardous equipment because these drugs usually cause drowsiness. • Check the urine output of patients who have an enlarged prostate gland because a side effect of these drugs is urinary retention. • Avoid giving these drugs to patients with glaucoma because the action can increase intraocular pressure. • Warn patients that many over-the-counter sleep aids contain first-generation antihistamines and taking these with an antihistamine could lead to overdose. • Watch for hyperexcitability and restlessness in children or older adults because they are more likely to have a paradoxical reaction to the drug. • Tell patients who are breast-feeding to avoid brompheniramine because it enters breast milk and will produce side effects in the infant. • Warn patients not to take these drugs with sedatives, opioids, anticholinergic drugs, or drugs that cause CNS depression because the CNS side effects will be more severe. • Warn patients to take these drugs for 2 weeks or less to avoid tolerance and long-term side effects.

Second-generation antihistamines: work by preventing histamine from attaching to the tissue receptor sites, thus decreasing allergic symptoms. The incidence of CNS depression is much less with these antihistamines.

DRUG/ADULT DOSAGE RANGE	NURSING IMPLICATIONS
fexofenadine (Allegra) 60 mg orally twice daily *or* 180 mg orally once daily loratadine (Claritin) 10 mg orally once daily levocetirizine (Xyzal) 2.5–5 mg orally once daily in the evening	• Teach patients not to take fexofenadine with grapefruit, orange, or apple juice because these products reduce the effectiveness of the drug. • Instruct patients taking the quick-dissolve tablets to place them under the tongue and not to eat or drink until they have dissolved to promote best absorption. • Ask whether the patient has any kidney problems before giving either fexofenadine or levocetirizine because poor kidney function allows the drug to remain in the system longer and can lead to overdoses. • Check the urine output of patients who have an enlarged prostate gland because a side effect of these drugs is urinary retention. • Use cautiously with other drugs that cause sedation or CNS depression because, although these drugs have fewer CNS side effects, they may worsen the CNS depression of other drugs. • Give levocetirizine in the evening because it has more sedating effects than other second-generation antihistamines.

Leukotriene inhibitors (modifiers): Zileuton (Zyflo) blocks production of leukotriene within white blood cells. Montelukast (Singulair) and zafirlukast (Accolate) block the leukotriene receptors on tissues. Both actions stop allergy symptoms and prevent the bronchoconstriction in asthma.

DRUG/ADULT DOSAGE RANGE	NURSING IMPLICATIONS
montelukast (Singulair) 10 mg orally once a day at the same time zafirlukast (Accolate) 20 mg orally twice a day zileuton (Zyflo) 1200 mg orally twice daily, within 1 hour after morning and evening meals	• Teach patients to take zafirlukast 1 hour before or 2 hours after a meal because the drug is best absorbed on an empty stomach. • Teach patients to report any yellowing of the skin or eyes, darkening of the urine, or white/gray stools because these drugs can impair the liver. • Warn patients and families to observe for changes in behavior or mood because all these drugs have been found to cause these problems in some patients. • These drugs are not to be used during an acute asthma attack because they require a long time to get to peak action. They are prevention rather than reliever drugs.

Continued

Table 7.1 Examples of Common Antihistamines, Leukotriene Inhibitors, and Mast Cell Stabilizers—cont'd

Mast cell stabilizers (cromones): work by preventing mast cell membranes from opening and releasing histamine and leukotriene.

DRUG/ADULT DOSAGE RANGE	NURSING IMPLICATIONS
cromolyn sodium (NasalCrom) 1 spray (5.2 mg/spray) in each nostril three to four times per day; may be increased to six times a day if needed *or* 20 mg oral inhalation by nebulizer every 6 hours nedocromil sodium (Tilade) 2 inhalations (1.75 mg each) four times a day	• Remind patients that there may be mild stinging or burning of the nasal lining with use, but this is an expected side effect, not an allergy. • Teach patients to rinse the mouth and gargle after using the nebulizer to minimize dry mouth or throat, throat irritation, and hoarseness. • Remind patients that these drugs must be used as prescribed daily to reduce symptoms because they are not rapid-acting.

in Chapter 13. Antihistamines also limit the release of acetylcholine, which produces a drying effect (anticholinergic), particularly in the bronchioles and the GI system. Table 7.1 lists common antihistamines, their actions, and nursing implications.

Uses

Antihistamine H_1-receptor blockers (antagonists) are used to treat almost any type of allergic reaction, including allergic rhinitis (nasal stuffiness and drainage). They are also used to treat asthma that is triggered by an allergic reaction. Histamine plays a central role in producing most of the typical eye and nasal signs and symptoms such as sneezing, nasal stuffiness, and postnasal drip.

Antihistamines are classed as either first-generation drugs or second-generation drugs. First-generation drugs are available over the counter (OTC). Most of these products cross the blood–brain barrier and cause sedation (sleepiness) along with the antiallergy and anticholinergic effects. These drugs are effective in helping reduce symptoms of sneezing, itching, and rhinorrhea (runny nose) when used for a short time.

Second-generation antihistamines are newer and usually have a more rapid onset of relief of sneezing, pruritus (itching), and rhinorrhea. These drugs do not cross the blood–brain barrier and thus do not cause significant sedation. Some are available by prescription and some are OTC. In general, they are less effective against nasal congestion than are first-generation drugs.

Expected Side Effects

Drowsiness is an expected side effect for most antihistamines. In fact many OTC sleep aids contain the antihistamine diphenhydramine. Patients should also expect dry mouth, increased heart rate, increased blood pressure, dilated pupils, and urinary retention to occur because of the anticholinergic effect of the antihistamines.

Adverse Effects

Most adverse effects are related to severe anticholinergic symptoms, such as cardiac dysrhythmias or dangerously high blood pressure. A rising intraocular pressure (pressure inside the eye) in patients with glaucoma can worsen the disease and could cause blindness. Symptoms of overdosage include nervousness, anxiety, fear, agitation, restlessness, weakness, irritability, talkativeness, and insomnia. These symptoms may progress to dizziness, light-headedness, tremor, and hyperreflexia, with progression to confusion, delirium, hallucinations, and euphoria. Antihistamines, especially first-generation drugs, should be used with great caution in children because responses can be unpredictable.

Problems with memory have been reported with continuous use of these agents, especially in older patients. Children and some older adults may have the opposite reaction (a *paradoxical* reaction) in which the patient has hyperexcitability, agitation, or confusion.

Lifespan Considerations
Older Adults

Older adults often have pronounced anticholinergic effects such as constipation, dry mouth, and urinary retention (especially in men).

Drug Interactions

The sedative effect often seen with antihistamines is increased when other central nervous system (CNS) depressants (such as hypnotics, sedatives, tranquilizers, depressant analgesics, and alcohol) are used along with the antihistamine. The sedative effect of antihistamines also adds to the effect of anticholinergic drugs, and they can strengthen the anticholinergic side effects of monoamine oxidase inhibitors (MAOIs), as well as tricyclic antidepressants.

When antihistamines are used along with *ototoxic drugs* (drugs that may damage hearing, such as large doses of aspirin or other salicylates, or streptomycin), the antihistamine may relieve some of the symptoms of ototoxicity, such as dizziness; as a result, these important symptoms may be masked. They may also interfere with the effects of anticholinesterase drugs.

❖ Nursing Implications and Patient Teaching

◆ *Assessment.* Ask the patient about the presence of drug allergy, other drug use, and the presence of asthma, glaucoma, peptic ulcer disease, prostatic hypertrophy, bladder neck obstruction, respiratory or cardiac disease, and the possibility of pregnancy. A patient with thyroid disease or migraine headaches may be unable to take antihistamines because of the *tachycardia* (rapid heartbeat) produced. These conditions are either contraindications or precautions for the use of antihistamines.

◆ *Planning and implementation.* Antihistamines for allergy should be taken only when needed. The type and dose should be chosen for the desired effect and the person being treated. For example, first-generation drugs make people very sleepy, and people who do tasks that require alertness probably should not use them. This also is a concern in older patients who are prone to falls.

Giving oral doses with food or drink can limit GI side effects; however, some antihistamines must be taken on an empty stomach. Check a drug reference guide to determine whether the drug can be given with food or certain liquids or if it needs to be taken on an empty stomach.

When an IM preparation such as diphenhydramine is used, inject it deep into the muscle to prevent tissue irritation. Intravenous (IV) injection of these agents is done slowly, with the patient lying down because of the risk of the drug causing low blood pressure. Long-term use of topical nasal antihistamines increases the risk for sensitization, often causing a rebound effect, or an increase in the symptoms you are trying to stop.

◆ *Evaluation.* Assess the patient to determine whether allergy symptoms are reduced. Watch for any side effects.

Assess older adults for side effects such as dizziness, *syncope* (light-headedness and fainting), and confusion. Problems with *dyskinesia* (difficulty in movements of the body), *bradykinesia* (slow movement), stiffness, and tremor are reactions that may also develop and must be reported to the prescriber.

◆ *Patient and family teaching.* Tell the patient and family the following:
- Unless you must restrict your fluid intake because of another health problem, drink extra fluids to help prevent the respiratory tract dryness that often occurs with antihistamine use.
- If any skin reactions occur, stop taking the drug at once and notify your healthcare provider. Do not increase the dose or drink alcohol while taking antihistamines because the CNS depressant effects of antihistamines may be increased.
- Avoid tasks such as driving or activities that require alertness until you know how antihistamines affect you because they cause drowsiness in many patients.
- If the drug causes stomach upset, take it with meals or milk to decrease this problem.
- You may develop tolerance to an antihistamine. If one drug seems to stop working over time, your healthcare provider may suggest trying another antihistamine for better control of symptoms.

- Do not take any drugs without the knowledge of your healthcare provider, especially sedative drugs, while taking an antihistamine.

LEUKOTRIENE INHIBITORS
Action
Leukotriene inhibitors, sometimes called *leukotriene modifiers*, are drugs that block the leukotriene response and lessen or prevent the symptoms of allergy and asthma. Different leukotriene inhibitors have different actions to reduce inflammation. Zileuton (Zyflo) blocks production of leukotriene within white blood cells. Montelukast (Singulair) and zafirlukast (Accolate) block the leukotriene receptors on tissues. As a result of either action the inflammatory response is reduced. Table 7.1 lists common leukotriene inhibitors, their actions, and nursing implications.

Uses
Some leukotriene inhibitors are used for allergic rhinitis. Use of these inhibitors can relax respiratory smooth muscle and increase airflow through the bronchial tubes because leukotriene can also trigger bronchospasms. Thus these drugs also are used for prevention and long-term treatment of asthma.

Expected Side Effects, Adverse Reactions, and Drug Interactions
Leukotriene inhibitors are generally safe and well tolerated. Headache, nausea, and diarrhea are the most common side effects.

Although adverse reactions to the leukotriene inhibitors are rare, liver dysfunction is possible with long-term use. The leukotriene inhibitors interact with drugs that stimulate liver metabolism such as phenytoin, phenobarbital, carbamazepine, and rifampin. Montelukast has the least amount of drug interactions.

❖ Nursing Implications and Patient Teaching
◆ *Assessment.* Ask the patient about the other drugs he or she takes. Ask about the possibility of pregnancy, breast-feeding, or liver disease.

◆ *Planning and implementation.* Leukotriene inhibitors are not started if the patient is having an acute asthma attack. They are drugs given as part of an asthma treatment regimen but will not relieve an acute attack of asthma. Watch to see whether there might be adverse drug interactions with other drugs the patient is taking. Some of these drugs are to be given either with food or on an empty stomach.

◆ *Evaluation.* Therapeutic effect is usually seen within 3 to 7 days with a reduction in the number and severity of allergic reactions or asthma attacks.

◆ *Patient and family teaching.* Tell the patient and family the following:
- Report any increase in asthma attacks or allergic symptoms to your healthcare provider.

- Consider not taking these drugs if you are pregnant or breast-feeding, although this is an individual decision to be made by you and your healthcare provider based on risk and benefit.
- These drugs are used to prevent (rather than stop) an asthma attack or allergic response; therefore do not suddenly stop taking the drug or decrease the dosage.

MAST CELL STABILIZERS (CROMONES)

Another type of drug that reduces the amount of histamine and leukotriene release and can be helpful for allergy or asthma is the class of **mast cell stabilizers (cromones)**. They work on the surface of mast cells and prevent them from opening to release the inflammatory mediators. For nasal allergies and asthma they are used as inhaled drugs. Common cromones and their nursing implications are listed in Table 7.1.

DECONGESTANTS

Actions and Uses

Nasal congestion occurs either because the nasal tissue is inflamed and swollen or because nasal secretions are thick and obstruct the nasal passage. **Decongestants** are drugs that reduce the swelling of nasal passages. There are two kinds of decongestants: sympathomimetic and corticosteroids.

Sympathomimetics are drugs that produce or mimic stimulation of the sympathetic (adrenergic) nervous system and have the same action as the body's own adrenaline. When blood vessels are stimulated by the sympathetic nervous system (alpha receptors), they shrink (*constrict*). Once the blood vessels shrink, the secretions in the membranes of the nose can drain better and stuffiness and pressure are relieved. These drugs may also be used to decrease congestion around the eustachian tubes with middle ear infections. Most of these products are now available OTC. They can be taken orally or by nasal spray. Saline nasal spray and saline irrigations using a Neti Pot™ are an effective alternative to nasal sprays and can be used routinely to relieve nasal symptoms. There are no side effects to the use of saline and it can be used as often as necessary.

Corticosteroids are drugs built on the structure of cholesterol that are able to prevent or limit inflammation and allergy by slowing or stopping production of histamine and leukotriene. Corticosteroid nasal sprays are effective at controlling nasal inflammation. They stabilize the membranes of the white blood cells that produce histamine and leukotrienes that cause inflammation. They work on the white blood cells that help to fight infection; therefore their use is not recommended for people with sinus infections, or who have immune diseases or are taking immune-suppressing drugs. If they are absorbed systemically, it is possible for people to become ill because of the lessening response of infection-fighting white blood cells. It takes up to 2 weeks for corticosteroid nasal sprays to begin working. Oral, IV, and IM corticosteroids can also be used for allergic reactions but have many side and adverse effects. They may be used orally for allergies and asthma but are more commonly given as inhaled drugs. Table 7.2 lists common decongestants, their actions, and nursing implications. See Chapter 12 for a complete discussion of the actions and uses of corticosteroids, as well as the nursing responsibilities.

Uses

Nasal decongestants are used to shrink nasal mucous membranes and relieve nasal congestion caused by allergies or cold symptoms.

Expected Side Effects

Topically applied nasal decongestants (sprays or drops) are well tolerated because the amount that enters the bloodstream is too small to cause side effects. Local effects include irritation and dryness of the mucous membranes. Sympathomimetic nasal spray that is overused can enter the bloodstream and cause nervousness, insomnia, tremors, and heart palpitations. Expected side effects of oral decongestants include headache, nervousness, dizziness, insomnia, and tremors. A slight nosebleed is common with corticosteroid nasal sprays, but if it becomes severe, it would be considered an adverse effect.

Adverse Reactions

Oral sympathomimetic decongestants can have adverse side effects related to mimicking the sympathetic nervous system response. The sympathetic nervous system (beta$_1$ receptors) increases heart rate, increases the force of contraction of the heart muscle, increases the speed of electrical conduction in the heart, and constricts the blood vessels. The adverse effects that can be seen are cardiac dysrhythmias, hypertension, and palpitations, which could lead to a heart attack.

Sympathomimetic nasal decongestants can cause rebound congestion if overused or used more than 3 to 5 days. Rarely a severe shocklike syndrome with hypotension and coma has been reported in children. Psychological dependence and toxic psychoses have been reported with long-term, high-dose therapy. The severity of overdosage varies, resulting in a variety of symptoms. The US Food and Drug Administration (FDA) stipulates that these products are not to be used in infants and toddlers because of problems with inadvertent overdosage in this age group.

Corticosteroid nasal sprays can reduce the protective immune responses in the nose and throat. This action increases the risk for upper respiratory infections and overgrowth of oral fungus (yeast). As a result, redness, sores, or white patches may appear in the mouth or throat.

Table 7.2 Examples of Common Decongestants

Nasal corticosteroids: work to decrease inflamed and swollen nasal membranes by preventing mast cells and white blood cells within the nasal mucosa from releasing histamine, leukotriene, and other mediators of inflammation.

DRUG/ADULT DOSAGE RANGE	NURSING IMPLICATIONS
fluticasone (Flonase, Sensimist) 2 sprays of 110 mcg once daily triamcinolone (Nasacort) 2–4 sprays of 55 mcg/spray once daily	• Remind patients that relief is not immediate because these drugs take time to build up an effect. • Caution patients not to swallow the spray to prevent absorbing the drug systemically and causing more side effects. • Remind patients to clean and dry the applicator after each use (and never to share the inhaler with another person) to prevent infection because these drugs reduce the local immune response. • Tell patients to watch for white patches in the nose or throat that may indicate a fungal infection because these drugs reduce the local immune response.

Sympathomimetic drugs: work to shrink swollen nasal membranes by activating the adrenergic receptors on the blood vessels within the nasal mucosa, causing them to constrict. Swelling is reduced and sinus drainage is improved.

DRUG/ADULT DOSAGE RANGE	NURSING IMPLICATIONS
oxymetazoline, nasal spray (Afrin, many others), 2–3 sprays in each nostril PRN every 10–12 hours phenylephrine, spray or drops (Neo-Synephrine, many others), 0.5%–1% solution sprayed or dropped into the nose every 6 hours phenylephrine, oral tablets or liquids (Nasop, Sudafed, many others), 10–20 mg every 6 hours PRN pseudoephedrine (Dimetapp, Sudafed, many others) 60 mg orally every 6 hours *or* 120 mg orally every 12 hours	• Tell patients that relief of nasal congestion is immediate because these sprays and drops work on contact with nasal membranes. • Remind patients to use the nasal sprays for only a few days because tolerance and rebound stuffiness occur quickly. • Caution patients not to swallow the spray to prevent absorbing the drug systemically and causing more side effects. • Warn patients with high blood pressure, heart disease, glaucoma, or prostate enlargement to use these drugs with caution and not to exceed the prescribed dose because the drugs increase blood pressure, cause urinary retention, and increase intraocular pressure. • Suggest that patients who are using the oral forms of the drugs take them at least 4 hours before going to bed because these drugs can cause insomnia.

Drug Interactions

Interactions for sympathomimetics include caffeine, MAOIs, amphetamines, ergotamine, selegiline, and linezolid, which can cause hypertension and increasing heart rate with dysrhythmias. These drugs should not be taken with beta-blocking eye drops used for open-angle glaucoma. Corticosteroid nasal sprays should not be used with antibiotics or immunosuppressive drugs.

❖ Nursing Implications and Patient Teaching

◆ *Assessment.* Monitor heart rate and blood pressure in people taking sympathomimetic drugs, especially in those with a history of cardiac disease. Notify the prescriber if rapid heart rate or irregular heart rate develops or if hypertension worsens. For people taking corticosteroid nasal spray, assess the nasal and mouth area for white patches or redness that may indicate a fungal infection. For people susceptible to infection, take their temperature and monitor any signs and symptoms that might indicate an infectious process rather than an allergy, that is, thick green nasal discharge, shortness of breath, or wheezing.

◆ *Planning and implementation.* Oral sympathomimetic drugs can decrease the effectiveness of some high blood pressure drugs and should not be used in persons with uncontrolled hypertension or cardiac insufficiency. Patients on antibiotics, antifungals, immunosuppressives, or HIV drugs or those who have a sinus infection should not use corticosteroid nasal sprays.

◆ *Evaluation.* Nasal stuffiness and inflammation should be relieved instantly with sympathomimetic nasal spray and within an hour if taking oral sympathomimetics. Nasal corticosteroids can take up to 2 weeks to reduce symptoms.

◆ *Patient and family teaching.* Tell the patient and family the following:
- Before using a decongestant, check with your prescriber if you have heart disease, high blood pressure, glaucoma, diabetes, an enlarged prostate, or thyroid disease because decongestants can make these problems worse.
- Avoid the use of caffeine, alcohol, or other stimulant drugs while using oral sympathomimetic decongestants because heart rate and blood pressure problems will increase.
- Avoid taking sympathomimetic drugs within 4 hours of bedtime because these drugs may cause insomnia.
- If you develop extreme restlessness, insomnia, tremors, and heart palpitations, stop using the drug and notify your healthcare provider.

- Do not take sympathomimetic drugs if you are pregnant or breast-feeding.
- Do not overuse sympathomimetic nasal spray or use it for more than 3 days because a rebound stuffiness and congestion are likely to occur.
- If you have high blood pressure or heart problems, check with the pharmacist before using OTC cold preparations that say they relieve nasal congestion or stuffiness because OTC cold preparations often contain sympathomimetic drugs.
- If you have glaucoma or cataracts, check with your healthcare provider before using corticosteroid nasal sprays.
- Contact your healthcare provider if white patches develop in the nose or mouth, you have worsening nasal discharge, or flu symptoms and fever develop while taking corticosteroid nasal sprays.

ASTHMA AND CHRONIC OBSTRUCTIVE PULMONARY DISEASE

ASTHMA

Asthma is a long-term condition of the airways that causes smooth muscle constriction and inflammation of the airways and lungs. As a result of airway narrowing, airflow to lung tissue, where oxygen is picked up by the blood, can be greatly reduced. Although the actual symptoms of asthma may occur from time to time rather than continuously (known as an intermittent problem), the disorder is chronic and the person is always at risk for an asthma attack. However, the symptoms of asthma are reversible, and between attacks the patient usually has no signs or symptoms.

Two different problems can make the airways smaller and become obstructed (Fig. 7.2). Internal airway obstruction occurs when inflammation, often caused by an allergy, causes the mucous membrane lining to swell and secrete extra mucus. In addition, when the smooth muscle surrounding the airway tightens (constricts), it narrows the outside structure of the airway through *bronchoconstriction*. Many patients with asthma actually have both types of airway obstruction because an allergy can irritate bronchiolar smooth muscle. Drug therapy for asthma usually requires more than one drug type to manage the two causes of the disorder.

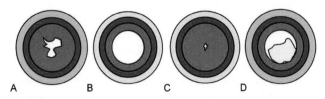

FIG. 7.2 Causes of narrowed airways: *(A)* Mucosal swelling. *(B)* Constriction of smooth muscle. *(C)* Mucosal swelling and constriction of smooth muscle. *(D)* Mucous plug. (From Workman ML, LaCharity LA, Kruchko SL: *Understanding pharmacology*, ed 1, St. Louis, 2011, Elsevier.)

> **Memory Jogger**
>
> Inflammation narrows airways from the inside, and broncho-constriction narrows airways from the outside.

Symptoms of an asthma attack are shortness of breath, wheezing (the whistling sound a vacuum makes when it becomes clogged), dry, hacking cough, or a feeling of tightness in the chest. Asthma episodes can occur frequently every day, a few times per week, during the day or night, with exercise, or on a seasonal basis. Management depends on the severity and frequency of symptoms.

CHRONIC OBSTRUCTIVE PULMONARY DISEASE

Chronic obstructive pulmonary disease (COPD) is a progressive disease that causes breathing difficulty. It obstructs airflow passages in the upper and lower airways, which includes the alveoli, where gas exchange takes place. The usual cause of COPD is cigarette smoking or exposure to secondhand smoke and air pollution that causes a constant inflammation of the upper airways known as *chronic bronchitis*. The inflammation causes large amounts of sticky mucus to be produced, which obstructs the upper airways, makes the work of breathing very difficult, and prevents air from flowing into the lungs and alveoli. Bronchitis affects only the airways, not the alveoli.

The same things that cause chronic bronchitis also cause the emphysema that is seen in COPD. Emphysema is damage to the lower airways and involves damage to the lung tissue and alveoli. When the alveoli become damaged, they can no longer stretch for oxygen to enter or shrink to force carbon dioxide out. The alveoli begin to collapse and die; the fewer alveoli that exist, the less oxygen is available to be moved into the bloodstream and the more carbon dioxide the body retains. COPD causes a chronic cough that produces clear, white, yellow, or green sticky mucus, wheezing, shortness of breath, chest tightness, and an enlarged chest.

Unlike with asthma, the person diagnosed with COPD always has symptoms, but these become worse with increases in inflammation from pulmonary infections and in response to pollution and other triggers. Unlike asthma, the lung damage with COPD is *not* reversible, although patients may have periods with less severe symptoms. Drug therapy for COPD involves most of the same drugs used for asthma because the symptoms are similar, although the actual causes differ.

DRUG THERAPY FOR ASTHMA AND CHRONIC OBSTRUCTIVE PULMONARY DISEASE

Drug therapy for both asthma and COPD includes bronchodilating and anti-inflammatory agents. Although both types of drugs are used, when used for COPD the dosage and delivery method may be different (some drugs are more often delivered by nebulizer rather than

Table 7.3 **The Step System for Drug Therapy in Asthma**

STEP 1	STEP 2	STEP 3	STEP 4	STEP 5
Daytime symptoms occur not more than twice per week and do not limit activity. Reliever drug needed not more than twice weekly.	Daytime symptoms occur not more than twice per week and do limit activity. Reliever drug needed not more than twice weekly.	Daytime symptoms occur more than twice per week, nighttime symptoms also are present. Symptoms limit activity. Reliever drug needed more than twice weekly.	Daytime symptoms occur more than twice per week, nighttime symptoms also are present. Symptoms limit activity. Reliever drug needed daily.	Daytime symptoms occur daily, nighttime symptoms also are present. Symptoms limit activity. Reliever drug needed daily or more than once daily.
As needed rapid-acting beta$_2$ agonist (relief inhaler)	As needed rapid-acting beta$_2$ agonist (relief inhaler)	As needed rapid-acting beta$_2$ agonist (relief inhaler)	As needed rapid-acting beta$_2$ agonist (relief inhaler)	As needed rapid-acting beta$_2$ agonist (relief inhaler)
No daily drugs needed	Daily treatment involves the use of *one* of these two options: Low-dose ICS Leukotriene receptor antagonist/inhibitor	Daily treatment involves the use of *one* of these four options: Low-dose ICS *and* long-acting beta$_2$ agonist Medium- to high-dose ICS Low-dose ICS and leukotriene receptor antagonist/inhibitor Low-dose ICS and low-dose theophylline	Daily treatment involves the use of the Step 3 option that provided the best degree of control and was well tolerated along with one or more of these two options: Medium-dose or high-dose ICS *and* long-acting beta$_2$ agonist Leukotriene receptor antagonist/inhibitor and sustained-release theophylline	Daily treatment involves the use of the Step 4 option(s) that provided the best degree of control and was well tolerated along with either of these two options: Oral glucocorticosteroid (lowest dose) Anti-IgE treatment

ICS, Inhaled corticosteroid; *IgE*, immunoglobulin E.
Data compiled from Global Initiative for Asthma (GINA). (2017). *Pocket guide for asthma management and prevention.* Retrieved from http://ginasthma.org/2017-pocket-guide-for-asthma-management-and-prevention/

as a sprayed inhalant). In addition, drugs that help thin secretions (mucolytics) are used more often in COPD therapy than in asthma therapy (discussed later in this chapter).

The goals of drug therapy for asthma are to: (1) prevent acute asthma attacks, and (2) stop an asthma attack as quickly as possible after it has started. Thus some drugs are **asthma controller drugs** (prevention drugs) that have the main purpose of preventing an attack. Controller drugs must be taken daily to be effective, even when the person has no symptoms of asthma. Controller drugs usually include longer-acting bronchodilators, as well as drugs that prevent excessive inflammation (anti-inflammatories). Drugs that have the main purpose of stopping an asthma attack are **asthma reliever drugs** (rescue drugs). They are usually short-acting bronchodilators that have no role in asthma prevention. The Global Initiative for Asthma has published guidelines for asthma diagnosis and drug management. These guidelines recommend a stepwise plan for using asthma drugs that takes into account asthma severity (Table 7.3).

Memory Jogger

Asthma controller drugs prevent asthma attacks and must be taken daily even when asthma symptoms are not present.

Asthma reliever drugs can rescue a person having an actual asthma attack. They are used only as needed and not on a schedule.

BRONCHODILATORS

Action

Bronchodilators are drugs that relax the airway smooth muscles, allowing the lumen of the airways to widen. The respiratory and cardiac systems have special receptors (alpha and beta receptors) in the muscle cells that help in speeding up or slowing down the respiratory and cardiac processes. The main action of bronchodilators in asthma and other respiratory diseases when the airways are constricted is to act like the body's own adrenaline, which binds to and stimulates the beta$_2$-adrenergic receptors within bronchial tube smooth muscle and allows them to relax. The most common class of drugs with this action are the beta$_2$-adrenergic agonists. (Recall from Chapter 3 that an agonist drug binds to its receptor and activates it.) Another class of drugs that allows relaxation of bronchial smooth muscle is the cholinergic antagonists. (Recall from Chapter 3 that an antagonist drug blocks a receptor rather than activates it.) Cholinergic drugs and agents (such as acetylcholine) have exactly the opposite action of adrenaline. So by giving a cholinergic antagonist, there is less acetylcholine present to interfere with the work of the body's adrenaline. This action allows natural adrenaline to bind to more beta$_2$-adrenergic receptors and causes relaxation of bronchial smooth muscle. They are also useful in decreasing the excessive thick and sticky secretions seen in chronic bronchitis.

Uses

The uses of bronchodilators in asthma and COPD depend on the drug's duration of action. **Short-acting beta$_2$-adrenergic agonists (SABAs)** are orally inhaled drugs that bind rapidly to beta$_2$-adrenergic receptors and can start smooth muscle relaxation within seconds to minutes. As a result, SABAs are used during an actual asthma attack and when the person with COPD has symptoms of bronchospasm. SABAs may also be used during other respiratory infections when patients experience bronchospasms. Thus SABAs are *reliever* drugs that act quickly. The effects also wear off quickly, and a person may need more than one dose to stop a bronchospasm or asthma attack. Examples of common SABAs are listed in Table 7.4.

> ### 🔝 Top Tip for Safety
>
> Teach patients with asthma to always have their SABA reliever drug with them at all times because an attack can occur anywhere and only an SABA can work fast enough to prevent a severe attack and death.

Some beta$_2$-adrenergic agonists are long-acting. Although they work in the same way as SABAs, they take time to build up an effect and the effect lasts longer. These **long-acting beta$_2$-adrenergic agonists (LABAs)** are orally inhaled drugs that bind over time to beta$_2$-adrenergic receptors and are used as asthma controller drugs that must be taken on a daily schedule to prevent bronchospasms and asthma attacks even when symptoms are not present. LABAs are not helpful during an acute attack because they take time to work. Examples of common LABAs are shown in Table 7.4. At times, so that patients have fewer drugs to take and remember, an LABA may be combined with an inhaled corticosteroid together in one inhaler. An example is Breo Ellipta, which is the LABA vilanterol combined with the inhaled corticosteroid fluticasone.

> ### 💡 Memory Jogger
>
> SABAs are reliever (rescue) drugs that are effective in stopping an actual asthma attack or bronchospasm. LABAs and cholinergic antagonists are controller (prevention) drugs and are not helpful during an asthma attack or bronchospasm.

> ### 💡 Memory Jogger
>
> Activated beta$_1$-adrenergic receptors and beta$_1$ agonist drugs increase heart rate, force of contraction, and speed of conduction (hint: you have only one [1] heart).
>
> Activated beta$_2$-adrenergic receptors and beta$_2$ agonist drugs cause bronchodilation (hint: you have two [2] lungs).
>
> Activated alpha-adrenergic receptors or alpha agonists cause vasoconstriction.

Cholinergic antagonists are also used as orally inhaled controller drugs. Their response is slower, but they work by relaxing the muscles around the airways so the airway can open wider and breathing is improved. Just like LABAs, cholinergic antagonists cannot stop an asthma attack or a bronchospasm once it has started. Examples of common cholinergic antagonists are shown in Table 7.4.

Xanthine-based drugs are an older type of bronchodilator that are given systemically and are rarely used because the dose that is effective is close to the dose that produces many dangerous side effects. This class of drug includes theophylline and aminophylline. They are used only when other types of management are not effective. Patients must have blood levels drawn frequently to ensure that the drug level is within the therapeutic range and not in the toxic range. The use of xanthines is not within the scope of this chapter.

Expected Side Effects

Orally inhaled bronchodilators usually have few and only mild side effects because most of the drug goes to the airways. The action of all types of bronchodilators results in the stimulation of both beta$_1$-adrenergic and beta$_2$-adrenergic receptors throughout the body, especially in the heart and blood vessels; therefore when bronchodilators are heavily used, common side effects include hypertension, tachycardia, headache, and insomnia. Some people feel "nervous" and may have tremors with these drugs. Dry mouth and a bad taste are common side effects. Cardiovascular side effects are more noticeable with the SABAs because the onset of action is so rapid.

Adverse Reactions

With inhalers that contain a preservative, patients may have allergic reactions (to the preservative). Also, if the bronchodilator is heavily used, it can be absorbed throughout the body and cause constriction of blood vessels in the heart muscle, leading to chest pain or even a myocardial infarction (heart attack).

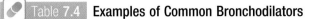 Table 7.4 **Examples of Common Bronchodilators**

Short-acting beta₂ agonists (SABAs): cause bronchodilation by rapidly binding to beta₂-adrenergic receptors in bronchial smooth muscle and stimulating muscle relaxation quickly, which widens the airways. These are *reliever/rescue* inhaled drugs used either during an asthma attack or just before engaging in activity that usually triggers an attack.	
DRUG/ADULT DOSAGE RANGE	**NURSING IMPLICATIONS**
albuterol (Apo-Salvent ✤, ProAir HFA, PMS-Salbutamol ✤, Respirol, Ventolin HFA, VoSpire ER) 1–2 inhalations (90 mcg each) every 4–6 hours PRN levalbuterol (Xopenex) 1–2 inhalations (45 mcg each) every 4–6 hours pirbuterol (Maxair) 2 inhalations (0.4 mg each) every 4–6 hours	• Teach patients to carry the drug with them at all times because it can stop or reduce a life-threatening asthma attack or bronchoconstriction. • Teach patient to monitor heart rate and other responses because excessive use causes rapid heart rate, nervousness, and tremors. • When taking this drug with other inhaled drugs, teach patients to use this drug first and wait at least 5 minutes before taking the other inhaled drugs to allow the bronchodilating effect to increase the movement of the other drugs into the lungs. • Teach patients to use the directions in Box 7.1 for correct technique to ensure the drug reaches the airways. • Instruct patients to use a spacer with the metered-dose inhalers (MDIs). If a spacer is not available, teach them to hold the mouthpiece 1–2 inches away from the mouth when the inhaler is activated and then to inhale the mist so that the drug reaches the airways and does not just stick to the back of the throat.
Long-acting beta₂ agonists (LABAs): cause bronchodilation by binding to beta₂-adrenergic receptors in bronchial smooth muscle over time and eventually stimulating continued smooth muscle relaxation. These are *controller/prevention* inhaled drugs used to prevent an asthma attack or bronchospasm. *LABAs are not to be used as a rescue drug.*	
DRUG/ADULT DOSAGE RANGE	**NURSING IMPLICATIONS**
arformoterol (Brovana) 15 mcg every 12 hours (1 vial) via nebulizer formoterol (Foradil, Oxeze, Perforomist) 12 mcg (one capsule) every 12 hours by DPI salmeterol (Serevent) 50 mcg (1 inhalation) every 12 hours by DPI	• Remind patients to use LABAs daily as prescribed, even when symptoms are not present, to prevent an asthma attack or bronchospasm. • Remind patients to *not* use LABAs as reliever/rescue drugs because their onset of action is too slow to help in an acute attack. • Teach patients using a dry-powder inhaler (DPI) to follow the instructions in Box 7.2 and the directions on the inhaler to ensure best effect of the drug.
Cholinergic antagonists: are inhaled controller drugs that cause bronchodilation by preventing the nervous system from releasing some acetylcholine, which then allows more of the body's own adrenaline to activate beta₂ receptors in bronchial smooth muscle.	
DRUG/ADULT DOSAGE RANGE	**NURSING IMPLICATIONS**
ipratropium (Atrovent) 2–4 inhalations (17 mcg each) over 6–8 hours tiotropium (Spiriva HandiHaler) 1 inhalation (18 mcg) every day by DPI tiotropium (Spiriva Respimat) 2 inhalations (2.5 mcg) daily by MDI	• Teach patients using an MDI to shake it well before using because the drug separates easily. • Teach patients to drink plenty of liquids because the drugs cause mouth dryness. • Teach patients about the expected side effects of stuffy nose, sore throat, and constipation because knowing the side effects helps relieve anxiety when they appear. • Instruct patients to report urinary retention or consistently increased heart rate to their healthcare provider because these are serious adverse effects of the drugs.

✤ Indicates Canadian drug.

Drug Interactions

Drug interactions may occur with MAOIs, tricyclic antidepressants, beta blockers (beta-adrenergic antagonists), other antihypertensive agents, digoxin, potassium-losing diuretics, and caffeine-containing herbs. The combination of two or more of these agents may produce an additive effect.

Many general anesthetics may cause dysrhythmias when they are used with these drugs. Nonselective beta blockers and beta-adrenergic blocking agents such as propranolol (Inderal) may block the bronchodilating effects of these beta₂ receptor–stimulating drugs. Bronchodilators can interfere with the action of some antihypertensive drugs.

❖ Nursing Implications and Patient Teaching

◆ *Assessment.* Ask whether the patient is pregnant, breast-feeding, or has a history of hyperthyroidism,

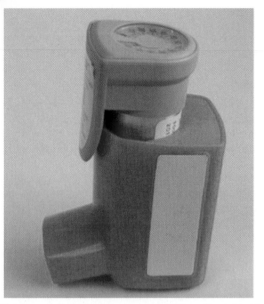

FIG. 7.3 Metered-dose inhalers with counter. (From Patel, M., Pilcher, J., Travers, J., et al. (2013). Use of Metered-Dose Inhaler Electronic Monitoring in a Real-World Asthma Randomized Controlled Trial. *The Journal of Allergy and Clinical Immunology: In Practice*, 1(1), 83–91.)

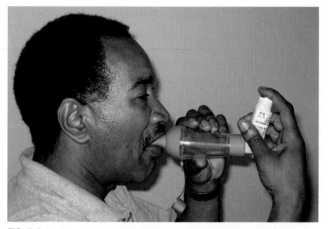

FIG. 7.4 Patient using an aerosol (metered-dose inhaler) with a spacer. (From Ignatavicius D, Workman ML, Rebar C: *Medical-surgical nursing*, ed 9, St. Louis, 2018, Elsevier.)

heart disease, hypertension, diabetes, glaucoma, seizures, or psychoneurotic disease. Ask whether the patient is taking other drugs that may interact with bronchodilators or has a history of allergy. Any of these conditions may present contraindications or precautions to the use of bronchodilators. Take a baseline set of vital signs to be able to assess for drug-related changes.

◆ *Planning and implementation.* Beta$_2$-adrenergic receptors in bronchial smooth muscle cells must be stimulated to relieve bronchial spasm. One of the drawbacks of bronchodilators is they may also stimulate receptors in the heart (beta$_1$), which increases the rate and force of cardiac contraction. Thus bronchodilators should be given with extreme caution to patients who already have cardiovascular, endocrine, or convulsive disorders that may be affected by these drugs.

The routes of administration of bronchodilators vary according to how ill the patient is (the diagnostic classification) and the preparation to be used. Drugs may be given parenterally, orally, or, most often, by oral inhalation (nebulizers or metered-dose inhalers [MDIs]). How well the orally inhaled drug works to control or relieve asthma and bronchospasm depends on correct use of the inhaler. Show a patient who is using an inhaler for the first time how to use the inhaler and give written instructions to refer to later. Research shows that many patients do not use inhalers correctly, so every time the patient comes in for a healthcare visit, ask for a demonstration of how the MDI is being used. Fig. 7.3 shows MDIs. Box 7.1 describes how to use an MDI, and Fig. 7.4 shows a patient using the inhaler with a spacer. Fig. 7.5 shows a typical dry-powder inhaler, and Box 7.2 describes how to use it. See Chapter 4 for instructions

regarding the use of a nebulizer to deliver orally inhaled drugs.

Irritation of the lung passages, mouth, and throat may occur with use of powdered drug forms or other inhaled agents. Rinsing the mouth with water after each treatment helps reduce this problem.

◆ *Evaluation.* Check the patient's pulse and blood pressure, and compare these findings with the baseline findings to assess whether the heart is affected by the drug. Response to therapy varies among patients. Assess for rate, depth, and ease of respiration to determine whether breathing problems have improved.

◆ *Patient and family teaching.* Tell the patient and family the following:

- Take the drug as directed by the healthcare provider and do not change the dose.
- Overuse of these drugs may result in severe side effects.
- Contact your healthcare provider if the drug is not helping your breathing problems.
- Contact your healthcare provider if bronchial irritation, dizziness, chest pain, insomnia, or any changes in symptoms occur.
- Drinking lots of fluid, especially water, makes the mucus thinner and helps the drug work better.
- Do not take any OTC drugs without first checking with your healthcare provider.
- To prevent exercise-induced bronchospasm, use your reliever bronchodilator inhaler 15 to 30 minutes before starting to exercise.
- Shake the inhaler well before using it.
- Follow the instructions for correct use of your inhaler.
- After using your inhaler, rinse your mouth with water to decrease dry mouth and bad taste.
- Keep a count of the total number of sprays used and discard the inhaler after 200 sprays or check the inhaler's counter to know when it is time to get a new one.
- For an MDI, clean the mouthpiece and dry it at least once a week.

Box 7.1   Teaching a Patient How to Correctly Use a Metered-Dose Inhaler

WITH A SPACER (PREFERRED TECHNIQUE)

1. Before each use, remove the caps from the inhaler and the spacer.
2. Insert the mouthpiece of the inhaler into the nonmouthpiece end of the spacer.
3. Shake the whole unit vigorously three or four times.
4. Fully exhale and then place the mouthpiece into your mouth, over your tongue, and seal your lips tightly around it.
5. Press down firmly on the canister of the inhaler to release one dose of the drug into the spacer.
6. Breathe in slowly and deeply. If the spacer makes a whistling sound, you are breathing in too rapidly.
7. Remove the mouthpiece from your mouth and, keeping your lips closed, hold your breath for at least 10 seconds and then breathe out slowly.
8. Wait at least 1 minute between puffs.
9. Replace the caps on the inhaler and the spacer.
10. At least once a day, clean the plastic case and cap of the inhaler by thoroughly rinsing in warm, running tap water; at least once a week, clean the spacer in the same manner.

WITHOUT A SPACER

1. Before each use, remove the cap and shake the inhaler according to the instructions in the package insert.
2. Tilt your head back slightly and breathe out fully.
3. Open your mouth and place the mouthpiece 1 to 2 inches away.
4. As you begin to breathe in deeply through your mouth, press down firmly on the canister of the inhaler to release one dose of the drug.
5. Continue to breathe in slowly and deeply (usually over 5–7 seconds).
6. Hold your breath for at least 10 seconds to allow the drug to reach deep into the lungs and then breathe out slowly.
7. Wait at least 1 minute between puffs.
8. Replace the cap on the inhaler.
9. At least once a day, remove the canister and clean the plastic case and cap of the inhaler by thoroughly rinsing in warm, running tap water.
10. Avoid spraying in the direction of your eyes.

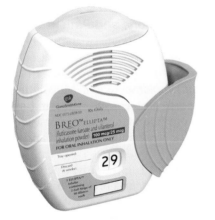

FIG. 7.5 Example of a dry-powder inhaler with a counter. (Courtesy GlaxoSmithKline.)

Box 7.2   Teaching a Patient How to Use a Dry-Powder Inhaler

FOR INHALERS THAT REQUIRE LOADING

First load the drug by:

- turning the device to the next dose of drug, or
- inserting the capsule into the device, or
- inserting the disk or compartment into the device.

AFTER LOADING THE DRUG AND FOR INHALERS THAT DO NOT REQUIRE DRUG LOADING

- Read your healthcare provider's instructions for how fast you should breathe for your particular inhaler.
- Exhale fully away from the inhaler.
- Place your lips over the mouthpiece and breathe in forcefully (there is no propellant in the inhaler; only your breath pulls the drug in).
- Remove the inhaler from your mouth as soon as you have breathed in.
- Never exhale (breathe out) into your inhaler. Your breath will moisten the powder, causing it to clump and not be delivered accurately.
- Never wash or place the inhaler in water.
- Never shake your inhaler.
- Keep your inhaler in a dry place at room temperature.
- If the inhaler is preloaded, discard it after it is empty.
- The drug is a dry powder and there is no propellant, so you may not feel, smell, or taste it as you inhale.

ANTI-INFLAMMATORY DRUGS

Anti-inflammatory drugs have a major role as controller drugs for asthma therapy and the inflammation associated with COPD. Leukotrienes and cromones are some of the drugs used, and they have been discussed earlier in this chapter. Corticosteroids work to slow or stop the inflammatory mediators histamine and leukotriene, and they work like the corticosteroid nasal spray discussed earlier in the Decongestants section. These are drugs that control asthma and COPD, and quite frequently they are combined with a long-acting inhaler. See Table 7.5 for commonly inhaled anti-inflammatory drugs used for asthma and COPD.

MUCOLYTICS AND ANTITUSSIVES

MUCOLYTICS

Action and Uses

Mucolytics, sometimes called *expectorants*, are drugs that decrease the thickness of respiratory secretions and aid

Table 7.5 Examples of Common Inhaled Corticosteroids

Inhaled corticosteroids: work to decrease inflamed airways by preventing mast cells and white blood cells within the respiratory mucosa from releasing histamine, leukotriene, and other mediators of inflammation. These drugs do *not* cause bronchodilation and should *not* be used as rescue drugs. An advantage is that the effects of inhaled corticosteroids are limited to the respiratory tract.

DRUG/ADULT DOSAGE RANGE	NURSING IMPLICATIONS
beclomethasone (QVAR) 1–2 inhalations (40 mcg each) twice daily by metered-dose inhaler budesonide (Pulmicort) 2 inhalations (180 mcg each) twice daily flunisolide (Aerospan HFA) 2 inhalations (80 mcg each) twice daily fluticasone (Flovent HFA, Flovent Diskus) 2 inhalations (80 mcg each) twice daily mometasone (Asmanex) 1 inhalation (220 mcg) once or twice daily	• Do not use in patients who have sputum that contains *Candida* or who have systemic fungal infections because these drugs reduce the immune responses. • Suggest that patients rinse their mouths after each use to minimize fungal infection of the mouth from immunosuppressive effects. • Warn patients that inhaled corticosteroids are not to be used to treat an acute asthma attack because they are not bronchodilators. • Teach patients to use these drugs daily as prescribed even when no symptoms are present because they are long-term controller drugs. • Advise patients to notify their healthcare professional if white patches in mouth or throat, or soreness and redness in mouth or throat appear because these are indications of infection. • Teach patients how to properly use the metered-dose and dry-powder inhalers (see Boxes 7.1 and 7.2) because improper use reduces drug effectiveness.

in their removal. It is believed they work by increasing the amount of fluid in the respiratory tract and may help break down or dissolve mucus, making removal of the secretions easier. Thinning the secretions promotes ciliary action and makes coughing more effective by increasing the amount of sputum available to spit out. Guaifenesin is a mucolytic drug contained in many combination OTC cough and cold products. It is available as a single agent both in OTC drugs (such as Mucinex, Robitussin, and Organidin NR) and in prescription-only products (such as Humibid LA and Touro EX tablets). The drug is available in immediate-release (e.g., oral solutions), extended-release, and combination immediate/extended-release formulations.

Guaifenesin is used to treat symptoms of productive cough. These drugs are also useful in COPD disease when thick mucus is a complication, and they are indicated in patients with coughs associated with viral upper respiratory tract infections. See Table 7.6 for a list of common mucolytic or expectorant drugs.

Lifespan Considerations

Pediatric

The FDA recommends that these products not be given to children younger than 2 years and some products not to children younger than 6 years because of cases of overdosage.

Expected Side Effects and Adverse Reactions

GI upset is a common adverse reaction to mucolytics. Dizziness, headache, and rash may also occur.

❖ Nursing Implications and Patient Teaching

◆ *Assessment.* Ask the patient about a history of cough, the presence of other respiratory disease or allergy, and the use of other drugs that may cause drug interactions.

◆ *Planning and implementation.* Mucolytics are not to be used for persistent cough without the advice of a healthcare provider. Chronic or persistent cough may be the result of a serious condition and should not be ignored.

In addition to drug therapy, teach patients to drink more fluid each day and breathe humidified air to help thin secretions. Suggest that they take the mucolytic with a full glass of water.

◆ *Evaluation.* Monitor the patient to ensure that secretions become thinner and are decreased. If the patient uses more than the recommended dosage, adverse reactions may occur.

◆ *Patient and family teaching.* Tell the patient and family the following:

• The purpose of mucolytics is to make the sputum more liquid and easier to spit out when you cough. The mucolytic drug alone will not make you stop coughing.

• Use a humidifier and drink at least 2 quarts of water daily while taking a mucolytic unless there is a medical reason for fluid restriction. These actions will help get the mucus out.

• Notify your healthcare provider if the cough is present with a high fever, rash, or persistent headaches, or if the cough returns once it has been under control.

• Use the drug only in the dosage recommended to decrease the odds of side effects.

• Take the drug with at least one full glass of water.

Table 7.6 Common Examples of Mucolytics and Antitussives

Mucolytics: thin respiratory secretions and reduce their stickiness. They also enhance the action of respiratory cilia. Both actions improve movement of mucus out of the airways.

DRUG/ADULT DOSAGE RANGE	NURSING IMPLICATIONS
guaifenesin (Mucinex; is also combined with many over-the-counter and prescription preparations for coughs and colds) 200–400 mg orally every 4 hours	• Ask patients with any side effects how much and how often they are taking the drug because when taken in recommended dosages, side effects are rare. • Ask patients about back pain and difficulty passing urine because high dosages are associated with the formation of kidney stones. • Instruct patients to notify the healthcare provider if symptoms have not improved within a few days or have worsened because these may indicate more serious respiratory problems.

Antitussives: suppress coughing by depressing the cough centers in the CNS, reducing the response to respiratory tract stretch receptor, or by reducing throat irritation.

DRUG/ADULT DOSAGE RANGE	NURSING IMPLICATIONS
benzonatate (Tessalon Perles, Zonatuss) 100 mg orally every 8 hours	• Tell patients to avoid driving or performing tasks that require concentration because this drug may cause sedation and dizziness. • Warn patients to swallow capsules whole because chewing them may result in an anesthetized throat that can make breathing and swallowing difficult and cause choking. • If using syrup, teach patients to avoid drinking water after swallowing because this action can dilute the drug and reduce its effectiveness. • Instruct patients to notify the healthcare provider if symptoms have not improved within a few days or have worsened because these may indicate more serious respiratory problems.
dextromethorphan (Delsym, Robitussin, Triaminic, many others) 10–20 mg orally every 4 hours PRN or 30 mg orally every 6–8 hours PRN	• Tell patients to avoid driving or performing tasks that require concentration because this drug may cause sedation and dizziness. • Warn parents not to give a child a higher dose or more often than prescribed because overdoses can cause dangerous CNS responses, respiratory depression, and seizures. • If using syrup, teach patients to avoid drinking water after swallowing because this action can dilute the drug and reduce its effectiveness. • Instruct patients to notify the healthcare provider if symptoms have not improved within a few days or have worsened because these may indicate more serious respiratory problems.
codeine-containing antitussives: promethazine and codeine (Pentazine with codeine, many others)	• Warn patients and families (especially of older adults) to check respiratory rate frequently because respiratory depression is possible. • Tell patients to watch for nausea and constipation because these are the most common side effects. • Tell patients to avoid driving or performing tasks that require concentration because this drug may cause sedation and dizziness. • Tell patients that physical addiction is rare, but possible, because codeine is an opioid. • Instruct patients to notify the healthcare provider if symptoms have not improved within a few days or have worsened because these may indicate more serious respiratory problems.

• To cough effectively, sit upright and take several deep breaths before trying to cough.
• Avoid driving or other activities that require alertness until you know how you respond to the drug because it may cause dizziness.

ANTITUSSIVES

Action and Uses

Antitussives are drugs that are used to relieve or suppress coughing. These drugs may act: (1) centrally on the cough center in the brain; (2) peripherally by anesthetizing stretch receptors in the respiratory tract; or (3) locally, primarily by soothing irritated areas in the throat. Products vary in their effectiveness. Antitussives are commonly combined with other drugs and are usually sold as OTC drugs. Antitussives containing controlled substances usually require a prescription, although some states may allow codeine combination products to be sold OTC if the patient signs for them.

The main action of an antitussive depends on whether an opioid antagonist is included. Narcotic or opioid antitussives suppress the cough reflex by acting directly on the cough center in the medulla of the brain. Nonopioid antitussives reduce the cough reflex at its source by anesthetizing stretch receptors in respiratory passages, lungs, and pleura, and by decreasing their activity.

Expected Side Effects, Adverse Reactions, and Drug Interactions

Common side effects of antitussives include drowsiness, dry mouth, nausea, and *postural hypotension* (low blood pressure resulting in dizziness when a person suddenly stands up). Some cough preparations contain a decongestant as well. Pseudoephedrine has been diverted for use as a substrate for the illegal synthesis of amphetamine and methamphetamine, so the sale and purchase of all OTC products containing pseudoephedrine or ephedrine, are controlled and must be signed for at the pharmacist counter. Those antitussives that contain codeine are also likely to cause constipation.

Opioid antitussives have an additive effect with other CNS depressants, so the dosage should be reduced.

❖ Nursing Implications and Patient Teaching

◆ *Assessment.* Ask the patient about allergy to antitussives, presence of COPD that may influence the patient's response to an opioid, possibility of pregnancy, and the use of other drugs or alcohol that may cause drug interactions. These conditions may be contraindications or precautions to the use of antitussives.

Ask about a history of a nonproductive cough or a prolonged and productive cough, which may keep the patient awake at night or cause muscular pain.

◆ *Planning and implementation.* Patients with allergy to these drugs or patients with COPD who have problems with breathing are not usually given opioid antitussives. Opioid antitussives may cause drug dependence. Some of the antitussives are schedule II controlled substances and thus will require a prescription written for no refills because the drugs may become abused.

These preparations may cause drowsiness, so teach the patient to avoid tasks that require alertness after taking the drug.

Antitussives are oral drugs that should be used only for short periods. Short therapy decreases the risk for rebound symptoms from prolonged use or the possibility of abuse.

◆ *Evaluation.* Check for therapeutic effects, including the cough stops or there is a decrease in frequency and duration of coughing spells, and the patient is able to sleep better at night. Also monitor the patient for adverse reactions and drug tolerance.

◆ *Patient and family teaching.* Tell the patient and family the following:

- Take the drug as prescribed and do not change the dose or frequency.
- Use caution when doing tasks that require alertness while taking an opioid antitussive because these drugs cause drowsiness.
- Overuse of the codeine-containing antitussives may cause severe constipation.
- Do not take opioid antitussives with alcohol or any other drugs that slow the CNS because the side effects will be intensified.
- Change positions slowly when getting up from a lying or sitting position because many antitussives occasionally cause light-headedness, dizziness, or fainting when you get up quickly.

Get Ready for the NCLEX® Examination!

Key Points

- Allergies can be caused by any substance (allergen) that is inhaled, swallowed, or touched. They are known as antigens by the immune system.
- IgE is the antibody that the immune system makes to counteract the allergen antigens; it releases histamine and leukotrienes to combat the antigens.
- Respiratory symptoms from the release of histamine and leukotrienes are runny nose, water, itchy eyes, rashes, sneezing, and wheezing caused by bronchoconstriction.
- Antihistamines, leukotriene inhibitors, and decongestants can ease the symptoms of allergies.
- Nasal decongestants (sympathomimetics) can cause rebound congestion and should not be used for more than 3 days.
- Asthma causes bronchoconstriction and difficulty breathing.
- Leukotriene inhibitors, bronchodilators, and anti-inflammatory drugs can help control asthma.

- COPD is a chronic disease involving upper and lower airways (bronchitis and emphysema).
- Short-acting bronchodilator agents (SABAs) are used as rescue drugs because they work immediately to relieve a bronchospasm or asthma attack.
- Patients with asthma should always carry an SABA.
- Long-acting bronchodilator agents (LABAs) are used to control the disease and must be used every day as directed to prevent an asthma attack.
- Bronchodilators should be used first when using multiple inhalers. There should be 5 minutes between the use of other inhalers.
- Teach patients the proper use of MDIs and DPIs as described in Boxes 7.1 and 7.2.
- Cortisone inhalers and nasal decongestants can cause fungal infections because they reduce the local immune responses.
- Cortisone inhalers are *not* rescue drugs and should be taken as prescribed every day to prevent asthma attacks and bronchospasms.

Get Ready for the NCLEX® Examination!—cont'd

- Mucolytic drugs thin secretions and must be taken with water and increased fluids.
- Teach patients to use cough suppressants only as needed to prevent secretions from building up.
- Cough suppressants can cause CNS depression.

Review Questions for the NCLEX® Examination

1. Which antibody is produced in response to an allergen?
   1. IgE
   2. IgG
   3. IgA
   4. IgM

2. Which antihistamine should be used only when necessary in the geriatric population?
   1. levocetirizine (Xyzal)
   2. diphenhydramine (Benadryl)
   3. fexofenadine (Allegra)
   4. loratadine (Claritin)

3. Which drug mimics the effect of the sympathetic nervous system?
   1. fluticasone furoate (Flonase Sensimist)
   2. nedocromil sodium (Tilade)
   3. phenylephrine (Sudafed PE)
   4. ipratropium (Atrovent)

4. Which drugs are most effective for an acute asthma attack? (Select all that apply.)
   1. beclomethasone (QVAR)
   2. albuterol (Ventolin)
   3. salmeterol (Serevent)
   4. levalbuterol (Xopenex)
   5. pirbuterol (Maxair)
   6. cromolyn sodium (Intal)

5. A patient received an albuterol (Ventolin) small-volume nebulizer treatment 15 minutes ago. Which symptom warrants a call to the healthcare provider?
   1. Increase in heart rate from 72 to 90
   2. Increase in oxygen saturation from 88% to 94%
   3. Increase in hand tremors
   4. Chest discomfort

6. Which drugs are considered long-acting beta agonists (LABAs)? (Select all that apply.)
   1. arformoterol (Brovana)
   2. cromolyn Sodium (Intal)
   3. formoterol (Foradil, Oxeze, Perforomist)
   4. levalbuterol (Xopenex)
   5. salmeterol (Serevent)
   6. albuterol (Ventolin)

7. Which symptoms can be expected when using a cholinergic antagonist like tiotropium (Spiriva)? (Select all that apply.)
   1. Constipation
   2. Dry mouth
   3. Diarrhea
   4. Watery eyes
   5. Dry eyes

8. A patient asks the nurse why he must use the bronchodilator inhaler before his corticosteroid inhaler. What is the nurse's best response?
   1. There is no risk of an allergic reaction occurring if the bronchodilator is used first.
   2. If the bronchodilator is not given first, a fungal infection of the mouth is likely to occur.
   3. Opening up the bronchioles with the bronchodilator first helps the corticosteroid inhaler be more effective.
   4. The side effects of the bronchodilator are reduced if it is given first.

9. Why should guaifenesin (Mucinex) be given with a full glass of water?
   1. To prevent the side effect of nausea and vomiting.
   2. To assist in liquefying secretions.
   3. To prevent the side effect of constipation.
   4. To prevent increased stomach acid from causing an ulcer.

10. The order reads: "diphenhydramine (Benadryl) 75 mg IM stat." Diphenhydramine (Benadryl) is supplied as 50 mg/1 mL ampules. How many mL of diphenhydramine should be given?

Case Study

Mary Brady, age 32 years, comes to the clinic today with an exacerbation of her asthma. She reports having coldlike symptoms for several days and has been using her albuterol inhaler every 4 hours. She is short of breath and has a nonproductive cough. Her controller drug is salmeterol (Serevent) 1 puff twice daily.

Mary is anxious, tremulous, and sitting on the edge of the chair as she leans forward. She has audible wheezes, and when she answers your questions, she does so at just four words at time before she has to take a breath.

Heart rate: 110
Respiratory rate: 34
SpO$_2$: 90% on FiO$_2$ 0.21 (room air)
Blood pressure: 140/90 mm Hg
Temperature: 37°C
Breath sounds: diminished with expiratory wheezes throughout all lung fields.

1. What is your priority concern for Mary Brady?

2. The healthcare provider orders oxygen via nasal cannula at 3 L and albuterol 2.5 mg small-volume nebulizer. The albuterol you have on hand is packaged as 1.25/3 mL. How many mL of albuterol will you give to the patient?

3. What nursing actions will you take before giving the albuterol?

Get Ready for the NCLEX® Examination!—cont'd

4. What nursing actions will you take during and after administration?

   One hour after she came to the office Mary's vital signs are:

   Heart rate: 88

   Respiratory rate: 22

   SpO$_2$: 95% on room air

   Temperature: 37°C

   Breath sounds: slightly diminished in the bases but clear throughout

   She is talking in full sentences and says she feels better.

   The healthcare provider gave Mary a prescription for oral prednisone to take for 2 weeks and a mometasone (Asmanex) inhaler 1 puff (220 mcg) once or twice daily. She is to continue her current long-acting and short-acting inhalers as prescribed.

5. Regarding Mary's salmeterol and albuterol, are there any questions you would want to ask Mary regarding her home regimen?

6. What patient education regarding mometasone will you give Mary?

7. What patient education regarding salmeterol will you give Mary?

8. What patient education regarding albuterol will you give Mary?

Drugs Affecting the Renal/Urinary and Cardiovascular Systems

http://evolve.elsevier.com/Visovsky/LPNpharmacology/

Learning Outcomes

1. List the names, actions, possible side effects, and adverse effects of diuretic drugs.
2. Explain what to teach patients and families about diuretic drugs.
3. List the names, actions, possible side effects, and adverse effects of drugs to treat benign prostatic hyperplasia and overactive bladder.
4. Explain what to teach patients and families about drugs to treat benign prostatic hyperplasia overactive bladder.
5. List the names, actions, possible side effects, and adverse effects of drugs for high blood cholesterol and drugs for high blood pressure.
6. Explain what to teach patients and families about drugs to treat high blood lipid levels and about drugs to treat high blood pressure.
7. List the names, actions, possible side effects, and adverse effects of drugs for angina and heart failure.
8. Explain what to teach patients and families about drugs to treat angina and heart failure.
9. List the names, actions, possible side effects, and adverse effects of drugs for dysrhythmias.
10. Explain what to teach patients and families about drugs to treat dysrhythmias.

Key Terms

adrenergics (ă-dră-NĔR-jĭks, p. 141) A category of drugs that affects nervous system control of various organs and tissues by activating or blocking receptors that respond to the body's natural adrenergic substances, epinephrine and norepinephrine.

alpha₁-adrenergic antagonist (ă-dră-NĔR-jĭk ăn-TĂ-gě-nĭst, p. 144) A type of adrenergic drug that lowers blood pressure by blocking the adrenergic receptor sites in blood vessel smooth muscle that, when activated, cause vasoconstriction and raise blood pressure.

alpha₂-adrenergic agonist (ă-dră-NĔR-jĭk Ă-gă-nĭst, p. 144) A type of adrenergic drug that works centrally (in the brain) to turn on special alpha2 receptors that, when normally activated, actually cause vasodilation and decrease blood pressure.

angiotensin-converting enzyme inhibitor (ACE-I) (ăn-jē-ō-TĔN(T)-sən kŭn-'VĔRT-ĭng ĔN-zīm ĭn-HĬ-bă-tĕrz, p. 139) A type of renin-angiotensin-aldosterone system drug that reduces high blood pressure by stopping the conversion of angiotensin I to angiotensin II (the hormone that causes the vasoconstriction and increased aldosterone).

angiotensin II receptor blocker (ARB) (ăn-jē-ō-TĔN(T)-sən rĭ-SĔP-tĕr, p. 139) A type of renin-angiotensin-aldosterone system drug that actually blocks the vasoconstrictor and aldosterone-secreting effects of angiotensin II to lower blood pressure by selectively blocking the binding of angiotensin II at receptor sites found in many tissues.

antidysrhythmic (ĂN-tī-dĭs-RĬTH-mĭk, p. 150) Drug that works to make heart rhythm more regular and reduce serious dysrhythmias.

antihyperlipidemic (ĂN-tī-hī-pĕr-lĭ-pă-DĒ-mĭk, p. 134) Drug that lowers blood lipid levels.

antihypertensive (ĂN-tī-hī-pĕr-TĔN(t)-sĭv, p. 139) Drug that has the main purpose of lowering blood pressure.

beta blocker (BĀ-tă, p. 141) Drug that works as an antagonist and blocks the activity of beta-adrenergic receptors. Its main action lowers blood pressure and slows heart rate.

calcium channel blockers (KĂL-sē-ĕm, p. 141) A class of antihypertensive drugs that lower blood pressure by reducing the effect of calcium in the heart muscle and in the smooth muscles of arteries.

diuretic (dī-yă-RĔ-tĭk, p. 126) Drug that has the main action of decreasing fluid volume by increasing urine output.

hydroxymethylglutaryl-coenzyme A (HMG-CoA) reductase inhibitors (statins) (rē-DŬK-tās ĭn-HĬ-bă-tĕrz, p. 135) Antihyperlipidemic drugs that lower blood low-density lipoprotein levels by slowing liver production of cholesterol.

inotropic drug (ĭ-nă-TRŌ-pĭk, p. 153) A drug that affects contractility of the myocardium. A positive inotropic drug increases contractility; a negative inotropic drug decreases contractility of the myocardium.

loop diuretic (lūp dī-yă-RĔ-tĭk, p. 127) Drug that increases urine output by blocking active transport of chloride, sodium, and potassium in the thick ascending loop of Henle.

nitrates (NĪ-trāts, p. 147) A class of drugs that relax (dilate) peripheral veins and reduce resistance to blood flow in the arteries.

potassium-sparing diuretics (pă-TĂ-sē-ĕm, p. 127) Drugs that increase the excretion of water and sodium through increased urine output without the loss of potassium in the urine.

renin-angiotensin-aldosterone system (RAAS) drugs (RĔ-nĕn ăn-jē-ō-TĔN(T)-sən ăl-dō-STĔR-ōn, p. 140) Drugs that include angiotensin-converting enzyme inhibitors and angiotensin II receptor blockers that have the effect of interfering with the action of angiotensin II and aldosterone.

thiazides and thiazide-like sulfonamides diuretics (THĪ-ă-zīds, p. 126) Drugs that increase urine output by preventing water, sodium, potassium, and chloride from being reabsorbed into the blood through the walls of the nephron.

urinary antispasmodic (YŪR-ă-nĕr-ē ĂN-tī-spăz-MĂ-dĭk, p. 132) Drug that reduces overactive bladder symptoms by relaxing the bladder muscle.

vasodilators (vă-zō-DĪ-lā-tĕrs, p. 145) A class of drugs that act directly on the smooth muscle in the blood vessel walls to cause them to dilate (widen or relax).

The renal/urinary system works together with the cardiovascular system to maintain adequate circulation to all parts of the body. The interactions between these two systems help to maintain fluid balance, delivery of nutrients, and removal of waste products from cells, tissues, and organs. Most drugs that affect one system have an effect on the functioning of the other system.

DRUGS THAT AFFECT THE RENAL/URINARY SYSTEM

The renal/urinary system consists of two kidneys, two ureters, the bladder, and the urethra (Fig. 8.1). The kidneys act as a filter for the blood that circulates throughout the cardiovascular system. The renal/urinary system (kidneys and bladder) controls how much blood is in the body and the content of the fluid portion of the blood because of its close connection with the cardiovascular system. Although the kidneys do not regulate what comes into the body, they balance all body fluids and the blood by carefully controlling which substances remain in the body versus which substances

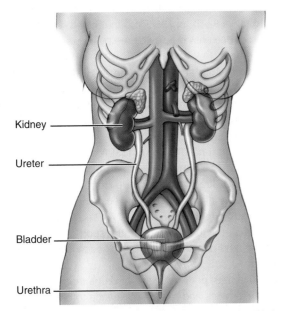

FIG. 8.1 The urinary system. (From Herlihy B: *The human body in health and illness*, ed 5, St. Louis, 2014, Elsevier.)

Labels: Kidney, Ureter, Bladder, Urethra

leave the body. In a sense, the kidneys act like a "washing machine" for the blood, removing wastes, excess substances, and extra fluid. Most drugs that affect the renal/urinary system change how much water and other substances are retained by the body or excreted in the urine.

DIURETICS

Diuretics are drugs that have the main action of decreasing fluid volume by increasing urine output. Although their site of action is the kidney, diuretics are chiefly used for cardiovascular problems such as high blood pressure (HBP; *hypertension*) and heart failure, rather than for kidney problems. Diuretics typically work well, are safe, are well tolerated by the patient, and are generally cost-effective.

Diuretics are usually classified into four groups: thiazides (e.g., chlorothiazide and hydrochlorothiazide), the thiazide-like sulfonamides (e.g., metolazone and indapamide), loop diuretics (e.g., furosemide and bumetanide), and the potassium-sparing diuretics (e.g., amiloride, triamterene, and spironolactone). The most effective diuretics are those that work at the ascending loop of Henle in the nephron (Fig. 8.2).

> ### Memory Jogger
> The four main categories of diuretics are:
> - thiazide diuretics
> - thiazide-like sulfonamide diuretics
> - loop diuretics
> - potassium-sparing diuretics

Actions

Thiazides and thiazide-like sulfonamide diuretics work at the end of the ascending loop of Henle and the beginning of the *distal convoluted tubule* in the nephron (see Fig. 8.2). This class of drugs increases urine output by preventing water, sodium, potassium, and chloride from going through the walls of the nephron to be reabsorbed back into the blood. They are not reabsorbed, so the water and electrolytes stay within the tubules, making their way through the renal system into the

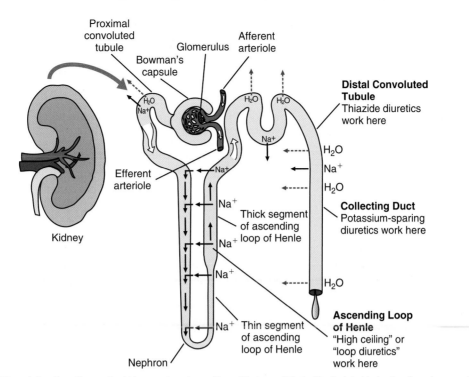

FIG. 8.2 Sites of diuretic action on the kidney and nephron. (From Workman ML, LaCharity LA: *Understanding pharmacology*, ed 2, St. Louis, 2016, Elsevier.)

bladder and then being excreted from the body. Thiazide and thiazide-like drugs are the most commonly used type of diuretic and often are first line in the management of HBP.

Over the long term, thiazides also act to dilate the smooth muscles in the arterioles, the smallest vessels in the arterial system. The heart does not have to work so hard to pump blood into the vascular system because the arterioles are dilated. See Table 8.1 for the dosages and nursing implications of selected thiazide diuretics.

> ### Lifespan Considerations
> **Pregnancy and Breast-Feeding**
>
> Thiazide diuretics are approved for use during pregnancy and may be used in low doses for breast-feeding mothers without adverse effects on the infant. More powerful diuretics are usually not recommended during pregnancy unless essential for the mother's health. High doses of diuretics for breast-feeding women may suppress lactation.

Loop diuretics are drugs that increase urine output by blocking active transport of chloride, sodium, and potassium in the thick *ascending loop of Henle* (see Fig. 8.2). Loop diuretics are widely considered the most powerful of the diuretics. Use can result in significant decreases in fluid volume and increase in urine output. Loop diuretics are used in a variety of conditions including heart failure, pulmonary edema, and cirrhosis of the liver with ascites. Potassium is one of the major electrolytes that can be lost after loop diuretic administration. Therefore monitor

potassium levels carefully because significant changes in potassium can result in cardiac dysrhythmias. See Table 8.1 for the dosages and nursing implications of selected loop diuretics.

> ### Memory Jogger
>
> Water always follows sodium. Diuretics that work by increasing sodium excretion in the urine always increase the water in urine output.

Potassium-sparing diuretics increase the excretion of water and sodium, leading to increased urine output without the loss of potassium. They are called *potassium-sparing* because they do not "waste" potassium, which often occurs with thiazide and loop diuretics. Potassium-sparing diuretics act by slowing the sodium pump in the *collecting duct* of the nephron so that more sodium and water are excreted as urine (see Fig. 8.2). See Table 8.1 for the dosages and nursing implications of selected potassium-sparing diuretics.

> ### Lifespan Considerations
> **Older Adults: Diuretics**
>
> Older adult patients are more likely to develop postural hypotension, confusion, low potassium levels (*hypokalemia*) (except with potassium-sparing diuretics), and increased serum glucose levels when on diuretics. Lower dosages may be required based on patient responses. Monitor older adults on diuretics more frequently for dehydration and symptoms of low potassium levels (*hypokalemia*), such as muscle weakness and irregular heartbeats.

Table 8.1   Common Diuretics

Thiazides: These drugs work to lower blood pressure by increasing urine output by preventing water, sodium, potassium, and chloride from going through the walls of the nephron to be reabsorbed back into the blood. They also dilate arterioles by relaxing the smooth muscle in these blood vessel walls.

DRUGS/ADULT DOSAGE RANGE	NURSING IMPLICATIONS
chlorothiazide (Diuril) 500–1000 mg orally once or twice daily hydrochlorothiazide (Esidrix, Ezide, Hydrodiuril, Oretic, Zide) 12.5–50 mg orally daily	• Weigh the patient daily while he or she is taking diuretics to monitor trends and prevent dehydration. • In the acute care setting, monitor intake and output to make sure that the patient achieves fluid balance. • Monitor potassium levels to assess that they are within normal levels because these drugs reduce blood potassium levels. • Monitor the patient's basic metabolic panel (BMP) to check for abnormal electrolytes, blood urea nitrogen (BUN), and/or creatinine. These laboratory tests can indicate fluid and electrolyte imbalance or kidney problems. • Report potassium levels below normal to the healthcare provider because low potassium levels can have serious effects on muscles and breathing. • Inform the healthcare provider if your patient has a history of gout because thiazide diuretics can cause a flare-up. • If the patient has diabetes, monitor his or her glucose level carefully because diuretics can cause elevated blood sugar. • Hold diuretics if patients have a blood pressure less than 90/60 mm Hg because this can be a symptom of dehydration or other adverse effects.

Thiazide-like sulfonamides: Like the thiazide diuretics, these drugs lower blood pressure by preventing water, sodium, potassium, and chloride from going through the walls of the nephron to be reabsorbed back into the blood. They also dilate arterioles by relaxing the smooth muscle in these blood vessel walls.

DRUGS/ADULT DOSAGE RANGE	NURSING IMPLICATIONS
indapamide (Lozol) 1.25–2.5 mg orally daily metolazone (Zaroxolyn) 2.5–5 mg orally daily	• Weigh the patient daily while he or she is taking diuretics to monitor trends and prevent dehydration. • Monitor potassium levels to assess that they are within normal levels because these drugs reduce blood potassium levels. • Report potassium levels less than 3.5 mEq/L or 3.5 mmol/L to the healthcare provider because low potassium levels can have serious effects on heart rhythm.

Loop diuretics: Loop diuretics work to increase urine output by blocking active transport of chloride, sodium, and potassium in the thick ascending loop of Henle.

DRUGS/ADULT DOSAGE RANGE	NURSING IMPLICATIONS
bumetanide (Bumex) 0.5–2 mg orally. 0.5–1.0 mg IM to maximum of 10 mg per day furosemide (Delone, Lasix) 20–120 mg orally daily; 20–40 mg IM	• Side effects are more severe with loop diuretics than other diuretics because drugs in this class are the most powerful diuretics. • Watch for symptoms of low potassium including dry mouth, increased thirst, muscle cramps, fatigue, weakness, and mood changes, because low potassium levels can have serious effects on muscles and breathing. • Report potassium levels less than 3.5 mEq/L or 3.5 mmol/L to the healthcare provider because low potassium levels can have serious effects on heart rhythm. • Remind the patient to stand up slowly to avoid orthostatic hypotension. • Notify the healthcare provider if the patient reports decreased hearing or a ringing in the ears because loop diuretics can be *ototoxic* (can damage hearing). Discontinuing the drug typically reverses the changes in hearing. • Monitor blood glucose in patients with diabetes because these drugs can cause hyperglycemia. • Check and record urine output to make sure the drug is working properly. You may need to empty the Foley catheter more frequently. • Urination typically occurs within 1 hour, so inform the patient that he or she will need to be close to a bathroom to avoid urinary urgency or incontinence.

Table 8.1   Common Diuretics—cont'd

Potassium-sparing diuretics: These drugs increase the excretion of water and sodium, leading to increased urine output without the loss of potassium. They act by slowing the sodium pump in the distal tubule of the nephron so more sodium and water is excreted as urine.

DRUGS/ADULT DOSAGE RANGE	NURSING IMPLICATIONS
amiloride (Midamor) 5–10 mg orally daily spironolactone (Aldactone) 50–100 mg orally once or in divided doses triamterene (Dyrenium) 50–100 mg twice daily	• Monitor potassium levels to assess whether they are within normal levels because higher-than-normal blood potassium levels can occur with these drugs. • Report potassium levels greater than 5.0 mEq/L or 5.0 mmol/L to the healthcare provider because high potassium levels can cause dangerous cardiac problems. • Teach patients signs of a high potassium level, including confusion, irregular heartbeat, nervousness, numbness or tingling in the hands or feet, unusual fatigue, and a heavy feeling in the legs. • Teach patients to stand up slowly to avoid orthostatic hypotension because these drugs decrease fluid volume and decrease blood pressure. • Teach the patient to avoid foods high in potassium (see Box 8.1) to prevent hyperkalemia. • Remind patients to avoid salt substitutes because they are often high in potassium.

Uses

Healthcare providers prescribe diuretics for a variety of conditions including HBP, heart failure, and cirrhosis of the liver. They are typically used in conditions that require a decrease in edema (decrease in fluid volume). Diuretics can sometimes increase the excretion of other drugs in cases of overdose (such as aspirin).

Expected Side Effects

Common side effects of diuretics include urinary urgency and urinary frequency. Other expected side effects include dry mouth, increased thirst, and light-headedness. Fluid and electrolyte imbalances are a common side effect of diuretics. Thiazide diuretics can cause an increase in uric acid, which can cause flare-ups of gout in certain patients. See Table 8.1 for specific dosages and nursing implications associated with each specific class of diuretics.

Adverse Effects

Diuretics increase urine output, so *dehydration* is one of the major adverse effects. Signs and symptoms of dehydration include increased heart rate, low blood pressure, decreased urine output or dark yellow urine, dry mouth with a sticky coating on the tongue, and tenting of the chest or the forehead (if you pinch the skin, the skin remains like a tent when you release the skin). Thiazides and loop diuretics can cause severe *hypokalemia* (low potassium), whereas potassium-sparing diuretics can cause *hyperkalemia* (high potassium). Signs of hypokalemia include muscle cramping, abnormal heart rhythm, and changes in reflexes. Signs of hyperkalemia include confusion, irregular heartbeat, numbness of the hands or feet, and a feeling of heaviness in the legs.

Loss of sodium can cause confusion, irritability, fatigue, and even seizures in some patients. A major adverse effect of all diuretics is severe low blood pressure that can result in falls, particularly in high-risk and older patients.

Drug Interactions

Increased loss of potassium can result from use of thiazide or loop diuretics if the patient is taking corticosteroids or certain antibiotics. For patients with bipolar illness using lithium, the loss of sodium caused by diuretics can increase the risk for lithium toxicity. Potassium-sparing diuretics with angiotensin-converting enzyme inhibitors (ACE-Is) or angiotensin receptor blockers (ARBs) can lead to hyperkalemia. Patients taking potassium-sparing diuretics should avoid salt substitutes to decrease the risk for hyperkalemia.

Top Tip for Safety

Potassium levels that are too high or too low can cause life-threatening dysrhythmias.

❖ Nursing Implications and Patient Teaching

◆ *Assessment.* Make sure to assess the patient for changes in vital signs (particularly a decrease in blood pressure). Assess the patient carefully for any signs of dehydration before giving any diuretic. Monitor daily weight for changes from a baseline weight (the patient's normal weight). If the patient's weight is below his or her normal weight, contact the healthcare provider before giving the diuretic. Check the patient's most recent potassium level. If the level is below the normal range (can be caused by thiazide or loop diuretics) or above the normal range (can be caused by potassium-sparing diuretics), make sure to contact the healthcare provider before you give the drug.

◆ *Planning and implementation.* Give the diuretics in the morning to avoid disturbing the patient's sleep at night. Be sure to tell patients that they will most likely experience urinary frequency and urgency, and thus should be near a bathroom or have access to a urinal or bedside commode after taking the drug. Also, make sure that they know to ask for help when getting up if needed. Tell patients to notify you if they have any weakness, muscle cramping, numbness or tingling in the extremities, or sensation of irregular heartbeat because these may be symptoms of a decrease in potassium level.

Continue to monitor trends in daily weight and blood pressure while the patient is taking diuretics. For thiazides and loop diuretics, teach patient to eat foods high in potassium (Box 8.1). For patients taking potassium-sparing diuretics, teach patients to *avoid* foods high in potassium (see Box 8.1).

◆ *Patient and family teaching.* Tell the patient and family the following:

• Take the drug exactly as prescribed. Do not skip or double doses.
• Doses are best taken early in the day to avoid affecting sleep at night.
• If you are taking a thiazide or loop diuretics, include several high-potassium foods in the diet every day.
• If you are taking a potassium-sparing diuretic, avoid foods high in potassium.
• Use sunscreen and protective clothing to avoid skin irritation and sunburn because of photosensitivity.
• Report any signs of abnormal potassium levels such as muscle cramping, weakness, numbness or tingling in the extremities, or sensation of irregular heartbeat to your healthcare provider.

• Daily weight will be helpful to monitor if there is any change in fluid levels above or below your normal weight. Notify your healthcare provider if you experience any unintentional weight loss or weight gain.
• If you are taking a diuretic for your blood pressure, remember that HBP is not cured by drugs, so do not stop taking the drug without consulting a healthcare provider.
• Avoid taking any over-the-counter (OTC) drugs without discussing with your healthcare provider to avoid a drug interaction.

DRUGS FOR BENIGN PROSTATIC HYPERPLASIA

Benign prostatic hyperplasia (BPH) is a noncancerous growth of the prostate gland frequently seen as men age. When the prostate gland becomes large enough, the patient can have problems urinating because the prostate puts pressure on the bladder and urethra (Fig. 8.3). Drugs used in the management of BPH are the alpha$_1$-adrenergic receptor blockers that relax the smooth muscle of the prostate and bladder outlet and the testosterone inhibitors that shrink the prostate. Both types of drug can help the patient pass urine more easily. See Table 8.2 for the dosages and nursing implications of selected drugs to treat BPH.

BLADDER ANESTHETICS

Bladder anesthetics are drugs that, when taken orally, are excreted into the urine and act as a local anesthetic on the mucous membranes of the urinary tract. The only drug in this class is phenazopyridine. Phenazopyridine can control symptoms of urinary irritation including burning, pain, and urinary frequency that often results from an acute urinary tract infection (like an "aspirin for the bladder"). The usual adult dosage is 200 mg

Box 8.1	Sources of High and Very High Potassium Foods	
CATEGORY	**HIGH (200–300 MG/SERVING)**	**VERY HIGH (>300 MG/SERVING)**
Fruits	Apricots (canned) Oranges (1 medium) Orange juice Peaches, fresh, 1 medium	Bananas, 1 small Mango, 1 medium Dried fruits, $\frac{1}{4}$ cup Prune juice
Vegetables	Asparagus, 4 spears Beets, fresh or cooked Brussel sprouts Okra	Beet greens, $\frac{1}{4}$ cup Black beans, cooked ($\frac{1}{2}$ cup) Potatoes with skin, baked potato, $\frac{1}{2}$ medium Baby carrots (10 pieces) Sweet potatoes, yams
Miscellaneous	Peanut butter, 2 tablespoons Nuts and seeds, 1 ounce Chocolate, 1.5 ounce bar Salmon, canned, 3 ounces	Bouillon, low sodium, 1 cup Milk, chocolate, 1 cup Pizza, 2 slices Salt substitute, $\frac{1}{4}$ teaspoon Yogurt, 6 ounce Milkshake, 1 cup Cappuccino, 1 cup

Modified from Mahan, L. Kathleen, Raymond, Janice: *Krause's food & the nutrition care process*, 14th ed. Elsevier, St. Louis (2017); also used list from USDA Food Composition Database https://ndb.nal.usda.gov/ndb/search/list

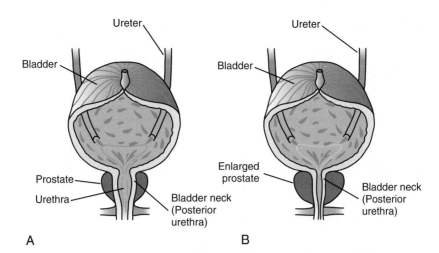

FIG. 8.3 (A) Normal prostate gland. (B) Enlarged prostate gland showing the narrowing of the urethra, decreasing urine flow. (From Workman ML, LaCharity LA: *Understanding pharmacology*, ed 2, St. Louis, 2016, Elsevier.)

Table 8.2   Common Drugs for Benign Prostatic Hyperplasia

Dihydrotestosterone (DHT) inhibitors: These drugs shrink the prostate by working as a "counterfeit" drug that looks like testosterone and binds to the enzyme that normally converts testosterone to DHT, its most powerful form. With less DHT in the prostate, the cells do not receive the signal to grow. As a result, the gland shrinks and puts less pressure on the urethra, allowing better urine flow.

DRUGS/ADULT DOSAGE RANGE	NURSING IMPLICATIONS
dutasteride (Avodart) 0.5 mg orally once daily finasteride (Proscar, Propecia) 5 mg orally once daily	• Teach patients that the most common side effect of these drugs is a decreased interest in sexual activity because knowing about the side effects reduces anxiety when they appear. • Instruct patients to report breast enlargement, nipple drainage, or pain in the testicles to their healthcare provider because these drugs may affect other hormones and sex tissues. • Warn patients and family members that pregnant women should not handle or touch these drugs because they can cause birth defects when absorbed through the skin. • Teach men who are having sex with a pregnant woman to wear a condom to prevent exposure to the fetus because this drug is present in seminal fluid.

Selective alpha₁ blockers: Relax smooth muscle tissue in the prostate gland, the neck of the bladder, and the urethra by binding to the alpha₁-adrenergic receptors in these tissues. When the receptors are activated, the smooth muscle constricts, tightening the prostate, which increases the pressure and squeezes the urethra. When these receptors are bound with selective alpha₁ blockers, the smooth muscle relaxes, placing less pressure on the urethra and improving urine flow.

DRUGS/ADULT DOSAGE RANGE	NURSING IMPLICATIONS
alfuzosin (Uroxatral) 10 mg orally once daily silodosin (Rapaflo) 8 mg orally once daily tamsulosin (Flomax) 0.4–0.8 mg orally once daily 30 minutes after a meal terazosin (Hytrin) 1—10 mg orally once daily at bedtime	• Ask patients who are taking tamsulosin whether they have an allergy to sulfa drugs because tamsulosin is made from a sulfonamide and may cause an allergic reaction in patients who are allergic to sulfa drugs. • Teach patients that the most common side effect of these drugs is a decreased interest in sexual activity because knowing about the side effects reduces anxiety when they appear. • Warn patients to change positions slowly because these drugs lower blood pressure and can cause dizziness.

orally three times daily after meals for 2 days. Warn patients that this drug turns the urine an orange-red color that can stain the toilet and clothing. Phenazopyridine does not treat the cause of the irritation to the bladder. It is not an antibiotic and cannot cure a urinary tract infection when used alone.

Top Tip for Safety

Phenazopyridine can be used a maximum of 2 days. If the patient is still having symptoms of bladder irritation after 2 days, notify the healthcare provider.

DRUGS FOR OVERACTIVE BLADDER

An overactive bladder (OAB) is a problem in which the person has a sudden, urgent need to urinate. In OAB, the *detrusor* muscle (bladder wall muscle) contracts before the bladder is full (Fig. 8.4). Often the person with OAB feels an urgent need to urinate (*urgency*) and may lose bladder control before reaching a toilet (*urinary incontinence*). Although OAB can occur in men and women, the problem is more common in women. Prevalence increases with age and can significantly affect quality of life.

Drugs prescribed for OAB are **urinary antispasmodics**, which improve symptoms and reduce incontinence by decreasing bladder muscle spasms. See Table 8.3 for the dosages and nursing implications of selected urinary antispasmodics.

DRUGS THAT AFFECT THE CARDIOVASCULAR SYSTEM

The primary purpose of the cardiovascular system is to supply oxygenated blood that includes water (plasma), nutrients, and hormones to tissues and organs, and remove carbon dioxide and waste products for elimination. Any breakdown in cardiovascular functioning can lead to uncomfortable symptoms, decreased quality of life, and even death if not managed carefully.

The cardiovascular system consists of the heart and blood vessels working together to move blood throughout the body. Using specialized cardiac muscle and nerve systems, electrical impulses cause the heart muscle to contract, pumping blood from the heart into the aorta

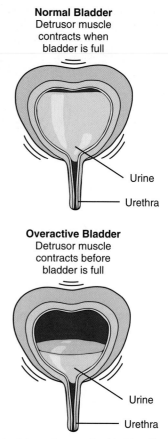

Normal Bladder
Detrusor muscle contracts when bladder is full

Urine
Urethra

Overactive Bladder
Detrusor muscle contracts before bladder is full

Urine
Urethra

FIG. 8.4 Pathophysiology of overactive bladder. (From Workman ML, LaCharity LA: *Understanding pharmacology*, ed 2, St. Louis, 2016, Elsevier.)

Table 8.3   Common Drugs for Overactive Bladder

Urinary antispasmodics: inhibit involuntary nerve-induced contractions of the detrusor muscle in the bladder wall, allowing the bladder to relax and hold more urine without the strong urge to urinate.

DRUGS/ADULT DOSAGE RANGE	NURSING IMPLICATIONS
oxybutynin (Ditropan) 5 mg orally two to three times daily oxybutynin (Ditropan XL) 5 mg orally once daily oxybutynin transdermal patch (Oxytrol) 3.9 mg/day applied transdermally every 3–4 days tolterodine (Detrol) 2 mg orally twice daily tolterodine (Detrol LA) 4 mg orally once daily solifenacin (Vesicare) 5–10 mg orally once daily darifenacin (Enablex) 7.5–15 mg orally once daily trospium chloride (Sanctura) 20 mg orally twice daily 1 hour before meals or on an empty stomach trospium chloride (Sanctura XR) 60 mg once daily 1 hour before breakfast	• Tell patients that common side effects include dry mouth, dry eyes, headache, and constipation because knowing the expected side effects reduces anxiety. • Teach patients to check their heart rates at least once daily and report irregularities or chest pain because these are symptoms of an adverse reaction. • Remind patients to avoid taking antihistamines with these drugs because the combination can cause urinary retention and/or constipation. • Teach patients to weigh themselves and report weight gain (more than 2 lb/day) or increased swelling to the prescriber because these drugs can cause urinary retention and heart failure. • Remind patients to avoid becoming overheated or dehydrated during exercise or hot weather because these drugs decrease sweating and increase the risk for heatstroke. • Teach patients to avoid consuming alcohol within 2 hours of these drugs because side effects such as drowsiness are increased. • Teach patients to avoid driving or any other activities that require clear vision until they know how the drugs will affect them because this class of drugs can cause blurred vision. • Teach patients using the transdermal patch system to remove the old patch before applying a new one to prevent drug overdoses.

to the arteries (Fig. 8.5). The oxygenated blood moves through the arteries to the arterioles, then to capillaries, where oxygen exchanges with carbon dioxide. The deoxygenated blood moves from the capillaries to the venules, then to the larger veins and back into the vena cava, where it returns to the heart.

Healthcare providers use a variety of approaches to prevent symptoms, manage symptoms, or treat abnormalities in the cardiovascular system. Some "cardiovascular" drugs help to prevent high cholesterol levels from narrowing arteries, others to treat HBP, and still others to manage symptoms associated with diseases of the heart itself.

We will address some of the most common cardiovascular drugs that you might see in practice to give you the best overview of how these drugs can help provide the best health and quality of life possible for your patients. As we do this, we will proceed from

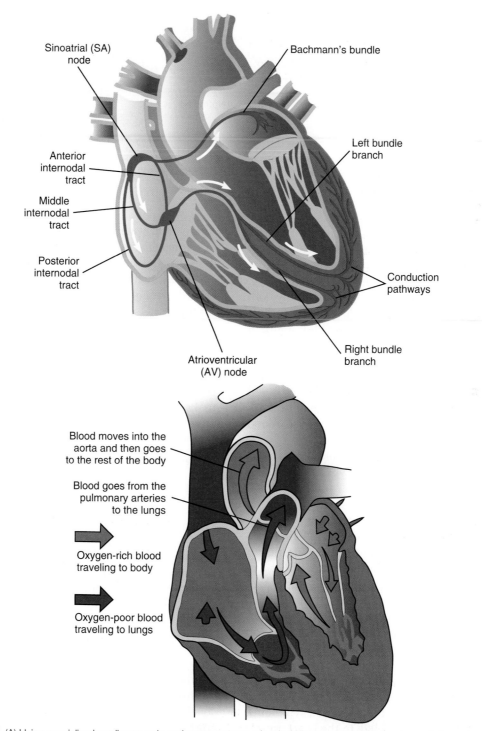

FIG. 8.5 (A) Using specialized cardiac muscle and nerve systems, electrical impulses cause the heart muscle to contract. (B) This results in blood pumping from the heart into the aorta to the arteries. (From Workman ML, LaCharity LA: *Understanding pharmacology*, ed 2, St. Louis, 2016, Elsevier.)

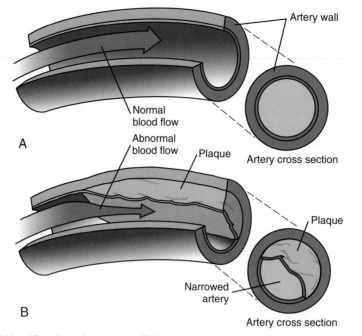

FIG. 8.6 (A) Normal blood flow through the artery. (B) Artery obstructed by atherosclerotic plaque. Note the restricted blood flow through the artery. (From Workman ML, LaCharity LA: *Understanding pharmacology*, ed 2, St. Louis, 2016, Elsevier.)

drugs typically used to reduce risk for cardiovascular disease to those drugs that treat cardiovascular disease.

Two major risk factors for cardiovascular disease are high levels of blood lipids (*hyperlipidemia*) and HBP (hypertension). Effective drug therapy can modify both of these risk factors. High levels of blood lipids, including cholesterol, can lead to thickening of the lining of arteries with fatty plaque, a condition called *atherosclerosis* (Fig. 8.6). Eventually atherosclerosis blocks some blood flow through the arteries. In combination with HBP, greater amounts of plaque occur with further blood vessel narrowing. As a result, the heart has to work harder to pump blood through the narrowed blood vessels.

Decreased blood flow through the coronary arteries that supply the heart muscle with oxygen can result in *ischemia* (lack of oxygen to the tissue) and pain called *angina*. To treat angina, select cardiovascular drugs can dilate (widen) the coronary arteries, thereby getting blood and oxygen to the heart muscle. If the blood flow is severely impaired through the coronary arteries or if a clot forms in a coronary artery, the patient can experience a *myocardial infarction* (heart attack) that results from a severe lack of oxygen to the heart muscle.

Over time, the ability of the heart to pump decreases in patients with prolonged HBP and/or changes in heart muscle resulting from a myocardial infarction. The decreased ability of the heart to pump effectively is called *heart failure*. Heart failure is managed by using a variety of cardiovascular drugs to improve the ability of the heart to pump and reduce the associated symptoms.

An additional result of damage to the heart muscle from HBP and atherosclerosis is changes within electrical conduction system of the heart. These changes can result in *dysrhythmias* (abnormal heart rhythms). The dysrhythmias can cause significant decreases in cardiac output and even death if not managed effectively. A number of cardiovascular drugs are used to restore normal heart rhythms.

In summary, the cardiovascular drug groups that we will discuss in this chapter include cholesterol-lowering drugs, blood pressure–lowering drugs, blood vessel dilators (antianginals), drugs to improve heart muscle contraction (positive inotropic drugs), and drugs to make electrical conduction through the heart more regular (antidysrhythmics). At times a patient may be taking drugs from a variety of cardiovascular drug categories.

> **Memory Jogger**
>
> The most common types of cardiovascular drugs are:
> - antihyperlipidemics
> - antihypertensives
> - drugs for angina
> - drugs for heart failure
> - antidysrhythmics

ANTIHYPERLIPIDEMICS

Hyperlipidemia is the condition of high levels of *lipids*, primarily cholesterol, and other fatty acids in the blood. **Antihyperlipidemics** are drugs that lower blood cholesterol levels. The body needs a certain amount of cholesterol for healthy cell membranes, hormones, vitamin D, and bile acids, so it is a normal and vital part of blood plasma.

The liver produces much of the body's cholesterol. Therefore when you think about cholesterol levels, you need to recognize that the levels are a combination of the cholesterol ingested in the diet and the cholesterol produced by the liver. It is important to note, though, that the liver contributes much more cholesterol to blood cholesterol levels than does the food you eat.

Blood lipids (cholesterol and other fatty acids) move through the body attached to protein carriers called *lipoproteins*. When considering cardiovascular disease and atherosclerosis, the most important lipoproteins are the high-density lipoproteins (HDLs), which are protective, and low-density lipoproteins (LDLs), which are harmful.

As you think about drugs for reducing cholesterol, you can consider the effect of the drug on the "good" cholesterol (the protective HDLs) or on the "bad" cholesterol (the harmful LDLs). HDLs remove cholesterol from the blood and transport it to the liver. If you have ever seen a catfish in action, you can see that it acts as a "scavenger" for food and cleans up the bottom of the fish tank. HDLs scavenge harmful lipids from the blood so that it does not stick to blood vessels and contribute to plaque. On the other hand, LDL cholesterols are major contributors to the onset and progression of heart disease and stroke.

For some patients, lipid levels are improved through diet, exercise, and lifestyle changes. Others may require lipid-lowering drugs (antihyperlipidemics). Most lipid-lowering drugs tend to reduce LDLs and other fatty acids. Some drugs can actually increase the scavenger HDLs.

> ### Memory Jogger
> LDLs are the "bad" cholesterol; HDLs are the "good" cholesterol.

Five classes of drugs are used to treat hyperlipidemia: statins (**HMG-CoA [hydroxymethylglutaryl coenzyme A] reductase inhibitors**), selective cholesterol absorption inhibitors, fibric acid derivatives, bile acid sequestrants, and niacin or nicotinic acid.

> ### Memory Jogger
> The five classes of antihyperlipidemics are:
> - HMG-CoA reductase inhibitors (most common)
> - cholesterol absorption inhibitors
> - fibric acid derivatives (fibrates)
> - bile sequestrants
> - niacin or nicotinic acid

HMG-COA REDUCTASE INHIBITORS (STATINS)

Actions

HMG-CoA reductase inhibitors (also called "statins") are antihyperlipidemic drugs that lower blood LDL levels by slowing cholesterol production by the liver.

They do not remove dietary cholesterol from the blood. The statins are the most effective drugs for lowering LDL levels and raising HDL levels. See Table 8.4 for the dosages and nursing implications of commonly prescribed HMG-CoA reductase inhibitors. Be sure to consult a drug reference source or handbook for information on other statin drugs.

Uses

The main use of statins is to lower blood LDL levels to reduce the risk for atherosclerosis, hypertension, heart attack, peripheral arterial disease, and stroke. Although other benefits have been described for statins, they are approved only to lower blood cholesterol levels.

Expected Side Effects

The most common side effects of statins include abdominal pain, headache, diarrhea, and muscle and joint discomfort. Other side effects are sore throat and heartburn. Patients with diabetes may experience an elevation of blood glucose. There is some evidence that long-term use of statins may be associated with cataract formation; however, the benefit of statin use outweighs the risk for cataracts.

Adverse Effects

The action of statins is in the liver and thus liver function is affected to some degree. Although rare, liver failure has been reported. With higher doses of statins patients may experience *rhabdomyolysis* (muscle breakdown). This is a very serious condition that can be life-threatening. Signs and symptoms of rhabdomyolysis include general muscle soreness, muscle pain, muscle weakness, stomach pain, and brown (tea-colored) urine. The brown urine results from the kidneys trying to filter out the products of muscle breakdown. Ultimately the patient experiences kidney failure.

Statins are dangerous if used during pregnancy. Cholesterol is important for normal brain development. If taken during pregnancy, statins can lower the cholesterol levels in the fetus, which results in brain deformities. For the same reason, statins are contraindicated in women who are breast-feeding.

> ### Lifespan Considerations
> #### Pregnancy and Breast-Feeding
> Statins are contraindicated during pregnancy and breast-feeding because of the effects of lower cholesterol levels on the developing brain.

Drug Interactions

Alcohol and acetaminophen increase the liver toxicity effects of statins. Aspirin and antacids decrease the effectiveness of statins. Grapefruit juice can increase the concentration of statins in the blood and should be avoided to reduce the risk for toxic side effects.

Table 8.4 Common HMG-CoA Reductase Inhibitors (Statins) Drugs

HMG-CoA reductase inhibitors (statins): antihyperlipidemic drugs that lower blood LDL levels by slowing liver production of cholesterol. They do not remove dietary cholesterol from the blood.

DRUGS/ADULT DOSAGE RANGE	NURSING IMPLICATIONS
atorvastatin (Lipitor) 10–80 mg orally once daily fluvastatin (Lescol) 20–40 mg orally once or twice daily fluvastatin extended release (Lescol XL) 80 mg orally once daily lovastatin (Altoprev) 20–80 mg orally once daily with evening meal lovastatin extended release (Altoprev) 20–60 mg orally once daily with evening meal pravastatin (Pravachol) 10–80 mg orally once daily rosuvastatin (Crestor) 5–40 mg orally once daily simvastatin (Zocor, FloLipid) 5–40 mg orally once daily in the evening	• Remind patients to remain on a low-cholesterol diet while taking statins because drugs do not reverse a high-cholesterol diet. • Check drug references for individual statins because some have best effects when taken in the evening and others can be taken without regard to meals for best effect. • Teach patients to avoid alcohol because drinking alcohol puts stress on the liver and adds to the stress of these drugs. • Tell patients to report severe muscle aches, changes in urine color, or decreased urine output because statins can cause rhabdomyolysis, a disorder resulting from broken muscle cells that damage the kidneys. • Teach patients that they should avoid grapefruit juice because it interacts with statins and can cause drug toxicity. • Remind patients to follow up with their healthcare provider for regular laboratory work because statins can cause liver problems. • Monitor patients for signs of liver problems, such as nausea, yellowing of the eyes or roof of the mouth, darkened urine, or light-colored stools, because these symptoms suggest damage to the liver. • Side effects are rare, but some patients experience GI symptoms including upset stomach, gas, constipation, and stomach cramps. Some patients experience mild muscle or joint ache. If patients experience these symptoms, remind them to contact their healthcare provider rather than stopping the drug.

❖ **Nursing Implications and Patient Teaching**

◆ *Assessment.* Carefully assess the patient's dietary patterns. Even though the patient is taking a drug to decrease cholesterol, it is not a good reason to continue eating foods high in saturated fats, such as fatty meats, fried foods, and baked goods made with *trans* fats such as donuts or cookies.

Review liver function tests in the medical record before giving statins. If you see any abnormalities or have any questions, contact the registered nurse (RN) or the healthcare provider. If you are working in a community setting, it will be important to know if women are pregnant or planning pregnancy because statins are very dangerous to the fetus. Furthermore, women must avoid statins while breast-feeding. In other adults, assess for any symptoms of impaired liver function. Ask patients about their use of alcohol before starting statin therapy. Heavy use of alcohol contributes to liver problems while taking statins, so the patient will need to understand this before he or she begins therapy.

◆ *Planning and implementation.* While on statin therapy patients may have scheduled blood lipid levels ordered by the prescriber. Patients will need to fast at least 12 hours before having cholesterol, HDL, LDL, and triglyceride levels drawn.

Timing of statin administration is very important to obtain the best result. A pharmacist or drug reference is helpful in determining the best time to give a specific statin. Some statins work best when given in the evening, some can be taken once a day without regard to meals,

and some may need to be taken twice a day. Do not give the drug with grapefruit juice because this juice inhibits drug breakdown, allowing higher drug blood levels that can cause toxic side effects.

◆ *Evaluation.* Monitor for expected side effects, including headache, upset stomach, sore throat, or diarrhea. These side effects are typically short-term and go away after time. Check patient for *jaundice* (yellowing of the skin and mucous membranes including whites of the eyes), as well as darkening of the urine or clay-colored stools. These are indications of liver toxicity (*hepatotoxicity*). All patients taking statins usually have regular liver function studies after starting the drug and then yearly or whenever symptoms occur. If the patient has any severe muscle aches or signs of liver problems, report these to the RN or healthcare provider immediately.

⌂ Top Tip for Safety

For patients who are taking statins, immediately report to the healthcare provider any severe muscle ache or signs of liver problems, such as jaundice or dark urine that the patient has noticed, because those symptoms can be signs of serious adverse effects.

◆ *Patient and family teaching.* Tell the patient and family the following:
• Lifestyle changes like exercise, a low-cholesterol diet, and good weight management are just as important

while you are taking the statins to help prevent cardiovascular disease.

- Make note of the recommended best time of day to take your statin and take it at the same time each day.
- Inform your healthcare provider if you might be pregnant or plan to become pregnant because statins can cause birth defects.
- Avoid grapefruit juice when you are taking statins because this can cause the drug to accumulate in the blood and increase the risk for toxic effects.
- If you have any signs of liver problems such as light-colored bowel movements, yellowish tinge to the skin or eyes, or dark urine, notify your healthcare provider immediately because these are indications of adverse drug effects.
- If you have severe muscle aches, notify your healthcare provider because this is an indication of a possible adverse drug effect.
- Expected side effects include headache, upset stomach, and mild achiness. These usually get better after a few weeks of starting the statin.
- Websites like the American Heart Association (http://www.heart.org) have resources to help you learn about cholesterol and low-cholesterol diets.

NONSTATIN ANTIHYPERLIPIDEMIC DRUGS

Nonstatin antihyperlipidemic drugs use a variety of actions to reduce blood cholesterol levels derived from ingested food. These drugs are used less often because they are not as effective as statins. They would most likely be prescribed if the person is not responsive to or unable to tolerate statins.

Selective Cholesterol Absorption Inhibitors

Selective cholesterol absorption inhibitors are the next most common drugs prescribed for lowering cholesterol. Ezetimibe was the first agent introduced in this category. The drug stays in the intestinal wall and acts on the intestinal epithelial cells to limit the absorption of cholesterol from food and from other sources in the body. Selective cholesterol absorption inhibitors are often combined with statins in pill form to give the patient the best chance of lowering LDL cholesterol and raising HDL cholesterol.

Fibric Acid Derivatives (Fibrates)

Gemfibrozil and fenofibrate are the preferred drugs of the fibric acid derivatives because they are more effective and have fewer adverse effects compared with some other drugs. Both are highly effective at lowering triglycerides and increasing HDL levels, but they have little effect on lowering LDL levels. Gemfibrozil and fenofibrate are generally well tolerated but can cause liver toxicity and *cholelithiasis* (gallstones). In general, these drugs are not recommended for patients with a history of gallbladder disease.

Bile Acid Sequestrants

Bile acid sequestrants, such as cholestyramine and colestipol, increase excretion of cholesterol and reduce LDL levels. They do this by forming a solid compound with bile salts, which increases bile loss through the feces (stool). Normal fat digestion is disturbed, so many patients do not tolerate these drugs because of uncomfortable GI side effects (e.g., constipation, bloating, and nausea). Bile acid sequestrants are not absorbed, so they do not have some of the severe systemic adverse effects that other antihyperlipidemics have.

Other drugs taken with the bile acid sequestrants may not get absorbed because they act by binding to substances in the intestinal tract. In particular, bile acid sequestrants reduce absorption of fat-soluble vitamins (A, D, E, and K), so the patient may show symptoms of vitamin deficiency especially if taking a high dose or the drugs are taken for a long time. Watch especially for bleeding problems that may result from vitamin K deficiency that affects the clotting cycle.

Niacin or Nicotinic Acid

You may have heard of niacin as one of the B-complex vitamins found in animal proteins, green vegetables, and whole wheat. In higher doses, it also can lower total cholesterol and LDLs, and can increase HDLs. Although recent guidelines suggest that niacin is not as effective as statins in reducing cardiovascular risk, you may see patients in your clinical practice who are taking niacin. One of the main problems with niacin use is the expected side effect of *flushing* (a sensation of warmth or "prickly heat" with redness that usually occurs on the face, neck, or trunk). The flushing occurs shortly after taking the drug and is very uncomfortable. Taking aspirin (30 minutes before) and increasing the niacin dosage very slowly over 3 to 4 weeks from 500 to 1000 mg three times daily may reduce the flushing. In addition, flushing may decrease over time while taking the drug. Other side effects include indigestion, gas, hot flashes, rapid heart rate, and sweating.

❖ Nursing Implications and Patient Teaching

◆ *Assessment.* Just as with the statins, it is very important to assess the patient's diet history, including his or her ability to adhere to lifestyle recommendations. These are just as important as the drug therapy because no cholesterol-reducing drug cures hyperlipidemia. Assess the patient's liver function tests; if there are any abnormal results, notify the RN or the healthcare provider. Assess the patient's use of alcohol because alcohol can increase the risk for damage to the liver.

◆ *Planning and implementation.* For those nonstatin antihyperlipidemic drugs that affect absorption of cholesterol from the GI tract, you will likely be giving supplemental doses of vitamins A, D, and K. Just as for the statins, carefully review the proper timing of these drugs in relation to meals. By themselves, selective cholesterol absorption inhibitors can be given without regard to meals. However, they are often combined with statins, so timing would be similar to statin drugs. For best results, fibric acid derivatives like gemfibrozil should be given 30 minutes before the morning and evening meals. Bile acid sequestrants are usually taken one or two times a day before meals. The drugs come in powder form and must be mixed with water, milk, or juice. Monitor how well the patient is tolerating the drug. If there are any signs of severe GI symptoms such as abdominal pain, severe bloating, or severe constipation, notify the RN or the healthcare provider.

◆ *Evaluation.* The healthcare provider will order follow-up blood tests to determine the patient's responses to cholesterol-lowering therapy. Compare these test results with those obtained before the drug was started to evaluate drug effectiveness and any changes in liver function.

◆ *Patient and family teaching.* Tell the patient and family the following:

* Take the drug at the time prescribed because timing is important for cholesterol-lowering drugs.
* Notify your healthcare provider and your pharmacist that you are taking a cholesterol-lowering drug so that they carefully review drug interactions with other drugs you are taking.
* Notify your healthcare provider if you have any significant side effects before you consider stopping the drug. Dosages may be adjusted by your healthcare provider or you may be switched to a different drug.
* Your drugs do not cure your high cholesterol problem. Continue making healthy lifestyle choices.

> **Bookmark This!**
>
> The American Heart Association has great information for you and your patients about heart health and heart disease: http://www.heart.org/HEARTORG.

ANTIHYPERTENSIVE DRUGS

Blood pressure is the pressure of circulating blood on the walls of arteries and veins as the blood moves through the body with each contraction and relaxation of the heart. A healthy blood pressure maintains circulation to major organs and all parts of the body during rest and during activity. Blood pressure that is too high or too low can cause critical problems that affect blood vessels, organs, and tissues. Many things can affect the blood pressure, including heart rate, how well the heart contracts, certain hormones, blood volume, physical activity, and stress.

Hypertension (high blood pressure) is a disorder in which the patient's blood pressure is consistently elevated above normal values. If left untreated, hypertension will damage major organs including the heart, brain, and kidneys. Managing hypertension dramatically reduces the odds of heart attack, stroke, and kidney failure. There are two kinds of hypertension. In *primary*

hypertension, the specific cause is unknown. In *secondary hypertension,* the blood pressure changes are a result of a specific cause. If the cause is treated or managed, the blood pressure naturally returns to normal. Most cases (about 90%) are primary hypertension. Primary hypertension cannot be cured but can be well managed with good drug therapy. We will focus our attention on managing primary hypertension.

Even though hypertension is the technical term, we will use the phrase *high blood pressure* (HBP) to discuss drugs and nursing management. In the past, use of the term *hypertension* created the impression that a person would be feeling "hyper" if his or her blood pressure was too high, when in fact HBP is often without symptoms. When patients felt calm, they believed their blood pressure was normal; therefore they did not think they needed drugs. This led to much confusion between patients and their healthcare providers. HBP is a much simpler term, and patients understand it better than hypertension.

According to the American Heart Association, HBP affects as many as one in three adults 20 years of age or older. Although the exact cause of HBP is unknown, there are a number of risk factors, including a family history of HBP, African American race, overweight or obesity, physical inactivity, current cigarette smoking or exposure to secondhand smoke, and too much alcohol consumption. People with diabetes, elevated blood lipids, or kidney disease also are at higher risk for HBP. Risk increases with age, so it is not surprising that as the population ages, there will be a need for a good understanding of HBP management. Whatever the cause, when HBP is untreated or poorly treated, people can develop serious health problems and even death.

Severity of HBP is classified according to the stages listed in Table 8.5. These stages were recently revised to recommend the elimination of the term "prehypertension" for the more accurate term "elevated" blood pressure. Accurate diagnosis is essential to determination

Table 8.5   Blood Pressure Classification

CLASSIFICATION	BLOOD PRESSURE MEASUREMENT	BLOOD PRESSURE READING
Normal	Systolic and diastolic	<120 mm Hg <80 mm Hg
Elevated	Systolic or diastolic	120–129 mm Hg <80 mm Hg
Stage 1 hypertension	Systolic or diastolic	130–139 mm Hg 80–89 mm Hg
Stage 2 hypertension	Systolic and diastolic	≥140 mm Hg ≥90 mm Hg

From Whelton PK, Carey RM, Aronow WS, et al. (2017). ACC/AHA/AAPA/ABC/ACPM/AGS/APhA/ASH/ASPC/NMA/PCNA Guideline for the prevention, detection, evaluation, and management of high blood pressure in adults: A report of the American College of Cardiology/American Heart Association Task Force on Clinical Practice Guidelines. *J Am Coll Cardiol* Nov 13:[Epub ahead of print].

of the best treatments for your patients. As an LPN, you will have an important role in using the proper technique for blood pressure screening. In addition, you will work with the health care team to reinforce recommended lifestyle changes (Box 8.2). If lifestyle changes alone are not effective in reducing the patient's blood pressure, healthcare providers begin drug therapy. Choices of prescribed drugs may depend on the patient's age, race, and whether the patient has diabetes or chronic kidney disease (which can complicate treatment). Do not hesitate to communicate with the health care provider if you are not clear about your patient's blood pressure goals.

Antihypertensives are drugs that have the main purpose of lowering blood pressure. A variety of drugs can lower blood pressure by different mechanisms. Not all patients respond to any one class of blood pressure–lowering drugs in the same way. Drug therapy for HBP often requires trial periods to establish the right drug or drug combinations to help any one patient achieve his or her blood pressure goal. For the general population, non-African American patients typically begin with thiazide diuretics. These drugs may be prescribed alone or in combination with **angiotensin-converting enzyme inhibitors (ACE-Is)** or **angiotensin II receptor blockers (ARBs)**. For African American patients, thiazide diuretics and calcium channel blockers are used alone or in combination for best management. For patients with diabetes and/or chronic kidney disease, ACE-Is and ARBs are used. Additional classes of drugs used in management of HBP most commonly include beta blockers, alpha blockers, alpha$_2$ agonists, combined alpha and beta blockers, and vasodilators.

Although the actions for the antihypertensives drugs differ, some nursing implications are the same for all of them. Box 8.3 describes these common nursing considerations for giving antihypertensive drugs. Nursing considerations and patient teaching issues specific to any single drug type are listed with the individual antihypertensive drug categories.

Many types of drugs are available to treat HBP. The drug selected for use depends on the severity of the disease. The drugs act at many sites in the body and through several different ways (Fig. 8.7). Patients may need several types of drugs to achieve the very best management of their blood pressure. Antihypertensive drugs have the following five main categories:

| Box **8.2** | **Recommended Lifestyle Changes for Patients With High Blood Pressure** |

Stop smoking.
Eat a well-balanced diet.
Decrease sodium (salt) intake.
Explore ways to reduce stressors in your life.
Maintain a healthy weight.
Try to get 40 minutes of moderate-intensity exercise three to four times each week.
Limit alcohol to no more than two drinks a day for men or one drink per day for women.
Avoid all over-the-counter drugs that can raise blood pressure.

| Box **8.3** | **General Nursing Implications for Antihypertensive Drug Therapy** |

ASSESSMENT

- Gather baseline vital signs before giving any drug for HBP.
- Get a complete list of all drugs that the patient is currently taking, including prescription, over-the-counter, and herbal drugs.
- Assess patient's use of alcohol and/or illegal drugs that might interfere with the drug therapy or increase risk for adverse effects.
- Review patient's laboratory work, particularly relating to kidney tests (blood urea nitrogen and creatinine levels), as well as serum sodium and potassium concentrations.
- Assess for fluid balance including the presence of edema or symptoms of dehydration.

PLANNING AND IMPLEMENTATION

- Teach patient to report all over-the-counter drugs, checking with the healthcare provider to avoid dangerous drug interactions.
- Remind patient to avoid sudden changes in position because most antihypertensive drugs cause orthostatic hypotension.
- Hold blood pressure drugs if patient has a blood pressure less than 90/60 mm Hg, and notify the healthcare provider.

- Monitor blood pressure every 4 to 8 hours and as needed at the beginning of therapy in case the patient has a significant drop in blood pressure.
- Monitor potassium levels to assess whether it is within normal levels. Report abnormal levels to the healthcare provider.
- Teach patient to avoid alcohol because it can cause hypotension in patients who are taking blood pressure drugs.
- Give the patient the drug at the same time every day. It is important to avoid missing doses because missed doses can cause rebound HBP.
- Teach patient to keep taking the drugs as prescribed because they do not cure HBP.
- Initiate fall risk precautions for older adult patients who are taking HBP drugs.

EVALUATION

- Monitor patient's blood pressure regularly to determine how well the patient is responding to the drug.
- Report any side effects or adverse effects to the healthcare provider.
- Track patient's response to the drugs to determine whether they are effective.
- Continue to reinforce healthy lifestyle changes (see Box 8.2).

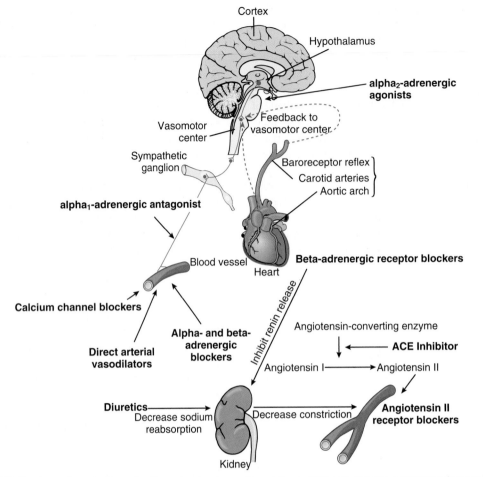

FIG. 8.7 Common sites of action of antihypertensive drugs. (From Lilley L, Collins S, Snyder J: *Pharmacology and the nursing process*, ed 8, St. Louis, 2016, Elsevier.)

1. Diuretics indirectly reduce blood pressure by producing sodium and water loss, thereby reducing fluid volume (see the Drugs That Affect the Renal/Urinary System section earlier in this chapter for the actions and nursing implications for diuretics).
2. **Renin-angiotensin-aldosterone system (RAAS) drugs** work by decreasing vasoconstriction and decreasing fluid volume to decrease blood pressure. These include:
   a. ACE-Is
   b. ARBs
3. Calcium channel blockers decrease blood pressure by relaxing vascular smooth muscle in the coronary and systemic arteries, leading to decreased peripheral resistance.
4. Adrenergic agents used for the treatment of HBP affect epinephrine and norepinephrine (neurotransmitters) in the nervous system. Depending on the receptor, these drugs can decrease vasoconstriction and decrease contractility of the heart, therefore decreasing blood pressure.
   a. beta blockers
      i. nonselective
      ii. selective

   b. alpha$_1$ antagonist
   c. alpha$_2$ agonist
   d. combined alpha/beta antagonists
5. Vasodilators directly affect the arterial and/or venous system to decrease peripheral resistance.

We discussed diuretics earlier in this chapter, so we will continue with the remaining four categories. Each class works a bit differently, so we will discuss them separately so that you can better understand how you will care for patients taking one or more HBP drugs at a time. In addition, you will see that several of the drug categories work well for patients with other cardiovascular illnesses.

ANTIHYPERTENSIVE DRUG ACTIONS

Renin-Angiotensin-Aldosterone System Drugs

RAAS drugs include ACE-Is and ARBs that have the effect of interfering with the action of angiotensin on blood vessels. When a person's blood pressure drops, cells in the kidney release a hormone called *renin* into the blood. Renin helps produce *angiotensin I*. Angiotensin I is converted to *angiotensin II* by an enzyme called the *angiotensin-converting enzyme* (ACE). Angiotensin II is a hormone that causes vasoconstriction and stimulates the adrenal cortex to increase *aldosterone* secretion. Aldosterone then can increase water and sodium reabsorption. This works very well in helping to raise blood pressure back to normal. A good understanding of this process is helpful when we discuss how ACE-Is and ARBs help to reduce HBP.

ACE-Is are a type of RAAS drug that reduce HBP by stopping the conversion of angiotensin I to angiotensin II (the hormone that causes the vasoconstriction and increased aldosterone). ARBs are a type of RAAS drug that actually block the vasoconstrictor and aldosterone-secreting effects of angiotensin II to lower blood pressure by selectively blocking the binding of angiotensin II at receptor sites found in many tissues. Both ACE-Is and ARBs decrease vasoconstriction and decrease the release of aldosterone. See Table 8.6 for the dosages and nursing implications of selected ACE-Is and ARBs.

> **Memory Jogger**
>
> ACE-I drugs typically use the suffix *-pril* (e.g., captopril, enalapril, and prinivil). ARBs typically end with the suffix *-sartan* (e.g., valsartan and losartan).

Calcium Channel Blockers

Calcium ions are very important in the contraction of heart and vascular smooth muscle cell membranes. **Calcium channel blockers** are a class of antihypertensive drugs that lower blood pressure by reducing the effect of calcium in the heart muscle and in the smooth muscles of arteries. They work in two main ways. First, calcium channel blockers help slow down the flow of calcium ions across cell membranes, reducing the amount of calcium available for arterial smooth muscle contraction. This leads to relaxation of coronary and systemic arteries. With the relaxation of the smooth muscle, blood flow improves and blood pressure decreases. The oxygen can then get to the heart muscle cells where needed. In addition, some calcium channel blockers slow the flow of electricity through the cardiac conduction system, slow heart rate, and can treat abnormal heart rhythms. As a result, you may see them used in patients with HBP, patients with angina, and patients with abnormal heart rhythms (dysrhythmias). See Table 8.6 for the dosages and nursing implications of selected calcium channel blockers.

> **Memory Jogger**
>
> Fluid retention is a common side effect of calcium channel blockers, and these drugs should be avoided in patients with heart failure.

Adrenergic Drugs

Adrenergics are a category of drugs that affect nervous system control of various organs and tissues by activating or blocking receptors that respond to the body's natural adrenergic substances, *epinephrine* and *norepinephrine*. To better understand how adrenergic drugs work, you need to understand the role of the sympathetic nervous system in blood pressure control. The sympathetic nervous system relies on two main neurotransmitters, epinephrine and norepinephrine (these neurotransmitters are also called *catecholamines*). The neurotransmitters carry impulses to receptors on the surfaces of the heart, lungs, and blood vessel smooth muscle that, once turned on, create a response. There are two main types of adrenergic receptors: alpha and beta receptors. Stimulation of these receptors turns on the response (called *agonists*); blocking the receptors prevents the expected response (called *blockers* or *antagonists*). (Recall the discussion of receptors, agonists, and antagonists from Chapter 3.)

Beta blockers. There are two main types of beta receptors: beta$_1$ receptors located primarily in the heart and beta$_2$ receptors located primarily in the lungs. An easy way to remember which type of receptor is affected by the drug is: beta$_1$, one heart; beta$_2$, two lungs. Stimulation of beta$_1$ receptors leads to increased heart rate and increased contractility of the heart. This is very helpful when you are healthy and need the fight-or-flight mechanism to work for you. In patients with HBP, these responses can be harmful, thus drugs are used to "block" the response.

Beta blockers are drugs that work as antagonists and block the activity of beta-adrenergic receptors. These drugs are classified into two groups: nonselective and selective beta antagonists. The *nonselective* agents block both beta$_1$ and beta$_2$ sites. This is important because you can see that the drug would not only affect beta$_1$ (heart) receptors, but also beta$_2$ (lung) receptors. Blocking beta$_1$ receptors will decrease heart contractility and heart rate (which can decrease blood pressure). On the other hand, blocking beta$_2$ receptors will cause bronchoconstriction—a problem especially if you have asthma. That is why the newer selective beta$_1$ blockers are better for patients with HBP and other heart problems (Fig. 8.8). The drugs do not have an effect on the lungs at normal doses.

Beta blockers typically end with the suffix *-olol*, such as in metoprolol, propranolol, or sotalol. The "olol" gives you the hint that the drug is a beta blocker. See Table 8.6 for the dosages and nursing implications of selected beta blockers.

> **Memory Jogger**
>
> You can use the terms *antagonist* and *blocker* interchangeably to describe a drug that turns off a receptor. For example, you can refer to metoprolol as a beta blocker or a beta antagonist.

Alpha$_1$-adrenergic antagonists. Stimulation of alpha$_1$-adrenergic receptors causes arterial vascular smooth

Table 8.6   **Common Antihypertensive Drugs**

Diuretics: reduce blood pressure by producing sodium and water loss, thereby decreasing fluid volume

DRUGS/ADULT DOSAGE RANGE	NURSING IMPLICATIONS
See Table 8.2 to review dosage ranges.	See Table 8.2 to review nursing implications.

Renin-angiotensin-aldosterone system (RAAS): drugs work by decreasing vasoconstriction and decreasing fluid volume to decrease blood pressure

DRUGS/ADULT DOSAGE RANGE	NURSING IMPLICATIONS
ACE-Is captopril (Capoten, Novo-Captopril) 12.5–50 mg orally two to three times daily enalapril (Vasotec, Epaned) 2.5–40 mg orally daily as single dose or two divided doses lisinopril (Prinivil, Zestril) 10–40 mg orally once daily quinapril (Accupril) 10–80 mg orally daily as single dose or two divided doses **ARBs** losartan (Cozaar) 25–100 mg orally daily as a single dose or in two divided doses valsartan (Diovan) 80–320 mg orally once daily irbesartan (Avapro) 150–300 mg orally once daily candesartan (Atacand) 8–32 mg orally daily as a single does or in two divided doses	• Avoid sudden changes in position because most antihypertensive drugs cause orthostatic hypotension. • Teach patients that these drugs can have a "first dose effect" leading to an increased risk for falls and dizziness. • Remind patients to keep taking the drugs as prescribed because they do not cure high blood pressure. • ACE-Is and ARBs can cause hyperkalemia (high potassium levels), so remind patients to avoid high-potassium foods (see Box 8.1), including salt substitutes. • Monitor patients' blood pressure regularly to determine how well the patients are responding to the drug. • Some patients may experience a dry cough while taking ACE-Is. If so, report this to the healthcare provider because an ARB usually does not cause a cough. • If the patient experiences any swelling of the eyes, mouth, face, or tongue, contact the healthcare provider immediately because this could be a sign of angioedema (Fig. 8.10), a potentially life-threatening condition. • These drugs can cause severe birth defects if taken during pregnancy, so they should not be taken by patients who are or may become pregnant. • Teach patients taking these drugs to avoid alcohol because it can cause hypotension. • Remind patients to avoid all over-the-counter drugs until checking with the healthcare provider to avoid dangerous drug interactions.

Calcium channel blocking agents: decrease blood pressure by relaxing vascular smooth muscle in the coronary and systemic arteries leading to decreased peripheral resistance

DRUGS/ADULT DOSAGE RANGE	NURSING IMPLICATIONS
amlodipine (Norvasc) 2.5–10 mg orally once daily diltiazem (Cardizem) 30–120 mg orally three to four times daily, up to 480 mg daily diltiazem extended release (Cardizem CD, Dilacor XR) 120–360 mg orally once daily felodipine (Plendil) 2.5–10 mg orally daily nicardipine (Cardene) 20–40 mg orally three times daily nicardipine sustained release (Cardene SR), may be given as 30–60 mg twice daily nifedipine (Adalat, Procardia) 10–30 mg orally three times daily, not to exceed 180 mg daily nifedipine extended-release (Adalat CC, Procardia XL) initially 30–60 mg orally once daily, not to exceed 90 mg daily verapamil (Calan, Isoptin) 80–120 mg orally every 8 hours verapamil extended-release (Calan SR, Isoptin SR) 120–480 mg once daily at bedtime	• Avoid sudden changes in position because most antihypertensive drugs cause orthostatic hypotension. • Remind patients to keep taking the drugs as prescribed because they do not cure high blood pressure. • Monitor patients' blood pressure regularly to determine how well the patients are responding to the drug. • Patients should avoid alcohol because it can cause hypotension in patients taking blood pressure drugs. • Remind patients to avoid all over-the-counter drugs until checking with the healthcare provider to avoid dangerous drug interactions. • Notify the provider if the patient experiences swelling in the legs because this can be a sign of fluid retention caused by calcium channel blockers. • Calcium channel blockers are avoided in patients with heart failure because of the potential for fluid retention. • Be alert for signs of Stevens-Johnsons syndrome (erythema multiforme), a life-threating skin condition that can be an adverse effect of calcium channel blockers. This condition is associated with skin lesions, fever, and joint aching. • Report heart rates less than 60 beats/min and blood pressures less than 90 mm Hg systolic to the healthcare provider before giving the drug, to avoid significant hypotension. • If you are caring for a patient who is receiving IV calcium channel blockers, check with the RN or healthcare provider regarding the need for a bed with a cardiac monitor.

Table 8.6 Common Antihypertensive Drugs—cont'd

Adrenergic agents: used for treatment of HBP. Affect the nervous system control of various organs and tissues by activating or blocking receptors that respond to the body's natural adrenergic substances, epinephrine and norepinephrine.

DRUGS/ADULT DOSAGE RANGE	NURSING IMPLICATIONS
Beta Blockers	**For All Adrenergic Agents**
acebutolol selective (Sectral) 400–1200 mg orally daily in two divided doses atenolol selective (Tenormin) 25–200 mg orally once daily betaxolol selective (Kerlone) 10–20 mg orally once daily labetalol (Normodyne, Trandate) 100–400 mg orally twice daily metoprolol (Lopressor, Toprol) 25–50 mg twice daily, up to 400 mg per day in 2 divided doses metoprolol (Toprol XL) 100 mg orally once daily, up to 400 mg once daily nadolol (Corgard) 40–240 mg orally once daily propranolol (Inderal) 10–20 mg orally 2–4 times daily, up to 160–320 mg daily in 2–4 divided doses propranolol extended release (Inderal LA, Inderal XL) 80 mg orally once daily, up to 160-320 mg once daily	• Avoid sudden changes in position because most antihypertensive drugs cause orthostatic hypotension. • Remind patients to keep taking the drugs as prescribed because they do not cure high blood pressure. • Monitor patients' blood pressure regularly to determine how well the patients are responding to the drug. • Patients should avoid alcohol because it can cause hypotension in patients who are taking blood pressure drugs. • Remind patients to avoid all over-the-counter drugs until checking with the healthcare provider to avoid dangerous drug interactions.
	Beta Blockers
	• Hold drug if heart rate is less than 60 beats/min or systolic blood pressure is less than 90 mm Hg to prevent adverse effects. • Teach patients that common side effects include decreased sexual ability, dizziness, drowsiness, difficulty sleeping, or weakness. Some patients may experience cold hands or feet. • Tell patients to report symptoms of depression to their healthcare provider. • Teach diabetic patients that beta blockers can mask signs of hypoglycemia (except for sweating). Remind them to check blood sugars regularly and treat low blood sugars. • Do not stop beta blockers suddenly, to avoid rebound HBP.
Alpha Blockers	**Alpha Blockers**
doxazosin (Cardura) 1–16 mg orally once daily at bedtime prazosin (Minipress) 1–5 mg orally two to three times daily at bedtime; do not exceed 20 mg daily terazosin (Hytrin) 1–5 mg orally daily at bedtime, may give in 1 or 2 divided doses. Maximum dose is 20 mg daily.	• A side effect of prazosin and terazosin is first-dose hypotension. As a result, these drugs may be given at night to prevent severe orthostatic hypotension. These effects diminish over time. • Monitor patients carefully for side effects, including dizziness, nervousness, fatigue, headache, and stuffy or runny nose, that can occur with alpha blockers. • Weigh patients at least two times a week because alpha blockers can cause fluid retention. • Tell patients to avoid driving or using heavy machinery until at least 24 hours after the first dose because alpha blockers can cause a sudden drop in blood pressure.
Alpha/Beta Blockers	**Alpha/Beta Blockers**
carvedilol (Coreg) 3.125–25 mg orally twice daily carvedilol extended release (Coreg CR) 10 mg orally once daily, up to 80 mg once daily labetalol HCl (Normodyne, Trandate) 100 mg twice daily (usual dosage range is 200–400 mg twice daily), up to 2400 mg orally in 2 to 3 divided doses	• Alpha/beta blockers have side effects and adverse effects common to both drugs.
	Alpha$_2$ Agonists (Also Known as Centrally Acting Adrenergic Agents)
Alpha$_2$ Agonists	• These drugs impact the CNS, causing decreased vasoconstriction and dilation of blood vessels; therefore they have a higher risk for side effects than other blood pressure drugs. As a result, they are used only in cases of difficult-to-manage high blood pressure.
clonidine (Catapres, Duraclon, Kapvay) 0.1 mg orally twice daily; usual maintenance dosage range is 0.2–0.6 mg twice daily clonidine transdermal patch (Catapress TTS-1) 3.5 cm^2, 7 cm^2, or 10.5 cm^2 patch applied to hairless site on body every 7 days methyldopa (Aldomet) 250 mg orally two to three times daily; may increase up to 3 g daily in divided doses	• Teach patients the common side effects, including dizziness, fatigue, dry mouth, and nasal congestion. • Rinses, good oral care, and sugarless gum may help decrease dry mouth in patients who are taking alpha$_2$ agonists. • Read the directions for applying the clonidine patch very carefully to ensure you are using the system correctly, then write the time and date on the patch before placing on the patient. • Do not stop alpha$_2$ agonists suddenly, to prevent rebound HBP.

Continued

Table 8.6	Common Antihypertensive Drugs—cont'd

Vasodilators: directly affect the arterial and/or venous system to decrease peripheral resistance

DRUGS/ADULT DOSAGE RANGE	NURSING IMPLICATIONS
hydralazine (Apresoline) 10 mg orally four times daily; may gradually increase up to 300 mg daily minoxidil (Loniten) 5 mg orally daily; usual dose is 10–40 mg daily in 1 to 2 divided doses	• Monitor blood pressure carefully at the beginning of therapy in case the patient has a significant drop in blood pressure. • Teach patients to weigh themselves every day and to report swelling of the hands or feet to their healthcare provider. • Remind patients to take the drug at the same time every day. It is important to avoid missing doses because missed doses can cause rebound HBP. • Teach patients to change position slowly to avoid orthostatic hypotension.

ACE-I, Angiotensin-converting enzyme inhibitor; *ARB*, angiotensin II receptor blocker.

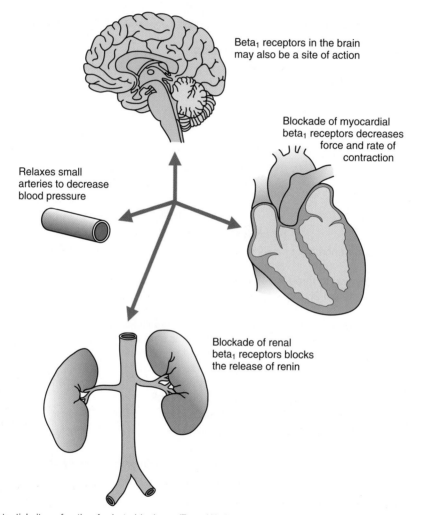

FIG. 8.8 Potential sites of action for beta blockers. (From Workman ML, LaCharity LA: *Understanding pharmacology*, St. Louis, 2011, Elsevier.)

muscle constriction (Fig. 8.9). For example, if the blood pressure is very low, certain drugs increase blood pressure by targeting the alpha$_1$ receptors. For patients with HBP, the alpha$_1$-adrenergic inhibitor drugs work through selective blocking of alpha$_1$-adrenergic receptor sites, leading to decreased peripheral vascular resistance and decreased blood pressure. So **alpha$_1$-adrenergic antagonists** are drugs that lower blood pressure by blocking the receptor sites in blood vessel smooth muscle that,

when activated, cause constriction and raise blood pressure.

Centrally acting alpha$_2$-adrenergic agonists. The **alpha$_2$-adrenergic agonists** work centrally (in the brain) to turn on special alpha$_2$ receptors that, when normally activated, cause vasodilation and decrease in blood pressure. These drugs can be very helpful in reducing blood pressure but have significant side effects, so they need

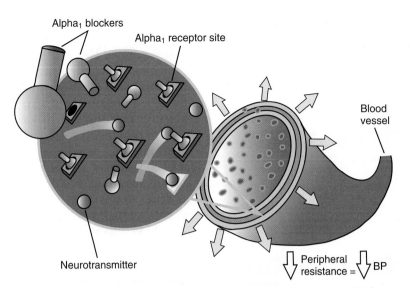

FIG. 8.9 Alpha₁ blockers fill alpha₁ receptor sites, preventing neurotransmitters from binding. With fewer receptors being stimulated, vasoconstriction is prevented or reversed and blood pressure is lowered. *BP*, Blood pressure. (From Workman ML, LaCharity LA: *Understanding pharmacology*, St. Louis, 2011, Elsevier.)

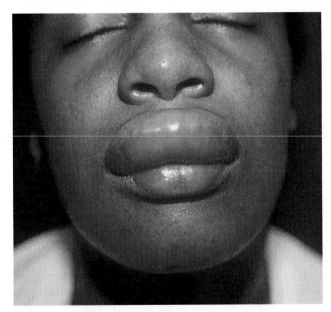

FIG. 8.10 Angioedema. (From Workman ML, LaCharity LA: *Understanding pharmacology*, St. Louis, 2011, Elsevier.)

to be used very carefully with regular blood pressure monitoring.

Combination alpha/beta blockers. Combination alpha/beta blockers have the benefit of affecting the responses of both types of adrenergic receptors. They relax the blood vessels like the alpha₁ blockers, and they slow the heart rate and contractility of the heart like the beta₁ blockers.

Vasodilators

Vasodilators dilate blood vessels in several ways. Some dilate both arteries and veins by preventing smooth muscle cell contraction. Others cause vasodilation by affecting the central nervous system. Some drugs work primarily on the arterial system, some more for the venous system, some work on both arteries and veins. Dilation of the blood vessels decreases blood pressure, improves blood flow to the major organs, and decreases the workload of the heart.

ANTIHYPERTENSIVE DRUG USES

Antihypertensives and diuretics are used alone or in combination to decrease elevated blood pressure to a desired level according to accepted guidelines. By maintaining normal blood pressure, these drugs help prevent complications of acute and chronic HBP. As you work with patients, you may see that the patients need several trials of different prescriptions before they get the right combination of drugs for the best control. Carefully monitoring will be essential.

EXPECTED SIDE EFFECTS OF ANTIHYPERTENSIVE DRUGS

All blood pressure drugs can cause *hypotension*, blood pressure that is too low to maintain adequate circulation. Most can cause *orthostatic hypotension*, that is, dizziness that occurs when changing positions. Symptoms associated with a blood pressure that is too low include dizziness, weakness, and confusion (particularly in older adults). These symptoms can lead to an increased risk of falls. As you study each class of drugs, remember to be able to recognize the difference between expected side effects and adverse reactions. When the blood pressure drops below 90/60 mm Hg or the patient is experiencing severe side effects, you will need to notify the healthcare provider to determine whether an alternative drug will work with fewer side effects.

ADVERSE REACTIONS OF ANTIHYPERTENSIVE DRUGS

Each class and each drug has many potential serious adverse reactions. The specific adverse effects are discussed in Table 8.6.

Lifespan Considerations

Older Adults: Antihypertensives

Older adults are particularly at risk for dizziness when taking these drugs. The orthostatic hypotension they experience places them at risk for falling when they rapidly change positions, such as getting up quickly from a chair or bed.

Top Tip for Safety

Antihypertensives

Teach patients who are taking antihypertensive drugs to stand up slowly to avoid dizziness and prevent falls.

DRUG INTERACTIONS WITH ANTIHYPERTENSIVE DRUGS

Frequently a patient with HBP has to take many different drugs because he or she has other medical problems as well. All of the antihypertensive drugs may have drug interactions. Check each drug the patient is taking; interactive effects that lower the blood pressure too much or make the blood pressure go even higher can occur. Be sure to consult a drug reference book or pharmacist for more information about drug interactions between the patient's prescribed antihypertensive drug and any other drug he or she is taking.

❖ Nursing Implications and Patient Teaching

◆ *Assessment.* As you assess your patient with HBP, remember to consider all modifiable and nonmodifiable risk factors. For example, knowing that African American individuals have a higher risk for HBP than white individuals will remind you to assess blood pressure in young adults, as well as older adults. Assessing patients for smoking, levels of physical activity, and high-sodium/high-fat diets will also be important. Lifestyle changes are critical whether the patient is taking blood pressure drugs or is in the prehypertension stage.

For all patients with HBP, it is critical to gather a thorough drug history. Certain prescription drugs, OTC drugs, herbal preparations, and even illegal drugs can actually cause HBP. Common prescription drugs, such as glucocorticoids, oral contraceptives, NSAIDs, and OTC drugs for cough and cold symptoms, may cause your patient to have elevated blood pressure. Patients who use illegal drugs, such as cocaine, anabolic steroids, and amphetamines, often are diagnosed with HBP when they are seen by healthcare providers for any reason. This can occur even in teenagers and young adults. As an LPN/VN, you may have the most contact with a patient in your care settings, so building a trusting relationship can help you screen for these and other risk factors for HBP.

Before giving any drug that affects blood pressure, baseline blood pressure checks are essential. Knowing the blood pressure before you give the drug will help you to evaluate the patient's response to the drug. Drugs such as beta blockers affect the blood pressure and the heart rate, so you will need to check the heart rate as well. If the heart rate is below 60, hold the drug and contact the healthcare provider. For several categories of drugs, you will need to know electrolyte levels such as potassium. If you are giving an ACE-I and the potassium level is above 5.0 mEq/L, hold the drug and contact the healthcare provider because ACE-Is can cause hyperkalemia. On the other hand, if you are giving a diuretic such as furosemide, you would be watching for hypokalemia (potassium levels less than normal).

◆ *Planning and implementation.* HBP has no cure; it can, however, be well managed. It will be important to involve your patient in planning care as much as possible so that he or she will better understand why taking a prescribed antihypertensive drug is important. For best results, patients will need both drug therapy and lifestyle changes. As mentioned earlier, HBP usually does not have symptoms, so the patient may not feel sick. It will be important for you to reinforce with the patient why treating the HBP is so important to maintaining good health even if he or she does not have any symptoms.

Top Tip for Safety

Ask patients about any herbal and OTC drugs they are taking because some may cause HBP and some may increase side effects of HBP drugs.

◆ *Evaluation.* It is important to evaluate the patient's response to the drug. Compare his or her current blood pressure with the baseline. Is the blood pressure improving? Is the patient tolerating the blood pressure drug without side effects? Evaluate how he or she is doing with lifestyle changes. Some patients are able to stop smoking but have difficulty with the dietary changes. Others may have made changes to diet but just have not been physically active.

The healthcare provider may order laboratory work including complete blood count, electrolytes, and blood urea nitrogen/creatinine to monitor renal function. This laboratory work helps identify adverse effects from the drug, as well as check for evidence of organ damage caused by chronic HBP.

Ask the patient about side effects the antihypertensive drug might be producing. Some of the drugs may cause impotence in men. If this is the case, men may want to discuss possible changes in the drug therapy with their healthcare providers. Always refer patients to their healthcare provider if they have stopped taking the HBP drugs because of side effects (see Box 8.3).

◆ *Patient and family teaching.* Tell the patient and family the following:

- Take this drug exactly as ordered. If a dose is missed, it should be taken as soon as it is remembered; if it is close to the next scheduled dose, skip the missed dose and return to the regular dosing schedule.
- Teach proper techniques for home monitoring of blood pressure and heart rate. If the blood pressure is less than 90/60 mm Hg or the heart rate less than 60, contact your healthcare provider.
- Keep a daily record of your blood pressure to bring to your appointments. This will help the healthcare provider make sure you are on the most effective drugs.
- Remember to get up slowly from a lying or sitting position to avoid dizziness from getting up too fast.
- Notify your healthcare provider of any new or uncomfortable symptoms that develop. These symptoms might indicate an adverse effect or may be relieved by simply changing to a new drug.
- Avoid alcoholic beverages while taking drugs for HBP.
- Keep with you a list of drugs that you take so that all healthcare providers are aware of the doses and types of drugs you are taking.

Bookmark This!

The National Institutes of Health has a wide variety of health information available to everyone in English (https://www.nih.gov/health-information) and in Spanish (https://salud.nih.gov).

DRUGS USED FOR ANGINA AND MYOCARDIAL INFARCTION

ANTIANGINALS

Coronary arteries supply blood, oxygen, and nutrients to heart muscle. For patients with atherosclerosis, plaque within the blood vessel leads to lack of blood flow and oxygen to the heart and potentially other areas of the body. Partial blood flow to the heart muscle can lead to lack of oxygen and chest pain known as angina. If the blood flow is significantly reduced, the heart muscle can die and the patient has a heart attack (myocardial infarction).

Major classes of drugs used to manage angina include nitrates, beta blockers, and calcium channel blockers. All of these drugs can improve circulation and reduce cardiac workload, therefore reducing *myocardial oxygen demand* (how much oxygen the heart needs).

NITRATES

Action

Nitrates are a class of drugs that vasodilate (widen blood vessels) by relaxing vascular smooth muscle in the peripheral venous system and reducing resistance to blood flow in the arterial system. Relaxing the smooth muscle in the veins helps increase pooling of venous blood, thereby decreasing the amount of blood returned to the heart (*preload*). Relaxing the arterial system decreases the pressures the heart has to pump against (*afterload*). These effects work together to help the heart receive more oxygen and pump more easily.

Uses

Rapid-acting nitrates (such as sublingual nitroglycerin [NTG] and intravenous NTG) are used to relieve pain in acute angina. The long-acting oral nitrates, topical NTG paste, and transdermal patches can prevent angina and reduce the severity and frequency of anginal attacks. Nitrates reduce the work of the heart after MI or in patients with heart failure.

Expected Side Effects

Throbbing headaches, caused by rapid blood vessel dilation in the head and face, occur in more than 50% of patients who take nitrates. The headaches usually occur very quickly after giving the drug and usually go away quickly if the patient is taking low doses. For patients who are taking high doses, acetaminophen or other analgesics may be needed to help reduce the pain. For patients who require long-term use of nitrates, headaches typically become less severe over time. It is common for patients to experience a slight drop in blood pressure after taking the drug because of venous dilation.

Adverse Effects

Some patients may have strong reactions to nitrates depending on the route of administration. Severe postural hypotension (low blood pressure when a person suddenly stands up), reflex tachycardia (rapid heartbeat) or paradoxical bradycardia, vertigo (feeling of dizziness or spinning), or severe weakness may occur.

Drug Interactions

Alcohol, antihypertensive drugs, opioids, and diuretics can increase the effect of nitrate drugs, causing tachycardia and severe hypotension. Caffeine, pseudoephedrine, methylphenidate, and certain antidiabetic drugs can decrease the effectiveness of nitrates. Drugs given for erectile dysfunction (e.g., sildenafil) can cause severe hypotension if given while the patient is taking nitrates.

❖ **Nursing Implications and Patient Teaching**

◆ *Assessment.* A good patient history including OTC and all prescription drugs is important to avoid drug interactions. It is important to get a baseline assessment of heart rate and blood pressure before giving any nitrate drug. For patients with acute angina, get a good description of the patient's symptoms, including onset, duration, and characteristics of the pain. Ask if they have ever had pain like this and if so, what have they done to relieve the pain. This will be very important as you

Box 8.4 | Patient Education for Taking Nitroglycerin Sublingual or Spray for Sudden Onset of Chest Pain

Step 1: Make sure to sit or lie down, then take 1 dose of NTG (sublingual or spray) right away after the start of the chest pain. *If the symptoms do not improve or get worse, call 911.*

Step 2: If the symptoms improve after the first dose but do not go away completely, you can take a second dose after 5 minutes. *If the symptoms do not improve or get worse, call 911.*

Step 3: If the symptoms continue to improve but do not go away completely, you can even take a third dose 5 minutes after the second dose. *If the symptoms do not improve or get worse, call 911. Do not take more than 3 doses in 15 minutes.*

Step 4: Call 911 if:
- Symptoms do not get better within 5 minutes or if they get worse after the first dose.
- Symptoms do not continue to get better after the second dose.
- Chest pain does not go away completely 5 minutes after taking the third dose.
- You feel that you have taken more than the required dose.

monitor the effectiveness of the nitrate. See Box 8.4 for the current recommendation for giving sublingual NTG to patients with acute angina.

◆ *Planning and implementation.* One of the advantages of NTG and other nitrates is that they come in a variety of forms. NTG tablets are easily absorbed under the tongue and are recommended in an emergency for quick action. However, swallowing the same tablets would destroy the NTG. On the other hand, certain forms, such as isosorbide, are given orally for longer action. NTG also is available as a paste or a transdermal patch so the NTG is absorbed into the bloodstream through the skin. Carefully titrating intravenous NTG relieves pain in severe angina.

Whatever the route, you need to be sure of the proper administration guidelines. Place sublingual NTG under the tongue for absorption into the bloodstream. Remind the patient that the drug is absorbed under the tongue and not chewed or swallowed. If the patient is prescribed NTG paste, measure the dosage carefully using the directions and the proper measuring paper. Remove all old NTG paste before applying the new paste to prevent dosage accumulation. Wear gloves when applying NTG paste because it is absorbed through the skin (on patients and on nurses!).

Top Tip for Safety

Teach patients not to chew or swallow sublingual NTG tablets because the drug is destroyed in the GI system and will not help the angina.

Top Tip for Safety

Wear gloves to apply NTG paste to avoid absorbing it through the skin into your bloodstream.

Carefully monitor the patient's response to NTG. Almost all patients who are taking NTG experience a drop in blood pressure because it is a vasodilator. Do not give NTG if the patient's blood pressure is less than 90/60 mm Hg. Patients often experience a headache after taking NTG. Administration of acetaminophen or other pain drug can help reduce the headache. These headaches typically go away within a few weeks as the patient begins to get used to the drug.

Patients develop a tolerance to NTG, so they must have time "off" of the drug so it does not lose effectiveness. For example, place NTG patches in the morning, then remove at bedtime as directed. If the patch was left on the body for 24 hours, the next dose would be less effective. The patient would no longer receive the benefit of the nitrate. That time off during the night ensures that the drug will continue to work. See Table 8.7 for additional information about NTG and nursing implications

◆ *Evaluation.* It is very important to evaluate the patient for effectiveness. Sublingual NTG is given in patients with a sudden onset of angina. It is fast and can be effective. For evaluation, does NTG relieve or reduce angina? If it does not, call 911. In any emergency situation, failure of the drug to relieve pain is an indicator that the patient may be having a heart attack and is likely to have heart muscle damage if they do not receive emergency care.

Evaluate the patient's blood pressure carefully after giving any nitrates until you are clear about their usual response. For sublingual NTG, you may monitor blood pressure every 5 minutes until the pain is relieved or until emergency providers have arrived to transport the patient to the acute care setting.

Top Tip for Safety

Anginal Attacks

For acute angina, teach the patient to put one NTG tablet under the tongue as soon as the pain begins and not to chew or swallow the drug. Tell the patient to let the drug dissolve under the tongue while he or she lies down and rests. If the pain is not relieved or reduced within 5 minutes, the patient should call 911 or report to the emergency room. The patient should not drive if he or she is having chest pain! While waiting for the ambulance, the patient may take a second pill. If the pain is not relieved within another 5 minutes, the patient may take a third pill. The patient should not take more than three sublingual tablets.

◆ *Patient and family teaching.* Tell the patient and family the following:
- Keep the NTG tablets in a dark, glass container to prevent breakdown of the drug.

Table 8.7   Common Antianginal Drugs

Nitrates: vasodilate by relaxing vascular smooth muscle in the peripheral venous system and reducing resistance to blood flow in the arterial system. These effects work together to help the heart get more oxygen and pump more easily.

DRUGS/ADULT DOSAGE RANGE	NURSING IMPLICATIONS

isosorbide mononitrate (Ismo, Monoket) 20 mg orally twice daily 7 hours apart
isosorbide mononitrate extended release (Imdur) 30–60 mg orally once daily (up to 240 mg/day)
nitroglycerin (many brand names)
  Sublingual or buccal: 0.3–0.6 mg; may repeat every 5 minutes three times
  Sublingual or lingual spray: 1–2 sprays; may repeat every 5 minutes three times
  Oral (sustained-release capsules) 2.5–6.5 mg every 6–8 hours
  Topical ointment: 1–2 inches every 6–8 hours; include up to 12-hour nitrate-free interval
  Transdermal patch 0.1–0.8 mg/h up to 0.8 mg/h; patch is worn 12–14 h/day; include 10–12-hour nitrate-free interval
	• Monitor blood pressure carefully while the patient is taking nitrates because a decrease in blood pressure is a common side effect of the drug.
	• Teach patients that they may experience a headache with nitroglycerin drugs because blood vessel dilation in the head and face causes pain. Mild headaches may be treated with a mild pain reliever such as acetaminophen (Tylenol).
	• Wear gloves when applying nitroglycerin ointment or paste to avoid absorption into your skin.
	• Make sure to remove used patches according to directions (most often removed at bedtime) because patients need a drug-free period to avoid tolerance to the drug.
	• Rotate sites when using paste or patches as directed to prevent skin breakdown.
	• If using paste or patch, choose a hairless area on the upper arms, back, or chest for best drug absorption.
	• For acute episodes of chest pain, give sublingual nitroglycerin or lingual spray (spray onto or under the tongue) for best drug absorption into the blood vessels of this area.
	• Store NTG tablets in a dark, glass container to prevent breakdown of the drug.
	• Make sure to check the expiration dates of NTG tablets because they deteriorate quickly and then are not effective in treating chest pain.
	• Teach male patients that drugs for erectile dysfunction, if taken with nitrates, can cause a severe drop in blood pressure.

Beta blockers: reduce sympathetic stimulation to the heart, decreasing heart rate and decreasing contractility of the heart muscle. As a result, they decrease myocardial oxygen demand.

DRUGS/ADULT DOSAGE RANGE	NURSING IMPLICATIONS
See Table 8.6 to review dosage ranges.	See Table 8.6 to review nursing implications.

Calcium channel blocking agents: decrease blood pressure by relaxing vascular smooth muscle in the coronary and systemic arteries leading to decreased peripheral resistance. This decreases myocardial oxygen demand.

DRUGS/ADULT DOSAGE RANGE	NURSING IMPLICATIONS
See Table 8.6 to review dosage ranges.	See Table 8.6 to review nursing implications.

• Carefully check the expiration dates of NTG tablets. Tablets that have expired are not effective in treating chest pain.
• Do not drink alcoholic beverages while taking nitrate products. If you have a special occasion, notify your healthcare provider before you decide to drink alcohol.
• If you are using NTG spray, do not smoke or use near an open flame because the drug is flammable.
• For transdermal patch application, select a hairless spot (or clip your skin hair) and apply the patch to the skin. Do not cut the patch because it will affect the dose of the drug. If the patch comes off, discard and replace with a new one in a different site. Rotate the sites each day to prevent skin irritation.
• Avoid drugs for erectile dysfunction such as sildenafil (Viagra) because they can cause a severe drop in blood pressure.

• Keep a record of every anginal attack. If you are having an increase in frequency of attacks or changes in the symptoms, notify your healthcare provider.

ANTIDYSRHYTHMICS

The heart has its own electrical conduction system made of specialized cells. These cells are able to automatically create, conduct, and respond to electrical impulses. Electrical impulses travel through the heart muscle, causing the heart to contract and pump blood through the heart and the rest of the body. The primary pacemaker of the heart is the sinoatrial node (Fig. 8.5). When working properly, the pacemaker of the heart automatically creates impulses that cause an orderly contraction of the atria and ventricles, which can be felt as a smooth and regular pulse. The heart muscle contracts and blood flows through the heart chambers into the lungs and the rest of the body. The pacemaker is able to respond to the needs of the body for increased oxygen. For example, during exercise, heart rate increases so that the muscles receive enough oxygen. If the patient has a drop in blood pressure, the heart usually responds by increasing the rate to restore blood pressure. If there are threats to the functioning of the pacemaker of the heart, the patient can experience an abnormal rhythm and cardiac output is reduced.

When the cells in the conduction system do not have enough oxygen, are damaged through disease, or if electrolytes are out of balance, irregular heart rhythm results. The abnormal heart rhythm (whether too slow or too fast) can have a significant impact on cardiac output. These abnormal rhythms may be *benign* (not requiring drugs) or life-threatening. You still may hear nurses in the clinical area using the term *arrhythmia* to describe abnormal heart rhythm. We use the term *dysrhythmia* (irregular rhythm) rather than arrhythmia (without rhythm) to describe abnormal heart rhythm.

Dysrhythmias may be fast or slow, with an irregular or regular pattern. Common causes of dysrhythmias include hypoxia (such as in a blockage of the coronary artery), fluid and electrolyte imbalances (such as high or low potassium levels), adverse effects of certain drugs, and interventions to the heart including cardiac catheterization or open-heart surgery.

Dysrhythmias are usually classified according to the site of origin and type of rhythm abnormality produced. For example, atrial dysrhythmias start in the atria, supraventricular dysrhythmias start above the ventricles, and ventricular dysrhythmias start in the ventricles. An example of an atrial dysthymia is atrial fibrillation (rhythm starts in the atria, irregular rate). Ventricular tachycardia is a rapid heart rate that starts in the ventricles. The primary question for you is: Does this rhythm affect how well the patient's heart can pump? The goal of any treatment plan or therapeutic regimen is for the patient's heart to regain a normal rate and rhythm so that normal circulation is restored. Most acute care settings offer specific courses to help nurses identify specific dysrhythmias.

Action

Antidysrhythmic drugs work to make heart rhythm more regular and reduce serious dysrhythmias. Even though many dysrhythmias require nonpharmacologic treatments (ranging from pacemaker insertion to giving the heart an electric shock), drugs play an important role in treating abnormal heart rhythms to help the heart achieve a more normal rhythm. Antidysrhythmic drugs affect the cells that are beating irregularly during different phases of electrical conduction. Some of the drugs used to help regulate heart rhythm are also used to treat HBP and other cardiovascular problems.

Antidysrhythmic drugs are classified using the Vaughan Williams classification system. This system helps organize the drugs according to where they act in the conduction cycle.

1. Class I drugs are sodium channel blockers (e.g., quinidine, procainamide, and disopyramide)
   a. Lengthen the period during which the cells cannot release or discharge their electrical activity
   b. Make the heart less excitable; slow the impulse conduction through the heart
2. Class II drugs are beta blockers (e.g., propranolol, esmolol, and acebutolol)
   a. Reduce sympathetic stimulation to the heart, decreasing heart rate
   b. Decrease contractility of heart muscle
3. Class III drugs are potassium channel blockers (e.g., amiodarone)
   a. Makes the cells less excitable
   b. Can slow the heart rate
4. Class IV drugs are calcium channel blockers (e.g., diltiazem and verapamil)
   a. Selectively block the ability of calcium to enter the heart muscle cells
   b. Slow the conduction through the sinoatrial and/ or atrioventricular node
5. Other (digoxin or magnesium sulfate)

Uses

The cause of the dysrhythmia determines which drug class will be most effective for treatment. Whatever the abnormal rhythm, the goal is to restore the rhythm to normal and maintain adequate cardiac output.

Digoxin is used primarily to treat heart failure but also plays a role in treating fast dysrhythmias, such as atrial fibrillation or supraventricular tachycardia. It slows the heart rate by slowing how fast the sinoatrial node fires and slowing conduction through the atrioventricular node. It also strengthens the contraction of the heart. Toxic levels of this drug also cause dysrhythmias. Other drugs that affect heart activity are the beta-adrenergic blockers such as sotalol or acebutolol. Drugs in this class act very much like quinidine on the heart, but they also decrease the response of the heart muscle to epinephrine and norepinephrine (other chemical neurotransmitters) by blocking the stimulation of the heart's beta receptors.

> **Memory Jogger**
>
> Learning the common suffixes can help you recognize the specific class of drugs.
> 1. Beta blockers often end with "olol."
> 2. ACE-Is often end with "pril."
> 3. ARBs often end with "sartan."

Many antidysrhythmic drugs are so powerful that they are given only in critical care units where the patients are closely monitored. As the patient's condition becomes more stable, oral versions of the drug or another antidysrhythmic may be used for long-term therapy. Table 8.8 lists drugs that may commonly be used in the treatment of acute and chronic dysrhythmias.

Adverse Reactions

Drugs that are given to control dysrhythmias may also cause other dysrhythmias. All patients who are receiving these drugs should have their heart carefully monitored by ECG for any change.

🔲 Top Tip for Safety

Drugs given to control dysrhythmias may also cause other dysrhythmias. Monitor the patient for symptoms of irregular heart beats.

❖ Nursing Implications and Patient Teaching

◆ *Assessment.* Ask about the patient's health history, including any drug allergies, other drugs taken that may cause drug interactions, and other medical problems. It is best practice to assess the apical heart rate using your stethoscope before giving the drug. Some irregular heart rates are very weak and are difficult to palpate with a radial pulse.

◆ *Planning and implementation.* The healthcare provider typically obtains an ECG before giving the drugs. This test will help the provider determine how well the drugs work. In addition, take baseline and follow-up vital signs when you are giving antidysrhythmic drugs. In some settings, you may have the responsibility of monitoring changes in blood pressure or pulse as the patient begins taking the drug. Any significant changes must be reported to the RN or healthcare provider. Hospitalized patients often continue their antidysrhythmic drugs when they go home, so you should take

---

💊 Table 8.8   Common Antidysrhythmic Drugs

Sodium channel blockers: increase the length of time the cells cannot discharge their electrical activity, making the heart less excitable. They slow the conduction of impulses through the heart. These drugs help to treat supraventricular and ventricular dysrhythmias. Some are used in life-threatening dysrhythmias

DRUGS/ADULT DOSAGE RANGE	NURSING IMPLICATIONS
quinidine (Quinora, Quinaglute) As quinidine sulfate 200–300 mg orally every 6–8 hours As quinidine sulfate extended release 300–600 mg every 8–12 hours As quinidine gluconate extended release 324–648 mg orally every 8–12 hours disopyramide (Norpace) 150–200 mg every 6 hours (range 400–800 mg in 4 divided doses); in some cases, may require a loading dose of 300 mg orally one time only flecainide (Tambocor) 100–200 mg orally every 12 hours; maximum is 400 mg daily propafenone (Rythmol) 150–300 mg orally every 8 hours propafenon sustained-release (Rythmol SR) 225–425 mg every 12 hours	• Carefully monitor the heart rate and blood pressure of the patient because these drugs can cause hypotension and dysrhythmias. • Teach patients to avoid any over-the-counter drug to prevent dangerous interactions. • Quinidine can cause significant GI side effects. Remind patient to take the drug with food to ease the symptoms. • Give the drug exactly as scheduled to avoid irregular blood levels. Patients may need to use timers to help remember to take the drug on schedule. • Monitor patient weight and intake and output because some of these drugs can cause urinary retention. • Older adult patients are more likely to experience dizziness and confusion, and thus are at greater risk for falls. • Teach family members to assess the patients for any confusion and report to the healthcare provider. • Carefully review your drug reference or manual before giving any sodium channel blocker to review additional side effects and adverse effects specific to each drug.

Beta blockers: reduce sympathetic stimulation to the heart, decreasing heart rate and decreasing contractility of the heart muscle. They are often used to treat rapid dysrhythmias that originate about the ventricle (supraventricular tachycardia).

DRUGS/ADULT DOSAGE RANGE	NURSING IMPLICATIONS
acebutolol (Monitan, Sectral) 200 mg orally twice daily (usual therapeutic range 600–1200 mg daily) propranolol (Inderal) 10–20 mg orally three to four times daily. May increase to 160–320 mg daily in 3–4 divided doses sotalol (Betapace, Sorine) 80 mg orally every 12 hours; average dosage 160–320 mg daily	• Monitor the patient's heart rate and blood pressure. Hold the drug if the heart rate is less than 60 beats/min or systolic blood pressure is less than 90 mm Hg. • Teach patients that stopping beta blockers can cause serious complications, including rapid heart rate, hypertensive crisis, and heart attack. • Monitor blood sugar regularly in patients with diabetes because beta blockers can increase or decrease blood sugar levels. They can also mask the signs of hypoglycemia (such as increased heart rate). • Teach patients that depression can be a side effect of taking beta blockers. If they experience symptoms of depression, contact their healthcare provider.

Continued

Table 8.8 **Common Antidysrhythmic Drugs—cont'd**

Potassium channel blockers: make cells less excitable and reduce the heart rate. They are often used to help convert atrial fibrillation and/or atrial flutter to a normal sinus rhythm. They can also be used to treat dangerous ventricular dysrhythmias.

DRUGS/ADULT DOSAGE RANGE	NURSING IMPLICATIONS
amiodarone (Cordarone). Usual dose 200–400 mg orally daily in one or divided dose. May begin with loading dosage: 800–1600 mg daily for 1–3 weeks, then increase to 600–800 mg for 1 month before beginning at the maintenance dose.	• Monitor for common side effects such as dizziness, fatigue, and hypotension. If you are caring for a patient on intravenous potassium channel blockers, side effects may be severe and include neurologic symptoms such as unsteady gait, numbness and tingling, and tremor. • Be sure to monitor the respiratory status of patients who are taking amiodarone because it may cause pulmonary complications. • Teach patients who are taking amiodarone that the drug causes sensitivity to light, so they may need to wear dark glasses when going outside. In addition, they should wear protective clothing and a sunscreen barrier. • Remind patients that they may not have side effects until they have taken the drug for several days or weeks. • Tell patients that long-term use of amiodarone may cause a bluish discoloration of the face, neck, or arms. Reassure them that the side effect is reversible and will fade away over several months. • Patients will need to schedule eye examinations every 6–12 months because amiodarone can cause corneal microdeposits or other eye changes. • Remind male patients to report any pain or swelling in the scrotum to the healthcare provider. The patient may need a decrease in drug dosage.

Calcium channel blockers: impede the ability of calcium to enter the heart muscle cells. They slow the conduction of electrical impulses through the sinoatrial and atrioventricular nodes. Calcium channel blockers are primarily used to treat supraventricular tachycardias.

DRUGS/ADULT DOSAGE RANGE	NURSING IMPLICATIONS
diltiazem (Cardizem, Diltzac, Tiazac) oral 30–120 mg three to four times daily diltiazem extended-release capsules (Cardizem CD, Cardizem, LA, Dilacor XR) 120–240 orally once daily; may go up to 240–480 mg once daily verapamil (Calan, Isoptin) 80–120 mg orally every 8 hours; may increase up to 480 mg daily in 3 to 4 divided doses verapamil extended release (Calan SR, Isoptin SR, Covera-HS) 180–480 mg orally once daily or in 2 divided doses. Some forms may be given at bedtime.	• Avoid sudden changes in position because most antihypertensive drugs cause orthostatic hypotension. • Remind patients to keep taking the drugs as prescribed because they do not cure high blood pressure. • Monitor patients' blood pressure regularly to determine how well they are responding to the drug. • Teach patients to avoid alcohol because it can cause hypotension in patients taking calcium channel blockers. • Avoid all over-the-counter drugs until checking with the healthcare provider to avoid dangerous drug interactions. • Notify the healthcare provider if the patient experiences swelling in the legs because this can be a sign of fluid retention caused by calcium channel blockers. • Calcium channel blockers are avoided in patients with heart failure because of the potential of fluid retention. • Be alert for signs of Stevens-Johnsons syndrome (erythema multiforme), a life-threating skin condition that can be an adverse effect of calcium channel blockers. This condition is associated with skin lesions, fever, and joint aching. • Report heart rates less than 60 beats/min and blood pressures less than 90 mm Hg systolic to the healthcare provider before giving the drug, to avoid significant hypotension. • If you are caring for a patient who is receiving intravenous calcium channel blockers, check with the RN or healthcare provider regarding the need for a bed with a cardiac monitor.

Table 8.8 Common Antidysrhythmic Drugs—cont'd

Cardiac glycosides: decrease the speed of conduction through the atrioventricular node, decreasing the number of atrial polarizations, and slow the ventricular rate.

DRUGS/ADULT DOSAGE RANGE	NURSING IMPLICATIONS
digoxin (Digitek, Lanoxicaps, Lanoxin) 0.125–0.375 mg daily orally (dose varies depending on drug form and patient response); older adults maximum dose 0.125 mg daily	• Calcium channel blockers such as verapamil and diltiazem are replacing use of digoxin for atrial dysrhythmias. Nevertheless, if you do have patients who are taking digoxin, monitor the patients very carefully for symptoms of digoxin toxicity, such as lack of appetite, nausea, vomiting, and vision changes. • Monitor potassium levels carefully because a low potassium level can cause dangerous dysrhythmias. • In rare cases, patients may receive a loading dose to begin therapy, then will be switched to a normal dose after 24 hours. This is becoming a much less common practice. • If patients experience any symptoms of digoxin toxicity, make sure to contact the healthcare provider. Optimal blood levels range between 0.5 and 0.8 ng/mL. • Take an apical pulse before giving digoxin. Do not give the drug if the pulse is less than 60 beats/min. • Give digoxin at the same time every day to prevent irregular drug blood levels. • Teach patients that a missed dose may be taken within 12 hours of the scheduled time and to never take double doses because of the high risk for drug toxicity.

advantage of every opportunity to teach patients about these drugs.

◆ *Evaluation.* In some settings, the patient is monitored using telemetry (24-hour-a-day cardiac monitoring). Specially trained staff (e.g., monitor technicians, nurses, and LPN/VNs with training) will monitor for changes in the ECG patterns. Monitor for changes in vital signs because improvement in rhythm often leads to improvement in vital signs.

◆ *Patient and family teaching.* Tell the patient and family the following:

- Take this drug exactly as ordered and do not skip doses or double the dose.
- Report any new or distressing symptoms to the nurse or other healthcare provider, especially any sudden weight gain, trouble breathing, or increased coughing.
- Return regularly for checkup visits to the healthcare provider to see how the drug is affecting your heart function.
- Do not take any other drugs before consulting with the healthcare provider to make sure the combination is safe. This includes aspirin, laxatives, cold and sinus products, or other OTC drugs.

INOTROPIC DRUGS

The term *inotrope* is used to describe contractility of the heart. An **inotropic drug** affects contractility of the *myocardium* (heart muscle). A drug that is a positive inotrope increases contractility; a negative inotropic drug decreases contractility of the myocardium. In heart failure, positive inotropic drugs increase contractility of the heart (in other words, they increase the ability of the heart to pump).

Memory Jogger

A *positive* inotropic drug *increases* contractility and the ability of the heart to pump.
A *negative* inotropic drug *decreases* contractility and the ability of the heart to pump.

Examples of positive inotropes include cardiac glycosides such as digoxin, phosphodiesterase inhibitors such as milrinone, and dobutamine. The major cardiac glycoside is digoxin. Between the 1960s and the early 2000s, digoxin was one of the main drugs used in heart failure to increase the contractility of the heart. As researchers learned more about the pathophysiology of heart failure, other drugs have replaced digoxin as a drug of choice. Digoxin is still used as an antidysrhythmic and an adjuvant agent in heart failure. Names, dosages, and nursing implications for common antidysrhythmics are listed in Table 8.8. For more information about specific antidysrhythmics, consult a drug reference book or a pharmacist.

Action

As a positive inotrope, digoxin activates contractile proteins in the heart muscle, increasing their ability to contract. This increase in contractility continues even if the patient is taking a beta blocker (negative inotrope as you remember that beta blockers can decrease contractility to decrease how hard the heart works). In patients with heart failure, an increased force of contraction may lead to an improvement in cardiac output.

In addition, digoxin affects the conduction system of the heart, decreasing heart rate. As a result, digoxin can effectively treat atrial fibrillation in some cases. Other inotropic agents that are used in patients with heart failure include milrinone and dobutamine. These agents are used in seriously ill, symptomatic patients. Both require extensive monitoring, so they are typically used in acute care or palliative care settings to reduce symptoms of heart failure.

Patients with heart failure are more likely to receive ACE-Is or ARBs, beta blockers, and/or diuretics to manage symptoms and decrease progression of the illness. Nevertheless, digoxin is still used in some cases and has significant implications for the LPN/VN who is monitoring a patient who is taking it.

Uses

Positive inotropic drugs are primarily used for symptom management in patients with advanced heart failure and in critical care areas to increase contractility of the heart muscle and improve cardiac output.

Adverse Reactions

Inotropic drugs are very powerful and can be toxic. Symptoms of digoxin toxicity include anorexia, nausea, vomiting, diarrhea, visual disturbances such as blurred or yellow vision, and irregular heart rate (at times with palpitations). At times patients may experience anxiety, depression, or confusion. Older adult patients are at particular risk for adverse effects of inotropic drugs, including digoxin.

A blood test that tells the level of digoxin (often called a "dig level") is a tool that determines the correct dose and protects the patient from toxicity. Some patients are more likely to develop high digoxin blood levels if they are older, have renal insufficiency, or have electrolyte imbalances caused by dehydration or drugs taken for other types of heart conditions. Treatment of digoxin toxicity begins by stopping the drug and beginning treatment of symptoms, as needed.

Adverse reactions in patients taking dobutamine include chest pain, palpitations, shortness of breath, bronchospasm, severe allergic reaction, and dysrhythmias. Adverse reactions associated with milrinone are similar and include chest pain, bronchospasm, severe allergic reaction, and dysrhythmias.

✖ Lifespan Considerations
Older Adults

Digoxin has a very narrow therapeutic range, which means that the effective dose is close to doses that can cause toxicity. Older adults are particularly at risk for digoxin toxicity. Symptoms of toxicity may begin slowly and are often easy to overlook. These symptoms include loss of appetite, nausea and vomiting, and changes in vision (blurred or with yellow-green).

Drug Interactions

Beta-adrenergic blocking agents, calcium gluconate, calcium chloride, succinylcholine, and verapamil increase both the therapeutic and the toxic effects of inotropic drugs. Any drug that changes the electrolyte balance may also lead to digoxin toxicity. In particular, patients who take drugs that reduce potassium levels, such as diuretics, are particularly susceptible to digoxin toxicity.

❖ Nursing Implications and Patient Teaching

◆ *Assessment.* Take vital signs before giving digoxin or any inotropic agents. While improving contractility of the heart, they can also affect the heart rate. For digoxin, make sure that the patient's heart rate is 60 or above. If you have a patient in an acute care setting who is taking digoxin for atrial fibrillation, it will be very important to have a skilled monitor technician available to monitor for any changes in the ECG. In addition you will need to assess whether the patient's potassium level is within normal limits because a low potassium level can increase the risk for digoxin toxicity. Should you have any questions about your assessment, notify the RN or the healthcare provider before giving these drugs. Assess for any potential adverse effects each time you give the drug.

If you are caring for a patient who is receiving intravenous milrinone or dobutamine, carefully monitor for a rapid heart rate and negative changes in the patient's condition (e.g., increased shortness of breath or chest pain) that may indicate adverse effects.

◆ *Planning and implementation.* Know about two different types of doses for patients taking digoxin: the initial loading dose and the maintenance (regular daily) dose. The healthcare provider may prescribe a higher and/or more frequent dose when a patient begins taking digoxin to reach a target blood level for a specific response. When the target blood level is reached, the smaller daily dose is given once a day to maintain the blood level.

👁 Top Tip for Safety

Digoxin lowers the patient's heart rate, so always measure the patient's apical heart rate for 60 seconds with a stethoscope before giving these drugs. This safety measure is essential to avoid an overdose. If the patient's pulse is irregular, you may not feel an accurate heart rate using the radial pulse alone.

👁 Top Tip for Safety
Digoxin

Remember the rules for the "leading" and "trailing" zeroes when giving digoxin. The usual dosages for digoxin in adults is very small compared with other drugs, ranging from 0.125 to 0.25 mg.

◆ *Evaluation.* Monitoring for drug toxicity is important for any patient who is taking a positive inotropic drug. If you notice any significant change in vital signs, notify the RN or the healthcare provider in charge of the patient. You may be caring for a number of patients with multiple chronic illnesses, so it is important to monitor for any adverse effects. The healthcare provider will order blood tests to measure the serum digoxin level. The therapeutic level of digoxin is 0.5 to 2 ng/mL (nanograms per milliliter). If the level is 2 ng/mL or above, hold the drug and notify the healthcare provider for best action.

Should a patient become severely digoxin toxic, the healthcare provider may prescribe digoxin immune fab (Digibind). This drug requires careful monitoring of the patient's vital signs and potassium levels, and special plans for slowly reducing the amount of drug that is given to avoid causing other life-threatening events.

◆ *Patient and family teaching.* Teach the family and patient the following:
- Let your healthcare provider know if you have any loss of appetite, nausea, vomiting, diarrhea, or any vision changes that can be an indication of digoxin toxicity.
- Do not skip a dose or stop taking the drug without discussing this with your healthcare provider.
- Keep appointments with your healthcare provider to make sure that the drug is still effective. Blood levels of the drug may be ordered.
- Do not take any other prescription drugs or OTC drugs without the approval of your healthcare provider.
- Notify your healthcare provider of any chest pain, shortness of breath, or peripheral edema that may indicate worsening heart failure.
- Include foods rich in potassium in your diet (unless contraindicated by your healthcare provider). Good sources of potassium include bananas, orange juice, green leafy vegetables, and baked potatoes.

Get Ready for the NCLEX® Examination!

Key Points

- Thiazide and thiazide-like drugs are the most commonly used type of diuretic and often are first line in the management of HBP.
- Loop diuretics are widely considered the most powerful of the diuretics. Use can result in significant decreases in fluid volume and increase in urine output.
- Potassium is one of the major electrolytes lost after loop diuretic administration. Monitor potassium levels carefully because significant changes in potassium can result in cardiac dysrhythmias.
- Potassium-sparing diuretics increase the excretion of water and sodium, leading to increased urine output without the loss of potassium.
- Monitor older adults taking diuretics more frequently for dehydration and symptoms of low potassium levels, such as muscle weakness and irregular heartbeats.
- Common side effects of diuretics include urinary urgency and urinary frequency.
- Diuretics can cause low blood pressure that can result in falls, particularly in high-risk patients.
- Patients who are taking potassium-sparing diuretics should avoid salt substitutes to decrease the risk for hyperkalemia.
- Potassium levels that are too high or too low can cause life-threatening dysrhythmias.
- Assess the patient carefully for any signs of dehydration before giving any diuretic.
- Warn patients and family members that pregnant women should not handle or touch dihydrotestosterone (DHT) inhibitors used for BPH because these drugs can cause birth defects if absorbed through the skin.
- Warn patients who are taking selective alpha$_1$ blockers for BPH to change positions slowly because these drugs lower blood pressure and can cause dizziness.
- Remind patients who are taking urinary antispasmodics to avoid becoming overheated or dehydrated during exercise or hot weather because these drugs decrease sweating and increase the risk for heatstroke.
- LDLs are the "bad" cholesterol; HDLs are the "good" cholesterol.
- All patients who are taking statins should have liver function studies shortly after starting the drug and then yearly, or if they experience any symptoms of liver problems.
- Statins are contraindicated during pregnancy and breast-feeding because of the effects of lower cholesterol levels on the developing brain.
- For patients who are taking statins, immediately report to the healthcare provider any reports of severe muscle ache or signs of liver problems, such as jaundice or dark urine, because those symptoms can be signs of serious adverse effects.
- One of the main problems for patients taking niacin is the expected side effect of flushing (red color in the face and neck).
- No cholesterol-reducing drug cures hyperlipidemia.
- Drug therapy for HBP often requires trial periods to establish the right drug or drug combinations to help any one patient achieve his or her blood pressure goal.
- You can use the terms *antagonist* and *blocker* interchangeably to describe a drug that turns off a receptor.
- ACE-Is and ARBs can cause hyperkalemia (high potassium levels), so remind patients to avoid high-potassium foods.
- Fluid retention is a common side effect of calcium channel blockers, so these drugs should be avoided in patients with heart failure.
- Beta blockers typically end with the suffix *-olol*, such as in metoprolol, propranolol, or sotalol.
- A side effect of prazosin and terazosin is first-dose hypotension. As a result, these drugs may be given at night to prevent severe orthostatic hypotension. These effects diminish over time.

Get Ready for the NCLEX® Examination!—cont'd

- Do not stop alpha₂ agonists suddenly, to prevent rebound HBP.
- Antihypertensives and diuretics are used alone or in combination to decrease elevated blood pressure to a desired level according to accepted guidelines and to prevent complications of acute and chronic HBP.
- All blood pressure drugs can cause hypotension, or too low of a blood pressure to maintain adequate circulation. Most can cause orthostatic hypotension, that is, dizziness that occurs when changing positions.
- Older adults are particularly likely to experience dizziness when taking these drugs. The orthostatic hypotension they experience places them at risk for falling when they rapidly change positions, such as getting up quickly from a chair or bed.
- Teach your patient to stand up slowly when taking drugs for HBP, to avoid dizziness and prevent falls.
- For all patients with HBP, it is critical to gather a thorough drug history. Certain prescription drugs, OTC drugs, herbal preparations, and even illegal drugs can actually *cause* HBP.
- Before giving any drug that affects blood pressure, baseline blood pressure checks are essential.
- HBP has no cure; it can, however, be well managed.
- Notify the healthcare provider of any new or uncomfortable symptoms that develop. These symptoms may indicate an adverse effect or may be relieved by simply changing to a new drug.
- Teach patients to avoid alcoholic beverages while taking drugs for HBP.
- Rapid-acting nitrates (such as sublingual NTG and intravenous NTG) are used to relieve pain in acute angina. The long-acting oral nitrates, topical NTG paste, and transdermal patches can prevent angina and reduce the severity and frequency of anginal attacks.
- Throbbing headaches occur in more than 50% of patients who take nitrates.
- Remember that all antidysrhythmic drugs can cause dysrhythmias.
- Positive inotropic drugs are primarily used for symptom management in patients with advanced heart failure and in critical care areas to increase contractility of the heart muscle and improve cardiac output.
- Digoxin has a very narrow therapeutic range, which means that the dose that is effective is close to the dose that causes toxic reactions. Older adults are particularly at risk for digoxin toxicity. Symptoms of toxicity may begin slowly and are often easy to overlook. These symptoms include loss of appetite, nausea and vomiting, and changes in vision.
- Digoxin lowers the patient's heart rate, so always measure the patient's apical heart rate for 60 seconds with a stethoscope before giving these drugs. If the patient's pulse is irregular, you may not feel an accurate heart rate using the radial pulse alone.
- Remember the rules for the "leading" and "trailing" zeroes when giving digoxin. The usual dosages for digoxin in adults can be from 0.125 to 0.25 mg.

Review Questions for the NCLEX® Examination

1. A patient with benign prostatic hypertrophy is receiving tamsulosin, a selective alpha₁ blocker, to help improve urine flow. Which of the following health factors would the LPN/VN report to the healthcare provider before giving the drug?
   1. The patient reports a history of allergy to sulfa antibiotics.
   2. The patient had a history of smoking 15 years ago.
   3. The patient is exercising three times a week.
   4. The patient's potassium level is 4.0 mEq/mL.

2. The LPN/VN is teaching a patient about his sublingual NTG tablets for an onset of chest pain. Which of the following statements by the patient shows that he or she understands the teaching?
   1. "I need to chew the NTG tablet thoroughly."
   2. "I will swallow the pill like all of my other heart pills."
   3. "I will place the NTG under my tongue when I have chest pain."
   4. "I like to take my NTG with applesauce so it tastes better."

3. The patient has a history of acute angina. Which of the following should the LPN/VN teach the patient regarding taking NTG tablets for chest pain? (Select all that apply.)
   1. Take one dose of NTG immediately at the onset of the pain. If the symptoms get a little better but do not go away, take the second dose 5 minutes later. You can even take a third dose 5 minutes after the second dose.
   2. Take no more than three doses in 15 minutes.
   3. Call emergency services if your symptoms do not improve or if they worsen after the first dose.
   4. You may feel a slight burning under the tongue when you take the NTG.
   5. Common side effects include light-headedness, muscle aches, and seizures.
   6. The NTG will work better if you also dissolve an aspirin under your tongue at the same time.

4. The patient has started taking niacin for her high cholesterol. Which of the following side effects is common in patients taking niacin?
   1. Hyperuricemia
   2. Glucose tolerance
   3. Flushing
   4. Constipation

5. The patient is taking digoxin 0.125 mg every morning with breakfast for atrial fibrillation. The LPN/VN checks the apical pulse and determines the rate to be 58 beats/min. Which of the following actions is appropriate by the LPN/VN?
   1. Ask the patient to drink a cup of coffee and return to the room in 1 hour to give the drug.
   2. Hold the drug and notify the healthcare provider.
   3. Give the drug and document in the medical record.
   4. Give the drug and notify the healthcare provider.

Get Ready for the NCLEX® Examination!—cont'd

6. Which of the following laboratory tests must be carefully monitored in a patient taking a loop diuretic?
   1. Potassium level
   2. Liver function studies
   3. Arterial blood gases
   4. Cholesterol level

7. Which of the following symptoms are associated with digoxin toxicity? (Select all that apply.)
   1. Nausea
   2. Anorexia
   3. Blurred vision
   4. Constipation
   5. Enlarged liver
   6. Diarrhea

8. A patient is receiving a new statin drug for elevated cholesterol level. Which of the following statements by the patient indicates a need for additional teaching?
   1. "I can eat anything I want since I am now taking this drug."
   2. "I will notify my healthcare provider if I have any severe muscle aches or changes in my urine."
   3. "I will need to have tests to make sure my liver is functioning properly as my doctor recommends."
   4. "I have to monitor my blood sugar daily because the drug can increase my blood sugar."

9. Which of the following side effects is seen in patients taking angiotensin-converting enzyme inhibitors but rarely seen in patients taking angiotensin II receptor blockers?
   1. Orthostatic hypotension
   2. Cough
   3. Dizziness
   4. Hypotension

10. Which of the following types of food should be avoided in patients taking angiotensin-converting enzyme inhibitors?
    1. Foods high in folic acid, such as lentils and avocado
    2. Foods high in vitamin K, such as green leafy vegetables
    3. Foods high in iron, such as red meat and salmon
    4. Foods high in potassium, such as bananas and orange juice

11. Match the drug action with the drug class.
    1. Slows the sodium pump in the distal tubule of the nephron
    2. Decreases heart rate and decreases contractility of the heart
    3. Blocks active transport of sodium, chloride, and potassium in the loop of Henle
    4. Blocks the formation of angiotensin II
    5. Causes vasodilation centrally by affecting receptors in the brain
       a. Angiotensin-converting enzyme inhibitor
       b. Loop diuretic
       c. Beta blocker
       d. Alpha$_2$-adrenergic agonist
       e. Potassium-sparing diuretic

Drug Calculation Review

1. A patient is receiving 0.125 mg of digoxin at 9:00 a.m. A 0.25 mg tablet (scored) is available. How many tablets will you prepare to give the patient?

Case Study

Mrs. Johnson is a 72-year-old African American woman with primary hypertension diagnosed 22 years ago after she went through menopause. According to her family history, her father had high blood pressure and her grandfather died of a stroke at the age of 63. She worked at an insurance office for about 40 years until she retired 5 years ago. She states she feels "pretty overwhelmed" since her husband was diagnosed with Alzheimer's disease 6 months ago. At this time she takes hydrochlorothiazide (Microzide) 50 mg twice a day and amlodipine (Norvasc) 10 mg a day. She tells you that she has missed doses lately because she has been so busy with her husband.

1. What are Mrs. Johnson's risk factors for hypertension?
2. What should you teach Mrs. Johnson about her antihypertensive drugs?
3. What strategies could you suggest to Mrs. Johnson to help control her hypertension?

Drug Therapy for Central Nervous System Problems

Learning Outcomes

1. List the names, actions, possible side effects, and adverse effects of drugs for Parkinson's disease.
2. Explain what to teach patients and families about drugs for Parkinson's disease.
3. List the names, actions, possible side effects, and adverse effects of drugs for Alzheimer's disease.
4. Explain what to teach patients and families about drugs for Alzheimer's disease.
5. List the names, actions, possible side effects, and adverse effects of drugs for epilepsy and other seizure problems.
6. Explain what to teach patients and families about drugs for epilepsy and other seizure problems.
7. List the names, actions, possible side effects, and adverse effects of drugs for multiple sclerosis.
8. Explain what to teach patients and families about drugs for multiple sclerosis.

Key Terms

antiepileptic drugs (AEDs) (ĂN-tī-ĕ-pǐ-LĔP-tǐk, p. 170) Drugs that reduce or prevent seizures.

biological response modifier (BRM) (bī-ĕ-LŎ-jǐ-kăl rǐ-SPŎN(t)s MŎ-dǐ-fīr, p. 179) Drug that modifies the patient's immune response to abnormal triggers for immunity and inflammation.

catechol-*O*-methyltransferase (COMT) inhibitor (KĂ-tĕ-kŏl-ō-MĔTH-ǐl-TRAN(t)s-fĕr-ās, p. 161) Drug that suppresses the activity of the COMT enzyme so that both naturally occurring dopamine and dopamine agonist drugs remain active in the body longer, helping to restore the acetylcholine–dopamine balance in the brain.

cholinesterase inhibitor (kō-lĕ-NĔS-tĕ-rās ǐn-HǏ-bǎ-tĕr, p. 167) Drug that delays memory loss by binding to the enzyme acetylcholinesterase and slowing its action, which allows any acetylcholine produced to remain functional longer.

delirium (dǐ-LǏR-ē-ĕm, p. 163) A distressed state of mind that causes irrational beliefs characterized by illusions and paranoia.

dopamine agonist (DŌ-pĕ-mēn Ă-gă-nǐst, p. 161) Drug that has the same chemical structure of natural dopamine and is used to increase the levels of dopamine in the brain and restore balance between acetylcholine and dopamine action.

dyskinesia (dǐs-kĕ-NĒ-zh(ē-)ă, p. 163) An abnormality and distortion in performing voluntary movements. It results in jerky motions and looks much like uncoordinated dance movements.

dystonia (dǐs-TŌ-nē-ă, p. 164) Abnormal involuntary movements such as chewing, grinding of the teeth, protrusion of the tongue, opening and closing the mouth, head bobbing, or jerky, constant movements of the feet or hands.

monoamine oxidase type B (MAO-B) inhibitor (mă-nō-ă-MĒN ŎK-să-dās, p. 161) Drug that suppresses the action of MAO-B, which allows dopamine levels to increase and reduce the symptoms of Parkinson's disease.

neurotransmitter (nyūr-ō-trănz-MǏ-tĕr, p. 159) Chemical that is released from the end of one nerve, crosses a space (cleft), and then binds to receptors on the beginning of the next nerve in the line (or a skeletal muscle) to transmit the electrical signal from one nerve to the next.

***N*-methyl-D-aspartate (NMDA) blocker** (p. 166) Drug that slows the progression of Alzheimer disease by blocking the entrance of calcium into neurons, which reduces or slows neuronal damage.

phenytoins (fĕ-NǏ-tĕ-wĕn, p. 170) Antiepileptic drugs that reduce or prevent seizures by binding to sodium channels on nerve membranes in the brain and making them less active, which prevents the spread of neuron excitation.

CENTRAL NERVOUS SYSTEM FUNCTIONS

The central nervous system (CNS) is the brain and the spinal cord (Fig. 9.1). The nerves coming from the spinal cord are part of the peripheral nervous system (PNS) and are controlled by the brain. The PNS nerves serve as a relay between the brain and the body by connecting the CNS to the organs, limbs, muscles, blood vessels, and glands. The CNS has many critical structures and actions that work together to ensure continued normal whole-body functioning. The brain monitors and regulates the coordination of body systems and activities, including movement, endocrine secretions, and the intellectual functions of thinking/decision making. It monitors body conditions by receiving sensory information from elsewhere in the body and by receiving sensory information from the environment from vision, hearing, smell, taste, spacial awareness, and touch. The brain interprets this information and then determines how the body should respond. For example, did you know that we do not actually see with our eyes? We "see" with our brain. The nerve endings (rods and cones) in the retina detect light and shape, then send these nerve signals as messages through the optic nerve to the brain. The brain translates the light image signals into what we "see" or think we see (perceive). Perception of vision is how optical illusions work. Magicians create illusions by taking advantage of how our brain interprets stimuli.

Many problems can occur inside or outside of the CNS that can affect brain function. This chapter focuses on drug therapy for CNS problems that mainly affect physical function. These problems include Parkinson's disease (PD), Alzheimer's disease (AD), epilepsy, and multiple sclerosis (MS). Drug therapy for problems that primarily affect behavior and mental health is presented in Chapter 10.

Movement is an important body motor function involving the brain, spinal cord, nerves, muscles, and bones. For example, your decision to move your arm deliberately first starts when you think about it, which excites nerve cells (*neurons*) in this part of the brain. This excitation is turned into an electrical signal that has to get to your arm muscles to actually move the arm in the direction you planned. Getting the signal from your brain to your arm muscles involves a relay of signals through a line of connected specific nerves. There is a space, or cleft, at each connection (Fig. 9.2). Electrical signals from neurons in the thinking area of your brain are sent (conducted) to the ends of these nerves, where the signal causes the release of neurotransmitters.

Neurotransmitters are chemicals that are released from the end of one nerve, cross a space (cleft), and then bind to receptors on the beginning of the next nerve in the line. This action transmits the signal that was started in your brain to the next nerve in the line. When the last nerve in the line gets to your arm muscles, the neurotransmitter binds to receptors on your arm muscles to trigger the muscle contractions needed to make your arm move.

Neurotransmitters can be excitatory or inhibitory. *Excitatory neurotransmitters* include acetylcholine (ACh), epinephrine, and norepinephrine. When the excitatory neurotransmitter ACh is released from the end of a nerve in response to thinking about moving your arm, it ensures this "action" signal gets transmitted to the next nerve in the line. At the point where the last nerve in the line is stimulated, the ACh it releases binds to receptors on the arm's skeletal muscles so they contract and move your arm as you intended.

Other neurotransmitters are inhibitory. *Inhibitory neurotransmitters* include dopamine, some types of serotonin, and GABA (gamma-aminobutyric acid). Smooth movement requires input from both an excitatory neurotransmitter (ACh) and an inhibitory neurotransmitter (dopamine). These inputs are balanced in such a way that when you decide to move your arm, you can control the direction of movement, the degree of movement, and the strength of the movement. After all, you do not need the same strength of arm movement to rub your eye gently as you do to throw a baseball 60 feet. Without dopamine modifying your arm muscle contractions, your arm movement would be fast, jerky, and wild. Think of how much hot coffee you would

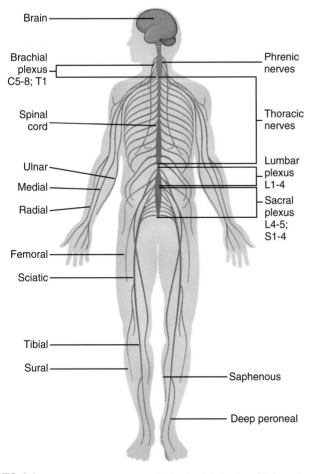

FIG. 9.1 Central nervous system. *C*, Cervical; *L*, lumbar; *T*, thoracic.

Brain

Brachial plexus C5-8; T1

Spinal cord

Ulnar

Medial

Radial

Femoral

Sciatic

Tibial

Sural

Phrenic nerves

Thoracic nerves

Lumbar plexus L1-4

Sacral plexus L4-5; S1-4

Saphenous

Deep peroneal

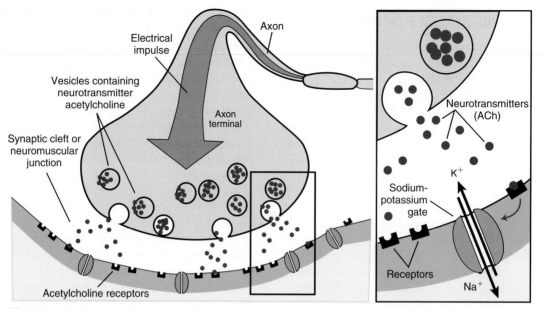

FIG. 9.2 Continuation of nerve signals by neurotransmitters. (From Fulcher EM, Fulcher RM, Soto CD: *Pharmacology,* ed 3, St. Louis, 2012, Saunders.)

spill moving a cup to your mouth if dopamine were not modifying this arm movement.

Some problems that occur within the CNS, such as PD, are a result of an imbalance of excitatory and inhibitory neurotransmitters. Others problems, such as epilepsy, result from conditions within the brain that allow neurons to become excited when the excitation is not needed. Still others, such as AD and MS, result from degenerative changes that occur within nerves or within the support cells of the brain.

DRUGS FOR PARKINSON'S DISEASE

PD is a CNS disorder in which there is not enough dopamine present to modify excitatory signals to skeletal muscles. Dopamine is an inhibitory neurotransmitter that is mostly produced deep in the midbrain area known as the substantia nigra part of the basal ganglia. When this brain area slows or stops production of dopamine, the balance between excitatory motor nerve signals and inhibitory motor nerve signals is reduced, causing mostly excitatory input (Fig. 9.3). Movements become hard to control and jerky, and some muscles are rigid because they fail to relax sufficiently. When the arms and legs move they "catch" at certain points in a "stop and go" fashion known as *cogwheel rigidity*. The neurologic problems also cause facial features to become "masklike" (Fig. 9.4). The gait becomes slow and shuffling with short steps. The risk for falls greatly increases. Other common symptoms of PD include tremors, stooped posture, difficulty stopping motion once it has started, difficulty chewing and swallowing, and drooling.

Depression, hallucinations, anxiety, and delusions are frequent complications of PD. Delusions and hallucinations can result from the changes in the brain that PD causes or they can occur from the adverse effects

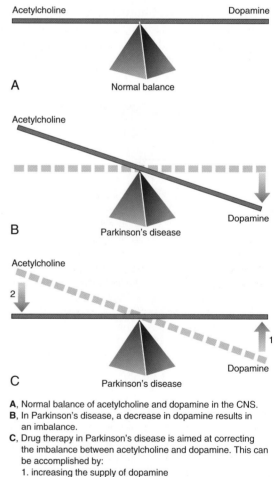

A, Normal balance of acetylcholine and dopamine in the CNS.
B, In Parkinson's disease, a decrease in dopamine results in an imbalance.
C, Drug therapy in Parkinson's disease is aimed at correcting the imbalance between acetylcholine and dopamine. This can be accomplished by:
  1. increasing the supply of dopamine
  2. blocking or lowering acetylcholine levels

FIG. 9.3 The neurotransmitter abnormality in Parkinson's disease. (From Lilley LL, Rainforth Collins S, Snyder J: *Pharmacology and the nursing process,* ed 8, St. Louis, 2017, Elsevier.)

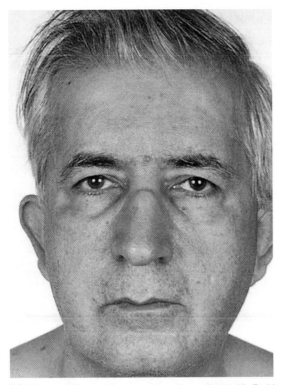

FIG. 9.4 The masklike facial expression of a patient with Parkinson disease. (From Perkin D: *Mosby's color atlas and test of neurology*, London, 1998, Mosby-Wolfe.)

Box 9.1 Symptoms of Parkinson's Disease

MOTOR SYMPTOMS	NONMOTOR SYMPTOMS
Slow movements (bradykinesia)	Constipation
Decreased arm swing when walking	Diminished sense of smell
Difficulty rising from a chair or turning in bed	Depression, anxiety, and irritability
Absence of facial expressions	Problems with focused attention and planning
Instability when standing up	Slowing of thought, language and memory difficulties
Freezing in place and having a rigid stance	Personality changes, dementia
Stooped, shuffling gait	Hallucinations and delusions
Tremors	Sleep disturbances
	Urinary frequency

of PD drugs themselves. The PD drugs increase the dopamine levels to improve the motor symptoms, but unfortunately at the same time, increasing the dopamine supply can cause hallucinations and delusions. Symptoms of PD worsen over time until finally the patient requires total care. See Box 9.1 for the motor and nonmotor symptoms of PD.

PD is the most common neurodegenerative disease, second to AD. The exact cause of PD is unknown but is thought to be caused from a combination of factors that include genetic, protective, and environmental reasons. The incidence of PD increases with age, but it

can occur before the age of 50 years. The disease strikes more men than women. The diagnosis of PD takes quite a while because there is no specific test for the disease. Diagnosis is made after all other neurologic disease processes have been ruled out. By the time the diagnosis of PD is made, most of the person's dopamine has been depleted.

Bookmark This!

Clinical trials and research into PD are ongoing and changing the face of the disease. Check out the Michael J Fox website: https://www.michaeljfox.org

Although drug therapy does not cure PD, it can delay the worsening of symptoms and allow patients to remain independent longer. Drug therapy for PD includes the drug classes of dopamine and dopamine agonists, **catechol-O-methyltransferase (COMT) inhibitors**, and **monoamine oxidase type B (MAO-B) inhibitors**. The common drugs in these classes are listed in Table 9.1.

At one time, the main drug category to manage PD was the anticholinergic drugs. These drugs attempted to balance the decreased dopamine levels by reducing the amount of ACh present. However, this action did not address the main problem of PD (lack of dopamine) and induced many side effects and adverse reactions. As a result, the anticholinergic drugs are not the most common therapy for PD.

Memory Jogger

The three classes of drugs to manage PD are:
- dopamine agonists
- COMT inhibitors
- MAO-B inhibitors

DOPAMINE AGONISTS

Action and Uses

Dopamine agonists are drugs that have the same chemical structure as natural dopamine and are given to increase the levels of dopamine in the brain to restore balance between ACh and dopamine action. The therapeutic effect of these drugs helps reduce muscle tremors and rigidity and improve mobility, muscular coordination, and performance. Dopamine agonists can be used alone or, as symptoms progress, can be used in combination. The National Parkinson Foundation recommends that carbidopa/levodopa (Sinemet, Rytary) be used as a first-line treatment for patients with PD who are older than 70 years and the newer dopamine agonists, such as pramipexole (Mirapex, Mirapex ER), ropinirole (Requip, Requip XL), and rotigotine (Neupro), be used as first-line treatment in patients between the ages of 50 and 70 years.

All patients will eventually require levodopa because dopamine is what is deficient in PD. Levodopa is synthesized in the brain and converted to natural dopamine.

Table 9.1   Examples of Common Drugs Used to Manage Parkinson's Disease

Dopamine and dopamine agonists: These drugs have the same chemical structure of natural dopamine and improve Parkinson symptoms by increasing the levels of dopamine in the brain to restore balance between acetylcholine and dopamine action.

DRUG/ADULT DOSAGE RANGE	NURSING IMPLICATIONS

carbidopa/levodopa (Rytary, Sinemet)
    Rytary (23.75 mg carbidopa/95 mg levodopa)
        orally initially three times per day and
        increase to a maximum daily dose of
        612.5 mg/2450 mg
    Sinemet (25 mg carbidopa/100 mg levodopa)
        orally three times a day and increase dosage
        to a total of 200 mg/2000 mg/day
pramipexole (Mirapex, Mirapex ER) initially,
    0.125 mg orally three times per day; dose is
    increased by 0.125–0.25 mg/dose every 5–7
    days to a maximum dosage of 1.5 mg orally
    three times per day (4.5 mg/day)
ropinirole (Requip, Requip XL) initially, 0.25 mg
    orally three times per day for the first week;
    gradually titrate at weekly intervals to a
    maximum of 24 mg/day
rotigotine (Neupro) apply transdermal patch at an
    initial dose of 2 mg/24 hours to a maximum of
    8 mg/24 hours
	• Carbidopa/levodopa tablets come in different dosages and are increased frequently from three times daily to up to five times daily according to improvement of symptoms. Tablets also come in extended-release form. Extended-release tablets are scored.
	• Do not crush or chew whole or half tablets; they must be swallowed intact.
	• Extended-release forms of the drugs that are not scored should not be halved, crushed, or chewed to retain the slow-release effect.
	• Give with 6–8 ounces of water at least 30–60 minutes before eating to maximize absorption. Give with nonprotein snack to avoid nausea.
	• Do not give with high-protein foods because they decrease absorption.
	• Instruct patients to get up slowly to avoid postural hypotension with all dopamine agonists.
	• Monitor blood glucose levels closely in diabetic patients to avoid hypoglycemia caused by increased sympathetic tone.
	• Closely monitor patients with a history of cardiac disease for hypotension and increasing dysrhythmias.
	• Monitor liver function studies because these drugs are metabolized in the liver and monitor complete blood counts because this drug can increase the risk for GI bleeding.
	• Notify the healthcare provider for any behavioral changes, hallucinations, or delusions.
	• Monitor for worsening dyskinesia and/or dystonia reactions and notify the healthcare provider if they occur because this can indicate a need for dosage change.
	• Skin reactions are common with the use of the rotigotine (Neupro) patch. Do not apply the patch in the same place for 14 days and, after removing the patch, gently clean the skin with mild soap and water.

COMT inhibitors: These drugs reduce the symptoms of Parkinson's disease by suppressing the activity of the COMT enzyme so that both naturally occurring dopamine and dopamine agonist drugs remain active in the body longer, helping to restore the acetylcholine–dopamine balance in the brain.

DRUG/ADULT DOSAGE RANGE	NURSING IMPLICATIONS

entacapone (Comtan) 200 mg orally given with
    each levodopa/carbidopa dose up to a
    maximum of 1600 mg/day
tolcapone (Tasmar) initially, 100 mg orally three
    times daily with the first dose given with
    carbidopa/levodopa; maximum dose is
    600 mg/day
	• Give entacapone with every dose of carbidopa/levodopa to enhance drug effect.
	• Give the first dose of tolcapone with the first dose of carbidopa/levodopa and subsequent doses 6–12 hours later.
	• Review liver function studies and monitor for liver failure in patients who are taking tolcapone.
	• Report signs of liver failure, such as abdominal pain, jaundice, and dark urine with nausea and vomiting, to the healthcare provider.
	• Remind patients that these drugs may cause a nondangerous side effect of turning the urine to orange-brown.
	• These drugs enhance the effect of dopamine, so symptoms of worsening dyskinesia or psychosis may occur. Notify the healthcare provider if these changes occur.
	• These drugs cannot be given with nonselective MAO inhibitors because of the increased cardiovascular risk.
	• Anticipate that the dose of carbidopa/levodopa may be decreased as these drugs take effect.

Table 9.1 Examples of Common Drugs Used to Manage Parkinson's Disease—cont'd

Selective MAO-B inhibitors: MAO-B breaks down dopamine in the brain and elsewhere in the body. These inhibitors allow existing dopamine to remain active in the brain longer.

DRUG/ADULT DOSAGE RANGE	NURSING IMPLICATIONS
rasagiline (Azilect) 0.5–1 g orally once daily safinamide (Xadago) 50–100 mg orally once daily selegiline (Eldepryl, Emsam, Zelapar) 5 mg tablet orally twice daily	• Give these drugs at the same time every day. Once-a-day doses can be taken at nighttime because they can cause drowsiness. • Teach patients to avoid foods and beverages that contain large amounts of tyramine when using all of these drugs and for 2 weeks after therapy is stopped. • Monitor vital signs, particularly blood pressure. • Teach patients and families to report severe headache, palpitations, nausea, and vomiting to the healthcare provider immediately because these are signs of a hypertensive crisis. • These drugs enhance the effect of dopamine, so symptoms of worsening dyskinesia or psychosis may occur. Teach patients and families to notify the healthcare provider if these changes occur. • Anticipate that the healthcare provider may decrease the dosage of carbidopa/levodopa as these drugs take effect.

COMT, Catechol-*O*-methyltransferase; *MAO-B*, monoamine oxidase type B.

For this reason, levodopa is the most important drug used to manage the symptoms of PD. Carbidopa is usually given in combination with levodopa because it enhances the levodopa so lower doses of levodopa can be used, thus preventing the nausea and vomiting that accompanies the continual increasing of the levodopa dose to control disease symptoms. Levodopa (Larodopa) is rarely given alone for this reason. "Wearing off" is an issue of the drug losing its effectiveness that can occur after levodopa is used for several years. Levodopa peaks in about 1 hour and wears off in 4 or 5 hours. This wearing-off effect causes rapid swings of symptoms. Symptoms improve when dopamine is present and worsen as the dopamine wears off. This can also be called an "on/off effect." The extended-release form of carbidopa/levodopa and the longer half-lives of dopamine agonists help to prevent this effect. Carbidopa/levodopa is also available as an intestinal infusion pump (Duopa). The pump is inserted directly into the small intestines via a small feeding tube and can deliver 16 continuous hours of carbidopa and levodopa to reduce motor symptoms.

Expected Side Effects/Adverse Reactions

The most common side effects of carbidopa/levodopa and all dopamine agonists include both postural and general hypotension, headache, GI disturbances, insomnia, dream abnormalities, impulse control, and confusion. The most common adverse reaction to carbidopa/levodopa (Rytary, Sinemet) is **dyskinesia** or involuntary muscle movements that look like uncoordinated dance movements. Dyskinesia is common in patients on long-term carbidopa/levodopa therapy (longer than 3 years). The effect of dyskinesia is minimized with the use of pramipexole (Mirapex, Mirapex ER), ropinirole (Requip, Requip XL), rotigotine (Neupro), and other dopamine agonists. Dopamine agonists can also cause **delirium**,

psychosis, and hallucinations. If these problems occur, the healthcare provider will need to determine whether the symptoms are related to the advancing disease process, depression, or the PD drug response.

Do Not Confuse

Risperidone is an antipsychotic sometimes used to combat psychosis in PD.
Ropinirole is used to treat symptoms of PD (stiffness, tremors, muscle spasms, and poor muscle control).

Carbidopa/levodopa dosages may be decreased as COMT inhibitors and MAO-B inhibitors are added to the drug regimen. This could precipitate *neuroleptic malignant syndrome*, with symptoms of agitation, coma, muscle rigidity, tremors, high fever, and an unstable blood pressure. Also, keep in mind that as COMT inhibitors and MAO-B inhibitors are added to the regimen of dopamine agonists, there will be an increase in available dopamine that can increase the adverse effects of the dopamine agonists until dosages of the dopamine agonists are adjusted by the healthcare provider.

When dopamine agonists are taken with protein, either as a meal or a snack, the effectiveness of the drug is reduced. These drugs are best absorbed on an empty stomach.

Drug Interactions

Using antihypertensive agents with dopamine agonists can cause severe hypotension. Using older, nonselective MAO inhibitors like phenelzine (Nardil) along with dopamine agonists can precipitate a hypertensive crisis. Phenytoin (Dilantin) reduces the effectiveness of dopamine agonists. Multivitamins that contain iron decrease the effects of carbidopa/levodopa. Vitamin

B₆ increases the metabolism of levodopa (Larodopa) without carbidopa. Metoclopramide (Reglan) can reduce the effectiveness of the dopamine agonists because metoclopramide is a dopamine antagonist and prevents the dopamine from combining with the dopamine receptors. Using dopamine agonists with sedatives will worsen drowsiness and can increase the risk for confusion, hallucinations, and delusions, especially in those persons already suffering from mental illnesses.

❖ Nursing Implications and Patient Teaching

◆ *Assessment.* Dopamine agonists frequently cause postural hypotension, so take a full set of vital signs, including orthostatic blood pressure readings (supine, sitting, and standing). Assessment of the patient's motor skills and functional ability for walking and eating is important to establish a baseline, as well as to ensure safety from falls and aspiration. Ask whether patients have had melanoma or closed-angle glaucoma. These conditions are contraindicated for dopamine agonist therapy because the drugs can worsen them. Closely monitor blood glucose levels because the sympathetic effects of levodopa can cause hypoglycemia. Observe for symptoms such as headache, anxiety, shakiness, weakness, and irritability that can indicate low blood glucose. Check blood urea nitrogen (BUN) and creatinine levels before starting pramipexole (Mirapex) to rule out renal impairment because 90% of the drug is excreted by the kidneys. Monitor liver enzymes before and at intervals during treatment because other drugs used in the treatment of PD are metabolized by the liver.

◆ *Planning and implementation.* Dopamine agonists are recommended to be given 30 to 60 minutes before meals, not only for better absorption but also to have maximum effect so the patient has less difficulty chewing and swallowing, which lessens the risk for aspiration. Never crush the extended-release tablets. When using rotigotine (Neupro) transdermal patches, apply at the same time every day and rotate application sites. Do not apply to the same site more than once every 14 days to avoid a skin reaction.

Dopamine agonists should be withdrawn slowly, because these drugs have a long half-life. When withdrawing one preparation and beginning a new preparation, the new drug is started in small doses and the old drug is withdrawn gradually. These agents are usually started at the lowest dose possible, and the dose is increased gradually until the maximum therapeutic effect has been obtained.

Dopamine agonists are available in patches, tablets, sustained-release capsules, syrups, and elixirs. They are generally well absorbed from the GI tract. Peak blood levels of carbidopa/levodopa (Sinemet), one of the main treatment drugs, is achieved in 1 to 6 hours, depending on the route of administration and the formulation of the drug given. Sustained-release capsules reach peak plasma blood levels in 8 to 12 hours. Sustained-release capsules are not recommended for initial therapy because they do not allow enough flexibility in dosage regulation.

◆ *Evaluation.* Tell the patient and family the following:
- Take care when using drugs for sleep, pain, to relax muscles, and to control bladder function along with your drugs for PD because the combination can lead to confusion, hallucinations, and other symptoms.
- Change positions slowly from lying down to standing up because low blood pressure can occur and cause you to fall.
- Contact your healthcare provider as soon as possible if you develop hallucinations or delusions.

Long-term use of dopamine agonists may lead to *akinesia* (loss of movement), *tardive dyskinesia* (abnormal and involuntary movements, especially of the lower face), and **dystonia** (impairment of muscle tone). The dosage is likely to be reduced to the minimum effective level to reverse these effects, and very slow and careful changes in dosages are made as necessary to avoid overmedication. Monitor all patients closely for behavior changes because these drugs can exacerbate depression and psychosis. Report abnormal involuntary movement such as chewing, grinding of the teeth, protrusion of the tongue, repeated opening and closing of the mouth, head bobbing, or jerky, constant movements of the feet or hands because this can indicate dystonia, which can be related to either progression of the disease itself or the wearing off of dopamine. If these appear, alert the healthcare provider because the drug dosage may need to be adjusted.

◆ *Patient and family teaching.* Tell the patient and family the following:
- Clinical improvements are cumulative (get better over time) and may take 2 to 3 weeks. Therefore continue to take the drug even if you see no changes at first.
- If possible, take the drug on an empty stomach 30 to 60 minutes before a meal or snack so the drug is absorbed well and can help you chew and swallow better.
- If the drug causes nausea, you can take it with some crackers or other carbohydrates. Do not take the drug with food containing protein because this can reduce the drug's effectiveness.
- Avoid taking levodopa (Larodopa) with vitamin B₆ (pyridoxine) because the vitamin accelerates the inactivation of the drug. This is not a problem if you are taking levodopa/carbidopa (Sinemet).
- Contact your healthcare provider immediately if symptoms suddenly become worse, if you have intermittent winking or muscle twitching, or if abdominal pain, constipation, distention, or urinary problems occur.
- Take care when using drugs for sleep, pain, to relax muscles, and to control bladder function along with your drugs for PD because the combination can lead to confusion, hallucinations, and other symptoms.

- Change positions slowly from lying down to standing up because low blood pressure can occur and cause you to fall.
- Contact your healthcare provider as soon as possible if you develop hallucinations or delusions.

CATECHOL-O-METHYLTRANSFERASE INHIBITORS

Action and Uses

Catechol-O-methyltransferase (COMT) is an enzyme that breaks down (metabolizes) naturally occurring catecholamine-based neurotransmitters, including dopamine. It also breaks down dopamine agonist drugs. Catechol-O-methyltransferase (COMT) inhibitors are drugs that suppress the activity of the COMT enzyme so that both naturally occurring dopamine and dopamine agonist drugs remain active in the body longer, helping to restore the ACh–dopamine balance in the brain. Levodopa is the main dopamine agonist drug used in PD. COMT is given with levodopa to allow blood levels of levodopa to stay high enough to enter the brain, where it is converted to dopamine. Entacapone (Comtan) and tolcapone (Tasmar) are two COMT inhibitors that are currently used for PD.

Expected Side Effects/Adverse Reactions

Both of these drugs can potentiate the dopaminergic adverse effects of levodopa and can cause dyskinesia and hypotension. The most common expected effects are GI upset and discoloration of the urine (brownish orange color). Both drugs are metabolized by the liver, but tolcapone (Tasmar) has a higher risk for causing severe liver failure, so it is not used unless other measures have failed. Tolcapone is not used in persons with existing hepatic disease. Liver function studies must be closely monitored every 6 months if tolcapone (Tasmar) is used.

Drug Interactions

Neither entacapone nor tolcapone should be taken with other MAO inhibitors like phenelzine (Nardil) because they reduce catecholamine metabolism and can cause cardiovascular problems such as severe hypertension, tachycardia, and dysrhythmias. Likewise, any direct catecholamine drugs like epinephrine or methyldopa may increase heart rates, cause dysrhythmias, and cause severely high blood pressures. The MAO-B inhibitors selegiline (Eldepryl, Zelapar) and rasagiline (Azilect) used in PD are considered safe to take with COMT inhibitor drugs because they are selective in blocking the breakdown of dopamine and not other catecholamines, so the adverse cardiac effects are avoided.

❖ Nursing Implications and Patient Teaching

◆ *Assessment.* The patient may experience orthostatic hypotension because COMT inhibitor drugs potentiate the action of carbidopa/levodopa. Take a full set of vital signs and orthostatic blood pressures, and remind patients to rise slowly to avoid falls. In addition, monitor for indications of dyskinesia and hyperkinesia, and notify the healthcare provider if they occur.

◆ *Planning and implementation.* Entacapone is given with every dose of carbidopa/levodopa; tolcapone is given with the first dose of carbidopa/levodopa, with subsequent doses being given 6 to 12 hours later. If tolcapone is used, monitor patients for liver failure and review liver function studies.

◆ *Evaluation.* Evaluate patients for akinesia, dystonia, and tardive dyskinesia as discussed earlier because these drugs are given with carbidopa/levodopa and increase the response of dopamine agonists. Also monitor patients for depression and psychosis.

◆ *Patient and family teaching.* Tell the patient and family the following:
- Take entacapone with each levodopa/carbidopa dose for best effect.
- The first dose of tolcapone is given with levodopa/carbidopa, and subsequent doses are given about 6 and 12 hours later.
- Notify your healthcare provider if you develop jaundice, abdominal pain, or swelling because these symptoms may indicate liver failure. This is especially important if taking tolcapone.
- Notify your healthcare provider if you have worsening depression, delirium, or hallucinations.
- Do not suddenly stop taking either of these drugs because they must be tapered off slowly to avoid a worsening condition.
- Your urine may have a brownish orange discoloration that is an expected side effect and is not dangerous.
- Rise slowly from a sitting or lying position to prevent faintness, dizziness, and falls caused by an unexpected drop in blood pressure.

MONOAMINE OXIDASE TYPE B INHIBITORS

Action and Uses

MAO is an enzyme made in many body areas that breaks down (metabolizes) many substances. MAO-A breaks down many neurotransmitters, including epinephrine, norepinephrine, serotonin, and dopamine. MAO-B is more specific for breaking down dopamine and serotonin. MAO-B inhibitors suppress the action of MAO-B, which allows dopamine levels to increase and reduce the symptoms of PD. It is sometimes used to help treat depression because this drug category also reduces the breakdown of serotonin. These drugs have fewer side effects than MAO-A inhibitors, which are nonselective. Three MAO-B inhibitor drugs—selegiline (Eldepryl, Zelapar), rasagiline (Azilect), and safinamide (Xadago)—are used in combination with carbidopa/levodopa. They are usually used early in the disease as monotherapy or in addition to dopamine agonist drugs. Adding MAO-B inhibitors to the drug regimen can allow the dose of levodopa to be decreased, thus lessening the side effects of higher levodopa levels.

Box 9.2 Foods That Contain Tyramine

- Cured or smoked meats, fish, and cheeses (e.g., salami, anchovies)
- Avocados, bananas, figs, and raisins
- Beer and red wine
- Sauerkraut
- Sour cream
- Soy sauce or soy-containing foods like miso soup
- Yeast extract found in some breads, canned foods, and snacks
- Yogurt
- Pickled herring

Expected Side Effects/Adverse Reactions

The usual side effects of MAO-B inhibitors are dry mouth, nausea, constipation, and light-headedness. Confusion and hallucinations can occur, especially in older adults. An adverse effect of severe hypertension can occur if MAO-B inhibitors are used in high doses, but they are unlikely to occur at lower doses. Tyramine-rich foods need to be avoided when taking any MAO inhibitor because these foods can cause a severe hypertensive crisis. See Box 9.2 for a partial list of foods to avoid when taking MAO inhibitors. Also, photosensitivity can occur and increase the risk for sunburn. These drugs cause drowsiness.

Drug Interactions

MAO-B inhibitors have interactions with some opiate drugs used for pain, such as meperidine, tramadol, and methadone, and can cause a hypertensive crisis. They should not be used with droperidol or cyclobenzaprine. Taking MAO-B inhibitors with tricyclic antidepressants, such as amitriptyline, or selective serotonin reuptake inhibitors, such as fluoxetine, or other MAO inhibitors can cause hyperthermia, tremors, seizures, or delirium. Drugs that stimulate the sympathetic (fight-or-flight) nervous system, such as amphetamines, phenylephrine (decongestant), and dextromethorphan (cough medicine), can cause a hypertensive crisis. Ginseng, ephedra, ma huang, and St. John's wort can also cause a hypertensive crisis and should be avoided with MOA inhibitors.

❖ Nursing Implications and Patient Teaching

◆ *Assessment.* Monitor vital signs, especially during dose increases. Alert the healthcare provider for any changes, especially in blood pressure and pulse, because orthostatic hypotension, hypertension, or tachycardia with new dysrhythmias may indicate adverse reactions to these drugs.

Monitor all patients closely for behavior changes because these drugs can cause hallucinations, delusions, depression, or confusion.

◆ *Patient and family teaching.* Tell the patient and family the following:

- These drugs can take several weeks to begin working.
- Do not exceed the prescribed drug dose because doing so can cause dangerously high blood pressure.
- Avoid foods that contain tyramine, such as beer, red wine, aged cheese, smoked meat, cheese, fish, soy, pickled herring, among others.
- Report symptoms of very high blood pressure, such as a severe headache, irregular pulse, or nausea and vomiting to your healthcare provider immediately.
- Very low blood pressure is possible, as well as dizziness, light-headedness, and fainting, so slowly rise from a sitting or lying position.
- Do not take over-the-counter drugs or herbs without checking with the pharmacist or your healthcare provider.
- These drugs cause drowsiness, so avoid driving or using dangerous machinery until you know how the drug affects you.
- Wear sunscreen, sunglasses and protective clothing when outside because this drug increases the risk for serious sunburn, even if you have dark skin.

DRUGS FOR ALZHEIMER'S DISEASE

AD is a common form of dementia. *Dementia* is the progressive loss of brain function. There are many causes and types of dementia, and AD is one that can be helped initially with drug therapy. In AD there is a familial tendency or genetic predisposition to develop problems within and around brain neurons that affect their function. The protein beta amyloid builds up and forms deposits in the brain. The nerves themselves also become tangled and form nonfunctional meshes within the brain. The excitatory neurotransmitter ACh is decreased in the brain, which results in more difficulty with memory and learning. In addition, blood flow throughout the brain decreases. Over time, these changes reduce the size of the brain and all aspects of brain function (Fig. 9.5). Unfortunately no single test can be used to diagnose AD, and drug therapy does not cure the problem. Drugs provide only temporary improvement in symptoms and include cholinesterase inhibitors and *N*-methyl-D-aspartate (NMDA) blockers. Research in the area of AD is ongoing, and help for family and professional caregivers is available.

The symptoms of early AD involve memory issues and can be mistaken for normal aging. The disease is progressive and memory problems become increasingly more challenging, such as getting confused regarding times and places or forgetting how to get home. Changes in mood, judgment, and personality eventually occur. Box 9.3 lists the 10 warning signs of AD.

More than 5 million persons suffer from AD. Risk factors include older age (65), a family history, and having the *APOE-e4* gene. Diagnosis is made based on symptoms, family interviews, physical examination, and neurologic and cognitive examinations. As previously mentioned, the drugs available for AD may simply

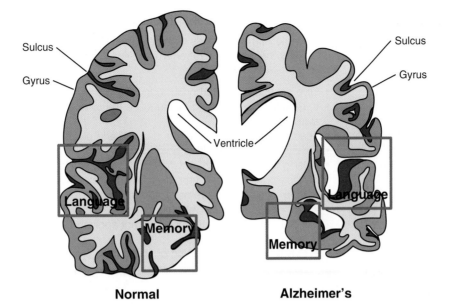

FIG. 9.5 Cross sections of a normal brain and a brain affected by Alzheimer's disease. Neurons die in areas of the brain that are important to memory and language. (From Workman ML, LaCharity LA: *Understanding pharmacology,* ed 2, St. Louis, 2016, Elsevier.)

| Box 9.3 | Ten Warning Signs of Alzheimer's Disease |

1. Memory loss that disrupts daily life
2. Challenges in planning or solving problems
3. Difficulty completing familiar tasks at home, at work, or at leisure
4. Confusion with time or place
5. Trouble understanding visual images and spatial relationships
6. New problems with words in speaking or writing
7. Misplacing things and losing the ability to retrace steps
8. Decreased or poor judgment
9. Withdrawal from work or social activities
10. Changes in mood and personality

offer a temporary improvement in symptoms. The effectiveness of the drugs is different from person to person, and the length of time that the drug is therapeutic is limited as well. Table 9.2 lists examples of the common names, adult dosages, and nursing implications for these drugs.

Bookmark This!

The Alzheimer's Foundation of America provides care and services to individuals living with AD and to their families and caregivers: https://alzfdn.org.

CHOLINESTERASE INHIBITORS

Action and Uses

Drug therapy attempts to increase ACh levels because the excitatory neurotransmitter ACh is reduced in the brain of patients with AD. Acetylcholinesterase is an enzyme that specifically breaks down ACh. **Cholinesterase inhibitors** are drugs that bind to acetylcholinesterase and slow its action, which allows any ACh produced to remain functional longer. This action appears to delay memory loss and improve the patient's ability to perform his or her activities of daily living. Unfortunately, the drug is useful only temporarily. As the disease progresses, fewer intact neurons are available to make ACh. When this occurs, the drug is no longer effective. Currently, three cholinesterase inhibitors are being used in the treatment of AD: donepezil (Aricept), rivastigmine (Exelon), and galantamine (Razadyne). Table 9.2 lists examples of the common names, adult dosages, and nursing implications for these drugs.

Expected Side Effects/Adverse Reactions

Expected side effects of cholinesterase inhibitors are mild diarrhea, especially when starting treatment. Drowsiness, headache, loss of appetite, GI discomfort, as well joint pain and muscle cramping, can occur. Adverse effects include hallucinations, dysrhythmias, GI bleeding, infection, and difficulty urinating or incontinence. These drugs increase ACh concentrations, so they are considered to be cholinergic agonists and can have adverse effects on other body systems that cause symptoms of overstimulation of the parasympathetic nervous system (rest and digest). Box 9.4 lists these adverse effects.

Drug Interactions

Cholinesterase inhibitors should not be given with other drugs that can prolong the QT interval on the ECG because this can cause a fatal dysrhythmia known as *torsade de pointes*, a form of ventricular tachycardia. Dextromethorphan found in over-the-counter cough

Table 9.2 Examples of Common Drugs for Management of Alzheimer's Disease

Cholinesterase inhibitors: work to delay memory loss in Alzheimer's disease by binding to the enzyme acetylcholinesterase and slowing its action, which allows any acetylcholine produced to remain functional longer

DRUG/ADULT DOSAGE RANGE	NURSING IMPLICATIONS

donepezil (Aricept) 5–10 mg orally once daily
rivastigmine (Exelon) 1.5–3 mg orally twice daily; 4.6/24 hours to 9.5/24 hours transdermal patch
galantamine (Razadyne) 4–8 mg orally twice daily; extended-release tablets 8–16 mg orally once daily
	• Give donepezil (Aricept) once a day in the evening.
	• If using the disintegrating tablet, place the tablet on the tongue before swallowing.
	• Teach patients and families to measure and give the oral solution with a syringe.
	• Rivastigmine (Exelon) must be given with food.
	• If using the transdermal rivastigmine (Exelon) patch:
	  • Apply once daily to clean, dry, hairless, intact healthy skin to the upper or lower back to avoid removal by the patient.
	  • Do not use on areas with recent application of lotions, creams, or powder.
	  • Rotate application sites daily. Do not apply to the same site more than once every 14 days.
	  • May be used while bathing or showering.
	  • Apply patch at about the same time every day.
	  • Always remove the old patch before applying a new patch.
	• Give galantamine (Razadyne) twice-a-day oral dosage with food and the once-a-day oral dosage in the morning with food.
	• If using the liquid oral form of galantamine (Razadyne), measure the ordered dosage from the enclosed pipette into 3–4 ounces of a nonalcoholic drink.
	• Monitor weekly weights because these drugs may cause weight loss.
	• Monitor laboratory work as ordered to ensure safety from adverse effects.

NMDA blockers: work to slow the progression of Alzheimer's disease by blocking the entrance of calcium into neurons, which reduces or slows neuronal damage

DRUG/ADULT DOSAGE RANGE	NURSING IMPLICATIONS
memantine (Namenda, Namenda XR) 5–10 mg orally twice daily; extended-release capsules 7–28 mg orally once daily	• Extended release can be opened and contents sprinkled on applesauce before swallowing. Do not divide the contents of the capsules because this will result in unequal dosing. • If the oral solution of the drug is used, do not mix it with other liquids. Use a syringe or dropper to measure and give directly in the mouth. • Monitor the patient's neurologic function, serum creatinine levels, blood urea nitrogen, and liver function studies and notify the healthcare provider for changes from baseline. • Weigh the patient weekly because this drug can cause weight loss.

Box 9.4 Common Adverse Effects of Cholinergic Agonists and Cholinesterase Inhibitors

Cardiac: slow heart rate, low blood pressure, heart blocks, fainting
CNS: convulsions, headaches, seizures, sweating
GI: increased secretions, increased salivation, abdominal cramps, vomiting, diarrhea
Respiratory: increased secretions and bronchospasm
Urinary: urinary incontinence

medication, quinidine, and fluconazole are three such drugs. Consult a drug reference or pharmacist to determine whether these drugs interact with any other drug(s) the patient is taking. Anticholinergic drugs decrease the effectiveness of cholinesterase inhibitors, and taking the drug with other cholinesterase inhibitors such as edrophonium (Tensilon) increases the risk for adverse effects.

❖ Nursing Implications and Patient Teaching

◆ *Assessment.* Obtain a baseline weight and reassess at weekly intervals because these drugs can cause a loss of appetite. Observe for signs and symptoms that may indicate a GI bleed, such as dark, tarry stools and decreasing hemoglobin and hematocrit levels. Monitor blood test levels and report abnormal baseline liver function studies and BUN/creatinine levels to the healthcare provider because abnormalities can affect the metabolism of the drugs. Assess the urinary patterns and reassess for any changes that can indicate side effects of the drugs. Before a patient starts a cholinesterase inhibitor, assess him or her using an Alzheimer's Disease Assessment Scale so that an objective evaluation can be made when evaluating for symptom improvement. The assessment tools evaluate cognition, functional capacity, behavior, general health, and quality of life. By using these tools, you can better gauge how and if the drug is actually helping the patient.

Assess for swallowing difficulties so that the proper drug formulation can be given (liquid, sublingual tablets).

◆ *Planning and implementation.* Monitor patients who have asthma carefully for worsening of symptoms. Check vital signs, especially heart rate, and look for adverse signs and symptoms indicating parasympathetic stimulation, as indicated in Box 9.3.

◆ *Evaluation.* Monitor for improvement using an Alzheimer's Disease Assessment Scale. Monitor for any changes in vital signs and/or adverse reactions.

◆ *Patient and family teaching.* Tell the patient and family the following:

* It may take several weeks for the drugs to have a therapeutic effect.
* These drugs will not cure AD.
* If difficulty breathing, fainting, or GI bleeding occurs, notify your healthcare provider immediately.
* Notify your healthcare provider if expected side effects are causing increased discomfort or if new symptoms develop.
* Use the bathroom every 2 hours to avoid urinary incontinence because these drugs increase urination.
* Take donepezil (Aricept) at bedtime.
* Take galantamine (Razadyne) and rivastigmine (Exelon) at the same time twice a day with food to avoid GI upset.
* Your risk for falls is increased because these drugs can cause dizziness and weakness.
* Keep all follow-up appointments so that the effects of these drugs can be evaluated.

> **Bookmark This!**
>
> A list of cognitive assessment and family informational tools can be found on the Alzheimer's Association website: http://www.alz.org/health-care-professionals/cognitive-tests-patient-assessment.asp.

N-METHYL-D-ASPARTATE BLOCKERS

Action and Uses

There are NMDA receptors in the brain. When activated, these receptors allow more calcium into the brain neurons, which appears to be important in memory and learning. However, too much calcium damages neurons. It is thought that excess calcium is one mechanism that causes neuronal "tangles" to form in the brains of patients with AD. NMDA blockers are drugs that block the entrance of calcium into neurons, which reduces or slows the neuronal damage in AD. Memantine (Namenda, Ebixa) is used with the drugs donepezil (Aricept), rivastigmine (Exelon), and galantamine (Razadyne) to increase the effects of these cholinergic agonists.

Expected Side Effects/Adverse Reactions

The expected side effects of memantine are headaches, dizziness, and constipation. Adverse side effects include hallucinations, worsening confusion, depression, somnolence, shortness of breath, incontinence, and weight loss. This drug can also cause hypertension in certain individuals.

Drug Interactions

Drugs that increase the urine pH (alkaline) or are also excreted by the kidneys can interfere with the renal excretion of memantine and cause an increase in expected and adverse side effects. Carbonic anhydrase inhibitors like acetazolamide, which are used in the treatment of glaucoma and high-altitude sickness, quinidine, and dextromethorphan are such examples.

❖ **Nursing Implications and Patient Teaching**

◆ *Assessment.* Memantine is eliminated primarily by the kidney and should be used with caution in patients with kidney disease, people with risk for renal impairment due to age, and those taking other drugs that also have a risk for renal impairment. Baseline creatinine and BUN, as well as liver enzymes, should be measured. Urinary tract infections can increase the levels of memantine by increasing the pH. If the patient has symptoms of a urinary tract infection, obtain a urinalysis and consult with the healthcare provider before starting drug therapy. Monitor the respiratory rate and vital signs, especially the blood pressure in patients with heart disease. Report symptoms such as ataxia, dizziness, and other adverse reactions to the healthcare provider.

◆ *Patient and family teaching.* Tell the patient and family the following:

* Take or give memantine at the same time every day.
* The extended-release capsule can be opened and all of the contents can be sprinkled on applesauce if swallowing is difficult.
* If using the liquid form of the drug, do not mix it with other liquids to avoid interactions.
* Report problems with vision, skin rash, shortness of breath, agitation or restlessness, confusion, dizziness, incontinence, and weight loss to your healthcare provider.
* Avoid driving or engaging in hazardous activities until you know how the drug affects you.
* Report symptoms of a urinary tract infection (acute changes in mental status, frequency in urination, pain or discomfort during urination, or concentrated and bad-smelling urine) to your healthcare provider.

DRUGS FOR EPILEPSY

Epilepsy is a common type of chronic seizure disorder in which neurons of the brain become hyperexcitable and trigger electrical signals when they are not needed. The unnecessary signals cause rapid and repeated refiring of nerves in the brain, leading to seizures. *Seizures* are the body's total responses to those inappropriate brain signals. When these signals reach the skeletal muscles, a *convulsion* may occur, which is the sudden contraction of many muscle groups without the person's conscious control. A convulsion is the part of a seizure that is seen as the motor response to these brain signals. Other parts of seizure activity include changes in or loss of consciousness; a variety of sensory changes in vision, hearing, touch, smell, and taste; and autonomic symptoms such as facial flushing, incontinence, nausea, and drooling. Symptoms of seizures vary with the area of the brain affected and the type of seizure experienced.

Seizures are classified first as partial or generalized. Each classification has subtypes based on symptoms, how long an episode lasts, whether convulsions occur, how widespread the response is, and the degree of change in consciousness. Box 9.5 lists the classifications of seizures.

A variety of problems can produce seizures. For example, high temperatures in infants and children, strokes, head trauma, brain tumor, meningitis, and poisoning (especially from excessive alcohol intake or drugs) may induce seizures. Epilepsy is one cause of chronic and recurring seizures.

Although other types of epilepsy management exist, most often drug therapy is used. **Antiepileptic drugs (AEDs)** are drugs that reduce or prevent seizures. AEDs are divided into traditional and newer categories. Some drugs categorized as AEDs have additional uses for other problems and disorders.

TRADITIONAL ANTIEPILEPTIC DRUGS

The traditional AEDs include phenytoins, carbamazepine, ethosuximide, phenobarbital, and valproic acid. Although these drugs have different actions, side effects, adverse effects, and drug interactions, some nursing implications are the same for all of them. In addition, many of the points to teach patients and families about these drugs are the same. Box 9.6 describes these common nursing considerations for AEDs, and Box 9.7 describes general patient teaching points. Nursing considerations and patient teaching issues specific to any single drug type are listed with the individual drug categories in Table 9.3. Although these older drugs have more side effects and other issues than do some newer drugs, they are still used effectively today for most patients, often in combination with newer AEDs.

> **Memory Jogger**
>
> Traditional antiepilepsy drugs are:
> - phenytoins
> - carbamazepine
> - ethosuximide
> - phenobarbital
> - valproic acid

Actions and Uses

Phenytoins are AEDs that prevent the spread of neuron excitation in the brain by binding to sodium

---

Box 9.5   Classification of Major Seizures Types

TYPE	SYMPTOMS
PARTIAL SEIZURES	
Simple	No loss of consciousness, isolated or discrete motor symptoms (e.g., twitching of one toe or foot), changes in one or more senses, one or more autonomic symptom (e.g., drooling, facial flushing, etc.), usually last 20 to 60 seconds
Complex	Consciousness altered or impaired and person does not respond to environmental stimulation, may have a fixed gaze stare and be motionless, automatism (performance of repetitive motions such as head-turning from side to side, foot peddling motions), usually last 45 to 90 seconds
Partial with secondary generalization	Begins as a partial seizure with the patient retaining consciousness and then progresses to loss of consciousness
GENERALIZED SEIZURES: ALL HAVE THE FEATURE OF LOSS OF CONSCIOUSNESS	
Absence (petit mal)	Consciousness loss is brief (10 to 30 seconds) without loss of posture, minimal or no change in motor activity
Tonic-clonic (grand mal)	Often preceded by an aura or cry, whole-body convulsions starting with muscle rigidity followed by powerful contractions, posture lost, urinary incontinence, confusion after muscle responses are over, usually lasts less than 90 seconds
Atonic	Muscle tone loss in one or more muscle groups, usually lasts 10 to 60 seconds
Myoclonic	Brief (1 to 2 seconds) contraction of one (focal) or more muscle groups (can involve the whole body)
Status epilepticus	Single seizure lasting 15 to 30 continuous minutes or a series of recurring seizures between which the patient does not regain consciousness; may be convulsive, absence, myoclonic, or generalized convulsive (life-threatening)
Febrile	Tonic-clonic seizures induced by temperature elevation (usually in children), last 15 to 30 seconds

| Box 9.6 | General Nursing Considerations for Antiepileptic Drugs |

ASSESSMENT
- Before giving any AED, obtain a complete list of drugs that the patient is taking, including over-the-counter and herbal preparations, because these drugs interact with numerous drugs, herbals, and supplements.
- Always consult a drug reference or pharmacist to determine possible interactions between AEDs and any other drug a patient is prescribed.
- Check baseline vital signs, level of consciousness, and gait, all of which can change as a result of AEDs.
- Assess adolescents for recent changes in height and weight because these changes affect the dosage needed to prevent seizures.
- Ask female patients of childbearing age if they are pregnant, planning to become pregnant, or breast-feeding because many of the AEDs have an increased risk for birth defects and/or enter breast milk and affect the infant.
- Ask patients whether an aura occurs before any seizure.
- Tell the patient to put on his or her call light if he or she feels that a seizure is about to occur.

PLANNING AND IMPLEMENTATION
- Be sure to place the patient's bed in the lowest position and raise the side rails to prevent injury.

- Remind the patient to call for help when getting out of bed and make sure that the call light is within easy reach because many AEDs cause dizziness.
- Make sure that oxygen and suction equipment are in the patient's room and in good working order in case a seizure does occur.
- Monitor the patient for seizure activity and be prepared to protect the patient from injury if one occurs.
- Monitor regularly scheduled blood levels of the drug(s) to determine whether they are in the effective range or could cause adverse reactions.
- Many AEDs increase the patient's suicidal ideation. Report to the healthcare provider immediately any patient statements or actions that indicate he or she may be considering self-harm.
- AEDs work in the CNS and depress its activity to some degree. They should not be taken with alcohol or any other type of CNS depressant.
- Suddenly stopping AED therapy can result in seizures. When changing drugs or discontinuing drugs, taper doses slowly to reduce the risk for seizures.

| Box 9.7 | General Patient and Family Teaching Points for Antiepileptic Drugs |

- Teach patients about the importance of keeping follow-up appointments with the healthcare provider to monitor drug effectiveness and drug blood levels.
- Instruct patients to take the drug exactly as prescribed and not to suddenly stop taking the drug, because seizures may occur.
- Teach patients to take a missed dose as soon as it is remembered, but not to take a double dose. Teach patients to immediately report any new, worsening, or unusual symptoms to the healthcare provider.
- Remind patients to avoid any over-the-counter drugs or supplements without checking with their healthcare provider to prevent possible interactions.

- Instruct patients to avoid alcoholic beverages or other drugs known to depress the CNS because severe CNS depression may occur. Also, for some patients, alcohol triggers seizure activity.
- Remind patients to avoid driving, operating dangerous equipment, or doing anything that requires mental alertness until they know how the AED affects their level of consciousness and reflexes.
- Tell patients and families that if signs of increasing depression are seen to notify the healthcare provider immediately because many of these drugs increase depression and suicidal ideation.

channels on nerve membranes and making them less active. These are among the oldest drugs used in the management of epilepsy and are available as tablets, capsules, liquid suspensions, and solutions for injection. A prodrug of phenytoin is fosphenytoin (Cerebyx), which is only available intravenously and used short term. It is converted to phenytoin in the body. Phenytoins are approved for use only with seizure disorders.

Carbamazepine is an AED that limits the spread of neuron excitation by altering the sodium channels of nerve membranes to prevent or slow the refiring of neurons. Its structure is similar to that of the tricyclic antidepressants. This drug is often used to control epilepsy in children. In addition, it is used as a mood stabilizer and to reduce skeletal muscle spasms.

Ethosuximide is an AED that raises the seizure threshold by altering calcium channels on the neuron membranes. The number of seizures is reduced because stronger excitation is needed to stimulate them. Although this drug can help reduce all types of seizures, it is most effective for absence seizures. Ethosuximide is used to reduce seizures during pregnancy because it is less likely to cause birth defects than the phenytoins or carbamazepine.

Phenobarbital is a drug from the barbiturate class that raises the seizure threshold by enhancing the action of the inhibitory neurotransmitter GABA, resulting in widespread CNS depression. It is the oldest drug used to control seizures and is also used as a sedating agent. Phenobarbital has the longest duration of action of all the traditional AEDs. It is used for all types of seizures except absence seizures and on a short-term basis for

Table 9.3   Examples of Common Traditional Antiepileptic Drugs

DRUG/ADULT DOSAGE RANGE	NURSING IMPLICATIONS

phenytoin (Dilantin, Phenytek)
   Loading dose: 15–20 mg/kg orally or
   IV given in divided doses
   throughout the day
   Maintenance dose: 4–7 mg/kg per
   day orally divided into 2–3 doses
	• Dosages for different forms of phenytoin are not interchangeable because the drug concentrations vary by type.
	• Warn patients that gum hyperplasia is a side effect of this drug and that good oral hygiene is needed to prevent tooth loss from gum disease.
	• Remind patients who take warfarin that closer monitoring is needed and the warfarin dose may need to be adjusted because phenytoin has mixed interactions on warfarin's effect.
	• Ask patients about all other drugs they take because phenytoin interacts with many, many other drugs. Check with a pharmacist and the patient's healthcare provider about the need for dosage adjustments with any drug.
	• Avoid giving this drug by the IM route because it is a severe tissue irritant.
	• Phenytoin is known to cause birth defects and is not used during pregnancy.
	• Teach patients to take their pulses daily and to report changes and irregularities to their healthcare provider because these drugs can cause bradycardia and other heart rhythm problems.

carbamazepine (Epitol, Tegretol, Tegretol XR) initial dose 200 mg orally daily; over time, increase to 100–400 mg orally every 6–8 hours; sustained-release forms: 200–800 mg orally every 12 hours	• This drug is known to cause birth defects and is not used during pregnancy. • Teach patients to take their pulses daily and to report changes and irregularities to their healthcare provider because these drugs can cause tachycardia, atrial fibrillation, and other heart rhythm problems. • Instruct patients to walk slowly and carefully, especially on stairs, because this drug may cause ataxia and increase the risk for falls. • Remind patients who take warfarin that closer monitoring is needed and the warfarin dose may need to be increased because carbamazepine reduces the effect of warfarin. • Ask patients about all other drugs they take because carbamazepine interacts with many, many other drugs. Check with a pharmacist and the patient's healthcare provider about the need for dosage adjustments with any drug. • Suggest that patients take the drug with meals or a substantial snack to decrease GI problems.

ethosuximide (Zarontin)
   Initial dose: 250 mg orally every 12
   hours
   Maintenance: 20–40 mg/kg/day
   orally in 2 divided doses
	• Ask patients about all other drugs they take because ethosuximide interacts with many, many other drugs. Check with a pharmacist and the patient's healthcare provider about the need for dosage adjustments with any drug.
	• If the patient has GI side effects, suggest that he or she take the drug with meals or a substantial snack to decrease these problems.
	• This drug may be used during pregnancy because it has a lower risk for birth defects than do other traditional AEDs.

phenobarbital 1–3 mg/kg/day orally or IV/IM, once or twice daily primidone (Mysoline) initially, 125–250 mg orally once daily at bedtime; gradually increase to 250–500 mg orally every 8 hours to a maximum of 2 gm a day	• This drug is known to cause birth defects and is not used during pregnancy. • Observe mental status and respiratory effectiveness carefully and often because this drug can cause profound CNS depression, respiratory depression, and cognitive impairment. • Check with a pharmacist before giving phenobarbital with any other drug because it has many incompatibilities. • Warn patients and families that there is an increased risk for falls, especially when first starting the drug, because of CNS depression and ataxia.
valproic acid (Depakote, Depakene, Depacon [injectable form]) 10–15 mg/kg per day orally or IV, divide doses if the total is more than 250 mg; may be increased up to 60 mg/kg per day in divided doses	• Remind patients who take warfarin that closer monitoring is needed and the warfarin dose may need to be decreased because valproic acid increases blood levels of warfarin. • Remind parents of young children who are taking this drug to check the child weekly for yellowing of the skin or whites of the eyes, darkening of the urine, or light-colored stools because severe liver toxicity can occur. If any of these changes are present, notify the healthcare provider. • Give intravenous infusions slowly, over 60 minutes, to avoid injection-site pain and severe dizziness. • This drug is known to cause birth defects and is not used during pregnancy.

insomnia and anxiety. This drug is available in tablet form, oral solutions, and solutions for injection. Primidone is a prodrug and is converted to phenobarbital in the body. It has the same actions, side effects, interactions, and precautions as phenobarbital.

Valproic acid is an AED that raises the seizure threshold by possibly increasing the activity of the inhibitory neurotransmitter, GABA. Not all of its actions are known. It is often combined with divalproex sodium to increase its duration of action and to reduce the frequency of dosing. In addition to most seizure types, valproic acid is also used to help manage manic types of bipolar disorders.

Expected Side Effects

The most common side effect of phenytoin is gum hyperplasia, especially with long-term use. Other common side effects include abdominal discomfort. Unlike many other AEDs, phenytoin does *not* cause drowsiness.

The most common side effects of carbamazepine are constipation, nausea and vomiting, and *ataxia* (unsteadiness when walking). Other side effects include itching, rash, muscle weakness, and an increased risk for sunburn.

Ethosuximide has fewer common side effects than other traditional AEDs. The most common side effects of this drug are heartburn (*dyspepsia*), nausea and vomiting, dizziness, drowsiness, and fatigue. Adverse effects of this drug are rare.

Phenobarbital and primidone have many CNS side effects, especially drowsiness and ataxia. Additional side effects include blurred vision, dizziness, and mental status changes. These problems are most apparent when therapy first begins and become less severe over time.

The most common side effects of valproic acid are drowsiness, muscle weakness, nausea, diarrhea, and menstrual irregularities. Additional side effects include anorexia, double vision, and blurred vision. Instead of drowsiness, some patients have insomnia.

Adverse Reactions

Phenytoin is a known *teratogen* causing birth defects. It should be avoided during pregnancy. Other adverse effects of phenytoin include blood cell problems of anemia, reduced white blood cell counts with increased risk for infection, and reduced platelet counts with increased risk for bleeding. Although not common, heart rhythm problems, especially *bradycardia* (slow heart rate), can occur. Skin rashes with phenytoin can progress to widespread serious problems known as Stevens-Johnson syndrome, which can result in skin sloughing and other problems.

🔖 Top Tip for Safety

Development of a rash in a patient who is taking phenytoin (Dilantin) may signify the onset of a severe adverse reaction. Notify the healthcare provider immediately.

Carbamazepine, like the phenytoins, affects the bone marrow, leading to anemia, reduced white blood cell counts with increased risk for infection, and reduced platelet counts with increased risk for bleeding. Heart rhythm problems leading to *tachycardia* (rapid heart rate), atrial fibrillation, and severe hypertension may occur.

Phenobarbital (and primidone) can cause severe CNS depression, especially when given parenterally. It can cause respiratory depression and should not be given to patients who have chronic obstructive pulmonary disease or any other severe respiratory impairment. Phenobarbital has an increased risk for physical and psychological dependency, especially with long-term use, and is classified as a schedule IV controlled substance. Other possible adverse effects include bone marrow depression, cognitive impairment, exfoliative dermatitis, liver impairment, bradycardia, and coma, among many others. In cases of acute overdose, the patient may show exaggerated CNS depression, slow and shallow respirations, small pupil size (*miosis*), tachycardia, *areflexia* (absence of reflexes), shock, or coma. Death may occur as a result of cardiorespiratory failure. Consult a drug reference for a more complete list of adverse reactions associated with phenobarbital.

Valproic acid has been known to cause amnesia and heart rhythm irregularities, especially tachycardia. Hearing loss and GI bleeding are also possible.

🔖 Lifespan Considerations
Pediatric

Serious liver toxicity may be seen in some children who are taking valproic acid, especially those younger than 2 years or those receiving multiple AEDs. The risk for liver toxicity decreases as the child ages.

🔖 Lifespan Considerations
Pregnancy

The phenytoins, carbamazepine, phenobarbital, primidone, and valproic acid are known teratogens that commonly cause birth defects. These drugs are not to be used during pregnancy unless epilepsy cannot be controlled any other way.

Drug Interactions

The list of drugs that interact with all of the traditional antiepilepsy drugs is very long and includes very common drugs such as aspirin, acetaminophen, oral contraceptives, proton pump inhibitors, and drugs for diabetes. Of particular note are the drugs used to manage psychiatric problems and warfarin. To prevent severe complications and adverse reactions, avoid other prescription drugs unless the benefit outweighs interaction risks. Instruct patients to avoid over-the-counter drugs and supplements unless prescribed by their healthcare provider. Always consult a drug reference or pharmacist to determine possible interactions between AEDs and any other drug a patient is prescribed.

NEWER ANTIEPILEPTIC DRUGS

More than a dozen drugs are considered newer AEDs. Some are drugs that have been used for many years for other conditions and have been found to have effectiveness in helping to control some types of seizures. However, most must be used along with or added to a regimen that includes traditional AEDs. This type of "added on" therapy is known as *adjuvant therapy*. Only four drugs have been approved for use as single-drug therapy (*monotherapy*) of epilepsy in place of a traditional AED. These drugs may also be used along with traditional AEDs. Table 9.4 lists the names, dosages, and nursing implications of the four newer AEDs approved as monotherapy for epilepsy: oxcarbazepine, lamotrigine, lacosamide, and topiramate. Table 9.5 lists the newer AEDs that are approved only for use as adjuvant therapy along with one or more traditional AEDs. For more information about the newer AEDs used as adjuvant therapy, consult a drug reference.

💡 Memory Jogger

The newer AEDs approved for use as monotherapy are:
- oxcarbazepine
- lamotrigine
- lacosamide
- topiramate

OXCARBAZEPINE

Action and Uses

Oxcarbazepine is an AED derived from carbamazepine (see earlier Traditional Antiepileptic Drugs section) that reduces seizures by blocking sodium channels on neuron membranes, requiring greater stimulation for them to depolarize (fire). Thus it raises the seizure threshold. Although the structure is similar to carbamazepine, it has fewer CNS side effects. It is approved for use to control partial seizures.

Expected Side Effects/Adverse Reactions

The most common side effects of oxcarbazepine are drowsiness, dizziness, headache, and nausea. Visual side effects of double vision and blurred vision may also occur.

The most common adverse effects are amnesia and low sodium levels (*hyponatremia*). Rare problems include bone marrow suppression and confusion. Just as with

traditional AEDs, depression and suicidal ideation are possible. Although oxcarbazepine is less likely than traditional AEDs to cause birth defects, it is still not recommended during pregnancy.

Drug Interactions

Oxcarbazepine lowers blood sodium levels; this effect is intensified when the patient also takes sodium-excreting diuretics. This drug interacts with many drugs, especially aspirin, acetaminophen, oral contraceptives, proton pump inhibitors, drugs for psychiatric problems, drugs for HIV disease, and drugs for diabetes. To prevent severe complications and adverse reactions, avoid other prescription drugs unless the benefit outweighs interaction risks. Consult a drug reference or pharmacist for possible interactions with other drugs the patient is prescribed.

❖ Nursing Implications and Patient Teaching

◆ *Planning and implementation.* In addition to the general nursing implications for patients who are taking AEDs that are listed in Box 9.6, the following issues and actions are important for patients who are taking oxcarbazepine. Ask the patient about changes in vision such as blurred vision or double vision, which are common side effects of therapy with oxcarbazepine. If these visual changes are present, instruct the patient not to drive or operate dangerous machinery, to avoid an accident or injury.

This drug can cause blood levels of sodium to be low. Check laboratory values for sodium levels whenever they are drawn. Report levels lower than 135 mEq/L (mmol/L) to the healthcare provider. Assess for symptoms associated with low sodium levels, such as headache, increased muscle weakness, and decreased deep tendon reflexes. If present, document these symptoms and report them to the healthcare provider.

◆ *Patient and family teaching.* In addition to the teaching points listed in Box 9.7, tell the patient who is taking oxcarbazepine and his or her family the following:
- Keep all appointments for laboratory testing because the drug can cause electrolyte problems and decrease blood counts.
- Do not drive or operate dangerous equipment if you are experiencing vision changes such as blurred vision or double vision.
- If you notice increased muscle weakness and persistent headache, notify your healthcare provider because these may indicate low sodium levels.
- If you are taking oral contraceptives, use an additional form of contraception to prevent an unplanned pregnancy because this drug reduces the effectiveness of hormonal contraceptives.

LAMOTRIGINE

Action and Uses

Lamotrigine is a newer AED with an unknown mechanism of action and is thought to reduce seizures by

Table 9.4 Examples of Common Newer Antiepileptic Drugs Approved as Monotherapy

DRUG/ADULT DOSAGE RANGE	NURSING IMPLICATIONS
oxcarbazepine (Trileptal): initial: 300 mg orally every 12 hours; gradually increase to 1200 mg orally every 12 hours Oxtellar XR: initial 600 mg orally once daily; gradually increase to 2400 mg orally once daily	• Monitor blood sodium levels because this drug can cause hyponatremia. • Assess patients for symptoms associated with low sodium levels, such as headache, increased muscle weakness, and decreased deep tendon reflexes, and report these to the healthcare provider. • To avoid falls, caution patients to walk carefully and use hand rails on stairs whenever they feel some muscle weakness. • Instruct patients not to drive or operate dangerous equipment when their vision is blurry or doubled, to prevent an accident and injury.
lamotrigine (Lamictal) Initial: 50 mg orally once daily for 2 weeks, then 50 mg orally twice daily for 2 weeks, gradually increasing maintenance Maintenance: 250 mg orally twice daily Lamictal XR: start at 50 mg orally once daily for 2 weeks, then 100 mg orally once daily for 2 weeks, then increase by 100 mg per week until maintenance dose of 400–600 mg once daily is reached	• Be sure to use the correct "starter kit" when drug therapy first begins to avoid complications and interactions. • Assess the patient daily for skin rash, which can signal the beginning of life-threatening skin reactions. If a rash is present, hold the dose and notify the healthcare provider immediately. • Teach patients to check themselves daily for skin rashes and tell them to notify their healthcare provider immediately. • Check with the healthcare provider to determine whether folic acid supplements are needed because this drug interferes with the final production of folic acid in the body and some patients may become folic acid deficient. • Carefully check the dosages prescribed for black patients because clearance rates are lower and lower dosages are often needed to prevent drug overdose. • Instruct patients not to drive or operate dangerous equipment when their vision is blurry or doubled, to prevent an accident or injury.
lacosamide (Vimpat) Initial: 100 mg orally twice daily *or* 100 mg IV infusion twice daily Maintenance: 150-200 mg/day orally, twice daily	• Monitor patients for orthostatic hypotension and take steps to prevent falls, such as accompanying the patient during ambulation. • Instruct patients to change positions slowly, especially when moving from a lying or sitting position to a standing position, because this drug can cause orthostatic hypotension and syncope. • Remind patients that even if they like the mood produced by the drug not to increase the dosage or how often they take the drug, to avoid psychological dependence. • Instruct patients not to drive or operate dangerous equipment when their vision is blurry or doubled, to prevent an accident and injury. • Give IV infusions slowly, over 30–60 minutes, to avoid injection-site pain and heart rhythm problems. • Monitor the patient's blood pressure and heart rate and rhythm before giving the drug IV, every 15 minutes during the infusion, and after the infusion is complete, to identify severe hypotension or heart rhythm problems.
topiramate (Qudexy, Topamax, Trokendi XR) Quick-release forms: initially, 25 mg orally twice daily; gradually increase over 6–7 weeks to 200 mg orally twice daily XR forms: initially, 50 mg orally once daily; gradually increase over 6–7 weeks to 400 mg orally once daily	• Monitor laboratory values, especially blood pH, electrolytes, and ammonia levels because this drug can cause metabolic acidosis, elevated ammonia levels, and encephalopathy. • Assess patients for symptoms of encephalopathy, such as the development of lethargy, vomiting, changes in mental status, or hypothermia, and report these immediately to the healthcare provider so prompt encephalopathy treatment can begin. • The risk for metabolic acidosis is greater if the patient is also taking metformin for diabetes control. • Assess patients for symptoms of metabolic acidosis (slow heart rate, hypotension, muscle weakness, and warm, flushed skin) and, if present, report these symptoms to the healthcare provider immediately. • Follow dose-increasing schedules exactly to avoid adverse reactions.

blocking sodium channels on neuron membranes. It is approved for use as monotherapy for partial seizures, tonic-clonic seizures, and seizures associated with Lennox-Gastaut syndrome. In addition, it is approved for some types of bipolar disorders. Table 9.4 lists the names, dosages, and nursing implications for lamotrigine.

Expected Side Effects
The most common side effects of lamotrigine are drowsiness, abdominal pain, and visual disturbances (e.g., double vision and blurred vision). Other side effects include ataxia, dry mouth, and dizziness. An unusual issue with lamotrigine is that its clearance rate is lower

Table **9.5**	Examples of Newer Antiepileptic Drugs Approved as Adjuvant Therapy	
DRUG NAMES	**ADULT MAINTENANCE DOSAGE RANGE**	**TYPE OF SEIZURE ACTIVITY**
ezogabine (Potiga)	200–400 mg orally three times daily	Partial
felbamate (Felbatol)	400–800 mg orally three times daily	Lennox-Gastaut syndrome and severe seizures that cannot be controlled with any other drugs
gabapentin (Horizant, Gralise, Neurontin)	300–800 mg orally three times daily	Partial
levetiracetam (Keppra, Spritam)	1500 mg orally twice daily	Myoclonic; partial; tonic-clonic
pregabalin (Lyrica)	200 mg orally three times daily	Partial
rufinamide (Banzel)	1600 mg orally twice daily	Lennox-Gastaut syndrome
tiagabine (Gabitril)	8–14 mg orally four times daily or 16–28 mg orally twice daily	Partial
vigabatrin (Sabril)	1500 mg orally twice daily	Complex partial
zonisamide (Zonegran)	100–600 mg orally once daily	Partial

among black patients, which can lead to symptoms of overdose even when using usual recommended dosages.

Adverse Reactions

Lamotrigine can cause life-threatening rashes (including Stevens-Johnson syndrome and toxic epidermal necrolysis). It has a black box warning that states to discontinue the drug immediately if any rash appears during treatment. Although this problem can occur at any age, it is more likely to occur in children. The drug interferes with the formation of folic acid, an important vitamin, and some patients may become folic acid deficient. Although lamotrigine is less likely than traditional AEDs to cause birth defects, it is still not recommended during pregnancy. Just as with traditional AEDs, depression and suicidal ideation are possible.

Top Tip for Safety

If any rash appears during therapy with lamotrigine, stop the drug and notify the healthcare provider immediately because this could signal the beginning of life-threatening skin problems.

Drug Interactions

Lamotrigine interacts with many drugs, especially aspirin, acetaminophen, oral contraceptives, proton pump inhibitors, cardiac drugs, drugs for psychiatric problems, drugs for HIV disease, drugs for tuberculosis, and drugs for diabetes. To prevent severe complications and adverse reactions, avoid other prescription drugs unless the benefit outweighs interaction risks. Consult a drug reference or pharmacist for possible interactions with other drugs the patient is prescribed.

❖ **Nursing Implications and Patient Teaching**
In addition to the general nursing implications for patients who are taking AEDs that are listed in Box 9.6, the following issues and actions are important for patients who are taking lamotrigine.

◆ *Planning and implementation.* When drug therapy with lamotrigine is first started, three different "starter kits" are available. The one prescribed is based on whether the patient will be taking lamotrigine as monotherapy or with other specific AEDs. Be sure to use the correct starter kit to avoid complications and interactions.

Assess the patient daily for skin rash, which can signal the beginning of life-threatening skin reactions. If a rash is present, hold the dose and notify the healthcare provider immediately.

Assess black patients very carefully for side effects and adverse reactions because the drug clearance rate is about 25% lower than for patients of other races.

◆ *Patient and family teaching.* In addition to the teaching points listed in Box 9.7, tell the patient who is taking lamotrigine and his or her family the following:

- Check yourself every day for skin rashes. If a rash appears, notify your healthcare provider immediately because this response may be the start of a life-threatening reaction.
- If you are taking the extended-release form of the drug, swallow it whole and do not crush, open, or chew it to keep the drug release even throughout the day.
- If your mouth becomes uncomfortably dry, chewing gum, sucking hard candy, and drinking more water may help the problem.
- Do not drive or operate dangerous equipment if your vision is blurred or if you have double vision.

LACOSAMIDE

Action and Uses

Lacosamide is an amino acid with an unknown mechanism of action that appears to control seizures by acting at sodium channels to stabilize neuron membranes and prevent repetitive excitation and firing. It is approved for use as monotherapy to control partial seizures and can be used as an "add-on" drug with some other AEDs. Table 9.4 lists the names, dosages, and nursing implications for lacosamide.

Expected Side Effects

The most common side effects of lacosamide are headache, dizziness, blurred vision, and double vision. Other side effects include fatigue, nausea, and ataxia.

Adverse Reactions

Many people who are taking lacosamide experience *euphoria*, a feeling of intense well-being and happiness. This is considered an adverse reaction because it can lead to psychological dependence (but not addiction). Orthostatic hypotension (low blood pressure on moving to a standing position) with brief *syncope* (loss of consciousness) have been reported, leading to an increased risk for falls and injury. Unlike other newer AEDs, lacosamide does not reduce the effectiveness of oral contraceptives. Intravenous infusions of lacosamide can cause pain at the injection site, rapid lowering of blood pressure, and heart rhythm problems, especially bradycardia. Although lacosamide is less likely than traditional AEDs to cause birth defects, it is still not recommended during pregnancy. Just as with traditional AEDs, depression and suicidal ideation are possible.

Drug Interactions

Lacosamide interacts with many drugs, especially cardiac drugs, antihypertensives, drugs for psychiatric problems, drugs for HIV disease, antifungal drugs, and drugs for tuberculosis. To prevent severe complications and adverse reactions, avoid other prescription drugs unless the benefit outweighs interaction risks. Consult a drug reference or pharmacist for possible interactions with other drugs the patient is prescribed.

❖ Nursing Implications and Patient Teaching

In addition to the general nursing implications for patients who are taking AEDs that are listed in Box 9.6, the following issues and actions are important for patients who are taking lacosamide.

◆ *Planning and implementation.* Assess the patient's blood pressure before and after giving this drug because it can cause severe hypotension. This problem is worse in patients whose blood pressure is normally low. If the blood pressure is lower than normal, walk with the patient during ambulation and instruct him or her not to walk alone.

Ask the patient about changes in vision such as blurred vision or double vision, which are common side effects of therapy with lacosamide. If these visual changes are present or if the drug makes the patient dizzy, instruct him or her not to drive or operate dangerous machinery, to avoid an accident or injury.

When giving this drug intravenously, infuse it slowly over 30 to 60 minutes. Faster rates increase the risk for pain at the injection site, severe hypotension, and heart rhythm problems. Monitor the patient's blood pressure and heart rate and rhythm before giving the drug, every 15 minutes during the infusion, and after the infusion is complete.

Observe the patient for mood changes after taking this drug. Some people feel euphoric, which can increase the risk for psychological dependency.

◆ *Patient and family teaching.* In addition to the teaching points listed in Box 9.7, tell the patient who is taking lacosamide and his or her family the following:

- Change positions slowly, especially when moving from a lying or sitting position to a standing position, because you may experience a sudden drop in blood pressure.
- Report any unexpected loss of consciousness to your healthcare provider because this is a possible adverse reaction to the drug.
- Do not drive or operate dangerous equipment if your vision is blurred, if you have double vision, or if you are dizzy, to prevent an accident or injury.
- Some people feel especially happy or even "high" when they take this drug and may be tempted to take it more often (i.e., become dependent on this feeling). Regardless of this mood change, do not take the drug more often than prescribed.

TOPIRAMATE

Actions and Uses

Although the exact mechanisms are not clear, topiramate appears to reduce seizures by preventing the spread of excitation in the brain rather than raising the seizure threshold. It seems to have three actions that produce this response. Topiramate acts at sodium channels to stabilize neuron membranes and prevent repetitive excitation and firing, enhances the inhibitory neurotransmitter GABA, and blocks some excitatory receptors. It is approved for use as monotherapy for partial seizures, tonic-clonic seizures, and seizures associated with Lennox-Gastaut syndrome. In addition, it is approved as an "add-on" drug for control of epilepsy. The drug has been used to treat migraines but is not approved for this use. Table 9.4 lists the names, dosages, and nursing implications for topiramate.

Expected Side Effects

Common side effects of topiramate are abdominal pain, nausea, dizziness, drowsiness, and fatigue. Additional side effects include taste changes, anorexia, and *paresthesias* (sensations of numbness, tingling, and "pins and needles").

Adverse Reactions

Topiramate can cause memory impairment and electrolyte imbalances, especially low levels of phosphorus and calcium. At higher doses, topiramate can cause metabolic problems, particularly acidosis and elevated ammonia concentrations. When ammonia levels become too high, they can causes encephalopathy, which leads to brain damage and death. Symptoms of elevated ammonia levels and encephalopathy are unexplained lethargy, vomiting, changes in mental status, and low core body temperatures (hypothermia). Topiramate is a known teratogen that can cause birth defects. It is not to be used during pregnancy unless epilepsy cannot be controlled any other way. Just as with other AEDs, depression and suicidal ideation are possible.

> 🕊 **Top Tip for Safety**
>
> If blood ammonia levels are high or if symptoms of encephalopathy are present, the drug is immediately discontinued and treatment for encephalopathy is started.

Drug Interactions

Topiramate interacts with many drugs, especially aspirin, acetaminophen, oral contraceptives, cardiac drugs, diuretics, antihypertensives, antifungals, drugs for psychiatric problems, drugs for HIV disease, drugs for tuberculosis, drugs that affect blood clotting, and drugs for diabetes. To prevent severe complications and adverse reactions, avoid other prescription drugs unless the benefit outweighs interaction risks. Consult a drug reference or pharmacist for possible interactions with other drugs the patient is prescribed.

❖ Nursing Implications and Patient Teaching

In addition to the general nursing implications for patients who are taking AEDs that are listed in Box 9.6, the following issues and actions are important for patients who are taking topiramate.

◆ *Planning and implementation.* Assess patients who are taking topiramate for the development of lethargy, vomiting, changes in mental status, or hypothermia (lower than normal core body temperature) because these may be symptoms of encephalopathy caused by high blood ammonia levels. Report any of these symptoms to the healthcare provider immediately. Be prepared to draw blood for an ammonia level (normal ammonia levels are 10–80 mcg/dL [6–47 mcmol/L]).

Monitor laboratory values, especially pH and electrolytes, because this drug increases the risk for metabolic acidosis. The risk is greater if the patient is also taking metformin for diabetes control. Symptoms of acidosis include slow heart rate, hypotension, muscle weakness, and warm, flushed skin. If the patient has several of these symptoms, notify the healthcare provider immediately.

◆ *Patient and family teaching.* In addition to the teaching points listed in Box 9.7, tell the patient who is taking topiramate and his or her family the following:

- If you suddenly become lethargic, confused, and have vomiting, or if your temperature falls below 95°F (or 35°C), call your healthcare provider immediately because these are symptoms of a life-threatening complication.
- Do not chew or crush capsules because this will ruin the slow-release feature, and the drug may be absorbed so quickly that the risk for side effects and adverse reactions is increased.
- Do not chew or break the tablet form of the drug because it is very bitter tasting.

DRUGS FOR MULTIPLE SCLEROSIS

MS is an autoimmune disease that affects the fatty tissue (*myelin*) in the brain and spinal cord. Myelin surrounds and protects neurons and is important in providing support to neuron function in the CNS. Immune system cells and their products attack myelin and destroy patches of it in the CNS, creating plaques, which reduce nerve function (Fig. 9.6). Although the nerves are not directly attacked, nerve transmission is interrupted, which causes the symptoms of MS. Specific early symptoms depend on where in the brain and spinal cord the myelin is destroyed. Box 9.8 lists common

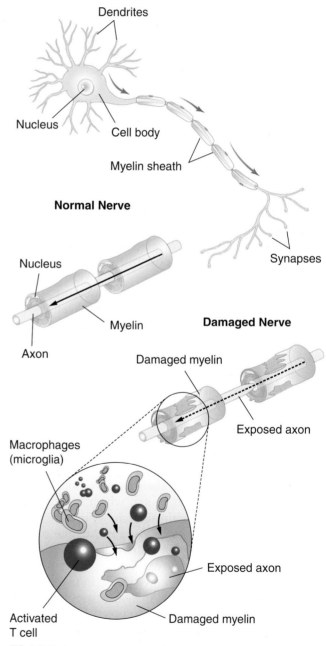

FIG. 9.6 Pathogenesis of multiple sclerosis. (From McCance K, Huether S, Brashers V, Rote N: *Pathophysiology: The biologic basis for disease in adults and children,* ed 7, St. Louis, 2014, Mosby.)

Box **9.8**	Common Early Symptoms of Multiple Sclerosis

- Fatigue
- Double vision/blurry vision
- Muscle weakness
- Numbness of arms and legs
- Difficulty walking
- Urinary tract infections
- Bowel and bladder dysfunction
- Depression
- Difficulty with concentration

symptoms of MS. The disorder develops in women twice as often as in men.

MS has a variety of types, with the most common being relapsing-remitting MS (RRMS). With RRMS, at first the patient has periods of worsening symptoms (*relapsing*) followed by periods in which symptoms are either not present or are very mild (*remitting* or *remissions*). The disorder is progressive with worsening symptoms, longer duration of symptoms, and fewer remission periods over time. Eventually symptoms are always present and most motor functions decline. Some patients with RRMS have lived more than 30 years with the disease; however, life expectancy is always decreased. MS cannot be cured, but drug therapy can slow progression and allow patients to remain functionally independent longer.

Management of MS is performed by neurologic healthcare providers and specialized clinics. First doses and drug regimens are started with this specialist. However, patients with MS can develop other acute problems and be hospitalized, where some drug therapy must continue. In addition, as motor function decreases, many patients with MS are placed in long-term care facilities. The drugs discussed in this chapter are primarily used for RRMS.

NONSPECIFIC ANTI-INFLAMMATORY DRUGS

For many years, treatment for MS consisted of generalized reduction of inflammation and immunity with powerful anti-inflammatories, such as corticosteroids. These drugs may relieve some symptoms but do not alter the course of the disease and have significant side effects. Corticosteroids may be used occasionally now at lower dosages, in addition to more specific drug therapies for MS. Chapter 12 discusses information about corticosteroids in detail.

SPECIFIC DRUGS FOR MULTIPLE SCLEROSIS

More therapeutic options are now available for MS. The three broad categories of drugs to reduce MS symptoms, slow progression, and increase the duration of remissions (for RRMS) are the **biological response modifiers (BRMs)**, monoclonal antibodies, and neurologic drugs. The names, dosages, and side effects/adverse

reactions to check for in patients who are receiving the drug are listed in Table 9.6.

Biological Response Modifiers

BRMs are drugs that modify the patient's immune response to abnormal triggers for immunity and inflammation. This drug class contains two drugs given by subcutaneous injection and two oral preparations. Both types of drugs are taken regularly. The two injectable BRMs are beta interferon (Avonex, Betaseron, Extavia, Plegridy, Rebif) and glatiramer (Copaxone, Glatopa). The oral drugs are fingolimod (Gilenya) and teriflunomide (Aubagio). The BRMs are prescribed by healthcare providers who are specialists in the care of patients with MS. These specialists and specialty nurses are responsible for patient teaching and managing side effects and adverse reactions. The names, dosages, and side effects/adverse reactions to check for in patients who are receiving BRMs are listed in Table 9.6.

Monoclonal Antibodies for Multiple Sclerosis

Monoclonal antibodies for MS are antibodies that attack and either inactivate or destroy lymphocytes involved in direct destruction of myelin or that produce chemicals (cytokines) that trigger the immune system to destroy myelin. The lymphocyte population in the periphery of the body is reduced along with lymphocytes in the CNS. All of these drugs increase the risk for infection by reducing general immunity and can trigger severe allergic reactions. These drugs are all given as intravenous infusions on a specific schedule that ranges from once monthly, to once every 6 months, to once yearly. They are given only in specialized centers or in offices of healthcare providers who are specialists in the care of patients with MS. These specialists and specialty nurses are responsible for monitoring patients during and after infusion, patient teaching, and managing side effects and adverse reactions. The names, dosages, and side effects/adverse reactions to check for in patients who are receiving these drugs are listed in Table 9.6.

Specific Neurologic Drugs for Multiple Sclerosis

Neurologic drugs approved specifically for MS are dimethyl fumarate (Tecfidera) and dalfampridine (Ampyra). Both are oral drugs that must be taken daily to help improve some symptoms of MS. Therefore they are likely to be part of the prescribed drug regimen for patients with MS when they are admitted to the hospital or another care facility. The benefits of the drugs require that therapy continue in all care settings.

Dimethyl fumarate (Tecfidera) reduces inflammation in the CNS, which helps protect neurons and myelin from damage. Dalfampridine (Ampyra) blocks potassium channels in unmyelinated nerves, helping them to continue to function. It is used to help improve the walking ability of patients with MS. The names, dosages, and side effects/adverse reactions to check for in patients who are receiving these drugs are listed in Table 9.6.

Table 9.6 **Examples of Drugs for Relapsing-Remitting Multiple Sclerosis**

Biological response modifiers: modify the immune response of patients with MS to abnormal triggers for immunity and inflammation, which slows progression of the disease, improves symptoms, and increases the duration of remission periods

DRUG/ADULT DOSAGE RANGE	EXPECTED SIDE/ADVERSE EFFECTS

beta-interferon (Avonex, Betaseron, Extavia, Plegridy, Rebif)
  Maintenance: depends on strength and formulation of the drug; given
    subcutaneously three times weekly, every other day, or once every
    14 days for long-duration formulas
fingolimod (Gilenya) 0.5 mg orally once daily
glatiramer (Copaxone, Glatopa) 20 mg subcutaneously daily of the
  20 mg/mL solution *or* 40 mg subcutaneously three times per week of
  the 40 mg/mL solution
teriflunomide (Aubagio) 7 or 14 mg orally once daily
	• Flulike symptoms
	• Headache
	• Injection-site reactions
	• Peripheral neuropathy
	• Elevated liver enzymes
	• Slow heart rate
	• Thinning scalp hair

Monoclonal antibodies for MS: slow progression of MS by attacking and either inactivating or destroying lymphocytes involved in direct destruction of myelin or that produce chemicals (cytokines) that trigger the immune system to damage myelin

DRUG/ADULT DOSAGE RANGE	EXPECTED SIDE/ADVERSE EFFECTS

Alemtuzumab (Lemtrada)
  Maintenance: 12 mg IV daily for 3 consecutive days (total dose of
    36 mg)
daclizumab (Zinbryta)
  Maintenance: 150 mg injected subcutaneously once monthly
natalizumab (Tysabri) 300 mg IV infusion given over 1 hour every 4
  weeks
ocrelizumab (Ocrevus)
  Maintenance: 600 mg IV infusion every 6 months
	• Increased risk for infection
	• Higher risk for severe allergic reactions
	• Infusion-site reactions
	• Flulike symptoms
	• Back pain
	• Hypotension
	• Edema
	• Patient should not be taking more than one
	  monoclonal antibody at a time

Neurologic drugs for MS: slow progression and reduce symptoms of MS using several different mechanisms to either protect nerves and myelin from destruction or improve impulse transmission of demyelinated nerves

DRUG/ADULT DOSAGE RANGE	EXPECTED SIDE/ADVERSE EFFECTS
dalfampridine (Ampyra) 10 mg orally every 12 hours dimethyl fumarate (Tecfidera) 240 mg orally twice daily	• Increased risk for infection • Headache, dizziness, muscle weakness • GI problems, heartburn, constipation • Confusion, seizure activity • Nausea, diarrhea, abdominal pain • Flushing, itching, rashes • Increased risk for infection

MS, Multiple sclerosis.

Get Ready for the NCLEX® Examination!

Key Points

- The symptoms of PD are caused by an imbalance in neurotransmitters in which the amount of ACh (an excitatory chemical) is normal, but there is too little dopamine (inhibitory chemical) in the brain. Motor and sensory symptoms are progressive and debilitating.
- Dopamine agonists are best absorbed on an empty stomach. When taken 30 to 60 minutes before a meal or snack, they help the patient be better able to chew and swallow.
- Taking dopamine agonists with food that is high in protein reduces the drug's effectiveness.
- Levodopa peaks in about 1 hour and wears off in 4 or 5 hours. This wearing-off effect causes rapid swings of symptoms. This can also be called an "on-off" effect.

- Long-term use of dopamine agonists may lead to *akinesia* (loss of movement), *tardive dyskinesia* (abnormal and involuntary movements, especially of the lower face), and *dystonia* (impairment of muscle tone).
- Dopamine agonists can exacerbate depression and psychosis.
- Monitor blood glucose levels closely when using dopamine agonists because the sympathetic effects can cause hypoglycemia.
- Teach people who are taking MAO-B inhibitors to avoid tyramine-containing foods such as beer, wine, or aged meats and cheeses (as examples).
- In AD, nerves become tangled and form nonfunctional meshes within the brain, and the excitatory neurotransmitter ACh is decreased in the brain. These changes result in progressive difficulty with memory and learning.

Get Ready for the NCLEX® Examination!—cont'd

- Cholinesterase inhibitors are drugs that bind to acetylcholinesterase and slow its action, allowing ACh to remain functional longer, possibly delaying memory loss and improving functional ability.
- Cholinesterase inhibitors are parasympathetic agonists, so they can cause adverse side effects in the entire body, such as bradycardia, hypotension in the cardiac system, and seizures in the neurologic system.
- Memantine (Namenda) is an NMDA blocker that can allow more available calcium to the brain neurons, possibly improving memory. It is given with the cholinesterase inhibitors to boost the effect of cholinesterase inhibitors.
- Patients with AD should be weighed weekly to monitor for weight loss that can be caused by all the drugs used to improve memory.
- Donepezil (Aricept) should be given at night.
- Phenobarbital is a schedule IV controlled substance with an increased risk for physical and psychological dependency.
- Stopping AEDs suddenly can trigger seizure activity. The drugs are tapered slowly to reduce this possibility.
- With any AED, depression and suicidal ideation are possible.
- The phenytoins, carbamazepine, phenobarbital, primidone, and valproic acid are known teratogens that commonly cause birth defects. These drugs are not to be used during pregnancy unless epilepsy cannot be controlled any other way.
- Always consult a drug reference or pharmacist to determine possible interactions between AEDs and any other drug that a patient is prescribed.
- Serious liver toxicity may be seen in some children who are taking valproic acid, especially those younger than 2 years old or those receiving multiple AEDs.
- If any rash appears during therapy with lamotrigine, stop the drug and notify the healthcare provider immediately because this could signal the beginning of life-threatening skin problems.
- Topiramate can increase blood levels of ammonia and cause encephalopathy with brain damage.
- There is no cure for MS.
- Monoclonal antibodies for MS have a high risk for severe allergic reactions.
- The monoclonal antibodies for MS all increase the risk for infection.

Review Questions for the NCLEX® Examination

1. Which foods or beverages does the nurse teach patients to avoid taking with the combination drug carbidopa/levodopa (Sinemet)?
   1. Grapefruit or grapefruit juice
   2. Pasta and carbohydrates
   3. High-fat meal
   4. Steak dinner

2. Which condition is considered a possible contraindication to the use of dopamine agonists in a patient with Parkinson's disease?
   1. Closed-angle glaucoma
   2. Diabetes
   3. Hypertension
   4. Tremors

3. Which nursing intervention is most appropriate to take when a patient is taking entacapone (Comtan)?
   1. Limit the intake of foods that contain tyramine.
   2. Notify the healthcare provider for orange-brown urine.
   3. Monitor for signs of abdominal pain, jaundice, dark urine, and yellowing of the eyes.
   4. Increase fluids to 3 liters a day to prevent hypotension.

4. Which dinner foods are most appropriate for a patient who is taking selegiline (Eldepryl)?
   1. Roast beef, baked potatoes, green beans, and beer
   2. Green salad with yogurt dressing, baked chicken, rice, and sparkling water
   3. Pizza with anchovies and mushrooms and a cola
   4. Fresh salmon, kale salad with oil and vinegar dressing, fried potatoes, and iced tea

5. Which laboratory results are most important to monitor for a patient on dopamine agonists? (Select all that apply.)
   1. Complete blood counts
   2. Liver function studies
   3. Glucose
   4. Potassium
   5. Urinalysis
   6. Ammonia levels

6. Which nursing interventions are most important before giving donepezil (Aricept)? (Select all that apply.)
   1. Obtain an accurate weight.
   2. Complete an Alzheimer's Disease Assessment Scale.
   3. Obtain a 12-lead ECG.
   4. Obtain a chest radiograph.
   5. Ask the patient about a history or symptoms of GI bleeding.
   6. Ask the patient whether he or she is sexually active.

7. Which neurotransmitter is thought to be deficient in Alzheimer's disease?
   1. Acetylcholine
   2. Dopamine
   3. Serotonin
   4. Norepinephrine

8. A patient with Alzheimer's disease has been prescribed rivastigmine (Exelon). Which expected side effect is most often associated with this drug?
   1. Erectile dysfunction
   2. Headaches
   3. Hallucinations
   4. Flulike symptoms

Get Ready for the NCLEX® Examination!—cont'd

9. Which cardiac side effects could be expected if a patient is on a cholinesterase inhibitor (Hint: cholinergic agonist) like donepezil (Aricept)? (Select all that apply.)
   1. Bradycardia
   2. Increased saliva
   3. Hypertension
   4. Hypotension
   5. Heart block
   6. Constipation

10. Which expected side effects are associated with memantine (Namenda)? (Select all that apply.)
    1. Headache
    2. Dizziness
    3. Diarrhea
    4. Constipation
    5. Hallucinations
    6. Weight gain

11. Which traditional antiepileptic drug is recommended for use during pregnancy?
    1. Carbamazepine
    2. Ethosuximide
    3. Phenytoin
    4. Valproic acid

12. A patient who is taking lamotrigine reports the appearance of a new rash. What is your best action?
    1. Report the rash to the healthcare provider immediately.
    2. Add the reaction to the patient's list of allergies in his or her record.
    3. Instruct the patient to take the drug with a substantial meal or snack.
    4. Suggest that the patient apply a cortisone-containing cream to the area.

13. Which patient taking lamotrigine is more likely to develop symptoms of overdose with recommended dosages?
    1. 15-year-old Asian male with asthma
    2. 22-year-old white female who is pregnant
    3. 48-year-old Mediterranean female who is hypertensive
    4. 52-year-old African American male who has type 2 diabetes mellitus

14. Which antiepileptic drugs have an increased risk for psychological dependency? (Select all that apply.)
    1. Carbamazepine
    2. Ethosuximid
    3. Lacosamide
    4. Phenytoin
    5. Phenobarbital
    6. Valproic acid

15. Which drug for multiple sclerosis is specifically prescribed to improve walking?
    1. Beta-interferon
    2. Daclizumab
    3. Dalfampridine
    4. Tecfidera

Case Study

Steven Moor is a 60-year-old male mechanical engineer who was referred to the neurology clinic for an intermittent resting tremor of the left hand that has progressed to the right hand. He has a history of type 2 diabetes. On assessment the patient has normal cognition, and an intermittent mild resting tremor was observed in both hands, as well as some stop and go movements (cogwheel rigidity) and slow movements (bradykinesia) when asked to reach for a pencil and hand it from the right hand to the left. Gait, balance, and reflexes were normal. The diagnosis of Parkinson's disease was considered by the healthcare provider.

1. What drug categories are available for Mr. Moor?
2. Because of his age, which dopamine agonists will the healthcare provider likely prescribe first?
3. Which drugs will be added to his regimen as his disease progresses?
4. What special considerations should be made as a result of Mr. Moor's history of diabetes?
5. Which adverse effects would you discuss with Mr. and Mrs. Moor as the dosing of dopamine agonists increases?
6. Can you list some nursing interventions for Mr. Moor as his symptoms progress related to:
   a. Impaired physical mobility
   b. Self-care deficit
   c. Impaired verbal communication
7. Mrs. Moor asks you about new research or clinical trials she might look into for her husband. Can you advise where she might begin educating herself?

Drug Therapy for Mental Health

10

Learning Outcomes

1. List the names, actions, possible side effects, and adverse effects of drugs for anxiety and sleep.
2. Explain what to teach patients and families about drugs for anxiety and sleep.
3. List the names, actions, possible side effects, and adverse effects of typical and atypical antipsychotic drugs.
4. Explain what to teach patients and families about typical and atypical antipsychotic drugs.
5. List the names, actions, possible side effects, and adverse effects of antidepressant drugs and mood stabilizers.
6. Explain what to teach patients and families about antidepressant drugs and mood stabilizers.

Key Terms

anxiolytic (p. 188) A description for any drug that can reduce anxiety.

atypical antidepressants (p. 196) Drugs that affect the neurotransmitters dopamine, norepinephrine, and/or serotonin to help reduce depression.

atypical antipsychotics (p. 193) These drugs are usually a combination of dopamine and serotonin (5-HT) blockers used to reduce positive symptoms and improve negative symptoms of some types of psychosis without causing severe extrapyramidal effects.

benzodiazepines (BNZs) (p. 185) A class of sedating-hypnotic drugs that depresses the central nervous system (CNS) by binding to benzodiazepine receptors, which then act with gamma-aminobutyric acid (GABA) receptors to enhance GABA effects. The results of these effects can reduce anxiety, induce sleep, and relax skeletal muscles depending on drug dose and concentration.

benzodiazepine agonists (p. 185) Drugs that have a different chemical structure from the benzodiazepines (BNZs) but still bind strongly to BNZ receptors and act in the same ways as BNZs to initiate sleep and promote longer sleep with less risk for dependence.

dopamine system stabilizers (DSSs) (p. 194) Drugs that affect dopamine and serotonin receptors slightly differently than other atypical antipsychotics. They partially activate dopamine 2 and $5\text{-}HT_{1A}$ receptors and block $5\text{-}HT_{2A}$ receptors. As a result, they have fewer motor side effects and adverse effects.

hypnotics (p. 185) Drugs that have the main purpose of promoting sleep by changing signals in the CNS and reducing responses to stimulation. Same as sedative.

monoamine oxidase inhibitors (MAOIs) (p. 188) Drugs that inhibit the enzyme monoamine oxidase that is responsible for breaking down certain neurotransmitters, including dopamine, norepinephrine, and serotonin. Blocking this enzyme increases the available neurotransmitters and results in reduction of depressive symptoms.

mood stabilizers (p. 204) Drugs used in treating patients with bipolar illness. They have a variety of actions that help to reduce the symptoms associated with mania, as well as improve the symptoms of depression. Several drugs in this category are also used as antiseizure drugs.

nonphenothiazines (p. 190) Drugs that are chemically different from the phenothiazines but have similar actions, side effects, and adverse effects.

phenothiazines (p. 190) Drugs that block transmission of dopamine at the dopamine receptors and other neurotransmitters at acetylcholine and alpha-adrenergic receptors. These actions allow patients to receive the benefits of reducing positive symptoms but have significant side and adverse effects.

sedatives (p. 185) Drugs that have the main purpose of promoting sleep by changing signals in the CNS and reducing responses to stimulation. Same as hypnotic.

selective serotonin reuptake inhibitors (SSRIs) (p. 188) Drugs that act by inhibiting the cellular reuptake of serotonin, increasing the concentration of active serotonin that is available to bind to postsynaptic receptors and improve a patient's sense of well-being and reduce depression.

serotonin norepinephrine reuptake inhibitors (SNRIs) (p. 188) This class of drugs inhibits the reuptake of both serotonin and norepinephrine, increasing the concentration of both neurotransmitters available to postsynaptic receptors. These actions can improve a patient's sense of well-being and reduce depression.

tricyclic antidepressants (TCAs) (p. 196) Older drugs used to reduce depression. The precise action is not known, but they are thought to interfere with the reuptake of norepinephrine and serotonin.

typical antipsychotics (p. 190) These drugs are thought to block dopamine 2 (D2) receptors in the brain. The blocking of dopamine receptors can help treat the positive symptoms of psychosis such as with schizophrenia (e.g., hallucinations and delusions). Blocking dopamine can also result in a variety of side and adverse effects, including pseudoparkinsonism and other extrapyramidal symptoms.

DRUG THERAPY AND MENTAL ILLNESS

Before we talk about mental illness, we need to think about the concepts of mental health and mental illness. According to the World Health Organization, mental health is a state of well-being and includes the ability to cope with normal life stresses, to work productively, to be aware of personal abilities, and to contribute to the community. A person's mental health is influenced by a variety of factors including environment, culture, economic status, as well as biological factors.

Mental illness is a condition in which an individual experiences significant changes in the ability to think, as well as changes in behaviors and emotions. The person often has difficulty in coping with normal stressors, interacting with others, and otherwise functioning within his or her own cultural norms.

> **Bookmark This!**
>
> The National Alliance for Mental Illness is a wonderful resource for caregivers, patients, and families: https://www.nami.org/. You can access information that can be helpful to you and your agency. You may even have a local group that provides support groups for your patients and their families.

Rather than categorizing any individual as having mental health or mental illness, it is important to consider the mental health/illness continuum (Fig. 10.1). At any given time, we may be coping very well with normal stressors, but at a later time a significant life event can trigger emotional problems or concerns. In contrast, some people experience far greater emotional problems or concerns to common normal stressors and have marked distress or impairment. This more severe impairment is consistent with mental illness.

According to the National Institute of Mental Health, nearly 18% of the adult population experiences some degree of mental illness, and about 4% suffer from serious mental health problems. Fortunately, as we learn more about the brain, drug therapy is able to reduce some of the suffering associated with living with mental illness.

As you learned in Chapter 9, chemical neurotransmitters have important roles in transmitting messages between the brain and other areas of the nervous system. A number of neurotransmitters are involved in memory, mood, and affect. A basic understanding of what these neurotransmitters do will help you to understand how drugs impact your patients. The main neurotransmitters affected by psychiatric drugs include serotonin, dopamine, norepinephrine, as well as gamma-amino butyric acid (GABA), acetylcholine, and histamine. Table 10.1 provides a basic description of these neurotransmitters and how they typically affect mental health and mental illness. This chapter focuses on drugs that are related to sleep, anxiety, depression, and other mood disorders, as well as psychosis.

DRUGS FOR SLEEP AND ANXIETY

SEDATIVES-HYPNOTICS

Sleep is a state of rest for the mind and body in which conscious awareness is reduced partially or completely.

Mental Health - Mental Illness Continuum

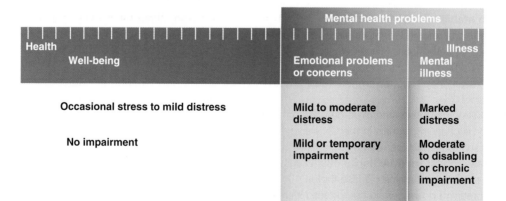

FIG. 10.1 The mental health and mental illness continuum. (From University of Michigan: Understanding U. In What is mental health? 2007. Retrieved from http://www.hr.umich.edu/mhealthy/programs/mental_emotional/understandingu/learn/mental_health.html.) https://hr.umich.edu/sites/default/files/resource_guide_final.pdf

Table 10.1	Examples of Neurotransmitters and Their Function in Mental Health	
NEUROTRANSMITTER	**AFFECTS**	**POSSIBLE CHANGES IN MENTAL HEALTH AND ILLNESS**
Norepinephrine	Sympathetic nervous system (fight-or-flight response) Alertness and arousal	Decreased in depression
Serotonin	Sleep, appetite, pain, mood	Decreased in depression
Dopamine	Learning, movement, motivation and drive, attention, pleasure and reward	Increased in schizophrenia
Gamma-Aminobutyric acid (GABA)	Inhibitory neurotransmitter Sleep, muscle tension, sedation	Decreased in anxiety
Acetylcholine	Parasympathetic nervous system (rest or repose)	Decreased in Alzheimer's disease

Sufficient amounts of sleep are needed daily to restore energy levels and promote optimum mental and physical functioning. Adults vary in how much sleep any one person needs daily, and whether it must occur over a 6- to 8-hour time or can occur over multiple shorter times throughout the day.

Most adults have experienced occasions when they either cannot get to sleep or do not remain asleep during an expected time period. This problem is known as *insomnia*. Many people have occasional insomnia, but others struggle with this problem almost daily. When sleep is insufficient for adequate rest, all aspects of functioning are affected. Areas of obvious impairment include learning, remembering, concentration, judgment, reaction time, coordination, and general social interactions. You probably have been around someone who is sleep-deprived or have had this problem on occasion yourself. People who suffer from sleep deprivation may feel irritable, impatient, or unable to concentrate.

People who have chronic insomnia usually require a more complex behavioral and pharmacologic approach to help the problem. For those who have intermittent problems with insomnia, drug therapy can be helpful. **Sedatives** are drugs that have the main purpose of promoting sleep by changing signals in the central nervous system (CNS) and reducing responses to stimulation. **Hypnotic** is another term for the same action as sedative. At times, people may also use or be prescribed one of many other drugs that have a side effect of sedation, such as antihistamines or muscle relaxants. This discussion is focused only on sedatives.

Action and Uses

The two main drug categories prescribed for sleep are the **benzodiazepines** (BNZs) and **benzodiazepine agonists** (BNZ agonists, also called *non-benzodiazepines*). BNZs are sedating-hypnotic drugs that depress the CNS by binding to BNZ receptors that act with gamma-aminobutyric acid (GABA) receptors to enhance GABA effects, resulting in sleep and muscle relaxation. Sleep begins in a shorter time after going to bed, and total sleep time is increased. Recall from Chapter 9 that GABA is an inhibitory neurotransmitter, so when GABA receptors are stimulated, CNS activity is reduced. Depending

on which type of BNZ receptor a specific BNZ binds to, other responses include reduced seizure activity and reduced anxiety. So depending on dose, drug concentration, and added chemicals, specific drugs from the BNZ class are approved for use as sedatives, but not to relieve anxiety. Others are approved to reduce anxiety but are not approved for sedation.

BNZ agonists have a different chemical structure from the BNZs but still bind strongly to BNZ receptors and act in the same ways. These drugs are more specific for sedative effects and have less muscle-relaxing or antiseizure actions. Table 10.2 lists the names, adult dosages, and nursing implications for the most common BNZ and BNZ agonists prescribed to induce sleep. Table 10.2 also lists the BNZs most commonly used to reduce anxiety. Check with a drug reference guide or a pharmacist for information about other sedative-hypnotic drugs.

Expected Side Effects and Adverse Reactions

Both classes of sedatives can cause mild daytime drowsiness and some memory loss. Both drug classes are metabolized by the liver and should not be used by anyone who has a liver disorder or impairment. The BNZs have a higher risk for addiction and dependency than do BNZ agonists. They also carry a black box warning for CNS depression. Overdoses are possible and serious. These drugs have a high risk for causing birth defects.

BNZ agonists have been found to induce physical activity during sleep for some people. Such activities include sleep-walking, sleep-eating, and even sleep-driving—all without the person's awareness or remembrance of the action!

Lifespan Considerations

Pregnancy

Pregnancy is an absolute contraindication for the BNZs because they have a high risk for causing birth defects. Although the chemical structure of the BNZ agonists is different, these drugs bind to the same receptors and have similar actions. As a result, they are not recommended during pregnancy.

Table 10.2   Examples of Common Drugs for Sleep and Anxiety

DRUGS FOR SLEEP

Benzodiazepines approved for sleep: drugs that induce and prolong sleep or reduce anxiety by binding to benzodiazepine receptors to enhance the inhibitory effects of GABA and make the CNS less responsive to stimuli

DRUG/ADULT DOSAGE RANGE	NURSING IMPLICATIONS
estazolam 0.5–2 mg orally at bedtime flurazepam 15–30 mg orally at bedtime temazepam (Restoril) 7.5–15 mg orally at bedtime. Maximum dose is 30 mg	• Teach patients not to take sedatives with alcohol or any other CNS depressant to avoid severe CNS depression, coma, or death. • Ask women if they are pregnant because these drugs have a high risk for causing birth defects. • Tell patients not to drive, operate dangerous equipment, or make serious decisions while under the influence of these drugs because impaired judgment and memory are possible. • Tell patients to only take the drug if they have sufficient sleep time available, to prevent confusion and other effects while awake.

Benzodiazepine agonists: drugs that have a different chemical structure from BNZs and act as agonists at the BNZ receptors to induce and prolong sleep or reduce anxiety by enhancing the inhibitory effects of GABA and making the CNS less responsive to stimuli

DRUG/ADULT DOSAGE RANGE	NURSING IMPLICATIONS
eszopiclone (Lunesta) 1–3 mg orally at bedtime lorazepam (Ativan) 2–4 mg orally at bedtime zaleplon (Sonata) 5–20 mg orally at bedtime zolpidem (Ambien) 5–10 mg orally at bedtime	• Suggest that patients have a family member or close friend with them when they first start taking the drug because incidences of sleep-walking, sleep-eating, and sleep-driving have occurred. • Tell patients not to drive, operate dangerous equipment, or make serious decisions while under the influence of these drugs because impaired judgment and memory are possible. • Teach patients that eszopiclone may cause a metallic taste in the mouth. • Teach patients not to take sedatives with alcohol or any other CNS depressant to avoid severe CNS depression, coma, or death. • Tell patients to only take the drug if they have sufficient sleep time available, to prevent confusion and other effects while awake. • Report agitation to the healthcare provider as this may be a side effect of eszopiclone. • Monitor patient's level of consciousness carefully because higher doses can lead to greater risk of daytime memory impairment and decreased alertness.

DRUGS FOR ANXIETY

Benzodiazepines approved for anxiety: drugs that induce and prolong sleep or reduce anxiety by binding to BNZ receptors to enhance the inhibitory effects of GABA and make the CNS less responsive to stimuli

DRUG/ADULT DOSAGE RANGE	NURSING IMPLICATIONS
alprazolam (Xanax) 0.25–0.5 mg orally two to three times per day; maximum of 4 mg/day in divided doses; often used PRN diazepam (Valium) 2–10 mg orally two to four times per day IM: 2–5 mg for moderate anxiety; for severe anxiety, 5–10 mg, may repeat in 3–4 hours if necessary lorazepam (Ativan) initially, 1–3 mg/day orally given in two to three divided doses; usual dose is 2–6 mg daily in divided dose; maximum dose is 10 mg/day	• These drugs may cause drowsiness, so advise patients to avoid driving, operating any heavy machinery, or making any important decisions while taking these drugs. • Provide patients with the call light and remind them to ask for help if getting out of bed because these drugs can cause dizziness and drowsiness. • Patients who are taking these drugs should be assessed using your agency fall risk protocols because these drugs increase the risk for falls. • These drugs are intended for short-term use because they can cause physical dependence. Notify the healthcare provider if you have a patient admitted to your facility who has been using these drugs for more than 2–4 weeks. • Teach patients who have been taking BNZs for more than 2–3 weeks not to stop them suddenly to avoid physical withdrawal symptoms. If they need to discontinue, they may require gradual and individualized taper. • BNZs should not be used in older adults because they are known to increase the risk for falls and mortality. • Assess your patients for any history of alcohol or other substance use disorder because they are at increased risk for BNZ dependence. • Teach the patient to avoid using nicotine products (such as cigarettes or chewing tobacco) or drinking caffeinated beverages (e.g., coffee, tea, and cola) because they can decrease the effect of anxiolytic drugs.

Table 10.2   Examples of Common Drugs for Sleep and Anxiety—cont'd

DRUGS FOR ANXIETY	
Miscellaneous benzodiazepine agonists approved for anxiety: newer drugs that reduce anxiety through a variety of actions that affect the serotonin and dopamine neurotransmitters	
DRUG/ADULT DOSAGE RANGE	**NURSING IMPLICATIONS**
buspirone (BuSpar) usual dose is 15–30 mg/day given in two to three divided doses; maximum dose is 60 mg/day	• Teach patients to avoid driving or operating machinery until they are certain that buspirone does not cause them to feel sleepy or dizzy. • Tell patients that the drug may be taken with or without food but should be taken the same way each time to avoid inconsistency in the dosage. • Remind patients to avoid eating grapefruit or drinking grapefruit juice while taking buspirone because it can increase the effect of the drug.

BNZ, Benzodiazepine; *GABA,* gamma-aminobutyric acid.

Drug Interactions

Caffeine reduces the effectiveness of sedative drugs from both classes. The BNZs interact with any drug that causes CNS depression and can make the depression deeper, which can lead to death. Other drugs known to increase the action of the BNZs and the BNZ agonists include cimetidine, fluoroquinolone antibiotics, some oral contraceptives, and many others. Be sure to consult a drug reference or a pharmacist to avoid possible drug interactions.

Top Tip for Safety

The drug flumazenil (Romazicon) is a BNZ receptor antagonist and is an antidote used to reverse an overdose of either a BNZ sedative or a BNZ agonist sedative. For adults, it is given intravenously with an initial dose of 0.2 mg. If there is no response after 45 seconds, the dose can be repeated. After that, it can be repeated every minute for a total of four doses.

❖ Nursing Implications and Patient Teaching

◆ *Assessment.* Ask the patient about all other drugs he or she takes, including over-the-counter drugs, to determine whether there are any other drugs that depress the CNS. Assess the patient's level of consciousness and ask whether he or she has a history of depression, confusion, falls, and pain. Also ask about common use of alcohol. These drugs should not be taken with any type of alcoholic beverage.

Ask whether a woman of childbearing age may be pregnant. These drugs should not be used during pregnancy.

◆ *Evaluation.* Usually, sedatives begin to take effect in 15 to 30 minutes. Check the patient (without waking him or her) at this time for drug effectiveness and for changes in respiratory rate and depth. If this is the patient's first time taking a sedative, recheck at least hourly for about 4 hours and assess for any unusual reactions, especially sleep-walking or other activity.

◆ *Patient and family teaching.* Tell the patient and family the following:
• Take these drugs for no longer than 2 to 3 weeks and only when needed, to avoid physical or psychological dependency.

• Only take a drug for sleep if you have at least 5 to 6 hours immediately available to sleep, to avoid excessive drowsiness when you are supposed to be awake.
• Do not drive, operate dangerous equipment, or make important decisions while under the influence of these drugs because they may alter your ability to reason clearly.
• Do not take a sedative with alcohol or any other drug that depresses the CNS, to prevent severe side effects, coma, and death.
• Do not take any other drug without the approval of your healthcare provider, to avoid dangerous interactions.
• When taking a BNZ agonist, be aware that drugs from this class can cause you to be physically active at night, even going for a drive, without your knowledge or memory of the event. It is best to have a family member or friend watch out for these effects when you first start taking the drug.
• Report any new or unusual side effects to your healthcare provider.
• Drinking excessive amounts of caffeinated beverages can reduce the effectiveness of the sedative.

ANTIANXIETY DRUGS

We can all identify with feelings of anxiety at certain times in our lives. We may describe it in terms of feelings of unease, worry, or apprehension. When we are anxious, we may experience both physical and behavioral symptoms. Perhaps our heart rate rises and we may feel a headache or breathe a little more rapidly. In some cases we may find ourselves being a little more irritable, pacing, or our muscles feel tense. These are all symptoms of anxiety. Anxiety is very common, particularly in times when you feel a little more stress. Anxiety can be mild, moderate, or severe depending on the situation. A person who has chronic or disabling anxiety may be experiencing an *anxiety disorder.* Advanced practice nurses or healthcare providers may diagnose the patient with the anxiety disorder. Examples include general anxiety disorder, social anxiety disorder, panic disorder, obsessive-compulsive disorder, or post-traumatic stress disorder. Although detailed discussion of each of these disorders is beyond the scope of this text, many can be well managed with a combination of nonpharmacologic strategies (including counseling) and pharmacologic therapy.

Major categories of antianxiety agents (also called **anxiolytics**) include BNZs, BNZ agonists, and certain antidepressants (**selective serotonin reuptake inhibitors [SSRIs]** and **serotonin norepinephrine reuptake inhibitors [SNRIs]**). In general, the choice of drug varies according to the need of the patient, including whether the anxiety is an acute or a chronic condition.

Action and Uses

The BNZ and BNZ agonist classes of drugs for sedation (discussed earlier) can also be used as anxiolytics. These drugs act with GABA receptors to enhance GABA effects leading to a reduction in anxiety and decrease in muscle tension. BNZs are recommended primarily for short-term use, such as during alcohol withdrawal before a patient has surgery. They generally should not be prescribed on a PRN basis because irregular use can actually cause an increase in anxiety with variation in blood drug levels. Long-term use of BNZs can result in physical dependence and withdrawal symptoms if the drug is stopped suddenly.

A newer drug from the BNZ agonist class, buspirone, reduces anxiety through a variety of actions that affect the serotonin and dopamine neurotransmitters. This results in a decrease of anxiety, muscle tension, sweating, and rapid heart rate. The onset of the anxiolytic effect is slower than with the BNZs and may take 1 to 2 weeks. Maximal effects of buspirone may take up to 3 to 6 weeks. This drug can reduce anxiety without the risk for physical dependence and the sedation that is often associated with BNZ drugs.

Certain drugs often considered antidepressants are commonly used to relieve symptoms of anxiety. A number of SSRIs and SNRIs are also effective in a variety of anxiety disorders. These drugs will be discussed in more detail in the section on mood disorders.

Expected Side Effects and Adverse Reactions

The expected side effects and adverse reactions are very similar to those presented in the section on sleep. BNZs and BNZ agonists may cause some drowsiness and memory loss when used for anxiety. Other side effects include dizziness, headache, or hypotension. Adverse effects include confusion, apnea, and seizures. Remember, the BNZs have a higher risk for addiction and dependency than the BNZ agonists.

Drug Interactions

Do not give BNZs to patients who are taking sodium oxybate (a drug specifically prescribed for narcolepsy, a sleep-wake disorder). This combination can result in serious respiratory depression, even coma. Avoid giving BNZs to patients who are taking opioids or any other drug that can result in CNS depression.

Do not give buspirone with **monoamine oxidase inhibitors (MAOIs)**, opioids, or drugs for tuberculosis. Drinking grapefruit juice can significantly increase the blood levels of buspirone, which increases the risk for adverse reactions.

❖ Nursing Implications and Patient Teaching

◆ *Assessment.* Check vital signs, including blood pressure, heart rate, and respiratory rate, before giving the drug. Patients with a history of lung, liver, or kidney problems may be more sensitive to the effects of the drug.

Assess the mental status of the patient before giving the drug. Is he or she oriented to time, place, and person? If not oriented, contact the healthcare provider before giving the drug.

Assess the patient for any history of alcohol or other chemical dependency because there is an increased risk for BNZ dependence. This is less likely with the BNZ agonists. Ask patients to describe their feelings of anxiety to determine effectiveness after you have given the drug.

🍂 Lifespan Considerations
Older Adults

BNZs are not recommended to treat insomnia, agitation, or delirium in patients 65 years or older, and they are avoided in all patients with cognitive impairment, dementia, or a history of falls or fractures.

◆ *Planning and implementation.* Many BNZs have a rapid onset and short duration of action, requiring multiple doses per day. They can be used very effectively for patients with acute anxiety or panic attacks. Buspirone, a BNZ agonist, and other antidepressants used for anxiety have much longer onsets of action and may take several weeks for the patient to notice an effect.

Monitor the patient for side effects of drowsiness or dizziness because these can cause an increased risk for falls. Report any changes in mental status, such as confusion or agitation, to the registered nurse (RN) or healthcare provider. If patients have respiratory depression after BNZ use, flumazenil (Romazicon), a BNZ receptor antagonist, can quickly reverse the effects.

For long-term mental health, nonpharmacologic therapies such as counseling, mindfulness training, yoga, or other interventions are essential. Provide the patient and their family with information for local resources including crisis lines, support groups, and websites such as the National Association of Mental Illness (NAMI).

◆ *Evaluation.* Ask the patient whether he or she has experienced any relief from anxiety. Explore how the drug affects the ability to focus, make decisions, and function. If the patient is still having symptoms, contact the healthcare provider for next steps. If the patient has been using BNZs for more than 2 to 4 weeks, suddenly stopping the drug will result in severe withdrawal symptoms including panic, vomiting, sweating, abdominal and muscle cramps, and even seizures. The risk for seizures is greatest during the first 24 to 72 hours after starting to withdraw the drug. Slow tapering of the drug dosage can decrease the risk of the withdrawal symptoms.

◆ *Patient and family teaching.* Tell the patient and family the following:

- Take this drug exactly as prescribed. Withdrawal symptoms can occur if the drug is used for longer than 2 to 4 weeks. If used for longer than that time, contact your healthcare provider because you will need to taper the dosage.
- Do not use this drug if you are pregnant or breast-feeding because the effects can be passed to the fetus or infant.
- Avoid drinking grapefruit juice while taking these drugs because it may cause an increase in effect.
- Avoid driving, operating hazardous machinery, or performing activities that require alertness until your response to the drug has been determined.
- Change positions slowly to minimize dizziness that may occur.
- Avoid drinking alcohol with these drugs to reduce the risk for severe sedation and respiratory depression.
- Do not use nicotine products (such as cigarettes or chewing tobacco) or drink caffeinated beverages (e.g., coffee, tea, and cola) because these can decrease the effect of anxiolytic drugs.

ANTIPSYCHOTICS

Before we discuss antipsychotic drugs, we need a good understanding about what we mean when we use the term *psychosis*. In general, psychosis involves a loss of contact with reality. How the psychosis occurs and the types of symptoms produced may vary. Psychosis may develop over a few hours or days (usually called *delirium*), or over months or years such as in schizophrenia.

It is important to distinguish between acute psychosis (as in delirium) and chronic psychosis (as in schizophrenia or bipolar illness) because you can see both conditions in your clinical practice. Delirium is considered an acute condition; patients experience a sudden change in their awareness and attention that is related to problems in the brain. Delirium can occur in a patient who has previously been alert and oriented but has come in for surgery or taken a new drug. It can also occur in a patient who has been diagnosed with dementia who suddenly has a change in symptoms after being moved from his or her home into a new setting. Family may notice before you do as a nurse that the patient is confused or "different." The previously calm patient may be trying to pull out tubes or get out of bed without help. The patient is suddenly agitated and confused, or may be unable to focus or may seem frightened. The patient's awareness can change over the course of the

day—sometimes oriented, sometimes confused. He or she often may have more symptoms at night. We may think that because it is often temporary that it is not a big problem. Unfortunately, delirium can increase patient length of stay, mortality, and the risk for falls.

Patients with chronic mental illnesses such as schizophrenia have symptoms that increase over a long period. In fact, it may be months or even years before the patient is accurately diagnosed. Families and friends may notice changes in behavior but may not be fully aware of the problems until the person has delusions and hallucinations. Many of these symptoms can be effectively managed with antipsychotic drugs and other therapies. This chapter predominantly reviews drugs that are used in patients with mental illness. Drugs that can be used in delirium may be mentioned, but the focus is on drugs for chronic mental illnesses.

In the past, antipsychotic drugs were used in patients with dementia. And while patients with dementia may exhibit confusion or agitation, use of antipsychotic drugs in these patients can cause an increased risk for stroke, a greater rate of *cognitive impairment* (decline in ability to think and remember), and even mortality.

Symptoms of psychosis are classified as *positive* symptoms and *negative* symptoms (Box 10.1). This can be a bit confusing because we often think of positive as "good" and negative as "bad." In mental health, the positive symptoms of psychosis are those that *add* to the person's normal behaviors. Positive symptoms include hallucinations (e.g., seeing things, hearing voices), delusions (e.g., ideas that they have special powers or are famous people), disorganized thoughts or speech (e.g., jumbled ideas or words that do not make sense to the listener). These are the conditions that we may think about right away when we hear the term *psychotic*. Negative symptoms are slightly different. These are the symptoms that *subtract* from the person's normal behavior. For example, negative symptoms include poor hygiene, difficulty with social relationships, lack of interest in activities, or lack of motivation.

Box 10.1	Examples of Positive and Negative Symptoms Associated With Schizophrenia
POSITIVE SYMPTOMS (SOMETHING THAT IS PRESENT THAT IS NOT NORMALLY PRESENT)	**NEGATIVE SYMPTOMS (SOMETHING THAT IS ABSENT THAT IS USUALLY PRESENT)**
Hallucinations (visual or auditory)	Lack of motivation
Delusions (holds a belief without any evidence)	Flat affect (decreased facial expression or tones with emotion)
Disordered thinking (unusual ways of thinking, speaking)	Decrease in personal hygiene
Agitation or other bizarre behavior	Lack of social interest

Drugs that treat symptoms of psychosis are grouped into two main categories: typical antipsychotics and atypical antipsychotics. These drugs are presented in reference for their use in the psychosis associated with schizophrenia.

TYPICAL ANTIPSYCHOTIC DRUGS

Action and Uses

The **typical antipsychotics** are the first generation of this drug type. In general, these drugs treat the *positive* symptoms of psychosis. They appear to block dopamine 2 (D2) receptors in the brain. Blocking of dopamine receptors helps treat the positive symptoms of psychosis such as hallucinations and delusions. They do not affect the negative symptoms.

Schizophrenia is considered to be a disease of over-stimulation of dopamine receptors from the presence of too much dopamine (remember, Parkinson's disease is too little dopamine). The typical antipsychotic blocks dopamine; thus it can treat the positive symptoms but also creates a series of side and adverse effects including pseudoparkinsonism and other extrapyramidal symptoms (EPSs). Normally the *extrapyramidal system,* the part of the nervous system involved in movement, helps ensure smooth or flowing movements of the body. EPSs, then, are associated with disordered movements.

The two main categories of typical antipsychotics are the phenothiazines and the nonphenothiazines. **Phenothiazines** block transmission of dopamine at the dopamine receptors. They also block acetylcholine and alpha-adrenergic receptors. By blocking these receptors, the patients receive the benefits of reducing positive symptoms but have risks for significant side and adverse effects. The **nonphenothiazines** have a similar action but are chemically different from the phenothiazines. Side effects and adverse effects are basically the same. Which drug type is prescribed long term depends on the patient's responses. Table 10.3 lists the names, adult dosages, and nursing implications for the most common typical antipsychotic drugs. Check a drug reference or with a pharmacist for information about other typical antipsychotics.

Expected Side Effects and Adverse Reactions

Expected side effects and adverse reactions of typical antipsychotics are primarily related to the blocking of key neurotransmitters. Examples of side effects include headache, drowsiness, nausea, constipation, and dry mouth.

The main adverse effects are described as EPSs. These symptoms are related to the decrease in dopamine; many are severe and some may be irreversible, so it is important to recognize them very early in treatment. They can occur in as many as 10% of patients who take these drugs. The main EPSs are pseudoparkinsonism, acute dystonia, akathisia, and tardive dyskinesia. Fig. 10.2 describes these symptoms.

Onset of EPSs varies, and treatment focuses on symptom management and altering the cause. *Acute dystonia* usually occurs within 1 to 4 days of the start of treatments. It is more common in younger men and patients who are taking large doses. It may be managed with anticholinergic drugs and BNZs. *Akathisia* usually

---

Table 10.3 **Examples of Common Antipsychotic Drugs**

Typical antipsychotics: These drugs are thought to block D2 receptors in the brain. The blocking of dopamine receptors can help treat the positive symptoms of psychosis such as with schizophrenia (e.g., hallucinations and delusions). Blocking dopamine can also result in a variety of side effects and adverse reactions including pseudoparkinsonism and other extrapyramidal symptoms (EPSs).

Phenothiazines: These drugs block transmission of dopamine at the dopamine receptors and other neurotransmitters at acetylcholine and alpha-adrenergic receptors.

DRUG/ADULT DOSAGE RANGE	NURSING IMPLICATIONS

chlorpromazine (Thorazine): for mild-to-moderate symptoms, 10 mg three to four times per day, or 25 mg two to three times per day orally, then adjusted to patients symptoms; IM: 25–50 mg every 4–6 hours. Higher doses may be required for severe symptoms.
fluphenazine (Prolixin)
  Oral dosage: 2.5–10 mg/day in divided doses; maximum dosage is 40 mg/day
  IM or subcutaneous dosage: the usual initial dose 12.5–25 mg IM or subcutaneously; maximum dosage is 100 mg as a depot injection; a single dose can last 3–6 weeks
	• Recognize the signs of EPSs because many are severe and some may be irreversible. They can occur in as many as 10% of patients who take these drugs.
	• Teach patients to avoid becoming dehydrated, participating in strenuous exercise, or extremes in temperature because these drugs may affect the body's ability to regulate core body temperature.
	• Report sudden increases in blood pressure; increase in temperature and confusion may indicate signs of neuroleptic malignant syndrome.
	• Know the specific onset of actions, peak effects, and durations when you are giving these drugs. Some injectable drugs are used for rapid treatment of symptoms, whereas others are designed for long-term management.
	• Monitor changes in mental status with the healthcare team to determine the effectiveness of these drugs.
	• Teach the patient to avoid activities that require alertness particularly when first using the drug. This usually improves over time.

Table 10.3   Examples of Common Antipsychotic Drugs—cont'd

Nonphenothiazines: These drugs have similar actions to the phenothiazines but are chemically different from the phenothiazines. Side effects and adverse effects are similar. Selection of drug is dependent on patient responses.

DRUG/ADULT DOSAGE RANGE	NURSING IMPLICATIONS
haloperidol (Haldol) 0.5–5 mg orally two to three times per day depending on symptoms IM: doses of up to 2–10 mg IM every 4–8 hours. May also be given as a depot injection.	• Recognize the signs of EPSs because many are severe and some may be irreversible. They can occur in as many as 10% of patients who take these drugs. • Teach patients to avoid becoming dehydrated, participating in strenuous exercise, or extremes in temperature because these drugs may affect the body's ability to regulate core body temperature. • Report sudden increases in blood pressure; increase in temperature and confusion may indicate signs of neuroleptic malignant syndrome. • Know the specific onset of actions, peak effects, and durations when you are giving these drugs. Some injectable drugs are used for rapid treatment of symptoms, whereas others are designed for long-term management. • Monitor changes in mental status with the healthcare team to determine the effectiveness of these drugs. • Teach the patient to avoid activities that require alertness particularly when first using the drug.

Atypical antipsychotics: The majority of these drugs are a combination of dopamine and serotonin (5-HT) blockers. These drugs can reduce positive symptoms and improve negative symptoms without the severe extrapyramidal effects characteristic of the typical antipsychotics.

DRUG/ADULT DOSAGE RANGE	NURSING IMPLICATIONS

risperidone (Risperdal)
   Initially 0.5–2 mg orally as a single or divided dose; Usual dosage is 4–16 mg/day orally
   IM as depot drug 25–50 mg every 2 weeks
ziprasidone (Geodon)
   Initially 20 mg orally twice daily with food. Maximum of 80 mg orally twice daily with food.
   IM: 10–20 mg per dose; do not give IM dosage for more than 3 consecutive days. Maximum dose is 40 mg daily
quetiapine (Seroquel) Initially 25 mg by mouth twice daily. May be increased to 300–400 mg in two to three divided doses daily. Maximum dose is 800 mg daily. Extended release form (Seroquel XR): Initially at 300 mg once daily in the evening. Maximum dose is 800 mg once daily.
	• Watch for signs and symptoms of extrapyramidal effects. This is less common with atypical antipsychotics but must be monitored.
	• Teach patient about good nutrition and physical activity because these drugs can cause weight gain.
	• Monitor blood sugars for patients with diabetes or those at risk for diabetes because these drugs can increase blood sugar.
	• Monitor vital signs because sudden changes in blood pressure or increase in temperature can indicate dangerous adverse effects.
	• Remind patients that they should not drink alcohol or take any sedating drugs without talking to the healthcare provider. These drugs can cause drowsiness or insomnia.
	• Encourage patients to keep a diet high in fiber to avoid constipation common with atypical antipsychotics.
	• For patients who have difficulty adhering to oral drug schedules, IM depot drugs may allow less frequent dosing up to 2 weeks or even longer.
	• Work with healthcare team members to maintain a safe patient environment while they are experiencing symptoms of their psychosis.
	• Teach patients to avoid extremes in temperature because these drugs can affect the body's ability to adjust to changes in temperature.

Dopamine system stabilizers: These drugs affect dopamine and serotonin receptors slightly differently than other atypical antipsychotics. They are partial D2 agonists and partial 5-HT_{1A} agonists, 5-HT_{2A} antagonists. As a result, they have fewer motor side and adverse effects.

DRUG/ADULT DOSAGE RANGE	NURSING IMPLICATIONS
aripiprazole (Abilify) 10–30 mg/day by mouth daily. IM: 30 mg/day for an immediate-release injection; 400 mg/month extended-release	• Teach patients that oral doses can be given with or without food. • Read drug information carefully when giving aripiprazole. In general the deltoid muscle can be used for IM doses ≤400 mg. Doses greater than 600 mg must be given in the gluteal muscles. Depending on the patient and dose, these drugs can be given every 6 weeks to 2 months. • See also nursing implications for atypical antipsychotics.

D2, Dopamine 2; *EPS,* extrapyramidal symptom.

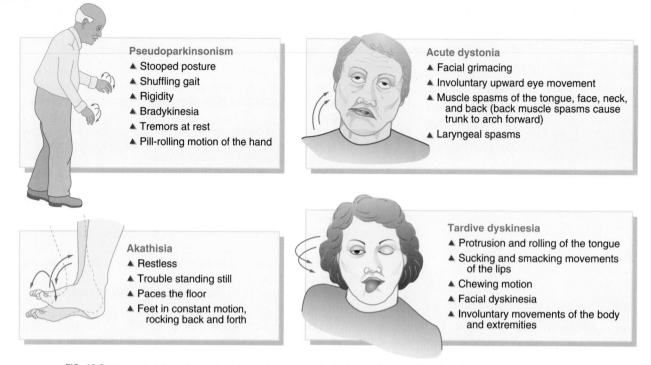

Pseudoparkinsonism
▲ Stooped posture
▲ Shuffling gait
▲ Rigidity
▲ Bradykinesia
▲ Tremors at rest
▲ Pill-rolling motion of the hand

Acute dystonia
▲ Facial grimacing
▲ Involuntary upward eye movement
▲ Muscle spasms of the tongue, face, neck, and back (back muscle spasms cause trunk to arch forward)
▲ Laryngeal spasms

Akathisia
▲ Restless
▲ Trouble standing still
▲ Paces the floor
▲ Feet in constant motion, rocking back and forth

Tardive dyskinesia
▲ Protrusion and rolling of the tongue
▲ Sucking and smacking movements of the lips
▲ Chewing motion
▲ Facial dyskinesia
▲ Involuntary movements of the body and extremities

FIG. 10.2 Characteristics of pseudoparkinsonism, acute dystonia, akathisia, and tardive dyskinesia. (From McCuistion LE, Yeager J, Winton M: *Pharmacology*, ed 9, St. Louis, 2017, Saunders.)

develops several days to several weeks into therapy. Management may include decreasing drug dosage and/or adding a BNZ or beta blocker. *Pseudoparkinsonism* usually occurs 1 to 2 weeks after beginning antipsychotic therapy. It is more common in women and older adults. Anticholinergics, antihistamines, and BNZs may be used to manage symptoms.

Unlike the earlier onset of other EPSs, *tardive dyskinesia* can occur during long-term therapy or after stopping therapy. It occurs more frequently in older women. The disorder is characterized by involuntary movements of the tongue, jaw, mouth, or face. The patient's lips may be smacking, cheeks puffing, or other bizarre movements of the arms and shoulders. It is more likely to occur in patients with bipolar disorder than in patients with schizophrenia.

These drugs may affect the body's ability to regulate core body temperature. The risk increases if patients become dehydrated, participate in strenuous exercise, or are in very hot environments. In rare cases, patients may experience *hypothermia*. This usually occurs in the presence of other risk factors such as hypothyroidism, brain injury, or cold environmental temperature.

Neuroleptic malignant syndrome (NMS) is a potentially fatal adverse effect. NMS is characterized by *hyperpyrexia* (an abnormally high body temperature above 104°F), confusion, changes in blood pressure (hypotension to hypertension), and EPSs, and can lead to coma and death. It occurs more often in men than women. Box 10.2 lists the common signs and symptoms associated with NMS.

Box 10.2 Signs and Symptoms of Neuroleptic Malignant Syndrome

- Sudden elevated temperature
- Increased white blood cell count
- Muscle rigidity
- Unstable blood pressure
- Elevated serum creatine kinase
- Hyperkalemia

Drug Interactions

Typical antipsychotic drugs interact with a wide range of drugs including acetaminophen, diuretics such as furosemide or hydrochlorothiazide, certain calcium channel blockers, and several antidiabetic agents. Make sure to consult a pharmacist or other healthcare provider if you have any questions.

❖ **Nursing Implications and Patient Teaching**

◆ *Assessment.* Determine baseline level of consciousness. Is the patient agitated? Hallucinating? If you are in a behavioral health setting, you may be working with the RN who conducts a formal mental status exam. Components of the mental status exam include factors such as the patient's appearance, behavior, mood, affect, and thought processes. This assessment is very helpful in determining a baseline to evaluate the effects of the drugs.

◆ *Planning and implementation.* Maintaining patient safety is vitally important in caring for patients who are experiencing psychosis. Whether the patient has acute delirium or chronic mental illness, the patient is at risk for injury to self or to others. Keeping the patient, caregivers, and others free from injury is a priority. As an LPN, you will work with other members of the healthcare team to keep the *milieu* (social environment or surroundings) safe and calm. Techniques for working with patients with psychosis is beyond the scope of this textbook, so make sure to consult professional resources in mental health, such as experienced mental health nurses, mental health nursing textbooks, or continuing education.

> ### 🔖 Bookmark This!
>
> The National Institute of Mental Health is a great resource for nurses, patients, and families to learn more about mental health disorders: https://www.nimh.nih.gov. You can print or order free brochures, booklets, posters, and fact sheets for your agency.

Monitor vital signs carefully for any significant changes. Increase in temperature or severe changes in blood pressure can indicate the severe adverse effect NMS.

Recognize the classic characteristics of EPSs (see Fig. 10.2). Early recognition is essential in reducing the risk for long-term consequences. Any changes in motor function such as in muscle tone, gait, or fine motor movement can be warning signs of EPSs, especially tardive dyskinesia. Report these symptoms to the RN or healthcare provider immediately. Treatment often requires discontinuing the drug. In some cases, these problems are irreversible.

> ### 🔼 Top Tip for Safety
>
> Recognize the classic characteristics of EPSs (see Fig. 10.2). Early recognition is essential in reducing the risk for long-term consequences.

Know the specific onset of actions, peak effects, and durations when you are giving these drugs. Some oral injectable drugs are used for rapid treatment of symptoms, whereas others are designed for long-term management. For example, an oral form of haloperidol may take 4 to 6 hours for peak effects, whereas an oral form of chlorpromazine may take 6 weeks to 6 months for peak effects. A good understanding of these facts will help you to plan your care and recognize whether the drug is effective.

◆ *Evaluation.* Has the patient had any changes in mental status after beginning this drug? Remember, these drugs affect only positive symptoms, so you may see a decrease in agitation, hallucinations, and delusions. Also note whether the patient has had any side effects from these drugs. For improvement in negative symptoms, the patient will need either addition of or substitution with atypical antipsychotics. In general typical antipsychotics are not used alone for an extensive period because of the possibility of EPSs.

◆ *Patient and family teaching.* Tell the patient and family the following:

- Continue to take the drugs as prescribed even if you do not start feeling better right away. It may take several weeks before significant changes occur. Suddenly stopping these drugs can result in nausea, dizziness, and tremors.
- Do not drink alcohol or use any sedatives while taking these drugs, to prevent deep sedation and other dangerous side effects.
- Avoid activities that require alertness, particularly when first using the drug because these drugs can reduce clear thinking and induce drowsiness. This usually improves over time.
- These drugs may affect your body's ability to adjust to changes in temperature. Avoid extremes of temperature, as well as situations that can affect your temperature, such as dehydration or strenuous exercise.
- If you or your family member has difficulty remembering to take these drugs, check with your healthcare provider about long-acting injectable drugs.
- These drugs may cause dryness of your mouth. You can try chewing sugarless gum, sucking on sugarless candy, or drinking sips of ice or water to reduce this sensation.
- If you develop unusual muscle spasms or other types of movement problems, contact your healthcare provider right away.
- Avoid getting liquid forms of these drugs on your skin because they can cause irritation.
- You can take many of these drugs with food to avoid GI upset.
- Avoid using any herbal or other over-the-counter drugs without first checking with your healthcare provider because these can interact with your prescription drugs.
- Wear a medical alert bracelet or carry a drug ID card to identify that you are taking these drugs.

ATYPICAL ANTIPSYCHOTIC DRUGS

Action and Uses

Atypical antipsychotics are also known as *second-generation antipsychotics*. Whereas typical antipsychotics block the dopamine type 2 receptors in the brain, atypical antipsychotic drugs work in a variety of ways. Many block dopamine 2 or other subtypes of dopamine receptor, as well as certain subtypes of serotonin. They are used primarily for schizophrenia but also can be used for bipolar illnesses and schizoaffective disorder.

The atypical antipsychotics have a lower risk for EPSs and have the benefit of treating the negative symptoms of psychosis, in addition to the positive symptoms (see Box 10.1) common in schizophrenia and some other mental illnesses such as bipolar disorder. Atypical antipsychotics are more commonly used for long-term management of chronic mental illnesses associated with psychosis. They are not recommended for any patient with psychosis from dementia.

The newest category is called **dopamine system stabilizers (DSSs)**. DSSs affect dopamine and serotonin receptors slightly differently than other atypical antipsychotics. They are partial dopamine 2 agonists and partial 5-HT1A agonists, 5-HT2A antagonists. As a result they have even fewer motor side effects and adverse reactions. The DSSs can be used in schizophrenia and bipolar disorders. These drugs can also be used to relieve symptoms in some autistic disorders and in Tourette's syndrome. Table 10.3 lists the names, adult dosages, and nursing implications for the most common atypical antipsychotic drugs. Check a drug reference or with a pharmacist for information about other atypical antipsychotics.

> **Memory Jogger**
>
> Atypical antipsychotics are also known as second-generation antipsychotics.

Expected Side Effects and Adverse Reactions

The most common side effects of atypical antipsychotics are both insomnia and drowsiness. Although many drugs have sexual side effects, these are less common than with the typical side effects. Other common side effects include dizziness, orthostatic hypotension, constipation, and dry mouth.

A major advantage of atypical antipsychotics is significantly lower rates of EPSs than the typical antipsychotics. This means a reduced risk for adverse effects such as acute dystonia, akathisia, tardive dyskinesia, and pseudoparkinsonism. Although the risk is not totally eliminated, the reduced risk makes atypical antipsychotic drugs preferable to the typical antipsychotics in most situations.

Weight gain is common with many of the atypical antipsychotics. Beyond the weight gain, *hypertriglyceridemia* (increase in blood triglycerides) and a risk for *insulin resistance* and diabetes type 2 are associated with these drugs. These changes can significantly increase the risk for cardiovascular problems, even death. Use caution in starting these drugs for patients with preexisting hypertension, heart or cerebrovascular diseases, heart failure, or any dysrhythmias.

Atypical antipsychotic drugs can also affect the ECG, prolonging the *QT interval* (part of the cardiac cycle). This is very important for any patients with heart disease because it can result in severe cardiac dysrhythmias.

One drug, clozapine, is associated with *agranulocytosis* (decreased white blood cell count). This can result in a significantly increased risk for infection, even death. As a result, clozapine is usually reserved for patients

Box 10.3	Signs and Symptoms of Serotonin Syndrome

- Confusion
- Agitation
- Restlessness
- Stomach disturbances/diarrhea
- Sweating
- Extremely high blood pressure
- Seizures
- Dilated pupils
- Tremors

who do not experience symptom relief from other antipsychotics.

Drug Interactions

Atypical antipsychotics interact with a wide range of drugs. Drugs that decrease dopamine, such as metoclopramide or any typical antipsychotics, increase the risk for EPSs. Use of these drugs with any SSRI or an SNRI can increase the risk for serotonin syndrome (Box 10.3).

Alcohol or other CNS depressants increase the sedating and nervous system side effects of these drugs. In addition, these drugs affect specific enzymes in the liver that metabolize drugs. Make sure to check your drug references and/or contact your agency pharmacist or the patient's healthcare provider for other interactions with additional drugs the patient takes.

❖ Nursing Implications and Patient Teaching

◆ *Assessment.* It is important to determine baseline level of consciousness for any patient prescribed an antipsychotic drug. Work with the RN and other healthcare team members to determine the patient's mental status. This includes assessment of appearance, behavior, mood, affect, and thought processes. A good baseline assessment is essential to determining whether the drugs are effective.

Determining baselines for vital signs, weight, and blood glucose is very important for patients beginning therapy with atypical antipsychotic drugs. These data are useful in looking for side or adverse effects the patient may experience.

Thorough assessment for any history of hypertension, diabetes, cardiovascular or cerebral vascular diseases, or dysrhythmia is needed. Also note if the patient is taking any prescriptions, over-the-counter drugs, or herbal drugs.

◆ *Planning and implementation.* As addressed above with typical antipsychotics, maintaining patient safety is very important. Make sure to work with members of the healthcare team to keep the patient, caregivers, and others free from injury.

Monitor the patient carefully for side effects and adverse effects. Sudden changes in vital signs such as drop in blood pressure or severe and sudden increase in temperature can be indicators of complications of drug therapy. For patients who are taking clozapine, monitor white blood cell counts. Fewer white blood cells can indicate a life-threatening complication of agranulocytosis. This significantly affects the patient's ability to fight infection.

Risk for EPSs is much lower with use of atypical antipsychotics than with the typical antipsychotics, but it can still occur. It is important to recognize any change in fine motor movement, gait, or muscle tone as potential adverse effects. Report these to the healthcare provider immediately.

Monitor the patient's weight on a regular basis because weight gain is a very common side effect of drug therapy. You may need to consult your agency dietician or RN to help patients find strategies for managing their weight.

Atypical antipsychotics can cause dry mouth, so make sure the patient has good oral hygiene. Sugar-free gums or candies, ice chips, or sips of water may be helpful in moistening the mouth. Remind the patient to avoid extremes of cold or heat, because the drug may affect the area of the brain responsible for temperature regulation.

◆ *Evaluation.* Determine whether the patient has had any changes in mental status since beginning this drug. Be sure of the individual drug's onset of action. Many of these drugs can take several weeks before they have significant impact on patient behaviors. Also remember that these drugs can impact both positive and negative symptoms. Assess whether the patient has an increase in the ability to interact with others, interest in activities and hygiene, as well as whether there has been a reduction in the positive symptoms of hallucinations and delusions.

◆ *Patient and family teaching.* Tell the patient and family the following:

- Continue to take the drugs as prescribed even if you do not start feeling better right away. It may take several weeks before significant changes occur. Suddenly stopping these drugs can result in nausea, dizziness, and tremors.
- Do not drink alcohol or use any sedatives while using these drugs, to avoid oversedation and other dangerous nervous system side effects.
- Avoid activities that require alertness, particularly when first using the drug, because the drug increases drowsiness and interferes with clear thinking. This usually improves over time.
- These drugs may affect your body's ability to adjust to changes in temperature. Avoid temperature extremes and situations that can affect your temperature such as dehydration or strenuous exercise.
- If you (or your family member) has difficulty remembering to take these drugs, check with your healthcare provider about long-acting injectable drugs.
- These drugs may cause dryness of your mouth. You can try chewing sugarless gum, sucking on sugarless

candy, or drinking sips of ice or water to reduce this problem.
- If you have unusual muscle spasms or other types of movement problems, contact your healthcare provider right away.
- You can take many of these drugs with food to avoid GI upset.
- Avoid using any herbal or other over-the-counter drugs without checking with your healthcare provider first because these can interact with your prescription drugs.
- Wear a medical alert bracelet or carry a drug ID card to identify that you are taking these drugs.

ANTIDEPRESSANTS AND MOOD STABILIZERS

ANTIDEPRESSANTS

Depression, whether mild or so severe that it interferes with activities of daily living (ADLs), has been recognized for centuries. Most people have days when they feel "down" or "blue." Sometimes depressive symptoms are triggered by difficult situations such as the loss of a loved one or by experiencing a sudden illness, which are normal responses to these life-changing events. However, intense and prolonged inability to interact with others, go to work, and keep up with the ADLs, as well as loss of interest in pleasurable activities, represent more significant depression (Box 10.4 lists common depressive symptoms). Depressive symptoms can go on for weeks, even months. Risk factors for depression include a family history of depression, substance abuse, history of abuse, certain drugs, or chronic illnesses. Fig. 10.3 shows some examples of people with depression.

Box 10.4	Symptoms of Depression

- Abrupt changes in eating habits
- Chronic fatigue; being slowed down
- Decreased ability to perform normal daily tasks
- Decreased appetite and/or weight loss, or overeating and weight gain
- Difficulty concentrating, remembering, or making decisions
- Feelings of hopelessness or pessimism
- Inability to experience pleasure in hobbies and activities that were once enjoyed
- Insomnia, early morning awakening, or oversleeping
- Irritability
- Numb or empty feeling, or absence of any feelings at all
- Persistent feelings of worthlessness, guilt, helplessness, or sadness
- Persistent physical symptoms that do not respond to treatment (e.g., headaches, digestive disorders, chronic pain)
- Recurrent thoughts of death or suicide
- Restlessness

From Workman M, LaCharity L: *Understanding pharmacology: Essentials for medication safety*, ed 2, St. Louis, 2016, WB Saunders, VitalBook file, box 27-1.

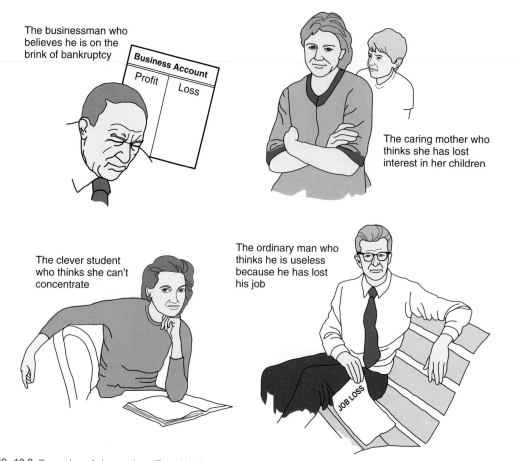

The businessman who believes he is on the brink of bankruptcy

Business Account
Profit   Loss

The caring mother who thinks she has lost interest in her children

The clever student who thinks she can't concentrate

The ordinary man who thinks he is useless because he has lost his job

JOB LOSS

FIG. 10.3 Examples of depression. (From Workman ML, LaCharity L: *Understanding pharmacology*, ed 2, St. Louis, 2017, Elsevier.)

There are several different categories of depression, including *dysthymic disorder* (a mild-to-moderate form of depression that lasts up to 2 years), major depressive disorder, and *bipolar disorder* (includes bipolar I and bipolar II). These are often referred to as *mood disorders*. Many types of therapy have been explored, but only in the last 50 years have drugs been discovered that significantly help reduce depressive symptoms.

Most patients require several trials of different drugs or drug combinations to determine which drug is most effective to manage their symptoms. This can be a time-consuming process for patients because most antidepressants take several weeks to take effect. Good communication between the patient and the healthcare provider is important through the process of finding the right drug with the fewest side effects.

MAOIs were the first drugs successfully used to treat depression. The **tricyclic antidepressants (TCAs)** became available in the 1960s. SSRIs were introduced in the 1970s, then SNRIs. One other category described as **atypical antidepressants** work slightly differently than the other antidepressants but do affect the neurotransmitters dopamine, norepinephrine, and/or serotonin.

Screen all patients who are taking antidepressants for thoughts of suicide or self-harm (known as suicide ideation). Observe your patients for any worsening of symptoms, suicidal thoughts, or unusual changes in behavior, particularly within the first few months of starting therapy or when dosage changes.

Bookmark This!

The Centers for Disease Control and Prevention has extensive resources for healthcare professionals on suicide: https://www.cdc.gov/violenceprevention/suicide/index.html. You can find risk factors, prevention strategies, and links to other helpful websites. This is a great resource for all nurses.

Antidepressants should not be stopped suddenly because this may cause withdrawal symptoms or a relapse of depressive symptoms. These drugs should be tapered or discontinued under the direction of the healthcare provider.

SELECTIVE SEROTONIN REUPTAKE INHIBITORS

Action and Uses

SSRIs act by inhibiting the reuptake of the neurotransmitter serotonin, increasing the concentration of serotonin that is available to bind to postsynaptic receptors (Fig. 10.4). These drugs are similar to TCAs but are prescribed more frequently because they are much safer and better tolerated. They can be used in a variety of conditions

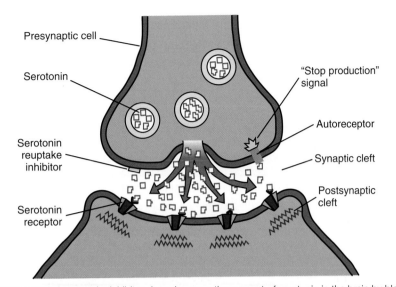

FIG. 10.4 Selective serotonin reuptake inhibitor drugs increase the amount of serotonin in the brain by blocking reuptake of neurotransmitters by neurons. (From Workman ML, LaCharity L: *Understanding pharmacology*, ed 2, St. Louis, 2017, Elsevier.)

including depression, premenstrual dysphoric disorder, posttraumatic stress disorder, obsessive-compulsive disorder, and general anxiety disorder. Table 10.4 lists the names, adult dosages, and nursing implications for the most common SSRIs. Check a drug reference or with a pharmacist for information about other drugs in this category.

> **Memory Jogger**
>
> The main categories of antidepressants are:
> - Selective Serotonin Reuptake Inhibitors (SSRIs)
> - Serotonin Norepinephrine Reuptake Inhibitors (SNRIs)
> - Tricyclic Antidepressants (TCAs)
> - Monoamine Oxidase Inhibitors (MAOIs)
> - Atypical Antidepressants

Expected Side Effects and Adverse Reactions

Expected side effects of SSRIs include nausea (especially during the first 2 weeks), drowsiness, insomnia, dry mouth, decreased appetite, increased sweating, and constipation. Sexual side effects are common in men and women. These range from decreased sex drive to decreased ability to orgasm and erectile dysfunction.

Adverse effects include increased risk for suicide, particularly in the first few months of therapy. This risk is slightly higher in young adults and children. In most cases the benefit of taking the SSRI to reduce symptoms of depression is greater than the risk for suicide. It is critically important for the healthcare provider to talk with the patient and his or her family about this risk in order to prevent this adverse effect.

Other adverse effects include bleeding, hyponatremia (low sodium level), and bone fracture, particularly in patients with osteoporosis. Skin reactions are rare but can be severe. These drugs can also cause changes in the electrical conduction system of the heart.

SSRIs should be avoided in pregnancy because the drugs affect the fetus. In fact, infants can experience neonatal abstinence syndrome, a condition associated with physical symptoms of drug withdrawal.

Suddenly stopping an SSRI can cause a flulike syndrome. Tapering the drug dosage can decrease the risk for these symptoms.

Drug Interactions

Any drug that affects serotonin can interact with SSRIs. This includes a variety of other antidepressants including MAOIs, SNRIs, and other SSRIs. Too much serotonin can lead to the adverse effect known as serotonin syndrome (see Box 10.3). Serotonin syndrome is a life-threatening adverse effect, so it must be avoided. Using the herbal drug St. John's wort (commonly used to treat mild-to-moderate depression) can significantly increase risk for serotonin syndrome.

Other potential drug interactions with SSRIs include drugs that can affect clotting such as anticoagulants, antiplatelet drugs, and NSAIDs. Caution should be used in giving SSRIs to patients with certain cardiac dysrhythmias.

❖ Nursing Implications and Patient Teaching

◆ *Assessment.* A thorough assessment of mental health status is important for patients who are beginning treatment with antidepressants. RNs or other healthcare providers typically perform the assessment. Baseline measurements of depression are often collected using questionnaires.

Assessment of suicide risk is essential before beginning antidepressant drugs. If you are practicing in a psychiatric setting, you may be trained to use specific questions or tools to assess risk (see Table 10.5 for an example of a screening device for suicide assessment). One simple way is to ask the patient if he or she has

Table 10.4   Examples of Antidepressant Drugs and Mood Stabilizers

ANTIDEPRESSANTS

Atypical antidepressants: These drugs work slightly differently than the other antidepressants but do affect the neurotransmitters dopamine, norepinephrine, and/or serotonin.

DRUG/ADULT DOSAGE RANGE	NURSING IMPLICATIONS
Bupropion (Wellbutrin, Zyban) 100–150 mg orally two to three times daily Extended release (Wellbutrin XL) 150 mg orally one to two times daily; may gradually increase to 450 mg/day	• Work with the RN or other healthcare provider to screen all patients who are taking antidepressants for thoughts of suicide because they are at increased risk, particularly when starting to take antidepressants. • Notify the healthcare provider if you assess the patient has a history of eating disorder because this may increase risk for seizure. • Do not discontinue these drugs suddenly because the patient may experience withdrawal symptoms. • Report any signs of agitation, irritability, or unusual behaviors to the RN or other healthcare provider because these drugs can trigger mania in some patients. • These drugs may be used in some cases to help patients to stop smoking. • Give the doses with food to decrease GI side effects. • Give the drugs in the morning to decrease the risk for insomnia. Do not give at bedtime.

Selective serotonin reuptake inhibitors: These drugs act by inhibiting the reuptake of serotonin, increasing the concentration of serotonin that is available to bind to postsynaptic receptors.

DRUG/ADULT DOSAGE RANGE	NURSING IMPLICATIONS
escitalopram (Celexa) starts with 20 mg orally once daily; may be increased to a maximum of 40 mg/day fluoxetine (Prozac) starting with 10 mg/day orally, may be increased to up to 80 mg/day. Delayed release form (Prozac Weekly) 90 mg once a week. paroxetine (Paxil) 10–20 mg orally usually in the morning; can be up to 60 mg/day. Controlled release form (Paxil CR) 12.5–75 mg daily. sertraline (Zoloft) 25–50 mg orally once daily; maximum of 200 mg/day	• Work with RN or other healthcare provider to screen all patients who are taking antidepressants for thoughts of suicide because they are at increased risk, particularly when starting to take antidepressants. • Do not discontinue these drugs suddenly because the patient may experience withdrawal symptoms. • Report any signs of agitation, irritability, or unusual behaviors to the RN or other healthcare provider because these drugs can trigger mania in some patients. • Teach patients to contact their healthcare provider before beginning any over-the-counter or herbal drugs, to avoid any harmful adverse effects including serotonin syndrome. • Remind patients that it may take several weeks for the drug to take effect, and they may not experience full benefit for 4–8 weeks after starting therapy. • Provide the patient with resources to treat their depression in the meantime by referral to community agencies or healthcare providers with expertise in treatment of depression, including a number for your local crisis line. • Teach patients that they may experience sexual side effects while taking these drugs and to contact their healthcare provider to discuss any alternative drugs that may be helpful. • Make sure to monitor for signs of dizziness or changes in gait that may lead to falls.

Serotonin and norepinephrine reuptake inhibitors: Drugs that inhibit the reuptake of both serotonin and norepinephrine increasing the concentration of both neurotransmitters available to postsynaptic receptors.

DRUG/ADULT DOSAGE RANGE	NURSING IMPLICATIONS
venlafaxine (Effexor) Immediate release: 75 mg/day orally given in two or three divided doses; may be increased to 375 mg/day given in three divided doses Extended release (Effexor XR) 37.5–75 mg orally once daily; maximum is 225 mg daily duloxetine (Cymbalta) initially, 20–60 mg by mouth daily as single or divided doses. Maximum dosage of 120 mg daily by mouth.	• Work with the RN or other healthcare provider to screen all patients who are taking antidepressants for thoughts of suicide because they are at increased risk, particularly when starting to take antidepressants. • Do not discontinue these drugs suddenly because the patient may experience withdrawal symptoms. • Report any signs of agitation, irritability, or unusual behaviors to the RN or other healthcare provider because these drugs can trigger mania in some patients. • Teach patients to contact their healthcare provider before beginning any over-the-counter or herbal drugs, to avoid any harmful adverse effects including serotonin syndrome. • Remind patients that it may take several weeks for the drug to take effect and they may not experience full benefit for 4–8 weeks after starting therapy. • Provide patients with resources to treat their depression in the meantime by referral to community agencies or healthcare providers with expertise in treatment of depression, including a number for your local crisis line. • Teach patients that they may experience sexual side effects while taking these drugs and to contact their healthcare provider to discuss any alternative drugs that may be helpful.

Table 10.4 **Examples of Antidepressant Drugs and Mood Stabilizers—cont'd**

ANTIDEPRESSANTS

TCAs: These drugs are thought to interfere with the reuptake of norepinephrine and serotonin. This increases the availability for these neurotransmitters for activation of the postsynaptic receptors.

DRUG/ADULT DOSAGE RANGE	NURSING IMPLICATIONS

amitriptyline (Elavil)
    Usual dose between
        50–150 mg/day orally at
        bedtime; hospitalized
        patients may need up to
        300 mg/day
imipramine (Tofranil) usual dose
    ranges between 30 and
    150 mg in single or divided
    doses. Maximum dose is
    200 mg/day for outpatients,
    300 mg/day for hospitalized
    patients.
	• Watch for side and adverse effects, especially as the dosage is being increased.
	• Remind patients that current use of marijuana can cause serious cardiac problems if given with TCAs.
	• Teach patients that using tobacco products can decrease the effectiveness of TCAs.
	• TCAs should be avoided with MAOIs, selective serotonin reuptake inhibitors, and serotonin norepinephrine reuptake inhibitors because they can cause an increased risk for serotonin syndrome.
	• Patients who are receiving TCAs for depression have often been through several trials of antidepressant agents without success. Make sure to assess the patient's history, current drugs, and mental status.
	• Give doses at bedtime because most patients have some drowsiness. This will also help prevent daytime sleepiness. In some cases, patients have difficulty sleeping after taking TCAs; if that is the case, the patient can take the drug in the morning.
	• Teach patients to contact their healthcare provider if they have any new or troublesome symptoms such as difficulty urinating, blurred vision, or shortness of breath because these can indicate adverse effects.

MAOIs: These drugs inhibit the enzyme monoamine oxidase that is responsible for breaking down certain neurotransmitters including dopamine, norepinephrine, and serotonin. Blocking this enzyme increases the available neurotransmitters and results in reduction of depressive symptoms.

DRUG/ADULT DOSAGE RANGE	NURSING IMPLICATIONS

phenelzine (Nardil) usually starts
    with 15 mg orally three times
    daily; may increase to 60 mg/
    day. Maximum dose is 90 mg/
    day
isocarboxazid (Marplan) begin
    with 10 mg orally twice daily;
    may increase to 60 mg/day
selegiline (Eldepryl, Zelapar)
    6–12 mg transdermal patch
    applied to the skin once a day
	• This drug is usually reserved for patients who have had multiple attempts at antidepressant agents without relief.
	• Provide the patient with information regarding foods/beverages high in tyramine (Box 10.5). These must be avoided because taking these while taking MAOIs can result in hypertensive crisis and even death.
	• Remind patient that it can take up to 4 weeks for the patient to feel the effect.
	• Monitor vital signs carefully because this drug can cause hypertensive crisis if taken with certain foods, drinks, or drugs.
	• To avoid serotonin syndrome, teach patients to wait at least 2 weeks after discontinuing the MAOI before taking any drugs with serotonin.

Mood stabilizers: These drugs are used primarily to treat patients with bipolar illness. They help to reduce the symptoms associated with mania, as well as improve the symptoms of depression. Several drugs in this category are also used as antiseizure drugs.

DRUG/ADULT DOSAGE RANGE	NURSING IMPLICATIONS

lithium carbonate (Lithobid)
    initially, 300 mg orally three
    times daily; maintenance
    dosage: 300–600 mg orally
    two or three times per day
valproic acid (Depakote,
    Stavzor) delayed release form
    for acute mania, 750 mg/day
    orally in divided doses; then
    can be increased to best
    effect; may be as much as
    60 mg/kg/day
carbamazepine (Tegretol,
    Carbatrol) initially, 200 mg
    orally daily; gradually
    increased; usual daily dosage
    range is 600–1600 mg/day
    orally in divided doses
	• Lithium has a narrow therapeutic range. Monitor carefully for side effects and adverse effects. See Table 10.6 for common symptoms of toxicity.
	• Teach the patient to avoid conditions that result in severe sweating or potential for dehydration because these can result in low sodium and increase the risk of lithium toxicity.
	• Teach patient to avoid reducing salt intake. Sodium is needed in the diet to prevent lithium toxicity.
	• Patients will need to have regular serum lithium levels drawn to help prevent lithium toxicity. Take first lithium level usually within 4 days of starting therapy (draw sample 12 hours after last dose given). Lithium level should range between 0.8 and 1.2 mEq/L initially, then 0.8 and 1.0 mEq/L. Lithium levels are typically needed every 2 months while on maintenance doses.
	• Risk factors for lithium toxicity include older age, kidney disease, low sodium levels, dehydration, heart disease, debilitated state, and taking certain drugs such as angiotensin-converting enzyme inhibitors, diuretics, or NSAIDs.
	• You can mix lithium oral solutions with fruit juice or flavored drinks to improve the taste. Do not mix the liquid with other drugs because they can form an insoluble salt.
	• Like lithium, carbamazepine serum blood level may be carefully monitored to avoid drug toxicity. Normal serum carbamazepine level is 8–12 mcg/mL.

GI, Gastrointestinal; *MAOI,* monoamine oxidase inhibitor; *NSAIDs,* nonsteroidal anti-inflammatory drugs; *RN,* registered nurse; *TCA,* tricyclic antidepressant.

Table 10.5	Columbia Suicide Severity Rating Scale

Ask questions 1 and 2:

1. Have you wished you were dead or wished you could go to sleep and not wake up?
2. Have you actually had any thoughts of killing yourself?

If Yes to 2, ask questions 3, 4, 5, and 6. If No to 2, go directly to question 6.

3. Have you been thinking about how you might kill yourself?
4. Have you had these thoughts and had some intention of acting on them?
5. Have you started to work out or worked out the details of how to kill yourself? Do you intend to carry out this plan?
6. Have you ever done anything, started to do anything, or prepared to do anything to end your life? If yes, ask: How long ago did you do any of these?

If the answer to question 1 or 2 on the scale is yes, information is also collected related to the intensity of ideation. Intensity is determined based on questions identifying most severe suicidal ideation on a scale of 1 to 5 (where 1 is least severe and 5 is most severe) for the past month and also over the lifetime of the individual. Other follow-up question topics related to suicidal thinking include frequency, duration, controllability, deterrents, reasons for wanting to die, and a description of suicide attempts.[a]

[a]Full Columbia Suicide Severity Rating Scales are available at http://www.cssrs.columbia.edu/scales_practice_cssrs.html.
(From Posner K, Brent D, Lucas C, Gould M, Stanley B, Brown G, Mann J: Columbia-Suicide Severity Rating Scale. 2009. Retrieved from http://www.cssrs.columbia.edu/scales_practice_cssrs.html; Halter MJ: *Varcarolis' foundations of psychiatric mental health nursing: A clinical approach,* ed 7, St. Louis, MO, 2013, WB Saunders Company, VitalBook file, p. 486.)

any thoughts of suicide or of "hurting themselves." If they do, immediately contact the RN or other healthcare team professional to further evaluate risk.

Ask the patient about current use of drugs including herbal and over-the-counter drugs. Knowledge of patients' drug use can help prevent serious complications of serotonin syndrome.

◆ *Planning and implementation.* After risk assessment, providing a safe environment for the patient is very important. Good communication and thorough monitoring will help you determine the effectiveness of therapy. Remind the patient that it may take several weeks for the drug to take effect. Provide the patient with resources to treat his or her depression in the meantime by referral to community agencies or healthcare providers with expertise in treatment of depression. Provide the patient with telephone numbers to the local crisis lines. Teach patients that they may have thoughts of suicide early in therapy. If they do, have them notify their healthcare provider or crisis line immediately. Considering suicide or self-harm is a side effect of the drug, not a logical action.

Most SSRIs can be given without regard to meals. Giving the drugs in the morning helps decrease the risk of difficulty sleeping. Some patients may experience sedation while taking SSRIs; if this is the case, the patients can take the drug in the evening.

Teach patients that it may take several attempts to get the best drug for their depression. Close work with healthcare providers will help the patient move toward best symptom relief.

◆ *Evaluation.* Patients typically begin to experience relief from symptoms within a few weeks of starting drug therapy. Maximum benefit may not occur until after the patient has taken the drug for 4 to 8 weeks after beginning therapy. Compare symptoms with baseline measurements. Ask the patient to describe any side effects he or she may be having. Ask whether they have had any thoughts of suicide or of self-harm. If so, report this immediately to the RN or the healthcare provider.

◆ *Patient and family teaching.* Tell the patient and family the following:

- Take the drugs exactly as ordered by your healthcare provider. It may take several weeks before you feel better.
- Some patients experience sexual side effects. Before you decide if you want to stop taking the drugs, make sure to contact your healthcare provider to discuss any alternative drugs that may be helpful.
- Take these drugs in the morning because many can cause insomnia.
- Symptoms such as nausea, loss of appetite, and headache typically go away after several weeks of treatment. Contact your healthcare provider if you have any questions.
- Do not take any herbal or over-the-counter drugs without talking to your healthcare provider. Herbal drugs, particularly St. John's wort, can cause a dangerous adverse effect if taken with SSRIs.
- Talk to your healthcare provider if you are pregnant or are considering becoming pregnant because these drugs can affect the fetus.
- Some patients have increased thoughts of suicide or of hurting themselves when they first start taking these drugs. These are side effects of the drug, not you. If you have these feelings, contact your healthcare provider or call your local crisis line immediately.

🔖 Top Tip for Safety

Selective Serotonin Reuptake Inhibitors

SSRIs may cause thoughts of suicide, most likely in children and young adults. Remind the patients and their families that this is just a side effect of the drug and should be reported to the healthcare providers immediately.

🔖 Lifespan Considerations

Older Adults

SSRIs can cause falls or fractures in older adults. Make sure to monitor for signs of dizziness or changes in gait that may lead to falls.

SEROTONIN NOREPINEPHRINE REUPTAKE INHIBITORS

Action and Uses

SNRIs inhibit the reuptake of both serotonin and norepinephrine, increasing the concentration of both neurotransmitters available to postsynaptic receptors. These drugs are very similar to the SSRIs. Response rates are very similar to the SSRIs as well. Examples of uses include depression, hot flushes, premenstrual dysphoric disorder, fibromyalgia, and chronic pain. They can also be used for some patients with diabetic neuropathy. Table 10.4 lists the names, adult dosages, and nursing implications for the most common SNRIs. Check a drug reference or with a pharmacist for information about other drugs in this category.

Expected Side Effects and Adverse Reactions

Expected side effects of SNRIs include nausea, dry mouth, loss of appetite, fatigue, and drowsiness. Some patients experience a condition called *hyperhidrosis* (increased sweating).

Sexual side effects are more common in men than women. These range from decreased sex drive to decreased ability to have an orgasm and erectile dysfunction. Some patients experience an elevation in blood pressure, particularly when starting an SNRI. Sudden discontinuation of an SNRI can cause withdrawal symptoms, so tapering is required.

Adverse effects include *epistaxis* (nosebleeds), GI bleeding, and liver damage. Like with SSRIs, patients can experience hyponatremia, severe skin reactions, and an increased risk for suicide. SNRIs are avoided particularly late in pregnancy because the drugs affect the fetus. Infants can experience neonatal abstinence syndrome.

Drug Interactions

Any drug that affects serotonin or norepinephrine can interact with SNRIs. This includes a variety of other antidepressants including MAOIs, SSRIs, and other SNRIs. These combinations can increase the risk for serotonin syndrome or neuroleptic malignant syndrome.

Using the herbal drug St. John's wort (commonly used to treat mild-to-moderate depression) can significantly increase risk for serotonin syndrome. Other potential drug interactions with SNRIs include drugs that can affect clotting, such as anticoagulants, antiplatelet drugs, and NSAIDs.

❖ **Nursing Implications and Patient Teaching**

◆ *Assessment.* A thorough assessment of mental health status is important for patients who are starting treatment with SNRIs. RNs or other healthcare providers typically conduct the formal assessment; however, you are a member of the team and can contribute your observations. Baseline measurements of depression are often collected using questionnaires.

Assessment of suicide risk is essential before beginning SNRIs. Ask the patient about current use of drugs including herbal and over-the-counter drugs. Knowledge of the patient's drug use can help prevent serious complications of serotonin syndrome.

◆ *Planning and implementation.* After risk assessment, providing a safe environment for the patient is very important. Good communication and thorough monitoring helps you determine the effectiveness of therapy. Remind the patient that it may take several weeks for the SNRI to take effect. Provide the patient with resources to treat his or her depression in the meantime by referral to community agencies or healthcare providers with expertise in treatment of depression. Provide the patient with telephone numbers to the local crisis lines.

Teach patients that it may take several trials of different drugs to find the best drug for their depression. Close work with healthcare providers helps the patient move toward the best relief of symptoms.

◆ *Evaluation.* Patients typically begin to experience relief from symptoms within a few weeks of starting therapy. Maximum benefit may not occur until after the patient has taken the drug for 4 to 8 weeks after beginning therapy. Ask patients if they have had any thoughts of suicide or of "hurting themselves." If so, report this immediately to the RN or the healthcare provider.

◆ *Patient and family teaching.* Tell the patient and family the following:

- Take the drugs exactly as ordered by your healthcare provider. It may take several weeks for you to feel better.
- Some patients experience sexual side effects. Before you decide if you want to stop taking the drugs, make sure to contact your healthcare provider to discuss any alternative drugs that may be helpful.
- Take these drugs in the morning because many can cause insomnia.
- Symptoms such as nausea, loss of appetite, and headache typically go away after several weeks of treatment. Contact your healthcare provider if you have any questions.
- Do not take any herbal or over-the-counter drugs without talking to your healthcare provider. Herbal drugs, particularly St. John's wort, can cause a dangerous adverse effect if taking with SNRIs.
- Talk to your healthcare provider if you are pregnant or are considering becoming pregnant because these drugs can affect the fetus.
- Some patients have increased thoughts of suicide or of hurting themselves when they first start taking these drugs. These are side effects of the drug, not you. If you have these thoughts, contact your healthcare provider or call your local crisis line immediately.

TRICYCLIC ANTIDEPRESSANTS

Action and Uses

TCAs are one of the older classifications of drugs first used in the 1950s. They are believed to affect the reuptake of norepinephrine and serotonin.

TCAs work as well as the SSRIs or SNRIs for treating mild-to-moderate depression, but they have more side effects. As a result, these drugs are usually reserved for severe depression or people who do not respond to other treatments. You might see TCAs used for patients with other illnesses such as migraine headaches, panic disorder, obsessive-compulsive disorder, or peripheral neuropathy. Table 10.4 lists the names, adult dosages, and nursing implications for the most common TCAs. Check a drug reference or with a pharmacist for information about other drugs in this category.

Expected Side Effects and Adverse Reactions

Common side effects of TCAs include dry mouth, drowsiness, constipation, nausea, and orthostatic hypotension. Some patients experience weight gain resulting from increased appetite; others may have weight loss. TCAs can cause mild-to-severe vision problems. If this happens, the patient should contact his or her healthcare provider.

Adverse reactions include cardiac dysrhythmias, heart failure, and seizures. TCAs can trigger a manic episode in patients who have an underlying bipolar disorder. They can also cause delirium in older patients with *cognitive impairment* (decreased memory, language, or thinking ability). Like other antidepressants, TCAs can increase the risk for suicide in younger patients. TCAs should not be used in patients with glaucoma because these drugs can increase intraocular pressure.

Drug Interactions

Avoid giving TCAs with drugs that depress the CNS, such as opioids, sedatives, or alcohol. These drugs can increase the risk for respiratory depression, sedation, and severe hypotension. TCAs can also interact with a wide variety of antidysrhythmic drugs, causing serious cardiac problems.

TCAs should be avoided with MAOIs, SSRIs, and SNRIs because of the risk for serotonin syndrome (see Box 10.3). Any drug that increases serotonin (including the herbal drug St. John's wort) can be dangerous in patients who are taking TCAs. Current use of marijuana can cause serious cardiac problems if given with TCAs. Use of tobacco products can decrease the effectiveness of TCAs.

❖ Nursing Implications and Patient Teaching

◆ *Assessment.* Patients who are taking TCAs for depression often have been through several trials of antidepressant agents without success. Make sure to assess the patient's history, current drugs, and mental status. A thorough history helps the healthcare provider make the best decisions for timing and dosages of the drugs. Assessment of suicide risk is essential before beginning or changing any antidepressant drugs.

Assess vital signs including baseline weight. TCAs can cause hypotension and weight gain. Report any history of drug abuse to the provider.

◆ *Planning and implementation.* Reassess the patient's symptoms to determine his or her response to the drugs. Remind patients that the effects may not take effect for several weeks. If the patient has a history of smoking, refer him or her to smoking-cessation resources in your community.

Teach patients about common drug side effects including dry mouth, constipation, and orthostatic hypotension. Some patients may experience an increase in blood pressure. If this occurs, report it to the healthcare provider.

◆ *Evaluation.* Evaluate your patient's response to the antidepressant because symptom relief may take several weeks. Always assess the patient for suicidal ideation. If a patient has thoughts of suicide, refer him or her immediately to the healthcare provider or to your local crisis line.

Patients who have taken TCAs for a long period will need to taper if they are going to be changing drugs. Tapering helps reduce the risk of withdrawal symptoms including headache, nausea, or diarrhea.

◆ *Patient and family teaching.* Tell the patient and family the following:

- Do not stop taking your drug suddenly because it can cause you to have symptoms such as nausea, vomiting, or diarrhea. Your healthcare provider can help you to taper your drug if you need to do so.
- Avoid alcohol, sedatives, opioid pain drugs, or any drugs that can cause drowsiness while you are taking TCAs.
- TCAs often cause dry mouth. Sugarless gum or candy, ice chips, or sips of water can help relieve this problem.
- You may be more sensitive to sunburn when taking these drugs and for several weeks after completing drug therapy. Make sure to use good skin protection including sunscreen and protective clothing.
- TCAs can cause dizziness or light-headedness with changes in position. Make sure to move slowly when you change from lying or sitting to a standing position.
- Most patients have some drowsiness, so you may want to take the drug at bedtime. That will help prevent daytime sleepiness. Some patients have difficulty sleeping after taking TCAs. If that is your experience, you can take the drug in the morning.
- Contact your healthcare provider if you have any new or troublesome symptoms such as difficulty urinating, blurred vision, or shortness of breath because these can indicate adverse effects.

- Wear a medical alert bracelet or necklace, or a wallet medical identification card listing this drug to inform healthcare providers that you are taking this drug.

MONOAMINE OXIDASE INHIBITORS

Action and Uses

Monoamine oxidases (MAOs) are enzymes located in cells throughout the body. The purpose of these enzymes is to break down neurotransmitters, including dopamine, norepinephrine, and serotonin. When MAOs are inhibited or blocked, there is an increase in the available neurotransmitters and then a decrease in depressive symptoms.

> ### Top Tip for Safety
>
> MAOIs may cause hypertensive crisis if the patient ingests foods or drinks that contain tyramine. Examples of these foods include aged cheese, overripe fruit, cured or smoked meat, beer, or wine.

MAOIs are typically used to treat severe depression that is not controlled with other categories of antidepressants. This is because of the serious interactions that can occur with certain drugs, foods, and beverages (see Box 10.5 for a list of high-tyramine foods and drinks). This can make taking MAOIs very challenging and risky.

Box 10.5   High-Tyramine Foods to Avoid If Taking Monoamine Oxidase Inhibitors

Alcoholic beverages
  Beer and ale
  Wine
  Alcohol-free beer
Dairy products
  Mature cheeses (e.g., cheddar, bleu cheese, mozzarella)
  Sour cream
  Yogurt
Fruits and vegetables
  Avocados
  Bananas
  Fava beans
  Canned figs
  Sauerkraut
Meats
  Bologna
  Liver
  Dried fish
  Meat tenderizer
  Pickled herring
  Sausages
  Salami
Other foods
  Caffeinated drinks (e.g., coffee, colas, and tea)
  Chocolate
  Licorice

Adapted from Keltner N, Steele D: *Psychiatric nursing*, ed 7, St. Louis, MO, 2015, Mosby, VitalBook file.

MAOIs can be used in cases of certain anxiety disorders that are not responsive to other drugs. Several can be used in treating patients with Parkinson's disease. Table 10.4 lists the names, adult dosages, and nursing implications for the most common MAOIs. Check a drug reference or with a pharmacist for information about other drugs in this category.

Expected Side Effects and Adverse Reactions

A number of side effects can occur while taking MAOIs. These include constipation, headache, dizziness, drowsiness, and dry mouth. Some patients experience orthostatic hypotension. Weight gain occurs in more than 10% of patients. This may be related to increased appetite and/or increased peripheral edema.

Adverse effects include the possibility of liver damage, a variety of blood disorders, and thoughts of suicide. Some patients who are receiving MAOI therapy may experience severe *hyponatremia* (severe loss of sodium).

Drug Interactions

The combination of MAOIs and certain drugs or foods can result in severe high blood pressure, even *hypertensive crisis* (extremely high blood pressure that can lead to stroke, heart failure, renal failure, and even death). Examples of drugs that can cause this dangerous interaction include SSRIs, SNRIs, St. John's wort, and any drug that has stimulant qualities such as beta agonists, epinephrine, and venlafaxine. Drugs that decrease blood pressure can increase the hypotensive side effects.

Use of MAOIs with drugs that depress the CNS, such as opioids, alcohol, and BNZs, can cause sedation, respiratory depression, and even coma. Patients who are taking insulin or oral hypoglycemic drugs may be at risk for hypoglycemic reactions.

> ### Top Tip for Safety
>
> Do not give MAOIs and SSRIs within 2 weeks of each other. Combining these drugs can cause serotonin syndrome, a life-threatening adverse effect related to too much serotonin.

Most problematic for patients who are taking MAOIs is the risk for hypertensive crisis from ingesting foods or drinks high in tyramine. Tyramine is an amino acid that is involved in the release of norepinephrine. Normally tyramine is broken down by monoamine oxidase (an enzyme). When the patient is taking an inhibitor of the enzyme (MAOIs), there is an increase in norepinephrine, which can then significantly increase blood pressure. This can cause sudden and severe hypertension. Patients must avoid caffeine-containing products that can cause an increase in blood pressure and irregular heart rhythms. These should be avoided for up to 2 weeks after the patient stops taking the MAOIs.

❖ Nursing Implications and Patient Teaching

◆ *Assessment.* Obtain a thorough drug history including the patient's history of drugs used for depression or other mental health issues. This is very important because MAOIs are usually prescribed after other drug therapies have failed. In addition, determine whether the patient has used any herbal drugs including St. John's wort. This is very important information for the healthcare provider in determining appropriate drugs and doses.

Obtain a diet history to assess food and drink preferences. Using MAOIs requires restricting certain types of food and beverage. Detailed diet histories may need to be determined by your agency's RN or registered dietician.

Assess baseline vital signs, weight, and laboratory work. These are important in assessing the patient's response to the drugs. Determine whether the patient has any suicidal thoughts (see Table 10.5).

◆ *Planning and implementation.* MAOIs are typically used in patients who do not respond to the other more commonly prescribed antidepressants. Remind patients that it may take up to 3 to 4 weeks to feel relief from depressive symptoms.

Patient teaching is vital to getting the best results from the drug and preventing adverse effects, particularly hypertensive crisis relating to eating foods high in tyramine. Beyond avoiding foods with tyramine, patients are at risk for weight gain while taking MAOIs. Refer patients to your agency dietician for follow-up.

Tell patients to use good oral hygiene while taking MAOIs because they can cause dry mouth. Sugar-free gums or candies or sips of water can also help to relieve symptoms.

Monitor vital signs and blood sugar levels carefully. Patients can experience hypotension while taking MAOIs. Diabetic patients who take insulin and/or other antidiabetic drugs are at increased risk for hypoglycemia.

◆ *Evaluation.* Ask patients regarding symptoms of depression. Have the symptoms decreased? Determine whether the patient has had any suicidal thoughts. If so, report it immediately to the RN or to the healthcare provider.

MAOIs continue to work on the body as long as 2 weeks after the drug is discontinued. Patients who have been taking these drugs should avoid drugs, foods, or drinks that can increase serotonin or tyramine.

◆ *Patient and family teaching.* Tell the patient and family the following:

- Take the drug as prescribed. It may take several weeks for you to feel the benefit.
- Do not drink alcohol or use any sedating drugs while using these drugs. They can cause severe sedation or a drop in blood pressure.
- Avoid coffee, colas, teas, and other drinks that have caffeine. These can cause a dangerous increase in your blood pressure.
- Do not take any herbal or over-the-counter drugs while taking MAOIs without checking with your healthcare provider, to avoid dangerous interactions.
- Remember that the effect of MAOIs can linger for up to 2 weeks after you stop taking the drug. Do not start eating any foods or drinking beverages that contain tyramine or caffeine. Do not take any new herbal or over-the-counter drugs without talking to your healthcare provider.
- Make sure to change positions slowly because these drugs can lower your blood pressure.
- These drugs can cause dizziness or drowsiness. Avoid driving, operating heavy machinery, or make important decisions. This feeling should improve with time.
- Notify your healthcare provider or call 911 if you experience a sudden fever, severe headache, nausea, vomiting, chest pain, or have a rapid heartbeat because these can be signs of severe adverse effects.
- Use a medical alert bracelet or keep a drug list to alert healthcare providers that you are taking this drug.

MOOD STABILIZERS

Mood stabilizers are drugs used mainly to treat patients with *bipolar illness.* This illness is characterized by extreme changes in mood. These extremes in mood can lead to an inability to work, difficulty in maintaining social relationships, and inability to function in basic ADLs. A challenging aspect of this illness is that many times patients may function very well early in the manic stage.

Once called "manic-depressive" illness, patients can exhibit symptoms of mania such as rapid speech, flight of ideas, excessive activity, staying awake for hours, and having feelings of elation or superiority. They may spend money recklessly, engage in sex with multiple partners, or engage in other high-risk behaviors (see Box 10.6 for a list of common symptoms of mania). On the other side, they may become extremely depressed, lose interest in events, feel sad or down, have feelings of hopelessness, and even consider suicide.

Box 10.6	Symptoms of Mania

- Abnormal or excessive elation
- Decreased need for sleep
- Grandiose notions
- Inappropriate social behavior
- Increased sexual desire
- Increased talking
- Markedly increased energy
- Poor judgment
- Racing thoughts
- Unusual irritability

From Workman M, LaCharity L: *Understanding pharmacology: Essentials for medication safety*, ed 2, St. Louis, 2016, WB Saunders, VitalBook file, box 27-2.

The mood stabilizers can help to manage or reduce the symptoms associated with mania, as well as improve the symptoms of depression. The main drugs include lithium and a variety of drugs considered antiepilepsy (also called "anticonvulsant") drugs (such as lamotrigine and carbamazepine). See Chapter 9 for more detailed information about antiepilepsy drugs.

Treatments are usually long term because the illness does not have a cure. Patients may have difficulty adhering long term to the therapies because of side effects, as well as the loss of some of the "highs" associated with the manic phase.

Action and Uses

Lithium is primarily used to treat patients with bipolar illness including acute mania and during long-term maintenance therapy. Although the exact mechanism of action in stabilizing mood is not known, it is believed that the drug inhibits the synthesis, storage, release, and reuptake of monoamine neurotransmitters. An advantage of lithium is that it does not cause sedation, depression, or *euphoria* (intense excitement or exhilaration). Onset of action for mania is usually about 1 week, but it may take up to 2 to 3 weeks for the patient to experience the full benefit.

Lithium has a very *narrow therapeutic range,* which means that the dosage that improves symptoms is close to the dosage that can causes toxic effects. Therefore it is important to regularly monitor the lithium blood levels of patients who are taking lithium. The first blood level of lithium is usually measured about 4 days into therapy. The healthcare provider then adjusts the patient's dosage accordingly. Regular serum lithium concentrations are required to keep the patient safe. Table 10.4 includes examples of mood stabilizers, including lithium, adult dosages, and nursing implications. Check a drug reference or consult a pharmacist for information about other mood stabilizers.

Expected Side Effects and Adverse Reactions

Expected side effects for lithium are mild weight gain, increased thirst, increased urine output, and dry skin. Some patients have mild drowsiness after starting lithium. Hand tremors occur in nearly 50% of patients but usually decrease with continued use of lithium. At first, patients may have some nausea, vomiting, or diarrhea after starting lithium therapy. This is important to assess, particularly because if it occurs later in therapy, nausea and vomiting can be signs of lithium toxicity.

It is very important to recognize the signs and symptoms of drug toxicity because of the narrow therapeutic range of lithium. Severity of symptoms increases with the lithium level. See Table 10.6 for detailed symptoms associated with lithium blood levels.

> **Top Tip for Safety**
>
> Early signs of lithium toxicity include increased nausea, vomiting, drowsiness, muscle weakness, coarse hand tremor, and incoordination. Later signs include *ataxia* (loss of control of body movements) and *tinnitus* (ringing in the ears).

Fluid balance is very important in patients who are taking lithium because any condition that leads to a drop in sodium levels or dehydration can increase the risk for lithium toxicity. Such conditions include reduced salt intake, intensive exercise, and very hot environments.

Adverse reactions include hypothyroidism, renal failure, and *diabetes insipidus* (severe imbalance of water in the body). Other adverse reactions include neuroleptic malignant syndrome and serotonin syndrome.

> **Top Tip for Safety**
>
> Lithium has a very narrow therapeutic range: knowledge of signs of lithium toxicity and careful monitoring of lithium levels are essential.

Table 10.6	Symptoms Associated With Elevated Lithium Levels		
THERAPEUTIC SERUM LEVELS (0.6–1.2 mEq/L)	**MILD-TO-MODERATE TOXICITY (1.5–2 mEq/L)**	**MODERATE-TO-SEVERE TOXICITY (2–3 mEq/L)**	**SEVERE TOXICITY (>3 mEq/L)**
Hand tremor (fine)	Diarrhea	Previous symptoms *and*	Previous symptoms *and*
Memory problems	Vomiting	Ataxia	Seizures
Goiter	Drowsiness	Giddiness	Organ failure
Hypothyroidism	Dizziness	Tinnitus	Renal failure
Mild diarrhea	Hand tremor (coarse)	Blurred vision	Coma
Anorexia	Muscular weakness	Large output of diluted urine	Death
Nausea	Lack of coordination	Delirium	
Edema	Dry mouth	Nystagmus	
Weight gain			
Polydipsia, polyuria			

From Keltner N, Steele D: *Psychiatric nursing,* ed 7, St. Louis, MO, 2015, Mosby, VitalBook file, p. 177.

Drug Interactions

Diuretics, NSAIDs, antidepressants, and antipsychotic drugs can interact with lithium. Any drugs that affect the electrical conduction of the heart also can cause dangerous interactions. Drugs that affect sodium intake or fluid balance can increase the risk for lithium toxicity.

❖ Nursing Implications and Patient Teaching

◆ *Assessment.* Laboratory work is usually required to determine whether the patient is a candidate for lithium therapy. Complete blood count, blood urea nitrogen and creatinine, serum electrolytes, and thyroid function tests provide baseline information to check patients for underlying health conditions.

A thorough assessment of mental status is important before beginning lithium therapy. In some cases, your patient may be having acute symptoms of bipolar illness including hyperactivity, irritability, pacing, and rapid speech. Work with the RN and other healthcare team members to determine the best way to give the drug.

Assess normal dietary history. Adequate sodium and fluid intake is important for decreasing the risk for lithium toxicity. Physical exertion or exposure to extreme heat can increase sweating and fluid loss, and increase risk for elevated serum lithium levels.

Determine whether the patient has a history of alcohol use, thyroid problems, cardiac disease, or renal problems because they can increase the risk for health problems from taking lithium. In most cases lithium is contraindicated in women who are pregnant or breast-feeding. Pregnant women with bipolar illness need to work very closely with their healthcare provider to choose the best alternatives to manage their symptoms.

◆ *Planning and implementation.* Monitor the patient for signs and symptoms of lithium toxicity, including nausea, vomiting, increased drowsiness, muscle weakness, severe hand tremor, and incoordination. Report these symptoms to the RN or healthcare provider immediately.

Serum lithium levels need to be monitored frequently while the patient is taking the drug. Blood levels are checked 4 days after the patient starts taking lithium. Desired level for acute mania is 0.8 to 1.2 mEq/L. Maintenance level is about 0.8 to 1.0 mEq/L. The healthcare provider adjusts dosages to keep the patient safe and to avoid toxicity. Any levels greater than 1.5 mEq are considered toxic. Levels greater than 3 mEq/L are associated with coma, organ failure, and even death.

Teach patients to avoid making any significant increases or decreases in salt intake or fluid intake. Patients may experience increased thirst or increased urination. In this case tell patients to contact their healthcare provider if these symptoms are severe.

Older adult patients are often more sensitive to lithium than younger patients. It is important to start these patients on lower doses and monitor the therapeutic and adverse effects closely while increasing dosage.

Lifespan Considerations

Older Adults

Older adults may show signs and symptoms of lithium toxicity at lower serum lithium levels. Dosages often start lower and are increased more slowly than with younger patients.

◆ *Evaluation.* Evaluate your patient's mental status regularly to determine the effect of the lithium. Emotional, cognitive, and behavioral symptoms of mania should diminish. As your patient is adjusting to the dose changes, evaluate for signs and symptoms of drug toxicity.

Blood levels will be drawn one to two times each week during the acute phase, then every 1 to 2 weeks until the patient's dosage and blood levels are stable. Then patients will need blood levels checked every 6 to 12 weeks.

◆ *Patient and family teaching.* Tell the patient and family the following:

* Take your lithium as prescribed. It may take several weeks before you notice a change in your symptoms.
* If you are taking the oral liquid, you can mix it with fruit juices or other flavored drink to improve the taste. Do not mix the liquid with other drugs.
* Avoid making any big increases or decreases in your salt and fluid intake. These can affect your drug levels and may increase the risk for adverse effects from your lithium.
* If you have excessive thirst or urination, notify your healthcare provider immediately because these can be related to adverse effects.
* Report significant nausea, vomiting, increased drowsiness, muscle weakness, severe hand tremor, and incoordination to your healthcare provider because these may indicate an adverse reaction.
* Do not use alcohol or any sedating drugs while you are on this drug to avoid serious CNS side effects.
* Contact your healthcare provider if you are thinking of becoming pregnant. Lithium may be toxic to your baby.
* Physical exertion or exposure to extreme heat can increase sweating and fluid loss, and increase risk for lithium levels.
* Keep all appointments to have your drug level monitored to avoid any adverse effects from lithium. This will be frequent when first starting to make sure you are getting the correct dosage and later every 6–8 weeks.
* Wear a medical alert bracelet or necklace and carry a medical identification card stating the name of the drug to ensure that all healthcare providers are aware that you are taking this drug.

Get Ready for the NCLEX® Examination!

Key Points

- Mental illness is a condition where the individual experiences significant changes in the ability to think, as well as changes in behaviors and emotions. Patients can have problems in coping with normal stressors, interacting with others, and functioning within their own cultural norms.
- The main neurotransmitters affected by psychiatric drugs include serotonin, dopamine, and norepinephrine, as well as GABA, acetylcholine, and histamine.
- All sedatives depress the central nervous system to some degree.
- Flumazenil (Romazicon) is a benzodiazepine receptor antagonist and is an antidote used to reverse an overdose of either a benzodiazepine (BNZ) or a BNZ agonist sedative.
- If a BNZ or BNZ agonist is taken with another CNS depressant, CNS effects are more severe and coma or death is possible.
- Major categories of antianxiety agents (also called *anxiolytics*) include BNZs, BNZ agonists, and certain antidepressants (selective serotonin reuptake inhibitors [SSRIs] and serotonin norepinephrine reuptake inhibitors [SNRIs]).
- BNZs act with GABA receptors to enhance GABA effects, leading to a reduction in anxiety and decrease in muscle tension.
- BNZs are recommended primarily for short-term use.
- Long-term use of BNZs can result in physical dependence and withdrawal symptoms if the drug is stopped suddenly.
- A newer drug from the BNZ agonist category, buspirone, reduces anxiety through a variety of actions that affect the serotonin and dopamine neurotransmitters.
- Certain drugs often considered antidepressants are commonly used to relieve symptoms of anxiety.
- BNZs should not be used to treat insomnia, agitation, or delirium in patients older than 65 years and should be avoided in all patients with cognitive impairment, dementia, or a history of falls or fractures.
- Symptoms of psychosis are classified as positive symptoms and negative symptoms. Typical antipsychotics treat positive symptoms, and atypical antipsychotics can treat both positive and negative symptoms.
- The main adverse effects for typical antipsychotics are extrapyramidal symptoms (EPSs). Early recognition can prevent long-term consequences.
- Neuroleptic malignant syndrome (NMS) is a potentially fatal adverse effect associated with antipsychotics and other drugs that affect dopamine.
- Atypical antipsychotics are also known as second-generation antipsychotics and have a lower risk for extrapyramidal effects.
- Patients who are taking atypical antipsychotics are at risk for weight gain, increase in blood triglycerides, and diabetes type 2.

- Most patients with depression require several trials of different drugs to determine which drug is the most effective to manage their symptoms.
- Screen for thoughts of suicide in all patients who are taking antidepressants.
- Patients should not stop taking antidepressants suddenly because this may cause withdrawal symptoms or a relapse of depressive symptoms.
- Maximum benefit of many antidepressants may take 4 to 8 weeks. Always make sure your patient has a referral to professional support services and information for local crisis lines.
- Teach patients not to take any herbal or over-the-counter drugs, particularly St. John's wort, because they can cause a dangerous adverse effect if taken with SSRIs, SNRIs, TCAs, or MAOIs.
- SSRIs may cause thoughts of suicide (*suicide ideation*) or self-harm; this occurs more often in children and young adults. Remind patients and their families that this is just a side effect of the drug and should be reported to the healthcare providers immediately.
- SSRIs and SNRIs can cause falls or fractures in older adults. Make sure to monitor for signs of dizziness or changes in gait that may lead to falls.
- Tricyclic antidepressants (TCAs) work as well as the SSRIs or SNRIs for treating mild-to-moderate depression but have more side effects. As a result, TCAs are usually reserved for severe depression or people who do not respond to other treatments.
- TCAs should be avoided with monoamine oxidase inhibitors (MAOIs), SSRIs, and SNRIs because of the risk for serotonin syndrome.
- MAOIs may cause a hypertensive crisis if the patient ingests foods or drinks that contain tyramine. Examples of these foods include aged cheese, overripe fruit, cured or smoked meat, beer, or wine.
- Do not give MAOIs and SSRIs within 2 weeks of each other. Combining these drugs can cause *serotonin syndrome*, a life-threatening adverse effect related to too much serotonin.
- Lithium is used mainly to treat patients with bipolar illness including acute mania and during long-term maintenance therapy.
- Lithium has a very narrow therapeutic range (patients easily can become toxic). Patients will need to have regular serum lithium levels assessed to keep the patient safe.
- Early signs of lithium toxicity include increased nausea, vomiting, drowsiness, muscle weakness, severe hand tremor, and incoordination. Later signs include ataxia (loss of control of body movements) and tinnitus (ringing in the ears).
- Fluid balance is very important in patients who are taking lithium because any condition that leads to lower sodium levels or dehydration can increase the risk for lithium toxicity.

Get Ready for the NCLEX® Examination!—cont'd

Review Questions for the NCLEX® Examination

1. Which precaution is most important to teach a patient who is prescribed temazepam (Restoril)?
   1. Take this drug with a full glass of water and remain upright for at least 30 minutes.
   2. Notify your healthcare provider if you become constipated or feel light-headed.
   3. Avoid driving within 6 to 8 hours of taking this drug.
   4. Do not take this drug for more than 1 week.

2. The patient is prescribed phenelzine (Nardil), a monoamine oxidase inhibitor, for depression. Which of the following foods should the patient avoid in his diet? (Select all that apply.)
   1. Cheddar cheese
   2. Apple juice
   3. Coffee
   4. Red wine
   5. Baked chicken
   6. Salami

3. A patient who started taking the antidepressant fluoxetine (Prozac) states he has not felt any relief from his depression and it has been 7 days. What is the best response?
   1. "I will tell the healthcare provider the drug is not working and you should be started on a new one."
   2. "Call your healthcare provider and tell them that you need a higher dose."
   3. "You need to start psychotherapy to get the effect you need."
   4. "This antidepressant can take up to 4 weeks to take effect."

4. While making rounds, an LPN/VN working in a psychiatric unit discovers the patient has a temperature of 104°F. The patient had recently started taking fluphenazine (Prolixin). Which adverse effect of typical antipsychotics is associated with a sudden high fever?
   1. Tardive dyskinesia
   2. Metabolic syndrome
   3. Serotonin syndrome
   4. Neuroleptic malignant syndrome

5. Which of the following is most important in assessing a patient newly diagnosed with depression?
   1. Suicidal ideation
   2. Drug history
   3. Family history
   4. Vital signs

6. A patient who is taking atypical antipsychotics reports a 10-pound increase since starting the drug. Which of the following recommendations is appropriate by the LPN/VN?
   1. "This is common for patients taking these drugs. There is nothing you can do about it."
   2. "You should talk to your healthcare provider about starting one of the drugs that just works on positive symptoms."
   3. "Let me talk to your healthcare provider about setting up an appointment to meet with a nutritionist to help you with your diet."
   4. "Usually people taking these drugs lose weight. You probably have a slow metabolism."

7. Which of the following neurotransmitters is commonly decreased by antipsychotic drugs?
   1. Dopamine
   2. Glutamate
   3. GABA
   4. Epinephrine

8. Which of the following symptoms are common in patients experiencing lithium toxicity? (Select all that apply.)
   1. Vomiting
   2. Dizziness
   3. Constipation
   4. Weight gain
   5. Tinnitus
   6. Ataxia

9. A 47-year-old woman states that she has been trying to treat her depression with exercise and "other things" for about 1 year. She is going to begin taking a new prescription of an SSRI. Which of the following is most important to ask the patient?
   1. "Are you taking any herbal drugs such as St. John's wort?"
   2. "How have the therapies worked so far?"
   3. "Which exercises are you using to treat your depression?"
   4. "Why did you wait so long to seek healthcare?"

10. A patient has a history of major depression and has tried many different types of drugs. She will now be starting a tricyclic antidepressant. Which of the following statements by the patient indicates a need for more teaching?
    1. "I will use sugar-free candy or gum to relieve my dry mouth."
    2. "I should let my healthcare provider know right away if I have any thoughts of suicide."
    3. "I will need to work carefully with my healthcare provider to get the right dosage for me."
    4. "If I have any nausea or a headache, I will stop taking my medication immediately."

Drug Calculation Review

1. A 36-year-old male patient with bipolar illness is to receive carbamazepine 200 mg by mouth twice daily in addition to lithium. The carbamazepine is available as 100 mg chewable tablets. How many tablets will the patient require each day?

2. A 23-year-old patient newly diagnosed with schizophrenia is to receive 2.5 mg of haloperidol IM for acute psychosis. Haloperidol is supplied in a vial of 5 mg/mL. How many mL will the patient receive?

Get Ready for the NCLEX® Examination!—cont'd

Case Study

Mr. Smith is a 42-year-old man with a history of schizophrenia. He has a history of using fluphenazine (Prolixin) injection to manage his symptoms but has not returned to the clinic for more than 2 months. His mother states that he has become increasingly irritable and has been hallucinating and paranoid. She is concerned for his safety. He is admitted to the psychiatric unit for observation and treatment.

1. What are your nursing priorities for a patient who is actively experiencing these symptoms?

2. The healthcare provider orders the typical antipsychotic haloperidol by mouth. What side effects will you be expecting for this patient?

3. The patient shows signs of acute dystonia. Describe the symptoms.

4. After the patient is stabilized, the healthcare provider gives the patient a prescription for the atypical antipsychotic risperidone. What will you teach the patient?

11

Drugs for Pain Management

Learning Outcomes

1. List the names, actions, possible side effects, and adverse effects of opioid agonists.
2. Explain what to teach patients and families about opioid agonists.
3. List the names, actions, possible side effects, and adverse effects of opioid agonist-antagonists.
4. Explain what to teach patients and families about opioid agonist-antagonists.

5. List the names, actions, possible side effects, and adverse effects of nonopioid centrally acting analgesics.
6. Explain what to teach patients and families about nonopioid centrally acting analgesics.
7. List five common types of miscellaneous drugs used to help manage pain and the types of pain they most commonly relieve.

Key Terms

acute pain (ă-KYŪT PĀN, p. 211) Pain that is usually related to an injury, such as recent surgery, trauma, or infection, and ends within an expected time frame.

addiction (ă-DĬK-shŭn, p. 216) A psychological dependence in which there is a desperate need to have and use a drug for a nonmedical reason. The addicted person has a limited ability to control this drug craving or use.

analgesic (ă-năl-JĒ-zĭk, p. 213) Drugs that have the specific purpose of relieving pain either by changing the patient's perception of pain or by reducing painful stimulation at its source.

chronic pain (KRŎ–ĭk PĀN, p. 211) Any pain that continues beyond the expected time frame of an acute injury process and that does not trigger the stress response.

corticosteroid (kŏr-tĭ-kō-'STĔR-oid, p. 220) Drugs with powerful anti-inflammatory actions that are chemically similar to the glucocorticoid hormones secreted by the adrenal glands.

dependence (dē-PĔN-dĕns, p. 216) A state in which the body shows withdrawal symptoms when the drug is stopped or a reversing agent is given.

miscellaneous analgesic (ă-năl-JĒ-zĭk, p. 220) Drugs that have specific purposes and actions for other health problems but can help provide relief for certain types of pain.

nonopioid centrally acting analgesic (Ō-pē-ŏyd, p. 218) Drugs that work in the CNS to help manage pain but do not interact with opioid receptors to do so.

opioid (Ō-pē-ŏyd, p. 214) Any substance either derived from natural opium or that is chemically similar to opium that alters the perception of pain and has the potential to induce dependence and addiction.

opioid agonist (Ō-pē-oid Ă-gă-nĭs, p. 214) Any drug that "turns on" (activates) the opioid receptors to change a patient's perception of discomfort and pain.

opioid agonist-antagonist analgesics (Ō-pē-ōīd Ă-gă-nĭst ăn-TĂ-gĕ-nĭst, p. 217) Pain-management drugs that have mixed actions at opioid receptor sites.

pain (PĀN, p. 210) An unpleasant sensation or emotion that produces or might produce tissue damage.

pain threshold (p. 211) The smallest amount of tissue damage that makes a person aware of having pain.

skeletal muscle relaxants (p. 221) Drugs that depress the CNS to reduce muscle spasms.

tolerance (TŎL-ŭr-ŭns, p. 216) A drug-related metabolism problem that causes the same amount of drug to have less effect over time.

withdrawal symptoms (wĭth-DRĂWL, p. 216) Changes in the body or mind, such as nausea or anxiety, that occur when a drug is stopped or reduced after regular use.

PAIN

PAIN DEFINITION

Pain is defined by the International Association for the Study of Pain as an unpleasant sensation or emotion that produces or might produce tissue damage. Pain is always a subjective experience; that is, pain is a sensation the patient feels and that cannot be felt or measured by someone else. This means that pain is personal to you. As a result, the important rule to remember is that *pain is whatever the patient says it is, occurring whenever the patient says it occurs and at the intensity the patient states.* All people experience pain a little differently because pain perception also includes behavioral, psychological, and emotional factors. Pain is a very common problem and a main reason why people go to a healthcare provider.

The smallest amount of tissue damage that makes a person aware of having pain is the **pain threshold**. It is the point that a person first feels any pain. The pain threshold is different for every person and varies from one body site to another. For example, a small blister on a fingertip usually is perceived as more painful than the same-size blister on the back. Factors such as age and the presence of other diseases also affect pain threshold. Most drugs used for pain management change (raise) the patient's pain threshold.

Pain is initially classified as either acute pain or chronic pain. **Acute pain** is usually related to an injury, such as recent surgery, trauma, or infection, and ends within an expected time frame. Accidentally hitting your thumb with a hammer is an example of acute pain. One of the main features of acute pain is your body's physical response to it. Acute pain triggers the stress response (sometimes called the *fight-or-flight response*), resulting in elevated heart and respiratory rates, increased blood pressure, sweating of the palms and soles, dry mouth, and dilated pupils. The person who has acute pain is often restless and unable to concentrate.

Chronic pain is any pain that continues beyond the expected time frame of an acute injury process. Some definitions of pain suggest that pain must exist for at least 6 months to be considered chronic, but that is a very long time to be in pain. People with cancer-related pain or chronic disorders (e.g., arthritis, shingles, or lower back pain [sciatica]) are experiencing chronic pain. It does not trigger the stress response because it has been present for so long that the body has adapted to it. As a result, the person with chronic pain does not have the physical responses seen with acute pain. Chronic pain may hurt less on some days than others but is usually always present. Causes may be difficult to find. This problem has often led to family members and healthcare workers not believing the patient's reports of pain presence and intensity. Chronic pain is often hard to relieve, may interfere with activities of daily living (ADLs), and greatly reduces quality of life.

Pain is also classified by time of presence, as well as by specific sensation and cause (Table 11.1). Some pain has a constant presence, and other pain comes and goes (is *intermittent*). Cancer pain has many causes and sensations that can influence the times when pain is felt. Thus cancer pain is complex and often requires more than one drug type to manage it.

HOW PAIN IS PERCEIVED

Pain is actually recognized (felt or perceived) in the brain rather than in the body area where it occurs. When a body part is injured, for example, when you drop a hammer on your toe, the toe is injured. This injury stimulates pain nerve endings in the toe that then send (transmit) electrical nerve impulses as a signal from the toe along nerves to the spinal cord. At the spinal cord the original signal is transferred to special pain nerve tracts up the spinal cord to the area of the brain where toe activity is located. At this point the signal is transferred to the brain and you now become aware of (perceive or "feel") the pain in your toe (Fig. 11.1). Then you can make and carry out plans to put ice on your toe and let someone else do the hammering.

You feel pain only in the brain, so anything that interferes with the transmission of the pain signal from

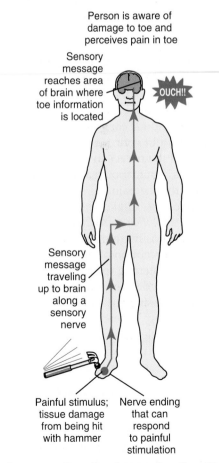

Person is aware of damage to toe and perceives pain in toe

Sensory message reaches area of brain where toe information is located

OUCH!!

Sensory message traveling up to brain along a sensory nerve

Painful stimulus; tissue damage from being hit with hammer

Nerve ending that can respond to painful stimulation

FIG. 11.1 A sensory pathway for pain perception. (From Workman ML, LaCharity LA: *Understanding pharmacology*, ed 2, St. Louis, 2016, Elsevier.)

Table 11.1   **Classification of Pain**

CATEGORY	CHARACTERISTICS	EXAMPLE
Acute	Sudden onset; has a specific cause; triggers the stress response with changes in breathing, heart rate, blood pressure; improves with time and healing	Postsurgical pain, traumatic injury, bone fracture, infection
Chronic	Continues beyond the usual course of an acute injury process; may not have an identifiable cause; does not trigger the stress response; is usually present continuously	Arthritis pain, sciatica, shingles
Continuous	Always present but may vary in intensity	Sciatica
Intermittent	Comes and goes	Abdominal cramping from constipation or intestinal irritation
Nociceptive	Specific to a body area that is easy to identify and describe; words used to describe often include aching and throbbing	Cuts, fractures, arthritis
Visceral	Hard to locate, may be referred to more distant sites than the cause of the pain; often described as continual aching	Pain under the right shoulder blade with gallstone disease
Neuropathic	Sharp, shooting, stabbing, and burning sensations	Diabetic neuropathy, trigeminal neuralgia, pain with shingles
Cancer pain	Often includes all specific types of pain with multiple causes (organ compression, tissue stretching, nerve compression, bone pain, etc.); complex; requires multiple types of agents for best relief	Usually advanced cancers that have spread beyond the originating site and are pressing on nerves and/or organs, putting pressure on the inside of bones, secreting chemicals that make pain receptors more sensitive, causing inflammation

your toe along the nerve to and in your brain can change if and how you perceive pain. So if you had a stroke that damaged the part of the brain where toe pain would be perceived, you would not feel that pain. If the pain nerve tracts in the spinal cord were severed, you would not "feel" the pain in your toe even though the injury is severe. Also, if the nerves in your leg were severed, the pain signals would not reach the brain and you would not feel the toe pain.

Anxiety, depression, fatigue, and other chronic diseases may increase the perception of pain. Activities that distract the patient, create positive attitudes, or provide support may reduce the perception of pain. Examples of these activities include listening to music, massage therapy, cold or hot packs, hydrotherapy, acupuncture, biofeedback, relaxation therapy, art therapy, hypnosis, therapeutic touch, Qigong or Reiki energy therapies, or use of transcutaneous electrical nerve stimulation units. Usually these nondrug therapy techniques are used with analgesics for optimum pain management.

PRINCIPLES OF PAIN MANAGEMENT

Although pain is a common problem, it is often poorly addressed. Based on the idea that pain is unpleasant and should be relieved, the Agency for Healthcare Research & Quality originally developed specific principles for pain management regardless of the source or type of pain. These principles are:

- *Ask* about pain on a regular basis. Drugs are to be given regularly and are more effective if given *before* the patient is in severe pain and miserable. Addiction is generally not a concern, especially for patients with chronic pain or terminal illness.
- *Assess* pain systematically. Use pain intensity scales (Figs. 11.2, 11.3, and 11.4).
- *Believe* the patient and family in their reports of pain and what relieves it.
- *Choose* pain-management options that are appropriate for the patient, family, and setting. The healthcare provider who makes this decision should be aware of the wishes of the family and the individual.
- *Deliver* interventions in a timely, logical, and coordinated fashion.
- *Empower* patients and their families.
- *Enable* them to manage their pain to the greatest extent possible.

ANALGESIC DRUGS FOR PAIN MANAGEMENT

Many nerve paths carry the sensation of pain from an injured part of the body to the brain. This means that there are different places to block or alter the sensation of pain. Some pain may be relieved by nondrug therapies such as exercise, heat, ice or cold compresses, music, massage, diversion techniques, sedation, and rest; changing the room to be quieter, darker, or cooler; or

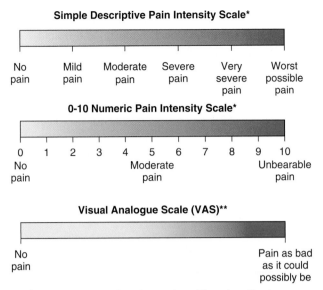

Simple Descriptive Pain Intensity Scale*

| No pain | Mild pain | Moderate pain | Severe pain | Very severe pain | Worst possible pain |

0-10 Numeric Pain Intensity Scale*

| 0 No pain | 1 | 2 | 3 | 4 | 5 Moderate pain | 6 | 7 | 8 | 9 | 10 Unbearable pain |

Visual Analogue Scale (VAS)**

No pain   Pain as bad as it could possibly be

* If used as a graphic rating scale, a 10-cm baseline is recommended.
** A 10-cm baseline is recommended for VAS scales.

FIG. 11.2 Common pain measurement scales. (From Black JM, Hawks JH: *Medical-surgical nursing: clinical management for positive outcomes*, ed 8, Philadelphia, 2009, Elsevier.)

other methods such as herbal poultices or acupuncture. Pain that is more severe often requires a management strategy of a combination of nondrug and drug therapies.

A wide range of drugs are used in managing pain. Some of these drugs are actual **analgesics**, which have the specific purpose of relieving pain either by changing the patient's perception of pain or by reducing painful stimulation at its source. The word *analgesia* means absence of the sensation of pain. The analgesic categories are *opioid agonists* (narcotics), *opioid agonist-antagonists, nonopioid centrally acting analgesics,* and *miscellaneous analgesics,* which include a variety of drug types with other purposes that also help reduce pain. Which specific type of drug is prescribed depends on the type of pain being experienced, the cause of the pain, pain intensity, expected duration of the pain, and the patient's perception of the pain.

> **Memory Jogger**
>
> The four main categories of drugs used for pain management are:
> - opioid agonists
> - opioid agonist-antagonists
> - nonopioid centrally acting analgesics
> - miscellaneous analgesics

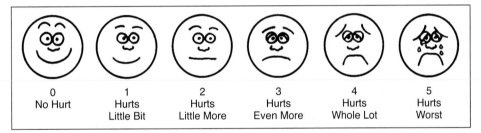

| 0 No Hurt | 1 Hurts Little Bit | 2 Hurts Little More | 3 Hurts Even More | 4 Hurts Whole Lot | 5 Hurts Worst |

Brief word instructions: Point to each face using the words to describe the pain intensity. Ask the child to choose the face that best describes own pain and record the appropriate number.

FIG. 11.3 Wong-Baker FACES pain rating scale. (Copyright 1983, Wong-Baker FACES Foundation, www.WongBakerFACES. org. Used with permission. Originally published in *Whaley & Wong's nursing care of infants and children.* © Elsevier Inc.)

Category	Score		
	0	**1**	**2**
Face	No particular expression or smile	Occasional grimace or frown, withdrawn, disinterested	Frequent-to-constant quivering chin, clenched jaw
Legs	Normal position or relaxed	Uneasy, restless, tense	Kicking, or legs drawn up
Activity	Lying quietly, normal position, moves easily	Squirming, shifting back and forth, tense	Arched, rigid, or jerking
Cry	No cry (awake or asleep)	Moans or whimpers, occasional complaint	Crying steadily, screams or sobs, or frequent complaints
Consolability	Content, relaxed	Reassured by occasional touching, hugging, or being talked to, distractible	Difficult to console or comfort

Each of the five categories–(F) Face, (L) Legs, (A) Activity, (C) Cry, (C) Consolability– is scored from 0-2, which results in a total score between 0 and 10.

FIG. 11.4 The FLACC pain rating scale for infants and patients who are not alert. (From Workman ML, LaCharity LA: *Understanding pharmacology*, ed 2, St. Louis, 2016, Elsevier.)

OPIOID AGONIST ANALGESICS

Many drugs used for managing severe pain are opioids. An **opioid** (also called a *narcotic*) is any substance either derived from natural opium (from the poppy plant) or that is chemically similar to opium that alters the perception of pain and has the potential to induce dependence and addiction. Opium includes many chemicals, such as morphine, codeine, and heroin. In addition to natural opioids, synthetic opioids have been developed by drug companies. Both natural and synthetic opioids are useful for pain management. Morphine is the basic chemical from which the synthetic opioid analgesics hydrocodone, hydromorphone, fentanyl, and oxycodone have been developed. All natural and synthetic opioids are *high-alert drugs* because they have an increased risk for causing patient harm if given in error.

Opioid agonists have a relatively high potential for abuse. In efforts to limit the abuse of these drugs, the federal government has regulations that describe who may prescribe or give opioids (see Chapter 2). You must learn and follow these rules to practice legally. Nurses usually have the responsibility for keeping opioids in a safe place, typically a locked cabinet, and account for their use in the hospital or nursing home setting.

As stated earlier, morphine is the main opioid agonist analgesic, and it is the drug with which all other pain-management drugs are compared for effectiveness. Table 11.2 shows the equianalgesic dosages needed for common opioid agonists to achieve equal pain relief. Although different opioid agonist analgesics vary by strength (some are stronger than morphine and some are not as strong as morphine), they all work in the same way and all have the same side effects and adverse effects. Morphine and other strong opioid agonists are used often in acute care and also in hospice settings for patients who have severe pain. Codeine, hydrocodone (Hydromet), and oxycodone (OxyContin) are weaker than morphine and are often used in combination with acetaminophen in the outpatient setting. On the other hand, hydromorphone (Dilaudid) is much stronger than morphine. Table 11.3 lists dosages and nursing considerations for common opioid agonists.

> **Memory Jogger**
>
> Strong opioid agonist analgesics such as hydromorphone and fentanyl require less drug (lower dosages given less often) to result in the same level of pain relief as weaker opioid agonist analgesics.

Action

Did you know you actually make your own internal morphine? Your brain has opioid receptors because you do make your own internal opioids to provide some pain relief and an increased sense of well-being when physically stressed. These internal morphine-like chemicals produced in the brain are *endorphins*, *enkephalins*, and

Table 11.2 Equianalgesic Adult Dosages of Common Opioid Agonists and Opioid Agonist-Antagonists

DRUG	EQUIANALGESIC[a] DOSE
Opioid Agonists	
morphine	30 mg (oral) 10 mg (parenteral)
codeine (many brand name combination drugs)	200 mg (oral) NOT RECOMMENDED 120 (parenteral)
fentanyl (Actiq, Apo-fentanyl ♣, Duragesic, Lazanda)	0.2 mg (transdermal patch) 0.1 mg (parenteral)
hydrocodone (Hycet, Lortab, Norco, Vicodin, and many brand name combination drugs)	30 mg (oral)
hydromorphone (Dilaudid, Apo-Hydromorphone ♣)	7.5 mg (oral) 1.5 mg (parenteral)
oxycodone (Endocodone, Oxaydo, OxyContin)	20 mg (oral)
oxymorphone (Numorphan, Opana)	10 mg (oral) 1 mg (parenteral)
Opioid Agonist-Antagonist	
buprenorphine (Buprenex, Probuphine)	0.4 mg (parenteral)
butorphanol (Stadol)	2 mg (parenteral)
nalbuphine (Nubain)	10 mg (parenteral)
pentazocine (Talwin)	150 mg (oral) 60 mg (parenteral)

[a]Equianalgesic means the dose that provides about the same degree of pain relief that is provided by 30 mg oral morphine.
♣ Indicates Canadian drug.

dynorphins. Think about the jogger who runs for 10 miles, looks terrible, and says, "I feel wonderful." How is this possible? With the physical stress and hard work of running 10 miles, the brain makes much more of these substances. They then bind to specific opioid receptors in the brain and activate the receptor to change your perception from discomfort and pain to comfort. So these internal opioids are **opioid agonists** because they "turn on" (activate) the opioid receptors to change the runner's perception of discomfort. External opioids that are given for pain relief also bind to opioid receptors as agonists to activate the opioid receptors. (You may need to review the action of agonists, antagonists, and receptors that was discussed in Chapter 3).

Morphine and all opioid agonist analgesics work by binding to opioid receptor sites in the brain and other areas. The main opioid receptors are mu (OP3), kappa (OP2), and delta (OP1). When a drug binds to and acts as an agonist at mu receptors, the responses include pain relief, some degree of respiratory depression with slower breathing, some sleepiness or sedation, decreased intestinal motility with constipation, pupil constriction,

Table 11.3 **Dosages and Nursing Implications for Common Opioid Agonists**

All opioid agonist analgesics work by binding to mu opioid receptor sites (activating them) in the brain and other areas, changing the person's perception of pain.

DRUG/ADULT DOSAGE RANGE	NURSING IMPLICATIONS
codeine 15–60 mg every 4 hours (oral and parenteral) fentanyl (Actiq, Apo-fentanyl ♣, Duragesic, Lazanda) 50–100 mcg IM or by slow IV over 1–2 minutes; 12–100 mcg/hr by transdermal patch hydrocodone (Hycet, Lortab, Norco, Vicodin, and many brand name combination drugs) 10–40 mg orally every 12 hours hydromorphone (Dilaudid, Apo-Hydromorphone ♣) 2–4 mg orally every 4–6 hours; 0.2–1 mg IV every 2–3 hours morphine 2–4 mg orally every 4–6 hours; 0.2–1 mg IV every 2–3 hours oxycodone (Endocodone, Oxaydo, OxyContin) 5–30 mg every 4 hours (immediate release); 10 mg every 12 hours (extended release) oxymorphone (Numorphan, Opana) 5–20 mg orally every 4–6 hours; 0.5–1.5 every 4–6 hours parenterally	• Reassess the patient's level of pain within an hour after giving an opioid to determine its effectiveness. • During periods of acute pain, encourage the patient to take the drug on the prescribed schedule for best pain relief. Assess elimination status daily because all opioids cause constipation. • Assess respiratory rate and pulse oximetry frequently because opioids can cause respiratory depression. • If patients cannot be aroused, have respirations below 8 per minute, have severe hypotension, or develop hypothermia, notify the healthcare provider immediately to prevent coma or death. • Patients may also be prescribed stimulant laxatives because of the high incidence of constipation common with opioids. • Instruct patients who are taking extended-release tablets or capsules not to chew, open, crush, bite, or cut them, to prevent rapid absorption of excess drug. • Instruct patients not drink alcohol or take other CNS depressants while on an opioid analgesic because the CNS effects are intensified. • Change fentanyl patches and rotate sites at least every 72 hours and wash the skin under the old patch to prevent excess drug absorption.

♣ Indicates Canadian drug.

lower blood pressure, and *euphoria* (a feeling of emotional happiness). When a drug binds to and acts as an agonist at kappa receptors, the responses include some pain relief, sedation, pupil constriction, and *dysphoria* (a state of feeling emotional or mental discomfort, restlessness, and anxiety). When a drug binds to and acts as an agonist at delta receptors, the responses include some pain relief, dysphoria, and hallucinations.

Morphine binds most tightly and best to the mu receptor, acting as an agonist. This activates the mu receptors and the person's perception of pain is changed. *Opioid agonists only change the perception of pain; they do nothing at the site of injured tissue to reduce the cause of pain.* Some drugs act as an agonist at one type of opioid receptor site and, at the same time, act as an antagonist at other opioid receptor sites, providing mixed responses. The opioids that provide the best pain relief bind most strongly (tightly) to the mu receptors. Pain drugs that are strong morphine agonists include morphine, hydromorphone, oxymorphone, and fentanyl. Those that bind moderately well to the mu receptors and provide some degree of pain relief include codeine, hydrocodone, and oxycodone.

Memory Jogger

Strong opioid agonist analgesics include:
• morphine
• hydromorphone
• oxymorphone
• fentanyl

Uses

Opioid agonists are used to manage moderate-to-severe acute pain and chronic pain. They may be used preoperatively (before surgery) to treat pain from injury or other disease processes, for constant cough (codeine), postoperatively for pain, and for labor. Opioids are available in oral tablets, capsules, lozenges, and liquids; intravenous and other parenteral solutions for injection; and some (such as fentanyl), as a continuous-release transdermal patch.

Some opioids are also commonly available as combination products along with drugs such as acetaminophen, aspirin, caffeine, and barbital. This allows a small dose of opioid to be combined with other chemicals to relieve symptoms or calm the patient.

Expected Side Effects

The two most common side effects of opioid agonists are sleepiness *(sedation)* and constipation. Other expected reactions to opioid agonist analgesics include *bradycardia* (slower heartbeat), hypotension, decreased respirations, *anorexia* (lack of appetite), dry mouth, and a sense of happiness *(euphoria)*. Most patients also have decreased pupil size *(miosis)*, especially older adults, and are at increased risk for falling.

Adverse Reactions

Serious adverse reactions include very slow, shallow breathing *(bradypnea)* also known as *respiratory depression*, severe hypotension, decreased urine output *(oliguria)*, below-normal body temperature *(hypothermia)*, excessive sedation or coma, and cool, clammy skin. These serious reactions may indicate overdose and require immediate medical attention. The drug dose should be lowered or the drug discontinued when any serious reaction occurs.

> **Top Tip for Safety**
>
> Serious adverse reactions and symptoms of overdose for opioid agonist analgesics that require immediate medical attention are:
> - respirations of 8 or less per minute
> - very low blood pressure
> - excessive sedation or coma
> - below-normal body temperature

If a serious adverse reaction or an overdose occurs with an opioid agonist, the effects can be reversed by giving an intravenous, IM, or subcutaneous opioid antagonist such as naloxone (Narcan) or naltrexone (Revia, Vivitrol). They work by binding tightly to the mu opioid receptors and blocking them so the opioid agonist cannot stay bound to them. In an emergency these drugs can be given without a prescription. Naloxone is also available as an intranasal spray, but this route is not as reliable as when given parenterally.

> **Lifespan Considerations**
>
> **Older Adult**
>
> Older adults are more likely to have some degree of liver and/or kidney impairment that reduces their ability to metabolize and excrete opioid agonists. This makes them more sensitive to the drugs, and normal doses can cause serious adverse reactions. Older adults may require dosages to be lower or the drugs given less frequently.

Tolerance, Dependence, and Addiction

Tolerance is a drug-related metabolism problem that causes the same amount of drug to have less effect over time. Although tolerance can happen with any drug type, it is most often seen with opioid agonists. This happens because the body gradually increases the rate at which it degrades and eliminates the drug. In the case of pain, higher dosages are needed for relief. **Dependence** is a state in which the body shows withdrawal symptoms when the drug is stopped or a reversing agent is given. **Withdrawal symptoms** are changes in the body or mind, such as nausea or anxiety that occur when a drug is stopped or reduced after regular use. Tapering off (slowly taking less of the drug) can reduce withdrawal symptoms. Psychological dependence, or **addiction**, is the desperate need to have and use a drug for a nonmedical reason. The addicted person has a limited ability to control this drug craving or use. Tolerance and dependence result from regular use of an opioid for a certain length of time and should not be confused with or labeled as addiction. Addiction is a problem; however, a patient in pain should not be denied pain relief because of fear of addiction. Before beginning opioid therapy for noncancer pain management, recent recommendations are to obtain thorough medical and social histories, including tobacco and alcohol use, and a family history of addiction. All opioid agonists have the potential to cause tolerance and dependence, which are not the same as addiction or abuse, when taken on a long-term basis.

Drug Interactions

The decreased pupil size, sedation, dry mouth, and euphoria are the central nervous system (CNS) effects of the opioid agonists along with pain relief. These effects can be intensified and made much worse when the patient also uses certain other substances or drugs that act on the CNS. These agents include alcohol, antianxiety drugs, skeletal muscle relaxants, barbiturates, many drugs used for psychiatric disorders, and other opioid agonists.

> **Top Tip for Safety**
>
> The sedating and slowed breathing effects of opioid agonist analgesics are intensified and made worse when the patient also drinks alcohol or uses antianxiety drugs, skeletal muscle relaxants, barbiturates, many drugs used for psychiatric disorders, and other opioid agonists. Be sure to determine which other drugs the patient also takes.

❖ Nursing Implications and Patient Teaching

◆ *Assessment.* Before a patient can be effectively helped with pain relief, it is important to determine the cause of the pain and its intensity. Do not simply give drugs prescribed for pain without understanding the source and intensity of the pain. Even in a patient with terminal cancer, assess each new pain for a specific cause that may have a more focused treatment.

Ask the patient to describe the pain and use a pain scale to assess pain intensity (severity). Fig. 11.2 shows several examples of pain rating scales for patients who are alert to indicate how much pain they are having. Fig. 11.3 shows an example of a pain rating scale for children and adults who may have trouble expressing their thoughts. Ask the patient whether he or she has ever received morphine (or other opioid agonist) in the past and what, if any, problems occurred with its use. When opioids are first prescribed, ask the patient about current tobacco and alcohol use, any past addiction to pain drugs, or a family history of substance abuse or addiction.

> **Lifespan Considerations**
>
> **Pediatric: Pain Assessment**
>
> Children experience pain in the same way as adults, but young children may have difficulty communicating their level of discomfort. Use an age-appropriate rating scale to assess pain in younger pediatric patients. When assessing pain in infants, pay attention to the infant's position (especially whether the legs are drawn up), facial expression, crying pattern, sleep/rest cycles, interest in eating, and how easily he or she can be consoled (see Fig. 11.4). Compare these observations with those obtained when the infant appears to be comfortable.

◆ *Planning and implementation.* Pain is best relieved when opioid agonists are given before the patient's pain becomes severe. This means they work better when given on a schedule rather than waiting until the patient asks for it. When the patient asks for another dose, check to see when the patient received his or her most recent dose of the prescribed opioid agonist to determine whether another dose can be given at this time. Also check the prescribed drug name and dose carefully. Opioid agonists are not interchangeable because drug strength varies. Only the prescribing healthcare provider can change the order. Be sure to sign out the dose as required by the Drug Enforcement Agency of the federal government.

If this is the first dose of an opioid agonist the patient is to receive, before giving the drug, check his or her respiratory rate and oxygen saturation because these drugs can cause respiratory depression. This action is important to perform on older patients and for those who are receiving higher doses.

Most patients become drowsy with opioid agonists; therefore it is important to ensure that the upper side rails are raised and the call light is in reach. If the patient is in a chair, remind him or her to call for assistance to avoid falls from drowsiness or low blood pressure.

◆ *Evaluation.* Usually, opioid agonist analgesics begin to take effect in 15 to 30 minutes. Check the patient at this time for pain relief and for changes in respiratory rate and depth. Recheck at least every hour. Opioid agonist analgesics may slow the respiratory rate and decrease the cough and sigh reflexes; thus patients who have had surgery, especially those who have smoked for a long time, may develop areas where the lungs do not inflate well (*atelectasis*) or collect fluid and develop pneumonia. If pain relief is not obtained or is not sufficient to keep the patient comfortable, report this to the prescriber so that changes in pain management can be made. Higher doses and/or more frequent dosing may be needed.

If the patient has been receiving an opioid agonist for 2 days or longer, ask him or her about constipation because this is a very common side effect of these drugs. If stool softeners or laxatives have been prescribed, give them as ordered. If they have not been prescribed and opioid agonist therapy is ongoing, remind the prescriber about the issue of constipation. The patient may need a laxative in addition to a stool softener.

◆ *Patient and family teaching.* Tell the patient and family the following:

- Take this drug as prescribed and do not change the dosage. For acute pain, it is most effective to take the drug before you have severe pain, if possible on a regular schedule. Write down the time when the drug was last taken to prevent taking too much by accident.
- Do not take any other drugs not prescribed by your healthcare provider.
- Alcohol increases the effects of the drugs, and taking both together may lead to serious adverse reactions.

- Report any new symptoms or problems to your healthcare provider.
- Change positions slowly to prevent dizziness and falling from a rapid drop in blood pressure.
- Do not drive, operate heavy machinery, or make important decisions while under the influence of the drug because your judgment may be impaired.
- Increase fluid and fiber intake to prevent constipation.
- Use prescribed stool softeners or laxatives to prevent severe constipation.
- Take oral opioids with food to prevent nausea.
- If the opioid agonist is an extended-release tablet or capsule, do not cut it in half, chew it, or crush it because the time-release feature will be ruined and too much drug may be absorbed too quickly and cause adverse reactions.
- Do not allow anyone else to use the drug.

OPIOID AGONIST-ANTAGONIST ANALGESICS

Opioid agonist-antagonist analgesics are pain-management drugs that have mixed actions at opioid receptor sites. Although not as strong as opioid agonist analgesics, they are thought to be at lower risk for addiction or abuse because of some of the side effects.

Action

Four opioid agonist-antagonists are available for pain relief (Table 11.4). Three of them (pentazocine, nalbuphine, and butorphanol) act as antagonists at the mu opioid receptors and as agonists at the kappa opioid receptors. This action makes them less effective for pain control than pure opioid agonists. They do still provide pain relief because, as described in the earlier Opioid Agonist Analgesics section, activation of the kappa receptors results in some pain relief, as well as sedation. The fourth drug, buprenorphine, is different because it acts as a partial agonist at mu receptors and as an antagonist at kappa receptors. This allows buprenorphine to have greater pain relief potential than the other three and less dysphoria. The sensation of dysphoria, which is a state of feeling emotional or mental discomfort, restlessness, and anxiety, is unpleasant and decreases the likelihood that patients would want to use these drugs when they are not in pain.

> 💡 **Memory Jogger**
>
> The opioid agonist-antagonist analgesics are:
> - pentazocine
> - nalbuphine
> - butorphanol
> - buprenorphine

Uses

The greatest use of the opioid agonist-antagonist analgesics is for relief of mild-to-moderate pain. They are less useful for severe pain. Pentazocine is available in an oral as well as a parenteral form. The three that

Table 11.4 Dosages and Nursing Implications for Common Opioid Agonist-Antagonists

Most opioid agonist-antagonists antagonize (block) the mu receptors and change the perception of pain by agonizing the kappa receptors. Buprenorphine is a partial mu agonist.

DRUG/ADULT DOSAGE RANGE	NURSING IMPLICATIONS
buprenorphine (Buprenex, Probuphine) 0.3 mg IM or IV every 6–8 hours butorphanol (Stadol) 1–4 mg IM or 0.5–2 mg IV every 3–4 hours nalbuphine (Nubain) 10 mg IM, IV, or subcutaneously every 3–6 hours pentazocine (Talwin) 30 mg IV or 30 mg IM/subcutaneously every 3–4 hours	• Reassess the patient's level of pain within an hour after giving an opioid agonist-antagonist to determine its effectiveness. • Assess the patient's emotional responses because butorphanol, nalbuphine, and pentazocine can cause dysphoria, anxiety, nightmares, and hallucinations. • Assess heart rate and rhythm frequently because these drugs can excite the cardiac system and cause dysrhythmias. • Avoid the use of butorphanol, nalbuphine, and pentazocine in a patient who is physically dependent on an opioid agonist because blocking the mu receptor can cause withdrawal symptoms.

are antagonists at the mu opioid sites have only limited problems with respiratory depression. Buprenorphine also has less respiratory depression than pure opioid agonists because it only partially agonizes the mu receptors.

Nalbuphine and butorphanol are sometimes used to manage pain during labor and delivery. Butorphanol may be prescribed as a metered-dose nasal spray for management of migraine headaches.

Expected Side Effects

Common mild side effects are similar to those for morphine. These include sedation, constipation, and constricted pupils.

Adverse Reactions

Higher doses of these drugs are associated with nightmares and hallucinations. The opioid agonist-antagonists can have serious cardiac reactions. Pentazocine, nalbuphine, and butorphanol excite the cardiac system, making the heart work harder and elevating blood pressure. They should not be used in patients who are suspected of having a heart attack, and they should be used carefully in those who have heart failure. Buprenorphine can cause serious cardiac dysrhythmias and should not be used for patients who have other serious dysrhythmias. Although respiratory depression is possible with these drugs, it is not common.

Use of pentazocine, butorphanol, or nalbuphine in a patient who is physically dependent on morphine or other opioid agonists will cause withdrawal symptoms. This occurs because they block mu receptor sites. The use of these three drugs in a patient who is physically dependent on opioid agonists is avoided.

Drug Interactions

The sedating effect of these drugs is made worse with alcohol, antianxiety drugs, skeletal muscle relaxants, barbiturates, many drugs used for psychiatric disorders, and pure opioid agonists. Be sure to determine which other drugs the patient also takes.

❖ Nursing Implications and Patient Teaching

◆ *Assessment.* Assess the patient's pain in the same way as for opioid agonists or any other type of pain-management drug. Ask the patient whether he or she has ever taken any of these specific drugs and whether any problems resulted from taking it. Also ask what other over-the-counter and prescribed drugs the patient has taken in the past 24 hours, especially any opioid agonist analgesics.

◆ *Planning and implementation.* Planning, implementation, evaluation, and patient and family teaching activities are the same as for opioid analgesics.

NONOPIOID CENTRALLY ACTING ANALGESICS

Nonopioid centrally acting analgesics are drugs that work in the CNS to help manage pain but do not interact with opioid receptors to do so. The two most commonly used drugs in this class are clonidine (Duraclon) and tramadol (Ultram, Ryzolt).

Memory Jogger

Two common nonopioid centrally acting analgesics are:
• clonidine
• tramadol

Action

Clonidine and tramadol have completely different mechanisms of action for pain relief. Clonidine is an antihypertensive drug most commonly used to lower blood pressure. It works for pain management by binding to specific receptors (alpha-adrenergic receptors) in the spinal cord and blocks their activity. This action keeps pain signals from the source of the pain from traveling to the level of the brain. As a result, fewer pain signals reach the brain to be "felt" as pain. Clonidine does not change the conditions at the source of the pain.

Although it has a chemical structure similar to codeine, tramadol has only weak effects at opioid receptors. Instead it works by blocking the action (inhibiting) some of the neurotransmitters in the spinal cord and areas of the brain. This action reduces pain signal transmission to brain sites that perceive pain. The usual adult dosage ranges for tramadol are 50 to 100 mg orally every 6 hours (immediate-release tablets) and 100 to 200 mg every 12 hours (extended-release capsules).

Uses

Clonidine formulated for pain management (Duraclon) is approved for severe pain (often cancer pain) and is given as a continuous epidural infusion. It is not a controlled substance because it is considered to have no potential for addiction or abuse. The oral formulation (Catapres) is only for blood pressure control and does not have a role in pain management.

Tramadol is an oral drug used for moderate or moderately severe acute pain. It is only as effective as codeine (not as effective as morphine) and is often used along with acetaminophen.

Expected Side Effects

Clonidine dilates blood vessels, which can lead to severe hypotension. It should not be used in patients who have low blood pressure. Tramadol has mild side effects of sedation, dizziness, dry mouth, and constipation.

Adverse Reactions

Tramadol can induce seizures and should not be used in any patient who has epilepsy or any other neurologic disorder.

Drug Interactions

Clonidine, because it is given by epidural, has no direct drug interactions. However, if a patient also takes another drug for blood pressure management, even epidural clonidine can make hypotension worse.

Tramadol has CNS and brain effects; therefore the sedating and other CNS effects are made worse with alcohol, antianxiety drugs, skeletal muscle relaxants, barbiturates, many drugs used for psychiatric disorders, and opioid analgesics. Be sure to determine which other drugs the patient also takes.

❖ Nursing Implications and Patient Teaching

◆ *Assessment.* Assess the patient's pain in the same way as for opioid agonists or any other type of pain-management drugs. Ask the patient whether he or she has ever taken any of these specific drugs and whether any problems resulted from taking it. Also ask what other over-the-counter and prescribed drugs the patient has taken in the past 24 hours. For tramadol, determine whether the patient has a known seizure disorder or any other neurologic problem. If such a disorder is present, hold the dose and notify the prescribing healthcare provider.

Planning, implementation, evaluation, and patient and family teaching activities are the same as for opioid analgesics.

ACETAMINOPHEN

Acetaminophen (Abenol, Atasol, Panadol, Tylenol, and many others) is a common drug used for pain relief. It can be purchased over the counter as a single drug or combined with other substances such as caffeine and aspirin (Excedrin). When combined with other pain-control drugs, especially opioid agonists, acetaminophen requires a prescription.

It can be given orally in tablets, capsules, or liquids, or rectally in a suppository. A special formulation (Ofirmev) is available as an intravenous infusion.

Action

Acetaminophen acts only in the brain to reduce the production of prostaglandins, a body chemical that can cause inflammation in other body areas. In the brain, prostaglandins increases the perception of pain. By reducing the amount of prostaglandins in the brain, perception of pain is reduced. Acetaminophen does not act at the site of an injury that is causing pain and does not have anti-inflammatory actions.

Uses

Acetaminophen alone is used to manage mild-to-moderate pain. It is often used for infants and children to reduce fever. In combination with other pain-control drugs, acetaminophen can help manage more severe pain. It is often used in place of aspirin or other NSAIDs for pain because acetaminophen does not increase the risk for bleeding. Also, children should not take aspirin because of its association with development of Reye syndrome. Acetaminophen comes in liquid, tablet, and capsule forms. The usual adult dose is 325 to 650 mg every 4 to 6 hours and should not exceed 3 g total daily. For children the usual dose is 7 to 15 mg/kg every 4 hours. The maximum total daily dose for children varies with the child's weight.

> 🔷 **Top Tip for Safety**
>
> Acetaminophen has a maximum daily total dose to prevent organ damage.

Expected Side Effects

Side effects of acetaminophen are rare when it is taken at the recommended dosages, although an allergic reaction is always possible. The most common side effects are nausea and skin rash.

Adverse Reactions

One problem with acetaminophen is that because it is available without a prescription, people often believe that it has no adverse effects, which is *not* true. When taken at higher doses or for prolonged periods, acetaminophen is toxic to the liver, which can be damaged or destroyed. This is why there is a maximum total daily dose for this drug.

Drug Interactions

Many common over-the-counter drugs for sleep, colds, headaches, and allergies contain acetaminophen as one of the ingredients. These additional sources of acetaminophen must be added when calculating the total daily dose of acetaminophen. Liver damage occurs more rapidly when acetaminophen is taken with alcohol.

> **Top Tip for Safety**
>
> Acetaminophen can be toxic to the liver and should not be taken by anyone who already has liver health problems.

❖ Nursing Implications and Patient Teaching

◆ *Assessment.* Assess the patient's pain in the same way as for any other type of pain-management drug. Ask the patient whether he or she has ever taken acetaminophen (you may have to use the most common brand name in your area, such as Tylenol) and whether any problems resulted from taking it. Also ask what other over-the-counter and prescribed drugs the patient has taken in the past 24 hours.

◆ *Planning and implementation.* Liquid oral acetaminophen comes in many strengths. Some liquid forms contain as few as 16 mg/mL, and others may contain as much as 70 mg/mL. *Carefully check the strength to ensure the correct dosage, especially with infants and children. If you are not sure of your dosage calculations, check with another nurse, healthcare provider, or pharmacist.* Acetaminophen can be given with or without food because it does not increase the risk for stomach ulcers.

◆ *Evaluation.* Within an hour after giving acetaminophen, assess the patient's pain level to determine effectiveness. Also ask the patient whether he or she noticed any other changes that may indicate a sensitivity to acetaminophen.

◆ *Patient and family teaching.* Tell the patient and the family the following:

- Take acetaminophen as prescribed by your healthcare provider and not more often or at higher dosages.
- Many over-the-counter drugs for colds, headache, allergies, and sleep aids also contain acetaminophen, as do some other drugs prescribed for pain. The acetaminophen in these drugs must be figured into the total maximum daily dose of 3 g for an adult along with any separate acetaminophen.
- Do not drink alcoholic beverages on days when you take acetaminophen or any drug that contains acetaminophen to prevent liver damage.

> **Lifespan Considerations**
>
> **Pediatric**
>
> An infant or young child should never receive an adult dose of acetaminophen because of its severe liver toxicity. Teach parents to read the label on liquid acetaminophen bottles for infants and small children very carefully to ensure the correct dose for the child's size. Teach parents to call the nearest pharmacy and talk with the pharmacist to ensure that the dose is correct if they are unsure what dose to give.

MISCELLANEOUS DRUGS FOR PAIN MANAGEMENT

Miscellaneous analgesics are drugs that have specific purposes and actions for other health problems but can help provide relief for certain types of pain. These drugs can help reduce a person's perception of pain and often enhance the pain-management effectiveness of other analgesics. They may be used alone or in combination with opioids. The most outstanding feature of nonopioid analgesics is that they are *not* chemically or structurally similar to opioids. As a result, they have less potential for dependence and addiction. Many of these nonopioid analgesics have other uses and are discussed in more detail elsewhere in this text. An overview of how they work and are used in pain control is provided in this section.

Regardless of category, nursing responsibilities when giving nonopioid analgesics are the same as those described for opioid agonists. Pain assessment and determination of effectiveness in managing pain are still necessary.

> **Memory Jogger**
>
> Common miscellaneous drugs and classes of drugs used for pain management include:
> - acetaminophen
> - corticosteroids
> - NSAIDs
> - skeletal muscle relaxants
> - antidepressants
> - anticonvulsants

CORTICOSTEROIDS

Inflammation usually causes pain. When tissue injury occurs, such as when you hit your thumb with a hammer or when you have a tooth pulled, the injured tissues release chemicals that start the inflammatory processes. These chemicals bind to pain receptors in the area and send pain signals along the nerve tracts to the brain. Also, these chemicals make the pain receptors more sensitive to any other stimulus. So even just touching the inflamed area can increase the pain.

Corticosteroids are drugs with powerful anti-inflammatory actions that are chemically similar to the cortisol hormones secreted by the adrenal glands. These drugs are able to greatly inhibit the production of mediators that result in the actions and symptoms of inflammation. However, they have many side effects and adverse effects that limit their use for pain. The two most common oral corticosteroids used for pain are prednisone and methyl prednisolone. Corticosteroids can be given intravenously, topically, and as an epidural injection (usually for acute back pain). Chapter 12 provides a complete discussion of the actions and uses of corticosteroids, as well as the nursing responsibilities.

NSAIDs

NSAIDs are nonopioid analgesics that have the main action of reducing inflammation. NSAIDs can help manage pain associated with inflammation, bone pain, cancer pain, and soft tissue trauma. Just like corticosteroids, NSAIDs drugs actually act at the tissue where pain starts and do not change a person's perception of pain.

NSAIDs help stop tissue production of the chemicals of inflammation and reduce the symptoms of inflammation (pain, warmth, redness, swelling, and reduced use) in the area of injury. With inflammation reduced, pain also is reduced. Many NSAIDs are available over the counter and are commonly used for mild-to-moderate pain. Some of these same NSAIDs at higher dosages per tablet or capsule, as well as the stronger NSAIDs, require a prescription and are used for pain for only a limited period. Mild NSAIDs include salicylic acid (aspirin), ibuprofen (Advil, Motrin), and naproxen (Aleve, Anaprox, Naprosyn). Stronger NSAIDs include oxaprozin (Daypro), indomethacin (Indocin), nabumetone (Relafen), ketorolac (Toradol), piroxicam (Feldene), celecoxib (Celebrex), and meloxicam (Mobic). All NSAIDs work in much the same way and have many of the same adverse effects. Chapter 12 provides a complete discussion of the actions and uses of NSAIDs, as well as the nursing responsibilities.

The most common NSAID in use today is salicylic acid, aspirin, which is available over the counter. A side effect of aspirin and many other NSAIDs is increased risk for bleeding. Aspirin affects blood clotting longer than do other NSAIDs. Other adverse effects include irritation of the stomach and intestinal tract, allergic reactions, and asthma. Stronger NSAIDs can raise blood pressure, cause water retention, and can damage the kidney. Aspirin should never be given to infants or children because of its association with the development of a very serious health problem known as Reye syndrome.

Lifespan Considerations

Pediatric

Aspirin should never be given to infants or children because of its association with the development of a very serious health problem known as Reye syndrome. This disorder often leads to mental deficits, coma, or death.

SKELETAL MUSCLE RELAXANTS

Skeletal muscles contract under nerve stimulation to allow you to move. So when you want to stand up from a sitting position, the motor area of your brain triggers the nerves that specifically control the muscles of your legs so that only those muscles contract for you to straighten your legs enough to lift you to a standing position. If for some reason the nerves connecting your brain to your leg muscles are not working, the muscles will not contract and no movement occurs.

A *skeletal muscle spasm* is an unwanted overcontraction of one or more muscles. This often occurs when nerves controlling contraction to a specific muscle send an inappropriate signal to that muscle. Common causes of inappropriate nerve signals include pressure on the nerve, swelling along the nerve path, and low blood calcium levels. Spasms also occur when a muscle is irritated or damaged. Pain from a spasm in a large muscle can be intense. If you have ever had a charley horse in your calf, you know how painful a muscle spasm can be.

Action

Skeletal muscle relaxants are drugs that act by depressing the CNS to reduce muscle spasms. This action slows signal transmission along motor nerves, which results in reduced muscle spasms and less muscle pain. The most commonly prescribed muscle relaxants are methocarbamol (Robaxin) and cyclobenzaprine (Flexeril) (Table 11.5).

Table 11.5 Dosages and Nursing Implications for Common Skeletal Muscle Relaxants

Skeletal muscle relaxants relieve the pain associated with muscle spasms by slowing contraction signal transmission in motor nerves.

DRUG/ADULT DOSAGE RANGE	NURSING IMPLICATIONS
methocarbamol (Robaxin) 1.5 g orally every 6 hours or 1 g IM/IV every 8 hours cyclobenzaprine (Flexeril) 5–10 mg orally every 8 hours	• Before giving the first dose of either of these skeletal muscle relaxants, ask whether the patient has a seizure disorder because these drugs lower the seizure threshold. • Check the dose of methocarbamol carefully because it is in grams, not milligrams. • Instruct patients who are taking extended-release tablets or capsules not to chew, open, crush, bite, or cut them, to prevent rapid absorption of excess drug. • Instruct patients not to drink alcohol or take other CNS depressants while on a skeletal muscle relaxant because the CNS effects are intensified.

Uses

Skeletal muscle relaxants are used for pain and insomnia when excessive skeletal muscle contractions or spasms contribute to these problems in adults. They are not usually used for children.

Expected Side Effects

Common side effects of methocarbamol are flushing, low blood pressure, slow heart rate, and fainting. Common side effects of cyclobenzaprine are dizziness, headache, dry mouth, blurred vision, and urinary retention.

Adverse Reactions

Serious adverse effects of methocarbamol are a high risk for allergic reactions and temporary memory loss (amnesia). It lowers the seizure threshold. Serious adverse effects of cyclobenzaprine are cardiac dysrhythmias and prolonged cardiac conduction. Cyclobenzaprine is not to be used in a patient who is recovering from a heart attack or who has a heart rhythm problem. It also should not be given to a patient who takes a monoamine oxidase inhibitor drug (which is usually used for psychiatric disorders) because of the risk for severe high blood pressure and high fever. Cyclobenzaprine also lowers the seizure threshold.

> ### ⌂ Top Tip for Safety
>
> Methocarbamol and cyclobenzaprine should not be given to anyone who has a seizure disorder because these drugs lower the seizure threshold.

Drug Interactions

The sedating and other CNS effects are made worse with alcohol, antianxiety drugs, skeletal muscle relaxants, barbiturates, many drugs used for psychiatric disorders, and opioid analgesics because skeletal muscle relaxants have CNS and brain effects. Be sure to determine which other drugs the patient also takes.

❖ Nursing Implications and Patient Teaching

◆ *Assessment.* Before giving a muscle relaxant to a patient for the first time, assess the level of consciousness, cognition, and skeletal muscle reactivity. Also ask the patient whether he or she has a seizure disorder or has ever had a seizure in the past because these drugs lower the seizure threshold.

Before giving the first dose of cyclobenzaprine, assess the patient's blood pressure and radial and apical pulses for any skipped beats, extra beats, or any other type of irregular heartbeat.

> ### ⌂ Top Tip for Safety
>
> Assess patients for irregularities before giving cyclobenzaprine. If you find any persistent heartbeat irregularity, notify the healthcare provider before giving the drug.

◆ *Planning and implementation.* After giving either muscle relaxant, assess for level of consciousness and degree of muscle relaxation or muscle weakness. Patients often become very drowsy and may fall. Raise the side rails and remind the patient to call for help to get out of bed.

Help the patient change position slowly because these drugs can cause a sudden lowering of blood pressure. Teach him or her to sit for a few minutes on the side of the bed before attempting to get up. Help the patient during walking to prevent falling.

Methocarbamol and cyclobenzaprine can both cause urinary retention. If a patient who is receiving one of these drugs has an enlarged prostate gland or is also taking a drug for overactive bladder, assess for signs or symptoms of urine retention. Symptoms include difficulty starting the urine stream, weak urine stream, and bulge in the lower abdomen.

◆ *Evaluation.* After giving the first dose of cyclobenzaprine, assess the patient's radial and apical pulses hourly for any skipped beats, extra beats, or any other type of irregular heartbeat. If you find persistent irregularity, notify the healthcare provider. Assess the patient's degree of comfort and muscle reflexes to determine effectiveness.

◆ *Patient and family teaching.* Tell the patient and family the following:

- These drugs are to be taken only on a short-term basis. Usually the drugs are prescribed for 2 to 3 weeks because of their potential for abuse.
- Just like for any substance that causes sedation, avoid operating any dangerous equipment, driving a car, or making critical decisions while under the influence of these drugs.
- Avoid alcohol because the sedation effect of these drugs is potentiated by alcohol.
- If you are taking cyclobenzaprine take your pulse daily and report new-onset, persistent irregularities to your healthcare provider. Go to the nearest emergency department or call 911 if you develop shortness of breath or chest pain.

ANTIDEPRESSANTS

Antidepressant drugs that improve long-term sense of sadness can reduce some types of chronic pain and cancer pain, especially *neuropathic* nerve pain with tingling and burning sensations. The most common antidepressants used for pain management are amitriptyline (Elavil), nortriptyline (Pamelor), paroxetine (Paxil), and sertraline (Zoloft). The oral doses of these drugs for pain management are often different than the doses used to manage depression. Antidepressants work for pain management by increasing the amount of natural opioids (endorphins and enkephalins) in the brain and also by reducing the depression that often occurs with chronic pain. Usually the patient must take an antidepressant for 1 or 2 weeks before he or she feels any relief from pain. Chapter 10 provides more discussion of the actions and uses of antidepressants, as well as the nursing responsibilities.

> **Memory Jogger**
>
> Common antidepressants used for pain management include:
> - amitriptyline
> - nortriptyline
> - paroxetine
> - sertraline

ANTICONVULSANTS

Anticonvulsants are drugs that work in the brain to reduce seizures. Some have been found to reduce neuropathic pain (nerve pain with tingling and burning)

and migraine headaches. The two most common anticonvulsants used for pain management are gabapentin (Neurontin) and pregabalin (Lyrica). They appear to work by reducing the rate of pain signal transmission along sensory nerves and may also affect pain perception. The doses for pain management are often higher than those used to manage seizure disorders. Chapter 9 discusses the actions and nursing responsibilities of anticonvulsants.

> **Memory Jogger**
>
> Two common antidepressants used for pain management are:
> - gabapentin
> - pregabalin

Get Ready for the NCLEX® Examination!

Key Points

- Pain is whatever the patient says it is, occurs whenever the patient says it occurs, and is the intensity the patient states.
- Opioid agonists only change the *perception* of pain; they do nothing at the site of injured tissues to reduce the cause of pain.
- Opioid agonist analgesics work by binding tightly to the mu opioid receptor in the brain and activating it.
- Strong opioid agonist analgesics (e.g., hydromorphone and fentanyl) require less drug (lower dosages) to result in the same level of pain relief as weaker opioid agonist analgesics.
- All opioid drugs are considered high-alert drugs because they have an increased risk for causing patient harm when given in error.
- Tolerance and dependence on opioid agonist analgesics are common and are not the same as addiction.
- Pain is best relieved when any type of analgesic is given on a schedule before the patient's pain becomes severe.
- Older adults may require opioid agonist dosages to be lower or the drugs given less frequently because of age-related changes in liver and kidney function.
- Do not give tramadol for any patient who has a seizure disorder (epilepsy) or any other neurologic disorder because this drug can induce seizures.
- A variety of drugs that are used as therapy for other health problems, such as inflammation, seizures, psychiatric disorders, and muscle spasms, can also help relieve some types of pain.
- Acetaminophen can be toxic to the liver and should not be taken by anyone who already has liver health problems.
- An infant or young child should never receive an adult dose of acetaminophen because of its severe liver toxicity.

- Corticosteroids have many side effects and adverse effects that limit their use in pain management.
- Aspirin and other NSAIDs interfere with blood clotting and increase the risk for excessive bleeding.
- Aspirin should never be given to infants or children because of its association with the development of a very serious health problem known as Reye syndrome.
- Methocarbamol and cyclobenzaprine should not be given to anyone who has a seizure disorder because these drugs lower the seizure threshold.
- Antidepressants and anticonvulsants can help reduce some types of pain, especially neuropathic pain.
- When antidepressants or anticonvulsants are used in pain management, the dosages are usually different from when they are used to manage depression or seizures.

Review Questions for the NCLEX® Examination

1. Which symptoms do you expect to find in a patient with chronic pain?
   1. Well-defined areas of burning, aching, or throbbing pain
   2. Symptoms are difficult to describe and are present continually
   3. Increased heart rate and blood pressure
   4. Sweating and dry mouth

2. Which side effects are expected with opioid agonist analgesics? (Select all that apply.)
   1. Aggression
   2. Slower breathing
   3. Constipation
   4. Drooling
   5. Euphoria
   6. Smaller pupils
   7. Sedation
   8. Hallucinations

Get Ready for the NCLEX® Examination!—cont'd

3. Which action will you suggest for a patient who reports feeling nauseated after taking an oral opioid agonist for pain?
   1. Tell the patient to take the drug with food.
   2. Ask the prescriber for a parenteral form of the drug.
   3. Tell the patient that the nausea will go away after a few doses of the drug.
   4. Remind the patient that nausea is less of a problem than is the sensation of acute pain.

4. In reviewing the health problems of a patient who is prescribed extra-strength acetaminophen for pain after a dental procedure, which problems may indicate a possible reason to avoid this drug? (Select all that apply.)
   1. Asthma
   2. Bruises easily
   3. Chronic alcoholism
   4. Diabetes mellitus
   5. Liver disease
   6. Patient is also taking oral contraceptives
   7. Patient is also taking a drug that disrupts blood clotting

5. The patient is prescribed to take an antidepressant for neuropathic pain. The patient tells you that this must be a mistake because he does not have depression. What is your best response?
   1. Explain that the antidepressant was prescribed because it is less likely that he will become addicted to it than to other painkillers.
   2. Remind him that all patients who are having significant pain are depressed to some degree even if he does not recognize it.
   3. Explain that the antidepressant works by increasing chemicals in the brain that are helpful in relieving pain.
   4. Reassure him that you will contact his healthcare provider and report that he is not depressed.

6. Which class of drugs for pain management controls pain by changing the cellular response at the site of the cause of pain?
   1. Opioid agonist-antagonists
   2. Skeletal muscle relaxants
   3. Opioid agonists
   4. NSAIDs

7. What is the most important question to ask a patient who is newly prescribed cyclobenzaprine for pain before giving the first dose?
   1. "Have you ever had a seizure?"
   2. "How often do you drink alcohol?"
   3. "When did you last have a bowel movement?"
   4. "Are you currently taking any over-the-counter drugs for pain?"

8. The patient taking a prescribed NSAID for chronic arthritis pain now has all of the following symptoms. Which one will you report to the prescriber immediately?
   1. Increased headaches
   2. Bloody stools
   3. Joint pain
   4. Difficulty sleeping

9. How much oral codeine would be needed for a patient to obtain the same degree of pain relief that 30 mg of oral morphine would provide?
   1. 20 mg
   2. 75 mg
   3. 150 mg
   4. 200 mg

10. What is the most important action to take after giving any analgesic for pain?
    1. Assess the patient's likelihood for addiction.
    2. Assess the patient for nightmares or hallucinations.
    3. Ask the patient to rate his or her degree of pain relief.
    4. Ask the patient to count backward by threes to assess cognition.

Drug Calculation Review

1. An infant is to receive 80 mg acetaminophen (Tylenol). The liquid you have on hand has a concentration of 100 mg/mL.
   1. How many mL is the correct dose for this infant? ___mL
   2. How many mL is the correct dose if the liquid has a concentration of 120 mg/5 mL? ___mL

2. A patient is to receive 15 mg morphine IM now for pain. The available drug is morphine sulfate 10 mg/mL. How many mL is the correct dose for this patient? ___mL

Case Study: Critical Thinking Activity

Mr. Blue is a 62-year-old man who lives alone. He was admitted 4 days ago to an extended care facility on his third postoperative day from a right total knee replacement for care and rehabilitation until he can safely care for himself at home. He is prescribed hydrocodone with acetaminophen (Vicodin) for pain control. The prescription reads: "Vicodin (5 mg hydrocodone; 300 mg acetaminophen) one to two tablets every 4 to 6 hours as needed for pain." He tells you that overall his pain is not bad except when he comes back from physical therapy. Then it is "really roaring." He also says he tries to take the drug just at that time so that he does not become addicted.

1. What type of pain is he having?
2. How will you know the severity of "really roaring" pain?
3. What specific type of drug is Vicodin?
4. What type of change(s) could be made in drug delivery with the current prescription to help relieve his pain more effectively?
5. What will you tell him about his potential for addiction?
6. If he were to receive two Vicodin tablets every 4 hours around the clock, what would be his total dose of acetaminophen for the day?

Learning Outcomes

1. List the names, actions, and possible adverse effects of NSAIDs.
2. Explain what to teach patients and families about anti-inflammatory drugs (NSAIDs).
3. List the names, actions, and possible adverse effects of corticosteroid-based anti-inflammatory drugs.
4. Explain what to teach patients and families about corticosteroid-based anti-inflammatory drugs.
5. List the names, actions, and possible adverse effects of disease-modifying antirheumatic drugs for management of arthritis and other inflammatory disorders.

6. Explain what to teach patients and families about disease-modifying antirheumatic drugs for management of arthritis and other inflammatory disorders.
7. List the names, actions, and possible adverse effects of antigout drugs.
8. Explain what to teach patients and families about antigout drugs.

Key Terms

antigout drug (p. 237) These drugs are used to prevent gout and shorten gout attacks. For gout prevention, they must be taken daily.

anti-inflammatory drug (N-tī-ĭn-FLĂ-mě-tōr-ē, p. 226) The primary purpose of these drugs is to reduce pain and prevent or limit the tissue and blood vessel responses to injury or invasion.

corticosteroids (kōr-tĭ-kō-'STĚR-oid, p. 230) These drugs, also known as glucocorticoids, prevent or limit inflammation by slowing or stopping all known pathways of inflammatory cytokine production. They are similar to the natural cortisol hormones secreted by the adrenal gland that are necessary for life.

disease-modifying antirheumatic drug (DMARD) (p. 235) These drugs reduce the progression and tissue destruction of the inflammatory disease process, especially rheumatoid arthritis, by inhibiting TNF.

nonsteroidal anti-inflammatory drug (NSAID) (nŏn-stě-RŌĬ-děl ĂN-tī-ĭn-FLĂ-mě-tōr-ē, p. 227) These drugs prevent or limit the tissue and blood vessel responses to injury by slowing the production of one or more inflammatory mediators. They are divided into two categories: (1) *nonselective NSAIDs* that inhibit the actions of both COX-1 and COX-2, and (2) *selective NSAIDs* that have more inhibitory effects on the COX-2 enzyme and fewer effects on the COX-1 enzyme.

INFLAMMATION CAUSES AND ACTION

Inflammation is a predictable set of tissue and blood vessel actions caused by white blood cells (WBCs; *leukocytes*) and their products as a response to injury or infection. These tissue and blood vessel actions cause the five major symptoms of inflammation: pain, redness, warmth, swelling, and loss of function. For example, think about having a severely sprained ankle. With the sprain, you can have redness, warmth, and pain. In addition, you cannot walk well on the ankle (loss of function). Although inflammation can be uncomfortable, it is a normal reaction of the body to tissue injury and is generally protective. However, when inflammation lasts a long time or occurs without tissue injury (or invasion by bacteria and other organisms), it is an overreaction that can damage and even destroy tissues over time.

> **Memory Jogger**
>
> The five main symptoms of inflammation are pain, redness, warmth, swelling, and loss of function.

When an injury occurs (continuing with the sprained ankle example), the damaged tissues and WBCs in the ankle release inflammatory chemical *mediators* that cause certain actions to occur. These mediators, which are important in starting and continuing inflammation, include kinins, prostaglandins (PGs), histamine, and tumor necrosis factor (TNF). Some mediators, especially histamine, act on blood vessels in the injured area,

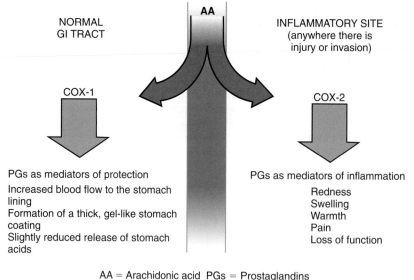

AA = Arachidonic acid PGs = Prostaglandins
COX-1 = Cyclooxygenase 1 COX-2 = Cyclooxygenase 2

FIG. 12.1 Arachidonic acid (AA) cascade resulting from injured cells. You can see the influence of the cyclooxygenase enzymes. (From Workman ML, LaCharity LA: *Understanding pharmacology*, ed 2, St. Louis, 2016, Elsevier.)

causing them to dilate and leak fluid from the capillaries. This results in redness and warmth of the tissues. Increased blood flow brings more WBCs to injured tissues, and the leaking capillaries cause swelling. Released kinins trigger pain receptors in nerve endings, which makes the area painful. This pain lets you know an injury has occurred so that you will take steps to protect your ankle from more harm.

As more WBCs come to the injured area, the arachidonic acid (AA) cascade increases the inflammatory response (Fig. 12.1). This begins by converting fat from injured cell membranes into AA. Then the enzyme *cyclooxygenase* (COX) converts AA into many mediators, especially different types of PGs. There are two forms of the COX enzyme: COX-1 and COX-2. COX-1 is present in all cells and makes PGs that are helpful and protective (think of COX-1 as "good COX"). For example, COX-1 in stomach lining cells makes PGs that produce thick mucus. The mucus protects the stomach lining from being harmed by the gastric acids needed for food digestion. In contrast, COX-2 is present mainly in areas of inflammation. COX-2 is responsible for the types of PGs and other mediators that start and continue the inflammation response (think of COX-2 as "bad COX").

Although uncomfortable, inflammation responses also help injured tissue to regain function. WBCs release *growth factors* that trigger repair of damaged tissues and cells by stimulating healthy cells in the injured area to divide and replace dead or damaged cells, and by promoting scar tissue formation in tissues that can no longer divide. It is important to remember that scar tissue does not act or function like normal tissue.

Although inflammation is mostly a protective process that helps prevent infection and promote healing, it can cause serious and sometimes painful tissue damage if it goes on for too long or occurs when it is not needed. For example, some people experience development of autoimmune diseases in which the immune system fails to recognize normal body cells and attacks some tissues continually with inflammation. One such disease is rheumatoid arthritis. The chronic inflammation in the joints with excessive and continual release of mediators (especially TNF) causes destruction of joint cartilage and other normal joint tissues, resulting in severe pain and greatly reduced joint function. Over time the person can lose all function in one or more joints and have very limited mobility along with chronic pain.

Bookmark This!

Here are some useful websites regarding inflammatory disorders and their treatment:
  National Institute of Arthritis and Musculoskeletal and Skin Disorders: https://www.niams.nih.gov
  Arthritis Foundation: http://www.arthritis.org
  Centers for Disease Control and Prevention Arthritis: https://www.cdc.gov/arthritis

INFLAMMATION MANAGEMENT

Many acute problems that cause inflammation, such as sprains, fractures, or tears, require short-term therapy with **anti-inflammatory drugs**. These drugs have as their primary purpose to reduce pain and prevent or limit the tissue and blood vessel responses to injury or invasion. On the other hand, a variety of chronic inflammatory disorders, such as arthritis, may require long-term therapy with anti-inflammatory drugs. The long-term therapy is prescribed to reduce symptoms of inflammation and prevent tissue-damaging complications. It is important to recognize that most of these drugs, whether used for short-term or long-term inflammation, can have serious adverse reactions, and patient response to therapy must be closely monitored.

A variety of drug categories—nonsteroidal anti-inflammatory drugs (NSAIDs), corticosteroids, disease-modifying antirheumatic drugs (DMARDs), and antigout drugs—are useful in managing acute and chronic inflammatory conditions. As mentioned in Chapter 11, one of the symptoms of inflammation is pain. Often when inflammation is managed, pain is also relieved to some degree. Thus anti-inflammatory drugs are also prescribed for pain management. For inflammation caused by gout, management also includes drugs that reduce the production of uric acid, the cause of gout.

NSAIDs

Actions

NSAIDs are able to prevent or limit the tissue and blood vessel responses to injury by slowing the production of one or more inflammatory mediators. NSAIDs are divided into two categories: (1) *nonselective NSAIDs* that inhibit the actions of both COX-1 and COX-2, and (2) *selective NSAIDs* that have more inhibitory effects on the COX-2 enzyme and fewer effects on the COX-1 enzyme (Fig. 12.2).

Nonselective COX inhibitors (e.g., aspirin, ibuprofen, and other NSAIDs) disrupt *both* COX-1 and COX-2 enzymes (see Fig. 12.2). So the nonselective COX inhibitors can block the protective and helpful cellular COX-1 effects (in other words, they block the "good COX"), as well as reduce the inflammation associated with activation of COX-2 (the "bad COX"). As a result, nonselective NSAIDs have more side effects than selective COX-2 inhibitor NSAIDs (those that affect only COX-2). Regardless of whether an NSAID is selective or nonselective, they all have the same anti-inflammatory action: reducing the production of PGs, kinins, histamine, TNF, and other inflammation mediators from AA. These effects produce the analgesic, anti-inflammatory, and *antipyretic* (fever-reducing) effects associated with NSAIDs.

The oldest NSAID still in use today is aspirin (acetylsalicylic acid [ASA]), which has a salicylate chemical structure. This chemical was first extracted from the bark and root of the white willow tree and has been used as an anti-inflammatory agent for centuries. More is known about aspirin from such longtime use, so it is considered the classic NSAID to which all other NSAIDs are compared. Aspirin is a salicylate, but different chemicals are used as the drug base in other NSAIDs. They work in the same way as aspirin but have different strengths and expected side effects and adverse effects.

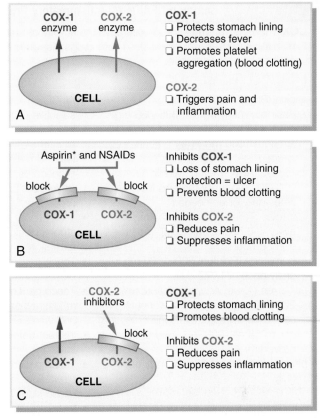

*Aspirin is only one of the NSAIDs.

FIG. 12.2 Basic actions of selective and nonselective NSAIDS. (A) Normally cells produce the enzymes cyclooxygenase 1 (COX-1) and cyclooxygenase 2 (COX-2). The enzymes cause chemical reactions with specific functions You can consider COX-1 enzymes as "good COX" such that they have the positive effects, whereas COX-2 (or "bad COX") enzymes have negative effects. (B) Aspirin and other nonselective NSAIDs block *both* the good COX (COX-1) and the bad COX (COX-2). While you reduce pain and suppress inflammation, you also can get the negative side effects. (C) Selective COX-2 inhibitors primarily block the COX-2 enzyme, so they have fewer side effects at normal doses. (From Kee JL, Hayes ER, McCuistion LE: *Pharmacology*, ed 8, St. Louis, 2015, Saunders.)

Some other earlier nonselective NSAIDs were more potent than aspirin but also had some very harsh side effects that limited their use. For example, colchicine and indomethacin are rarely prescribed today. Newer NSAIDs and other types of targeted therapies have also reduced the need to use these drugs. Table 12.1 lists the most common NSAIDs in use today.

Uses

NSAIDs are used as first-line therapy to treat a variety of illnesses, often associated with pain and/or fever. Pain in the muscles, nerves, and joints (myalgias, neuralgias, and arthralgias, respectively), as well as headache and dysmenorrhea, are commonly treated with NSAIDs. Various forms of arthritis, such as rheumatoid arthritis, osteoarthritis, and psoriatic arthritis, may be responsive to NSAIDs for pain and other symptoms of inflammation. NSAIDs are also used short-term for pain management from dental extraction,

Table 12.1   Common NSAIDs for Inflammatory Problems

COX-1 inhibitors: These drugs decrease the activity of both COX-1 and COX-2 to reduce the formation of inflammatory mediators from arachidonic acid. These drugs disrupt the normal functions of other products from arachidonic acid that are helpful and protective.

DRUGS/ADULT DOSAGE RANGE	NURSING IMPLICATIONS
aspirin (Bayer aspirin, Ecotrin, Aspirtab, many others) 325–650 mg every 4–6 hours as needed; extra strength 1000 mg every 6 hours as needed ibuprofen (Advil, Motrin, Midol) 200–800 mg orally three to four times daily or as needed ketorolac (Toradol) oral: 10–20 mg every 4–6 hours; IM: 15–30 mg every 6 hours. nabumetone (Relafen) 500–1000 mg orally once or twice daily naproxen (Aleve, Anaprox, Naprosyn) 220-500 mg orally every 12 hours; controlled release tablets initial dose 750 or 1000 mg orally once daily. piroxicam (Feldene) 20 mg orally once daily	• All COX-1/COX-2 inhibitors have more side effects at lower doses than do selective COX-2 inhibitors. • Warn patients that these drugs all increase the risk for bleeding because they all interfere with the platelet function of the clotting process. • Remind patients to stop taking aspirin 1 week before dental or surgical procedures, and other COX-1/COX-2 inhibitors at least 2–4 days before dental or surgical procedures because of the increased risk for bleeding from the procedure. • Tell patients to report stomach/abdominal pain or any signs of blood in the stool to their prescriber because these drugs all increase the risk for GI ulcer formation. • Teach patients not to take NSAIDs while taking warfarin because the risk for bleeding is then so severe that hemorrhage and strokes are likely. • Teach patients who are taking any NSAID except aspirin to weigh themselves at least twice weekly and keep a record because these drugs increase salt and water retention, which can worsen heart failure and raise blood pressure. • Instruct patients to take any NSAID with food to help prevent stomach irritation. • Teach patients to drink 2–3 L of fluid daily while on NSAIDs to ensure good blood flow to the kidneys because all of these drugs, except aspirin, can cause kidney damage. • Instruct patients who have diabetes to check blood sugar levels more often because these drugs increase the risk for hypoglycemia (low blood sugar) in patients who take oral antidiabetic drugs. • Teach patients to take the prescribed NSAIDs on a regular schedule because inflammation is better relieved when there is a stable blood level of the drug.

COX-2 inhibitors: These drugs are more selective and mostly inhibit the COX-2 arachidonic acid production of inflammatory mediators. Although the same side effects are possible as with the COX-1/COX-2 inhibitors, they usually occur only at higher dosages or with prolonged use.

DRUG/ADULT DOSAGE RANGE	NURSING IMPLICATIONS
celecoxib (Celebrex) 100–400 mg orally daily. May be in one to two divided doses meloxicam (Mobic) 7.5–15 mg orally once daily; capsules 5–10 mg orally once daily	• Before the first dose of celecoxib, ask whether the patient has an allergy to sulfa-based antibiotics because a patient allergic to sulfa is likely to also be allergic to celecoxib (it contains a chemical similar to sulfa). • Suggest to the patient that they should take these drugs with a full glass of water or a small amount of food to reduce GI upset. • Teach patients to take a COX-2 inhibitor exactly as prescribed because higher doses will result in the same side effects and adverse reactions as the COX-1/COX-2 inhibitors. • Avoid giving these drugs to anyone who has angina, who smokes, or who has severe coronary artery disease because they increase clot formation and the risk for heart attacks.

COX-1, Cyclooxygenase 1; *COX-2,* cyclooxygenase 2.

minor surgery, and soft tissue athletic injuries. Although many NSAIDs are available over the counter, they are still potentially dangerous drugs, and great care should be taken to avoid overdose. Larger doses must be obtained from a licensed prescriber and monitored very carefully.

As a side note, nonselective NSAIDs, particularly aspirin, inhibit platelet clumping or aggregation. This effect is very helpful when used in low doses for patients with coronary heart disease. Nevertheless, the effect on platelets can also lead to an increased risk for bleeding, particularly at higher doses. For NSAIDs other than aspirin, platelet inhibition is dose related and reversible. Patients who take aspirin must be monitored for bleeding because of irreversible platelet inhibition for the lifespan of the platelet, for as long as 7 to 8 days. This is very important if a patient is scheduled for an invasive procedure or surgery, so make sure to notify the prescriber if the patient has an upcoming surgery.

Nonselective NSAIDs inhibit both the COX-1 and COX-2. Selective NSAIDs primarily inhibit the COX-2 and thus have fewer side and adverse effects.

Expected Side Effects

Common side effects of nonselective NSAIDs are heartburn, nausea, vomiting, dizziness, headache, and increased risk for bleeding and bruising. The GI effects may be minimized or avoided if the drug is taken with at least a full glass of water. If the drug does cause mild GI upset, the patient may take the drug with a small amount of food or milk. All NSAIDs except aspirin can cause some degree of fluid retention, edema formation, and even raise blood pressure. This is particularly important to note in that NSAIDs should be avoided in patients who have high blood pressure, heart failure, or renal failure. Selective NSAIDs (the COX-2 inhibitors) have fewer GI effects because they do not impact the protective effects associated with the COX-1 enzyme.

Adverse Reactions

Although expected side effects are often bothersome to the patient, they typically can be managed and the patient can continue taking the drug. Adverse reactions, however, must be recognized and reported to the prescriber immediately, and the drug will most likely be discontinued. Several adverse reactions may occur in patients who are taking NSAIDs. These reactions include allergy (from mild symptoms of rash and shortness of breath to anaphylaxis), renal failure, GI bleeding (upper or lower), and blood disorders. Patients who are taking COX-2 inhibitors may have an increased risk for myocardial infarction and stroke, so it is important to recognize symptoms associated with those disorders. It is important to note that patients allergic to one nonaspirin NSAID may be allergic to another because of cross-sensitivity. Although this is generally rare, it is very important to note all allergies in the medical record and report to the prescriber before giving the drug.

Aspirin has been associated with the occurrence of *Reye syndrome* when given to children suffering from a viral infection such as varicella (chickenpox) or influenza. In Reye syndrome, symptoms may affect all organs of the body, but most seriously affected are the brain and liver. It can even lead to permanent brain damage and death. Thus the use of aspirin is avoided in children, especially those who have an acute illness.

🍁 **Lifespan Considerations**

Pediatric

Aspirin should not be given to infants or children who have an acute illness because of its association with the development of a very serious problem known as Reye syndrome. This disorder can lead to mental deficits, coma, or death.

Too much aspirin can lead to toxicity and can even be life-threatening. Symptoms of aspirin toxicity may progress from mild to severe, beginning with tinnitus (ringing of the ears), hyperventilation, diaphoresis (sweating), thirst, headache, drowsiness, skin eruptions, and electrolyte imbalance. These progress to central nervous system (CNS), depression, stupor, convulsions and coma, tachycardia (rapid heartbeat), and respiratory insufficiency. If patients exhibit any of these symptoms, it is very important to notify the prescriber early.

🍁 **Lifespan Considerations**

Older Adults

Older adults who are taking NSAIDs have a higher incidence of excessive bleeding and even perforated ulcer than younger adults. Those older adult patients who have some degree of renal impairment are at higher risk for damage to the liver and kidney caused by NSAIDs. These drugs should be avoided in older adults. If prescribed, they should be given with a proton-pump inhibitor, such as misoprostol (Cytotec), to reduce risks for GI effects.

Drug Interactions

Alcohol taken with any of the NSAIDs increases the risk for GI bleeding. There is an increased effect of anticoagulants, sulfonylureas, and sulfonamides if they are used at the same time as aspirin. NSAIDs interact with each other, which increases the risk for side effects, adverse effects, and toxicities. Thus the patient should not be taking more than one type of NSAID at any one time. Different NSAIDs interact differently with other drugs, and interactions are common. Consult a pharmacist or drug handbook for a complete discussion of the interactions associated with a particular NSAID. Examples of common interactions include:

- Aspirin and other NSAIDs should not be given to treat vaccination-associated fever and pain because they can prevent the immune response and its protection.
- NSAIDs (except for aspirin) decrease the effectiveness of many antihypertensive drugs, especially the angiotensin-converting enzyme inhibitors, angiotensin receptor blockers, beta blockers, and most diuretics.
- All NSAIDs increase the risk for bleeding for patients who take any type of anticoagulant.
- All NSAIDs increase the risk for hypoglycemia (low blood sugar) in patients with diabetes who take oral antidiabetic drugs.

❖ Nursing Implications and Patient Teaching

◆ *Assessment.* Do not be afraid to ask patients directly if they are using any other over-the-counter or prescribed NSAIDs because patients sometimes do not report or even forget occasional use of aspirin or other over-the-counter NSAIDs. So many different forms of NSAIDS are available over the counter, so it is important to assess whether patients are taking more than one kind.

Make sure to check for the presence of allergy to aspirin or other NSAIDs, history of asthma, blood disorders, GI problems or ulcer disease, or other liver or kidney problems. These conditions are precautions or contraindications to the use of NSAIDs and thus should be reported to the prescriber before giving the drug. Assess which other prescribed and over-the-counter drugs the patient takes daily because NSAIDs interact with many other drugs. Check with the pharmacist to determine whether or how the NSAID is expected to interact with the patient's other drugs.

◆ *Planning and implementation.* The dosages for different NSAIDs vary widely, so make sure that you know the correct dosage range for the specific drug you are giving. There are many forms of NSAIDS, including tablets, capsules, eye drops, chewable preparations, suppositories, and injectable. Several NSAIDs may even be applied topically. This is very helpful when the prescriber considers the best form for the patient's individual needs.

Give any NSAID with a full glass of water to reduce risk for GI disturbances. If the patient has any stomach upset, try giving with food or milk to reduce the symptoms. If the patient continues to have GI upset, notify the prescriber. If in suspension form, make sure to shake well so that the dosage is accurate. The patient should be well hydrated before taking the drug to reduce the risk for kidney damage.

◆ *Evaluation.* Monitor the patient to see that symptoms resolve (e.g., pain level decreased and temperature is reduced to 101°F or lower). Pain relief typically decreases after administration of the drug. Reduction of inflammation may take longer, even 1 to 2 weeks in some cases. The dosage should be reduced or the drug stopped if tinnitus (ringing in ears) develops. Observe for symptoms, such as pain or fever, that do not respond to the drug that suggest that the patient is getting worse, and notify the healthcare provider. The patient may need a larger dose, more potent drug, or alternative therapy.

Assess the patient for any signs of increased bleeding, especially of the gums and mucous membranes. Check skin for large bruises or those that flow together. Also assess for the presence of *petechiae* (pinpoint purple and reddish spots) on the torso or extremities. Examine stool, urine, and vomitus for the presence of obvious blood. When blood counts are performed, assess whether the number of red blood cells and platelets is normal or low. Report low counts to the healthcare provider immediately.

◆ *Patient and family teaching.* Tell the patient and family the following:
- These drugs may cause stomach upset, so NSAIDs should be taken with a full glass of water. If symptoms do occur, try taking the drug with food or milk.
- Contact your healthcare provider right away if ringing in the ears, abnormal bleeding or bruising, or bloody or black, tarry stools are noted.

- For some chronic problems you may need to take your prescribed NSAID for more than a week or two before noticing a decrease in symptoms.
- Make sure to drink at least 8 to 10 glasses of water a day to stay well hydrated while taking the NSAID.
- For best effect to reduce inflammation, take the prescribed NSAIDs on a regular schedule to keep a stable blood level of the drug.
- Do not take any other drugs, including over-the-counter drugs (especially aspirin or another NSAID), at the same time without informing your healthcare provider.
- Contact your healthcare provider if your fever does not come down within 24 to 48 hours.
- Keep aspirin and all other NSAIDs out of the reach of children because wrong doses may be toxic to a child.
- If you are unable to take the drug in the form prescribed (such as difficulty swallowing), contact your healthcare provider so that another form of the drug may be prescribed.

CORTICOSTEROIDS

Corticosteroids, also known as glucocorticoids, are drugs built on the structure of cholesterol that are able to prevent or limit inflammation by slowing or stopping all known pathways of inflammatory cytokine production. The corticosteroids are similar to the natural cortisol hormones secreted by the adrenal gland that are necessary for life. As a matter of fact, these drugs may be given to replace missing or low hormone levels in cases of adrenal insufficiency (Addison disease). They are most commonly used, however, to reduce the inflammatory response. Common systemic corticosteroid drugs include prednisone, methylprednisolone, hydrocortisone, and dexamethasone (Table 12.2).

> **⮂ Do Not Confuse**
>
> Do not confuse prednisone with prednisolone. Although both drugs are corticosteroids, their strengths, dosages, and some routes of administration differ.

Actions

Corticosteroids are very useful in managing severe or chronic inflammation. They are very powerful in decreasing the production of all known mediators that trigger inflammation. Corticosteroids inhibit enzymes and proteins that allow the COX-1 and COX-2 enzyme systems to start and continue the AA production of inflammatory mediators. They also slow the production of WBCs in the bone marrow. This action also helps reduce inflammation because WBCs usually are the source of the mediators that trigger inflammation. The actions of corticosteroids occur in all cells, not just those involved in inflammation. As a result, their therapeutic effects, side effects, and adverse effects are widespread. These problems limit how and when they can be used.

Table 12.2   Common Corticosteroid Drugs

Corticosteroids: These drugs inhibit enzymes and proteins that allow the COX-1 and COX-2 enzyme systems to start and continue the arachidonic acid production of inflammatory mediators. They are very powerful in decreasing the production of all known mediators that trigger inflammation. The systemic forms of these drugs disrupt the normal functions of other products from arachidonic acid that are helpful and protective.

DRUG/ADULT DOSAGE RANGE	NURSING IMPLICATIONS
dexamethasone (Decadron, Maxidex) 0.75 to 9 mg daily orally, IM, or IV given in 2 to 4 divided doses. Doses are adjusted according to patient response. prednisolone (Millipred, Econopred, Pred-Forte) 5–60 mg daily by mouth as a single dose or in divided doses prednisone (Deltasone, Predone, Sterapred) 5–60 mg orally daily in single or divided doses hydrocortisone sodium succinate (Solu-Cortef) 100–500 mg IM or IV. Repeat doses at 2-, 4-, or 6-hour intervals as ordered. methylprednisolone (Medrol, Solu-Medrol) 4–48 mg orally daily in divided doses according to patient condition and response; 10–120 mg IM, frequency of doses determined by patient condition and response betamethasone (Beta Derm, Del-Beta) Topical: apply a thin film of a 0.1% as directed hydrocortisone (Dermacort, Lanacort) Topical: 0.1%–1% apply as directed triamcinolone (Kenalog, Triderm) Topical: 0.025% to 0.5% apply to affected area as directed	• Check the order carefully because different types of corticosteroids come in different strengths and are not interchangeable. • Doses must be tapered rather than stopped suddenly to avoid adrenal insufficiency • Oral drugs should be taken with food or milk to reduce the risk for gastric ulcers. • Check the patient's blood pressure and weight when giving oral or parenteral corticosteroids because these drugs cause water retention and raise blood pressure. • Assess for infection because these drugs reduce the immune response and increase the susceptibility to infection. • When patients are taking these drugs long term, be sure to handle the patient carefully and not apply tape to the skin because these drugs increase bruising and thin the skin. • Never apply a topical corticosteroid cream, ointment, or lotion to a skin area that has indications of infection because the infection can spread. • Make sure to monitor blood sugar regularly for patients with diabetes or prediabetes because corticosteroids reduce the sensitivity of insulin receptors and increase blood glucose levels. They may need adjustments in oral antidiabetic drugs or insulin. • Patients may experience a change in mood while on corticosteroids; make sure to notify the prescriber if the patient has significant mood changes to reduce the risk for psychotic reactions. • For topical forms such as lotions, creams or ointments, make sure to apply a thin layer to the affected area as directed to avoid giving too large of a dose of corticosteroid.

COX-1, Cyclooxygenase 1; *COX-2*, cyclooxygenase 2.

Uses

Corticosteroids are most commonly given to reduce inflammatory, allergic, or immunologic responses. Examples of when corticosteroids might be used are acute adrenal emergencies, allergic states, acute brain injury, severe asthma, and any condition in which chronic inflammation could lead to tissue damage, such as osteoarthritis, rheumatoid arthritis, inflammatory bowel diseases, and systemic lupus erythematosus, among a wide variety of inflammatory and autoimmune diseases.

Local injection of corticosteroids can be used for intraarticular (into joints), soft tissue, or intrabursal (into bursae) problems, or for intralesional (into lesions) or subcutaneous dermatologic problems. Corticosteroids might also be used topically for acute and chronic dermatoses (see Table 12.2), rectal problems, and some eye (ophthalmic) or ear (otic) problems. Inhaled corticosteroids are commonly used to manage inflammation associated with asthma.

Expected Side Effects

The side effects of systemic corticosteroids in pharmacologic doses are predictable exaggerations of the actions of the corticosteroids that are normally produced by the adrenal glands, or the results of reduced function of the hypothalamic-pituitary-adrenal axis. Table 12.3 lists the short-term and long-term effects of corticosteroid use. Common side effects of corticosteroids that occur even when used for relatively short periods include sodium retention, increased blood pressure, weight gain, bruising, and reduced immunity. It is not unusual for patients, particularly patients with diabetes, to have an elevated blood sugar level, so doses of insulin or oral hypoglycemic agents may need to be adjusted while the patient is on steroid therapy. Patients may experience a change in mood while on corticosteroids; some patients may experience mild euphoria, whereas others may experience some depression. These drugs also increase the risk for bleeding in general and especially in the

Table 12.3	Common Side Effects of Systemic Corticosteroids
Side Effects That Can Occur as Soon as 1 Week of Therapy	
• Acne • Sodium and fluid retention • Elevated blood pressure • Sensation of "nervousness" • Difficulty sleeping • Emotional changes, crying easily	
Side Effects That Can Occur Within a Month After Therapy	
• Weight gain • Fat redistribution (moon face and "buffalo hump" between the shoulders) • Increased risk for GI ulcers and bleeding • Fragile skin that bruises easily • Loss of muscle mass and strength • Thinning scalp hair • Increased facial and body hair • Increased susceptibility to colds and other infections • Stretch marks	

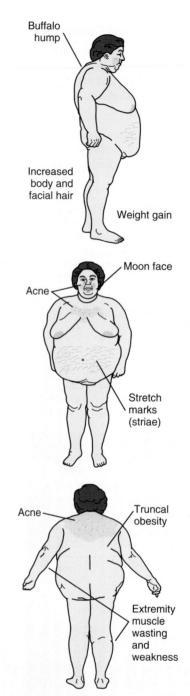

FIG. 12.3 Physical changes from long-term corticosteroid therapy, known as a "cushingoid" appearance. (From Workman ML, LaCharity LA: *Understanding pharmacology*, ed 2, St. Louis, 2016, Elsevier.)

GI tract. Although many of these effects may be considered expected, if they become severe, it is very important to notify the prescriber. Fig. 12.3 shows physical changes associated with long-term corticosteroid use known as cushingoid syndrome. Changes may reverse after the patient stops taking the drug, but that may take several months to a year.

Adverse Reactions

Many effects of systemic corticosteroids can cause serious problems if not carefully managed. The most important problems are associated with long-term use and include adrenal gland suppression and reduced immunity. Thus long-term use of corticosteroids is limited to more severe inflammation that cannot be managed any other way.

Adrenal suppression occurs when circulating blood levels of corticosteroids are higher than the amount of cortisol normally made by the adrenal glands (Fig. 12.4). This causes the adrenal glands to quit making and secreting natural cortisol because the body appears not to need the natural cortisol. Therefore the adrenal glands cells shrink (*atrophy*) and cannot quickly start making cortisol again. This becomes a problem if the patient suddenly stops taking corticosteroids because it may take weeks or even months for the adrenal glands to produce normal levels of cortisol again.

Cortisol is necessary to maintain life; therefore the patient who suddenly stops taking systemic corticosteroids has no circulating cortisol and could die of *acute adrenal insufficiency*. Symptoms include anorexia, nausea and vomiting, lethargy, headache, fever, joint pain, skin peeling, myalgia (widespread muscle pain), weight loss, and hypotension. Abruptly stopping the drug may also result in a rebound of symptoms of the condition being treated. So the patient who has been taking any corticosteroid daily for a week or longer needs to slowly decrease the dose over time (*tapering*) instead of just stopping the drug suddenly. Tapering of the drug allows the atrophied adrenal gland cells to gradually begin producing cortisol again and prevents acute adrenal insufficiency. Fig. 12.5 provides an example of a "dose pack" to assist the patient with dosing days 1 to 6, with each day tapering the dose.

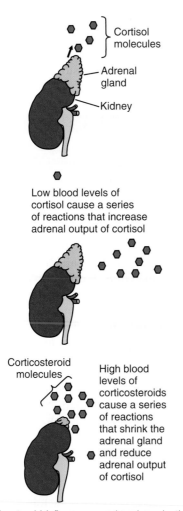

FIG. 12.4 Corticosteroid influence on adrenal production of cortisol. (From Workman ML, LaCharity LA: *Understanding pharmacology*, ed 2, St. Louis, 2016, Elsevier.)

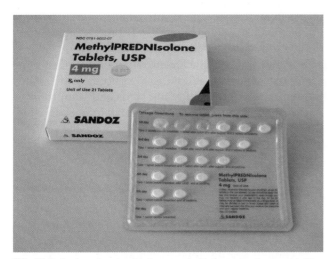

FIG. 12.5 Oral corticosteroid dose pack. Patients begin day 1 taking six tablets. Then, as the patient goes through the week, the drug dosages taper down daily until the sixth day. (Courtesy Sandoz International GmbH.)

Any use of corticosteroids also reduces the number of WBCs, which can decrease inflammation but also decrease immune response. The longer the patient has been taking a corticosteroid and the higher the dose, the more the immunity is reduced. This greatly increases the patient's risk for infection. Also, because inflammation is reduced, the usual symptoms of infection, especially fever and pus formation, may not be present. It is especially important to monitor the patient for other signs of infection such as cough, changes in color of any sputum or other drainage, and even symptoms such as headache or behavior changes.

Other adverse effects associated with long-term corticosteroid use include osteoporosis, cataract, hypertension, and ocular hemorrhage. Delirium or extreme changes in behavior such as mania may warrant reduction of dose or even cessation of the corticosteroid in affected patients.

> **Memory Jogger**
>
> Doses of systemic corticosteroids must be tapered rather than stopped abruptly, to prevent adrenal insufficiency.

Drug Interactions

Corticosteroids increase the effects of barbiturates, sedatives, narcotics, and anticoagulants. They decrease the effects of insulin and oral hypoglycemics, isoniazid, and broad-spectrum antibiotics. Drugs that increase the effects of corticosteroids include other NSAIDs and oral contraceptives, especially estrogen. Drugs that decrease the effects of corticosteroids include ephedrine, phenytoin, antihistamines, rifampin, and propranolol. The effect of corticosteroids on warfarin anticoagulants is variable; in some cases it may increase effect, whereas other cases decrease effect. Some drugs produce exaggerated side effects when given with corticosteroids. These include alcohol, NSAIDs, amphotericin B, thiazides and other potassium-wasting diuretics, anticholinergics, cardiac glycosides, and stimulants such as adrenaline, amphetamines, and ephedrine. The use of aspirin or any other NSAID should be avoided while taking corticosteroids because they also can cause GI distress.

❖ Nursing Implications and Patient Teaching

◆ *Assessment.* The use of corticosteroids has many contraindications and precautions, so it is very important to obtain a good drug history, including over-the-counter drugs, herbal agents, and any topical or inhaled drugs. The most important contraindication is infection that is not also being managed with anti-infective drug therapy. Assess the patient for any signs or symptoms of local or systemic infection before starting the drug. These include fever, drainage, foul-smelling urine, productive cough, or redness around a wound or other open skin area. Steroids tend to thin the skin and so their use increases the risk for skin tears. Steroids can also slow wound healing, so they must be carefully assessed in patients who are to have any kind of surgery. Report any symptoms of infection to the prescriber because corticosteroids reduce immunity and can make any existing untreated infection worse.

◆ *Planning and implementation.* Steroids come in many forms. Corticosteroids may be given by many different routes including oral, inhalation, intranasal, subcutaneous, IM, and IV. Topically, they can be given as creams or gels or as opthalmic or otic (ear) preparations. Only corticosteroid preparations with specific labels should be used for ophthalmologic or otic (ear) administration. Topical steroids should not be applied to open wounds. They should be avoided if there are any signs of infection because they may increase the risk of the infection spreading because of their effect on the immune/inflammatory response.

It is vitally important to confirm the proper form of the drug and the proper route of administration of corticosteroids. State practice acts will guide which route of drug administration is appropriate for the LPN/VN. Even if you do not give the drug, it will be important to monitor for expected side effects, adverse effects, and effectiveness.

Dosages vary a lot; the dose will be determined for each patient and each problem, based on the diagnosis, severity, prognosis, and estimated length of treatment. The general rule is that the patient will receive as high a dose as necessary initially to get a favorable response and then a decreasing amount until reaching the lowest level that will maintain the therapeutic effect but not produce complications. It is critical to check the dose, the route, and the specific drug name carefully because the strength of each drug may differ. *Do not exchange one type of systemic corticosteroid for another because the dosages may not be equivalent.*

It is recommended that doses of oral corticosteroids be taken with meals or a light snack to help reduce the chance of GI distress and peptic ulcer. Systemic corticosteroids are typically given orally, except in patients who are acutely ill or when the patient is unable to take them orally. The onset of action is typically 2 to 8 hours, and the effects are anywhere from 12 to 24 hours, depending on the drug. Oral corticosteroids are almost completely absorbed in the GI tract. For corticosteroids injected into a muscle or joint, effects may take several days to weeks for onset and duration of effects.

When corticosteroids are given orally to patients with functioning adrenal glands, the total dose should be taken first thing in the morning. This is the time when the adrenal glands are normally secreting the most cortisol, so the corticosteroid dose more closely mimics the body's usual actions.

◆ *Evaluation.* All patients who are receiving systemic corticosteroids should be carefully monitored, and the dosage may be adjusted by the prescriber to reflect reduced or increased symptoms, the patient's response, and any periods of stress in the patient's life (e.g., injury, infection, surgery, and emotional crisis). Patients who require high-dose or long-term treatment should be carefully monitored for symptoms of adrenal insufficiency for up to 1 year after stopping the drug.

Top Tip for Safety

Make sure to carefully protect the skin of patients who are taking corticosteroids while transferring or positioning to prevent skin tears.

Corticosteroids can hide the usual symptoms of infection and also increase the patient's risk for infection. This makes it essential for you to monitor for any unusual symptoms that the patient may be having that might suggest infection. For example, corneal fungal infections are particularly likely to develop with extensive ophthalmologic corticosteroid use. Therefore if the patient has any new blurred vision, discoloration of the eye, or tearing, they should contact their healthcare provider. Corticosteroids are particularly dangerous in patients with a history of tuberculosis, because the disease can be reactivated, so it is important to monitor for cough or shortness of breath.

◆ *Patient and family teaching.* Tell the patient and family the following:
* Keep all appointments to monitor therapy while taking this drug.
* Heavy smoking may add to the expected action of a corticosteroid because nicotine raises the blood level of naturally secreted cortisol.
* Avoid alcohol during the course of therapy because it enhances the risk for GI ulcers.
* Report any signs and symptoms of infection (e.g., fever, cough, pain or burning on urination, foul-smelling drainage, generally feeling unwell) to your healthcare provider immediately because corticosteroids reduce resistance to infection.
* Inform other healthcare providers, including your dentist, that you are taking a corticosteroid.
* Report any of the following signs and symptoms to the healthcare provider immediately because they indicate a life-threatening problem of the adrenal glands: malaise, weakness, hypotension, anorexia, nausea and vomiting, aching of bones and muscles, headache, increased temperature, and diarrhea.
* Do not stop taking the steroids suddenly.
* During and after corticosteroid treatment, wear a MedicAlert bracelet or necklace or carry a medical identification card with the name of the drug.
* Do not receive any immunizations without consulting the nurse or other healthcare provider first.
* Take oral corticosteroids with a meal or light snack to minimize stomach upset.
* Eat a diet rich in potassium and low in sodium to replace lost potassium and prevent excessive water retention.

- If you forget to take a prescribed dose, take a dose as soon as possible and then follow the prescribed schedule.
- Call the healthcare provider if rapid weight gain, black or tarry stools, unusual bleeding or bruising, or signs of hypokalemia (decreased potassium in the blood), such as anorexia, lethargy, confusion, nausea, and/or muscle weakness, develop.

DISEASE-MODIFYING ANTIRHEUMATIC DRUGS

Disease-modifying antirheumatic drugs (DMARDs) reduce the progression and tissue destruction of the inflammatory disease process, especially rheumatoid arthritis, by inhibiting TNF. They are prescribed primarily by specialists to prevent or limit bone destruction and are used only in diagnosed cases of rheumatoid arthritis or other chronic inflammatory disorders that have been getting worse despite other types of treatment. You need to know about these drugs because none of these agents is without significant risk and toxic effects. Patients who are taking these drugs need constant follow-up and regular evaluation, and may be admitted to the hospital or seen in offices for other problems.

Actions

DMARDs work through a variety of actions to decrease or suppress the inflammatory response and, in cases of rheumatoid arthritis, slow down the progression of disease and preserve joint function. The most commonly used DMARDs inhibit the inflammatory mediator TNF. They do this by binding to the TNF molecules produced by WBCs and prevent them from binding to TNF receptor sites on inflammatory cells and other cells. This prevents the cells with TNF receptors from continuing to produce even more TNF and other substances that enhance the inflammatory responses and cause direct tissue destruction. As a result, pain is relieved, physical function improves, and tissue damage is reduced or delayed. Most DMARDs are given by injection, although there are a few oral drugs as well. The two most common DMARDs are adalimumab and etanercept (Table 12.4).

Table 12.4   Disease-Modifying Antirheumatic Drugs

Disease-modifying antirheumatic drugs: These drugs reduce the progression and tissue destruction of the inflammatory disease process by inhibiting tumor necrosis factor. As a result, pain is relieved, physical function improves, and tissue damage is reduced or delayed.

DRUG/ADULT DOSAGE RANGE	NURSING IMPLICATIONS
adalimumab (Humira) 40 mg subcutaneously every other week. etanercept (Enbrel) 50 mg subcutaneously once to twice weekly	• The first dose of an injectable DMARD should be given by the healthcare provider or the registered nurse because of the risk of severe allergy. Monitor the patient every 15 minutes for the first 2 hours to detect adverse reaction. • Tell patients that injection-site reactions including redness, pain, swelling, and itchiness may occur but typically subside in a few days. • Make sure to rotate injection sites on the front of the thighs and the abdomen to ensure best absorption and prevent skin problems. Avoid giving within 2 inches of the umbilicus because this area has many blood vessels and absorption can be too rapid. • Read administration directions very carefully before giving to avoid improper dosing or damage to the drug. These drugs often must be refrigerated before giving. • Do not rub the site after giving the injection, to prevent bleeding and bruising of the site. • For patients with psoriasis, make sure not to inject in any lesions because drug absorption is delayed in these areas and the lesions may mask skin reactions to the drug. • Do not give these drugs to any patients with an active infection, including local infections, because the drug reduces the immune response and can make infections worse. • Teach patients to report any signs of infection to the healthcare provider immediately because the drug reduces the immune response and can make infections worse. • Patients who take these drugs before surgery may have greater risk for infections postoperatively because the drug reduces the immune response. • Instruct patients to avoid vaccination with live viruses while taking disease-modifying antirheumatic drugs because they may not be fully effective because of a reduced immune response. • Teach patients that it is not unusual to experience a mild headache while taking these drugs so that they will not be alarmed by this side effect.

TB, Tuberculosis.

Uses

DMARDs are used to treat many different types of chronic inflammatory disorders that involve severe tissue destruction caused by excessive amounts of TNF. In addition to rheumatoid arthritis, other autoimmune disorders that respond to DMARDs include ankylosing spondylitis, psoriasis, psoriatic arthritis, Crohn's disease, and ulcerative colitis.

Expected Side Effects

The most common side effect from the injected drugs are injection-site reactions. These include pain, swelling, itching, and redness at the site for about 1 week. Many patients also have headache and nausea. Patients may develop anemia and have an increased risk for bleeding because these drugs reduce bone marrow production of red blood cells and platelets.

Adverse Reactions

Severe adverse reactions are possible and relatively common in patients who are taking DMARDs, so it is important to monitor patients very carefully and teach patients the symptoms to report. All DMARDs reduce the patient's immune response to some degree, increasing his or her risk for infections. In fact, if a patient has had tuberculosis or viral infections (such as shingles or hepatitis) in the past, he or she is at high risk for reactivating these old infections. Even though reduced immunity is an expected result of therapy with DMARDs, it is considered an adverse reaction that must be monitored for severity. If reduced immunity is severe enough or severe infection develops, the DMARD therapy must be stopped.

> **Memory Jogger**
>
> All DMARDs reduce immunity and increase the risk for infection.

Heart failure can occur with these drugs. The heart failure may be new or, if the patient already has heart failure, it can become more severe while taking DMARDs. DMARDs should not be used in anyone who has severe heart failure.

Patients who are taking injectable DMARDs may be at greater risk for allergic reaction, even anaphylaxis, because the solutions may contain some animal proteins. Fortunately these reactions are not common.

Drug Interactions

If the patient is taking any other type of drug that reduces immunity, the suppression will be more severe if taken with a DMARD, greatly increasing the risk for infections. It is not recommended to give two different DMARDs that interfere with TNF at the same time.

Some immunizations contain live vaccines. For the patient who is receiving DMARDs, live vaccine immunizations are avoided because the patient may actually develop the disease the immunization is supposed to prevent.

DMARDs reduce immunity, so the patient may not have an accurate response to tuberculosis testing with the PPD (purified protein derivative) test. The response could be negative even if the person has active tuberculosis.

❖ Nursing Implications and Patient Teaching

◆ *Assessment.* Before giving the drug, ask the patient to list every drug he or she is currently taking. Ask about symptoms of infection such as fever, cough, foul-smelling drainage, pain or burning on urination, general malaise, and any recent exposure to people who are ill. Also ask whether the patient has received an immunization within the past month. All patients must be tested for tuberculosis before starting a DMARD.

> **Top Tip for Safety**
>
> Always ask patients whether they have a current infection or have had any of these infections in the past: tuberculosis, hepatitis, shingles, HIV infection, pneumocystis pneumonia, or any type of opportunistic infection.

◆ *Planning and implementation.* The first dose of an injectable DMARD must be given by either a healthcare provider or a registered nurse in a setting that can handle severe allergic reactions. It cannot be started in an extended care facility or in the home. Take the patient's vital signs, especially pulse, blood pressure, and oxygen saturation, before giving the first dose. Use this information as a baseline to assess for an adverse drug reaction.

Keep an emergency cart close to the patient during and for 2 hours after the first injection. After the first dose is given, observe the patient every 15 minutes for any type of allergic or adverse reaction for at least 2 hours. These observations include respiratory rate, ease of respirations, blood pressure, pulse oximetry, and rash or hives at the injection sites.

After the first therapeutic dose is given and no adverse reactions have occurred, LPN/VNs can give subsequent dosages. Some patients can be taught to self-inject subcutaneous doses. It is very important to carefully read specific directions for administration of the drugs before giving them. For example, adalimumab should not be shaken before giving because damage to the drug may occur. The drug can be left at room temperature for 15 to 30 minutes before injecting, but the cap or cover must be left on the drug bottle while allowing it to warm to room temperature.

◆ *Evaluation.* Closely monitor the injection site and the whole patient for signs of an adverse reaction. Document the patient's responses, even if no problems occur. Also document any symptoms or injection-site responses that do occur.

◆ *Patient and family teaching.*

- Check for and report the signs and symptoms of infection (e.g., fever, cough, malaise, foul-smelling drainage, pain or burning on urination) to your prescriber immediately.
- If you have learned how to inject the drug, make sure to always use the proper technique and contact your healthcare provider if you have any questions.
- Report any nausea, vomiting, loss of appetite, severe fatigue, or changes in color of the urine because they may be symptoms of problems with the liver.
- Avoid any over-the-counter drugs without contacting the prescriber to avoid dangerous drug interactions.

GOUT

Gout is a metabolic disorder that causes a person to either make too many uric acid crystals from the proteins he or she eats or to not eliminate the crystals in the urine. These crystals then deposit into the joints, causing arthritis symptoms of pain, redness, and swelling (gouty arthritis), and also causing progressive joint damage with function loss. Although the metabolic disorder is always present, the symptoms of gout come and go.

MANAGEMENT OF INFLAMMATION AND GOUT PAIN

About 10% of people who have gout can control the problem with lifestyle changes that involve eating less of the foods that produce uric acid (e.g., shellfish and fish such as herring, sardines, salmon, haddock, and anchovies; red meat, organ meats, and pork; beer and wine). For the other 90% of people with gout, diet is not the cause. Rather, they are unable to eliminate uric acid well through the kidneys. Weight loss if obese, avoidance of alcohol, and including low-fat dairy products and complex carbohydrates in the diet may also reduce the risk for flare-ups.

When symptoms of gout are present, general anti-inflammatory drugs can help to reduce the pain and inflammation but do not address the uric acid problem. These drugs also do not prevent the progressive joint damage. Specific drugs for pain management may also be prescribed during acute attacks (see Chapter 11). Drugs that actually lower uric acid levels can prevent gout attacks as well as reduce the symptoms during an attack.

ANTIGOUT DRUGS

The most common drugs used to reduce the uric acid levels associated with gout are uric acid synthesis inhibitors. The two drugs in this class are allopurinol and febuxostat (Table 12.5).

Actions

Allopurinol and febuxostat help prevent gout attacks by reducing the amount of an enzyme that converts the purines in protein into uric acid. So there is less uric acid available to form irritating and inflammatory deposits in joints. These drugs help patients to maintain a lower blood uric acid level.

Uses

The main use of **antigout drugs** is to prevent gout and shorten gout attacks. For gout prevention, they must be taken daily. Allopurinol (but not febuxostat) is also used to lower uric acid levels that occur when rapid cell destruction (such as with cancer chemotherapy) results in a huge release of the purines from proteins inside the cancer cells.

Table 12.5   Common Antigout Drugs

Uric acid synthesis inhibitors: prevent gout and reduce gout symptoms by lowering blood uric acid levels through inhibiting the enzyme that converts the purines of proteins into uric acid.

DRUG/ADULT DOSAGE RANGE	NURSING IMPLICATIONS
allopurinol (Aloprim, Zyloprim) 100–800 mg orally daily. Dosages higher than 300 mg must be given in divided doses. febuxostat (Uloric) 40–80 mg orally daily. Dose may increase if the patient's uric acid level remains high.	• Take allopurinol after a meal to prevent GI side effects. • Wait at least 3 hours after taking an aluminum-based antacid before taking allopurinol because the antacid inhibits its absorption. • If patients also take warfarin, they will need more frequent monitoring of international normalized ratios (INRs) because allopurinol interferes with warfarin metabolism. • Do not give either drug to a breast-feeding woman because the drugs do enter breast milk and their effects on the baby are not known. • Febuxostat can be taken any time of day regardless of meals. • Teach patients to drink plenty of fluids to dilute uric acid and prevent kidney complications of the drug. • Teach patients to keep all appointments for laboratory tests to monitor for drug effectiveness and toxicities.

Expected Side Effects

The most common side effects of allopurinol and febuxostat are headache, rash, and minor nausea. Rare side effects include breast development in men and erectile dysfunction. There is a risk for gout flare with the start of therapy, so teach patients to report increased gout symptoms. Gout flare may be managed with NSAIDs or colchicine.

Adverse Reactions

Adverse reactions with allopurinol and febuxostat are rare and occur only with very long-term use. Examples of adverse effects include kidney stone formation, liver failure, heart failure, and stroke. Rarely, depression and cardiac dysrhythmias have been reported.

Drug Interactions

Aluminum-based antacids inhibit absorption of allopurinol. Antigout drugs also interfere with the metabolism and action of warfarin. Febuxostat interacts with many chemotherapy drugs to form other metabolic products that can damage kidneys. This is why it is not used for the hyperuricemia associated with cancer therapy.

❖ Nursing Implications and Patient Teaching

Patients are rarely hospitalized for gout. The most important action is to teach patients how to take these drugs to prevent and control gout.

◆ *Patient and family teaching.* Tell the patient and family the following:

- Take allopurinol after a full meal to avoid an upset stomach.
- Drink 8 to 16 glasses of liquids, especially water, throughout the 24-hour day.
- Wait at least 3 hours to take allopurinol after using an aluminum-based antacid.
- Febuxostat can be taken with or without meals and is not affected by antacids.
- Avoid foods that are high in purines, such as beer or organ meats, because those foods may precipitate an acute attack.
- Keep all appointments for laboratory tests of uric acid levels, as well as for liver and kidney function while taking these drugs.
- Many drugs can trigger gouty flare-ups, so it is important to let your healthcare provider know if you have gout.

Get Ready for the NCLEX® Examination!

Key Points

- Acute inflammatory reactions are uncomfortable but are often helpful or protective.
- Chronic inflammatory reactions are uncomfortable and can cause tissue damage and destruction.
- All NSAIDs have the same mechanism of action, although the chemical structure, strengths, interactions, and adverse effects may vary.
- All NSAIDs increase the risk for bleeding in patients who also take any type of anticoagulant.
- NSAIDs (except for aspirin) decrease the effectiveness of many antihypertensive drugs, especially the angiotensin-converting enzyme inhibitors, angiotensin receptor blockers, beta blockers, and most diuretics.
- Patients who take corticosteroids must not suddenly stop the drug but rather taper the dose as directed to avoid adrenal insufficiency.
- Corticosteroids have a wide range of side and adverse effects, so patients must be very carefully monitored.
- Always ask patients who are to receive a DMARD about whether they have a current infection or have had any of these infections in the past: tuberculosis, hepatitis, shingles, HIV infection, pneumocystis pneumonia, or any type of opportunistic infection.
- Anti-inflammatory drugs do not prevent gout or the associated joint damage of gout.
- Use of drugs for gout should be combined with patient teaching about avoiding high-purine foods, weight loss, and avoiding alcohol.

Review Questions for the NCLEX® Examination

1. A patient taking an NSAID tells you that the drug causes an upset stomach. What is your best response?
   1. "Always take this drug with food or with milk."
   2. "Stop taking the drug and notify your prescriber."
   3. "Chew the drug instead of swallowing it whole."
   4. "Take the drug at night so you will sleep through the upset."

2. Which problem is a common side effect of long-term corticosteroid use?
   1. Acne
   2. Sodium and fluid retention
   3. Loss of muscle mass
   4. Difficulty sleeping

3. A nursing home resident has been prescribed 20 mg prednisolone orally immediately. The facility does not have prednisolone, only prednisone. What is your best action?
   1. Substitute prednisone for prednisolone because they are both corticosteroids.
   2. Hold the dose until the pharmacy opens the next day.
   3. Notify the prescriber immediately about this problem.
   4. Give the parenteral form of the drug.

4. What is the main goal of therapy with uric acid synthesis inhibitors for gouty arthritis?
   1. Reducing pain
   2. Curing the disease
   3. Preventing gout attacks
   4. Reducing uric acid levels

5. The patient prescribed an NSAID contacts the clinic to say that he has noticed that his bowel movements have become very dark, like tar. What will the LPN/VN say to the patient?
   1. "This is an adverse effect of the drug, you need to come to the clinic today."
   2. "This is an expected side effect of the drug. You can try taking an antacid when you take the NSAID."
   3. "You should stop taking NSAIDs. You are probably allergic."
   4. "The healthcare provider will switch the drugs to a less irritating type."

6. A 37-year-old woman diagnosed with rheumatoid arthritis has been managing her symptoms with NSAIDs and now is to start a DMARD. Which of the following statements suggests a need for more teaching?
   1. "I will monitor the injection site for redness or swelling because these are side effects of the injection."
   2. "I should avoid large crowds during flu season to decrease my risk for infection."
   3. "If I have any signs of infection, I will call my healthcare provider immediately."
   4. "I should avoid high-purine foods in my diet."

7. What is the main difference between a nonselective COX inhibitor and a COX-2 inhibitor?
   1. COX-2 inhibitors have fewer GI side effects than nonselective COX inhibitors.
   2. COX-2 inhibitors are less effective than nonselective COX inhibitors.
   3. COX-2 inhibitors can be taken with any over-the-counter drugs without risk.
   4. COX-2 inhibitors are safe in children with Reye syndrome.

8. A 72-year-old patient has been on prednisone for an autoimmune disease for 10 weeks. She is concerned about the side effects and tells the LPN/VN that she has decided to stop taking the drug. What is the LPN/VN's best response?
   1. "Make sure to notify your healthcare provider that you stopped taking the prednisone."
   2. "Call the prescriber first because it is very important that you do not stop prednisone suddenly, but rather taper the drug."
   3. "There are very few side effects to prednisone, so it must be another drug."
   4. "Do not stop taking the drug because you will increase your risk of infection."

9. Which of the following symptoms is associated with aspirin toxicity?
   1. Tinnitus
   2. Respiratory depression
   3. Constipation
   4. Abdominal pain

10. What category contains the drugs that reduce the progression and tissue destruction of the inflammatory disease process, especially rheumatoid arthritis, by inhibiting tumor necrosis factor (TNF)?
    1. Corticosteroids
    2. Nonsteroidal anti-inflammatory drugs
    3. Disease modifying antirheumatic drugs
    4. Purine reducing drugs

11. You are to give 6 mg dexamethasone IM. You have available dexamethasone vials 4 mg/mL. How many milliliters will you give? ____mL

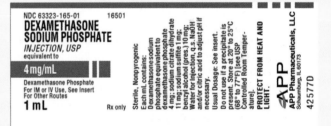

(Courtesy Fresenius Kabi USA, LLC)

Learning Outcomes

1. List the names, actions, possible side effects, and adverse effects of antiemetics and promotility drugs.
2. Explain what to teach patients and families about antiemetics and promotility drugs.
3. List the names, actions, possible side effects, and adverse effects of antacids and histamine H₂ receptor blockers.
4. Explain what to teach patients and families about antacids and histamine H₂ receptor blockers.

5. List the names, actions, possible side effects, and adverse effects of proton pump inhibitors and cytoprotective drugs.
6. Explain what to teach patients and families about proton pump inhibitors and cytoprotective drugs.
7. List the names, actions, possible side effects, and adverse effects of laxatives and antidiarrheals.
8. Explain what to teach patients and families about laxatives and antidiarrheals.

Key Terms

antacids (ănt-Ă-sĕd, p. 251) A category of drugs used to help neutralize gastric acid and reduce symptoms of indigestion and heartburn.

antidiarrheal (ĂN-tē-dī-ă-RĒ-ĕl, p. 259) Drug that reduces or stops loose, watery stools (diarrhea) and helps restore normal bowel movements.

antiemetic drugs (ĂN-tē-ĭ-MĚ-tĭk, p. 242) A category of drugs used to prevent and treat nausea and vomiting.

cannabinoids (kă-NĂ-bă-nōĭd, p. 247) Drugs that are either natural or synthetic forms of tetrahydrocannabinol (THC) that reduce nausea and vomiting by binding to both cannabinoid receptors in the chemoreceptor trigger zone (CTZ) and by preventing serotonin (5-HT₃) from binding to its receptors in the CTZ.

cytoprotective drugs (SĪ-tō-prō-TĔK-tiv, p. 253) A class of drugs that protects the lining of the stomach and prevents further damage to the lining from stomach acid.

histamine H₂-receptor antagonists (HĬ-stă-mēn, p. 252) A class of drugs that inhibits the binding of histamine to H₂ receptors on the parietal cells in the stomach, thereby decreasing gastric acid secretions.

laxatives (LĂK-sĕ-tĭv, p. 254) A class of drugs that promotes bowel movements by stimulating peristalsis, increasing the bulk of the stool, or by softening the stool. They are typically used to relieve constipation.

opioid agonists (Ō-pē-oid Ă-gă-nĭst, p. 260) A class of antidiarrheals that reduces GI motility and increases the ability of the intestine to absorb water. They do not have the analgesic or opioid-like effects of the drugs discussed in Chapter 11.

phenothiazine (fē-nō-THĪ-ĕ-zēn, p. 246) A type of antiemetic drug that reduces nausea and vomiting by blocking dopamine receptors in the CTZ. These drugs are also called *dopamine antagonists*.

promotility drugs (PRO-mō-tĭl-ĭ-tē, p. 248) A class of drugs that increases contraction of the upper GI tract, including the stomach and the small intestines, to move contents more quickly through the tract. They do this by blocking dopamine (D₂) receptors in the CTZ and the intestinal tract.

proton pump inhibitors (PRŌ-tŏn pŭmp ĭn-HĬ-bă-tĕrz, p. 248) A class of drugs that binds to the proton pump of the parietal cells in the stomach, which blocks acid secretion into the stomach.

serotonin (5-HT₃) receptor antagonists (sĕr-ă-TŌ-nĕn, p. 243) A class of antiemetic drugs that reduces or halts nausea and vomiting by blocking (5-HT₃) receptors in the intestinal tract and the CTZ so serotonin cannot activate these receptors.

substance P/neurokinin₁ (NK₁) receptor antagonists (NYŪR-ō-KĬ-nĕn, p. 245) A class of antiemetic drugs that blocks the substance P/neurokinin₁ (NK₁) receptors in the CTZ, preventing the substance P and neurokinin that are released from cells exposed to chemotherapy and from tissues that are traumatized during surgery from binding to and triggering the CTZ.

THE DIGESTIVE SYSTEM

The digestive system is composed of the mouth, esophagus, stomach, intestines, and accessory structures (Fig. 13.1). This system performs the mechanical and chemical processes of digestion, absorbs nutrients, and eliminates waste (Fig. 13.2). Although it is located inside the body, the digestive system is in constant contact with the external environment. After all, it is open at both ends and, unlike other internal body areas, substances placed in it do not need to be sterile. In addition to problems that arise within the digestive system itself, being open to the environment increases the number and type of problems that can occur anywhere along the GI tract.

Digestion begins in the mouth by chewing and mixing food with enzyme-rich saliva secreted by salivary glands. The food passes from the mouth to the anus through the digestive tract. Here is where the complex compounds that enter the mouth as food are reduced to smaller dissolvable particles and their carriers (see Fig. 13.2). Usable food particles are absorbed while indigestible pieces and waste materials are eliminated. *Accessory digestive glands* (salivary glands, gallbladder, and pancreas) secrete enzymes and other chemicals that are required to break down food substances and promote absorption into the bloodstream.

In the stomach, digestion requires a strong acid to break down protein or other substances. This acid is strong (has a low pH) and could erode the cells lining the stomach and form open sores (ulcers). Think of the burning sensation you feel in your mouth, throat, and nose when you vomit. Fortunately, several factors work together to protect the GI tract mucosa from injury. A

protective substance secreted by stomach-lining cells is one type of prostaglandin. This substance triggers the production of a thick mucus that forms a gel-like layer in the stomach that helps prevent stomach acid and enzymes from coming into direct contact with and

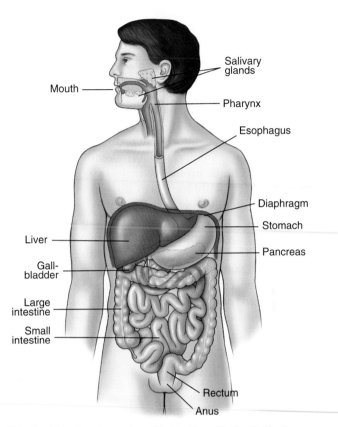

FIG. 13.1 The digestive system. (Modified from Herlihy B: *The human body in health and illness*, ed 5, Philadelphia, 2014, Elsevier.)

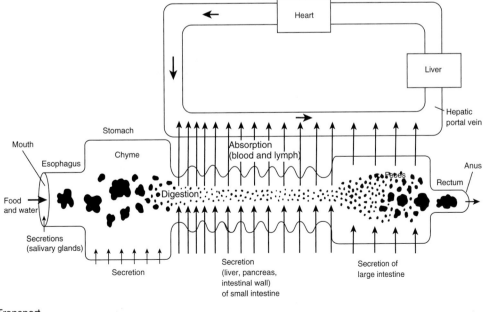

FIG. 13.2 Actions within the digestive system from ingestion of food and water, absorption of water and nutrients, secretion of aids to digestion, and removal of waste products. (From Vander AJ, Sherman JH, Luciano DS: *Human physiology*, ed 5, New York, 1990, McGraw-Hill. Used with permission.)

damaging the lining. *Prostaglandins* also maintain good blood flow to the stomach, which keeps these tissues well oxygenated and allows the immune system to help keep them healthy.

As partially digested food and liquid leave the stomach and enter the *duodenum* (the first 12–18 inches of the small intestine), these stomach contents are still very acidic. The duodenum does not have the mucous protection that the stomach has. So the duodenum could easily develop ulcers from this exposure to acid and digestive enzymes. However, the pancreas produces a lot of bicarbonate and secretes it into the duodenum to neutralize the acid in the contents from the stomach.

We have just mentioned two of the problems that the digestive system can have: vomiting and ulcer formation. Other problems include the movement of stomach contents back into the esophagus (*gastric reflux*), abnormally slow movement of contents through the intestinal tract (*constipation*), and abnormally fast movement of contents through the intestinal tract (*diarrhea*). This chapter focuses on drug therapy to prevent or manage these problems. In addition, the digestive tract can become infected with bacteria, viruses, fungus, and parasites. Drug therapy for conditions related to infectious agents is presented in Chapters 5 and 6.

ANTIEMETIC DRUGS

Nausea and vomiting are common GI problems that occur as a result of infection, fever, motion, certain foods, anesthesia, and exposure to many drugs, including cancer chemotherapy. Very often, nausea and vomiting occur together or vomiting follows nausea. However, nausea can occur without vomiting and is still an unpleasant sensation. Vomiting also can occur without the sensation of nausea.

Although we tend to think of nausea and vomiting as just problems of the digestive tract, they result from a complex set of interactions that involve the brain, nervous system, inner ear, and the stomach and intestines (Fig. 13.3). Messages from the cerebral cortex (e.g., fear or anxiety), the sensory organs (e.g., sights, odors, or pain), or the vestibular apparatus in the inner ear (e.g., motion sickness) can be sent to the vomiting center in the brain. These are called *direct-acting stimuli* because the message goes directly to the vomiting center. *Indirect-acting stimuli* involve the chemoreceptor trigger zone (CTZ). For example, opioids, alcohol, certain antibiotics, and types of anesthesia can stimulate the CTZ. The CTZ then sends messages to the vomiting center. Signals from the stomach or small intestine can send messages to the CTZ (such as after a big meal or a food that "does not agree" with you). Think of the last time you felt nauseated and had vomiting. Was it a direct or indirect stimuli that caused your nausea and vomiting?

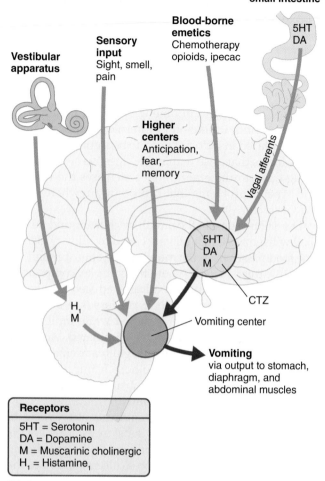

FIG. 13.3 Vomiting is a complex reflex. It involves stimuli to the vomiting center (VC) directly or indirectly through the chemoreceptor trigger zone (CTZ). You can see that many types of receptors are involved in vomiting. By understanding that there are different types of receptors, you can understand different types of antiemetics and how they work. For example, some affect dopamine, some serotonin, some histamine, and some acetylcholine.

🔰 **Top Tip for Safety**

Patients with nausea and vomiting are at risk for dehydration, weight loss, and electrolyte imbalance. Monitor and report any changes in fluid balance, food intake, and laboratory abnormalities.

Antiemetic drugs are used to prevent and treat nausea and vomiting that occur with any problem. There are many classes of antiemetic drugs, including serotonin receptor antagonists, substance P antagonists, phenothiazines, cannabinoids, promotility drugs, butyrophenones, and anticholinergics. Most of these drugs work in the brain, stomach, and intestinal tract, to change the sensation of nausea and to reduce the stomach contractions that make vomiting occur. Which class of drug is used depends on the severity of the problem and the patient's individual response. Some patients may require a combination of two or more types of antiemetic drugs for effective management of nausea and vomiting. We will discuss the first five categories of drugs. The butyrophenones and anticholinergic drugs are discussed in Chapter 9.

> ### Memory Jogger
>
> The major categories of antiemetic drugs are:
> - serotonin (5-HT$_3$) receptor antagonists
> - substance P antagonists
> - phenothiazines (dopamine antagonists)
> - cannabinoids
> - promotility drugs
> - butyrophenones
> - anticholinergics

SEROTONIN (5-HT$_3$) RECEPTOR ANTAGONISTS

Action and Uses

A major *neurotransmitter* (chemical that transmits signals from one nerve to the next nerve in the pathway or to the brain) that causes nausea and vomiting when it binds to its receptors in either the CTZ or to its receptors in the GI system is one particular form of serotonin. This specific form of serotonin is serotonin 5-hydroxytryptamine type 3 (5-HT$_3$). The **serotonin (5-HT$_3$) receptor antagonists** are a class of antiemetic drugs that reduces or halts nausea and vomiting by blocking serotonin (5-HT$_3$) receptors in the intestinal tract and the CTZ so serotonin cannot activate these receptors. The major uses of this class of antiemetics are to reduce or prevent the nausea and vomiting resulting from cancer chemotherapy, radiation therapy, and anesthesia-induced nausea and vomiting after surgery. They may be called *setrons* for short because they typically end in "setron." Table 13.1 lists the names, dosages, and nursing implications for common serotonin (5-HT$_3$) receptor antagonists. Be sure to consult a drug reference book for more information about specific drugs.

> ### Memory Jogger
>
> All of the serotonin (5-HT$_3$) receptor antagonists have the suffix *-setron* in their generic names.

Expected Side Effects

Common central nervous system (CNS) side effects for serotonin (5HT$_3$) receptor antagonists include dizziness, headache, and drowsiness. Some patients experience changes in taste, heartburn, constipation, or diarrhea. Rarely, a patient may experience chills with shivering.

Adverse Reactions

Adverse reactions include allergic reactions, dysrhythmias, and renal or liver damage. Serotonin syndrome can occur if the patient is taking other drugs that increase serotonin (e.g., certain antidepressants, St. John's wort). For more information about serotonin syndrome, see Chapter 10.

Table 13.1   Examples of Common Antiemetics

Serotonin (5-HT$_3$) receptor antagonists: reduce or halt nausea and vomiting by blocking (5-HT$_3$) receptors in the intestinal tract and the CTZ so serotonin cannot activate these receptors

DRUG/ADULT DOSAGE RANGE	NURSING IMPLICATIONS

dolasetron (Anzemet)
   100 mg orally given 1 hour before chemotherapy
ondansetron (Zofran, Zuplenz)
   8 mg orally 30 min before chemotherapy, then every 8 and 16 hours after the initial dose. May give doses every 12 hours 1–2 days after chemotherapy completed
palonosetron (Aloxi) 0.5 mg orally as a single dose 1 hour before chemotherapy
	• Make sure the patient has a call light available because these drugs can cause dizziness.
	• Give the drug before the patient has an episode of vomiting because they can prevent or relieve nausea before the patient vomits.
	• Contact the healthcare provider if the patient is also taking any drugs that affect serotonin levels because the interaction can cause serious adverse effects.
	• These drugs may be given for postoperative nausea and vomiting but are typically given intravenously rather than orally.

Substance P/neurokinin$_1$ receptor antagonists: reduce or prevent immediate and delayed nausea and vomiting by blocking the substance P/neurokinin$_1$ receptors in the CTZ, preventing both of these substances from binding to and triggering the CTZ

DRUG/ADULT DOSAGE RANGE	NURSING IMPLICATIONS
aprepitant (Emend-oral): on day 1, give 125 mg orally 1 hour before chemotherapy; on days 2 and 3, give 80 mg orally 1 hour before chemotherapy, or if no chemotherapy is scheduled on days 2 and 3, give in the morning. Available as capsule or as oral suspension. rolapitant (Varubi) 180 mg orally on day 1, given 1–2 hours before chemotherapy	• Always double-check doses of substance P/neurokinin$_1$ receptor agonists because protocols vary according to the potential of the chemotherapy drugs to cause nausea and vomiting. More "emetogenic" chemotherapy drugs may require more frequent dosing. • In some cases this drug may be combined with a corticosteroid agent to reduce symptoms of nausea and vomiting even further.

Continued

Table 13.1   **Examples of Common Antiemetics—cont'd**

Phenothiazines: reduce nausea and vomiting by blocking dopamine (D$_2$) receptors in the CTZ

DRUG/ADULT DOSAGE RANGE	NURSING IMPLICATIONS
prochlorperazine (Compazine, Compro) 5–10 mg orally three to four times daily; IM 5–10 mg every 3–4 hours PRN; rectal 25 mg twice daily; sustained release 10–15 mg every 12 hours promethazine (Phenadoz, Phenergan, Promethegan) 12.5–25 mg orally every 4–6 hours as needed; 12–25 mg IM every 4–6 hours as needed; rectal 12.5–25 mg by rectum every 4–6 hours as needed	• Teach patients to change position slowly because these drugs can cause orthostatic hypotension. • Remind patients that alcohol may increase drowsiness and increase risk for injury. • Watch carefully for side/adverse effects relating to these drugs and their effects on dopamine. Contact the healthcare provider for any Parkinson's disease–like tremors or gait changes, any muscle spasms, or any changes in motor movement such as tongue rolling or lip smacking because these are serious adverse effects. • Monitor the patient carefully for any sudden increase in temperature because this can be an indication of neuroleptic malignant syndrome, a rare but life-threatening adverse effect.

Cannabinoids: are either natural or synthetic forms of THC that reduce nausea and vomiting by binding to both cannabinoid receptors in the CTZ and by interfering with serotonin 5-HT$_3$ from binding to its receptors in the CTZ

DRUG/ADULT DOSAGE RANGE	NURSING IMPLICATIONS
dronabinol (Marinol, Syndros) as liquid-filled capsules 5 mg/m^2 orally given 1–3 hours before chemotherapy and then every 2–4 hours afterward for a total of four to six doses per day; 4.2 mg/m^2 as oral solution (rounded to the nearest 0.1 mg), given 1–3 hours before chemotherapy and then every 2–4 hours after chemotherapy, for a total of four to six doses per day nabilone (Cesamet) 1–2 mg orally twice daily; the initial dose is given 1–3 hours before chemotherapy; a dose of 1–2 mg the night before chemotherapy may be useful	• Cannabinoids are typically reserved for patients who continue to have nausea and vomiting who do not respond to other categories of antiemetics. • These drugs are typically given as solution or in liquid-filled capsules with the dosage individualized according to *body surface area*. For example, a person who is 6 feet tall and weighs 225 pounds would receive 11.2 mg of the drug. The dosage will be determined using body surface area calculations by the healthcare provider in conjunction with the pharmacist. • For liquid drugs, always make sure to use the proper measuring device (such as an oral syringe) to ensure accuracy. • The first dose should be taken on an empty stomach 30 minutes before meals. After the first dose, these drugs can be taken with food. • Advise patients to avoid alcohol, sedatives, or other CNS depressants because they may increase the risk for sedation. • Monitor the patient carefully for changes in mental status. Cannabinoids can cause confusion, sedation, and at times feelings of euphoria or a "high." These typically decrease after a few days of use.

Promotility drugs: a class of drugs that increases contraction of the upper GI tract including the stomach and the small intestines; they do this by blocking dopamine (D$_2$) receptors in the CTZ and the intestinal tract

DRUG/ADULT DOSAGE RANGE	NURSING IMPLICATIONS
metoclopramide (Reglan) 10–15 mg orally four times daily 30 minutes before meals and at bedtime trimethobenzamide (Tigan) 300 mg orally three to four times daily PRN; IM 200 mg three to four times daily PRN	• Monitor the patient carefully for any mood changes or restlessness because these are common side effects. • Check vital signs regularly to assess for changes in blood pressure (decrease) because there is a risk for orthostatic hypotension. • Give these drugs at least 30 minutes before meals and at bedtime because these are times of increased potential for nausea.

CTZ, Chemoreceptor trigger zone.

Drug Interactions

As mentioned earlier, these drugs can interact with a variety of drugs that contain the neurotransmitter serotonin or drugs that are like serotonin. Examples include monoamine oxidase inhibitors, morphine, and serotonin reuptake inhibitors. When combined with phenothiazine drugs, the patient may experience cardiac dysrhythmias.

❖ Nursing Implications and Patient Teaching

◆ *Planning and implementation.* In addition to the general nursing considerations related to care of the patient with antiemetic drugs described in Box 13.1, the following issues and actions are important. Follow protocols very carefully to ensure adequate timing before the patient receives chemotherapy. Monitor vital signs before and after giving the drug. In addition, ask your patient

Box 13.1 General Nursing Considerations for Antiemetic Drug Therapy

- Assess heart rate, blood pressure, respiratory rate, and level of consciousness before giving any antiemetic agent.
- Remove any foods, smells, or images that may make nausea worse.
- Ask the patient to describe his or her nausea, and if the patient vomits, record the color, consistency, and amount.
- Give the antiemetic drug for nausea rather than waiting until the patient vomits.
- Vomiting can result in dehydration and electrolyte imbalance, so make sure to monitor weight, skin turgor, and intake and output. Review serum electrolytes and report abnormal results to the healthcare provider.
- If the patient is taking an antiemetic for chemotherapy, carefully review the prescribed protocol to ensure good timing of drug administration.
- Determine the effectiveness of the antiemetic by monitoring the patient's report of relief from nausea and no further vomiting.
- Tell the patient to ask for help when getting out of bed or out of the chair because these drugs can cause dizziness and drowsiness. Be sure to have the call light within the reach of the patient.
- Report any symptoms of severe abdominal pain or signs of abdominal distention to the healthcare provider immediately because these may be signs of complications.
- Report emesis that looks like coffee grounds or is red-tinged to the healthcare provider immediately because this may indicate bleeding in the GI tract.
- Tell the patient to avoid driving or use of heavy machinery while taking antiemetics because they can cause dizziness and drowsiness.
- Teach the patient to contact the healthcare provider before adding any over-the-counter drugs or herbal drugs because they can increase risk for drug interactions.
- Remind the patient to avoid alcohol, sedatives, or tranquilizers unless specifically advised by the healthcare provider.
- Many of these drugs cause increase in sun sensitivity, so patients must avoid direct sunlight without sunscreen and/or protective clothing.
- Teach the patient to rinse his or her mouth carefully with clear liquids after vomiting. Ice chips or mild-flavored popsicles may be soothing to the patient.
- Teach the patient to contact his or her healthcare provider if nausea and/or vomiting lasts more than 2 days or if the patient is unable to take any fluids or has fever.

- Do not take any herbal agents without checking with a pharmacist or other healthcare provider while taking the serotonin (5-HT$_3$) receptor antagonists, to avoid possible interactions.
- Tell your healthcare provider if you are taking serotonin (5-HT$_3$) receptor antagonists because these drugs interact with a variety of other drugs.
- Avoid driving, operating any machinery, or participating in critical decision making while taking this drug because it may impair your judgment and reflexes.
- It is best to take the drug before you have vomited rather than waiting until after you have had an episode of vomiting.
- Do not use any alcohol or drugs with sedating effects while taking this drug.

SUBSTANCE P/NEUROKININ$_1$ RECEPTOR ANTAGONISTS

Action and Uses

Another receptor in the CTZ that can cause nausea and vomiting when activated is the substance P/neurokinin$_1$ (NK$_1$) receptor. *Substance P* is produced by many normal cells all over the body when they have been traumatized with inflammation and pain or exposed to noxious stimuli. Substance P enters the bloodstream and crosses into the brain, where it can bind to the substance P/NK$_1$ receptors that are present in many areas of the brain, including the CTZ and areas that perceive pain. Activating these receptors in the CTZ stimulates immediate and delayed nausea and vomiting. **Substance P/neurokinin$_1$ (NK$_1$) receptor antagonists** are drugs that block the substance P/NK$_1$ receptors in the CTZ. This prevents both substance P and neurokinin that are released from cells exposed to chemotherapy and from tissues injured during surgery from binding to and triggering the CTZ.

The most common uses for drugs in this class are to reduce or prevent the nausea and vomiting that result from cancer chemotherapy and after surgery. These drugs are especially effective at managing the delayed nausea and vomiting that often starts 24 to 72 hours after chemotherapy. The first drug in this class is aprepitant (Emend). These drugs are most effective when used in combination with the serotonin (5-HT$_3$) receptor antagonists. Table 13.1 lists the names, dosages, and nursing implications for the substance P/NK$_1$ receptor antagonists. Be sure to consult a drug reference book for more information about specific drugs.

Expected Side Effects

Fatigue, diarrhea, headache, and dizziness are side effects of the substance P/NK$_1$ receptor antagonists. In addition, the patient may experience mild hiccups, flatulence, and sweating.

Adverse Reactions

Neutropenia is one of the most common adverse reactions associated with substance P/NK$_1$ receptor

about any abdominal pain. Severe pain may indicate infection, bleeding, or other severe problems in the GI tract. Follow up with your patient to make sure they are getting relief from their nausea.

◆ *Patient and family teaching.* Tell the patient and family the following:

antagonists. Angioedema, severe allergic reactions, and respiratory depression may occur. Other blood abnormalities include anemia and thrombocytopenia, so monitor laboratory values carefully.

Drug Interactions

Substance P/NK$_1$ receptor antagonists interact with a variety of drugs. In particular, these drugs interact with opioid drugs, causing increased dizziness, drowsiness, and sedation. Use of these drugs with certain benzodiazepines can increase the effect of the benzodiazepines so should be used together with caution.

❖ Nursing Implications and Patient Teaching

◆ *Planning and implementation.* In addition to the general nursing considerations related to care of the patient with nausea and vomiting listed in Box 13.1, the following issues and actions are important. Carefully review the drug instructions to make sure it is prepared properly. For example, the oral form of aprepitant should not be opened until ready to prepare. At that time, the mixing cup provided in the drug kit should be filled with room temperature drinking water. Once you have added the precise amount of water to the mixing cup as directed, pour the contents of the drug into the cup and then snap the lid shut. Gently swirl the solution 20 times to mix it, then invert the cup. Do not shake the cup or foaming may occur. Be sure there are no clumps or foam in the solution. At that time, you can measure the solution to give to the patient. Discard any remaining solution.

Just as for the oral liquid aprepitant, injectable fosaprepitant must be carefully prepared. Do not shake the drug. You may gently swirl the drug or invert the solution to gently mix. Follow directions specifically for proper mixing and rate of administration.

◆ *Patient and family teaching.* Tell the patient and family the following:

- If you are taking the oral solution, avoid shaking the mixture. You can gently swirl and turn over the measuring cup or syringe.
- After the drug is mixed, it can be stored in the refrigerator for up to 30 days.
- Avoid alcohol and any sedating drugs while you are taking these drugs, to prevent side effects.
- Do not take any over-the-counter or herbal drugs without checking with your healthcare provider or pharmacist because drugs from this category can interact with other drugs.

PHENOTHIAZINES

Action and Uses

Phenothiazines are a type of antiemetic drug that reduces nausea and vomiting by blocking dopamine (D$_2$) receptors in the CTZ of the brain. For this reason drugs in this class are also called *dopamine antagonists.* Dopamine receptors are present in many other areas of the brain and the body. As a result, these drugs have many other effects in the body in addition to the antiemetic effects. Dopamine antagonists are approved to reduce nausea and vomiting from many problems except for the morning sickness associated with pregnancy. Table 13.1 lists the names, dosages, and nursing implications for the phenothiazines. Be sure to consult a drug reference book for more information about specific drugs.

Expected Side Effects

Common side effects include drowsiness, blurred vision, dry mouth, and dizziness. Some phenothiazines can cause urine to change to a pinkish red color. Sensitivity to sun exposure is common.

Adverse Reactions

Adverse reactions to phenothiazine drugs are most common at higher doses. As a result of blocking dopamine, the patient can experience extrapyramidal symptoms (EPS) as discussed in Chapter 10. These effects include tardive dyskinesia, acute dystonia, and even neuroleptic malignant syndrome. Blood abnormalities are also possible while the patient is taking phenothiazines. These drugs should be avoided in patients with cardiovascular disease because they can cause patients to experience angina, tachycardia, and/or orthostatic hypotension.

Drug Interactions

Phenothiazines interact with a wide variety of drugs. They should not be given with metoclopramide (Reglan), which also affects dopamine levels. Phenothiazines can increase the effects of any other drug that affects dopamine, including monoamine oxidase inhibitors and several other antidepressants. Benzodiazepines can cause increased drowsiness. Phenothiazines should be avoided in patients who are taking levodopa/carbidopa for Parkinson's disease.

❖ Nursing Implications and Patient Teaching

◆ *Planning and implementation.* In addition to the general nursing considerations related to antiemetic drug therapy listed in Box 13.1, the following issues and actions are important. Make sure to carefully assess the vital signs in patients who are taking phenothiazines because they can cause a decrease in blood pressure and an increase in heart rate in some patients. Avoid giving the phenothiazine antiemetic to any patient who has low blood pressure or is dehydrated. Make sure the patient has the call light available to ask for help when getting out of bed after receiving this drug because it can cause orthostatic hypotension.

Assess for any occurrence of EPS as discussed in detail in Chapter 10. If the patient demonstrates any unusual muscle movements or has any abrupt changes in temperature, heart rate, or blood pressure, notify the healthcare provider immediately.

◆ *Patient and family teaching.* Tell the patient and family the following:

- You may experience dizziness, drowsiness, or blurred vision while taking this drug. Avoid driving or using any heavy equipment or participating in any dangerous activity.
- Change position slowly to avoid dizziness.
- Do not drink alcohol while taking this drug. Alcohol may increase the side effects.
- You may notice a slight change in the color of your urine to a pinkish red. This is an expected side effect.
- If you have any muscle spasms (particularly of the neck muscles); involuntary movements of the face, tongue, or upper or lower extremities; or any unusual restlessness, notify your healthcare provider immediately.
- The drug may decrease your ability to sweat, so make sure to avoid becoming overheated during physical activity or very hot weather.
- For relief of dry mouth, try sugarless gum or candy, or use ice chips to moisten your mouth.
- These drugs can cause your skin to be more sensitive to light, so avoid direct sunlight and, if needed, wear protective eyewear and clothing. Wear sunblock while outside to avoid sunburn.

CANNABINOIDS

Action and Uses

Marijuana, a common street drug recently approved in some states for use in the medical treatment of certain health problems, has been used to help control the nausea and vomiting associated with cancer chemotherapy. Although many chemicals are present in marijuana, the ingredient that has antiemetic actions is tetrahydrocannabinol (THC). All humans have THC receptors in many areas of the brain, including in the CTZ and in pleasure centers. **Cannabinoids** are drugs that are either natural or synthetic forms of THC that reduce nausea and vomiting by binding to both cannabinoid receptors in the CTZ and by preventing serotonin 5-HT$_3$ from binding to its receptors in the CTZ. Use of cannabinoids as antiemetics is typically reserved for patients with severe nausea and vomiting that has not been relieved by other antiemetics because of the potential for addiction (rare but possible) and other side effects. Table 13.1 lists the names, dosages, and nursing implications for the cannabinoids. Be sure to consult a drug reference book for more information about specific drugs.

Expected Side Effects

The most common side effects are related to the effect of cannabinoids on the CNS. Some patients experience a dose-related "high" (easy laughing, elation, and increased awareness). Other CNS effects are dizziness, anxiety, insomnia, difficulty concentrating, and mood changes. Some patients may experience *emotional lability* (wide swings in emotion). These side effects may decrease after 2 weeks of treatment. Some patients have GI side effects such as nausea, vomiting, and abdominal pain. Orthostatic hypotension is more common in older adults.

Adverse Reactions

Acute confusion, hypersensitivity, and seizure-like activity have occurred in some patients. Rarely, hallucinations, excessive sweating, or fainting can happen, so it is important to carefully monitor the patient. Cannabinoids should be used with caution in patients who have a history of substance abuse (including alcohol) because of the increased risk for abuse of the drug.

Drug Interactions

Cannabinoids can interact with a variety of drugs. Examples include warfarin, calcium channel blockers, opioid agonists, and a variety of antiretroviral drugs used to treat HIV. Patients who take dronabinol should avoid grapefruit juice because it can increase adverse effects.

❖ **Nursing Implications and Patient Teaching**

◆ *Planning and implementation.* In addition to the general nursing considerations related to antiemetic drug therapy listed in Box 13.1, the following issues and actions are important. These drugs can be given using standard tablets and capsules or can be given as a liquid or in liquid-filled capsules with the dosage individualized according to *body surface area* (measure of the total external surface area of the body). The dosage is determined using body surface area calculations by the healthcare provider in conjunction with the pharmacist.

If you are giving a dose of the liquid drug, use the proper measuring device (such as an oral syringe) to ensure accuracy. Give the first dose on an empty stomach 30 minutes before meals. After the first dose, these drugs can be given with food.

Carefully monitor the patient for changes in mental status. Cannabinoids can cause confusion, sedation, and at times feelings of euphoria or a "high." These typically decrease after a few days to weeks of use. Advise patients to avoid alcohol, sedatives, or other CNS depressants because they may increase the risk of sedation

◆ *Patient and family teaching.* Tell the patient and family the following:

- Avoid using alcohol, sedatives, or any antianxiety drugs with these drugs without talking to your healthcare provider.
- Take the dose as prescribed; do not increase without talking to your healthcare provider.
- This drug may cause you to feel slightly "high," with feelings of easy laughing, mood changes, elation, and increased awareness. These feelings decrease in a few days to a few weeks.
- Do not drive, operate any machinery, or participate in important decision making while taking this drug.

- Ask family members to stay with you when you first start taking the drugs in case you have some confusion or dizziness.

PROMOTILITY DRUGS

Action and Uses

Promotility drugs (also called *prokinetic* drugs) are used to increase contraction of the upper GI tract including the stomach and the small intestines, which move contents more quickly through the tract. These drugs do this by blocking dopamine (D_2) receptors in the CTZ. They work similarly to the phenothiazines but do not have the sedating side effect. The promotility drugs may be used in patients with postoperative nausea and vomiting, chemotherapy-induced nausea and vomiting, and gastroesophageal reflux disease (GERD). They may also be used in patients who have difficulty emptying their stomach, such as a patient with diabetic gastroparesis. Table 13.1 lists the names, dosages, and nursing implications of common drugs from the promotility class. Be sure to consult a drug reference book for more information about specific drugs.

Expected Side Effects

The most common side effects are drowsiness, fatigue, and restlessness. Others are visual impairment, urinary incontinence, and insomnia.

Adverse Reactions

These drugs should be used with caution in patients with a history of depression because they can cause depression and even suicidal ideation, as well as seizures, blood disorders, cardiac dysrhythmias, and heart failure. Other adverse effects are related to the decrease in the neurotransmitter dopamine. This can result in symptoms similar to Parkinson's disease including tremor, bradykinesia (slow movement), and masklike facies. These symptoms decline in 2 to 3 months after stopping the drug. More severe adverse effects include tardive dyskinesia, akathisia, and acute dystonia. Neuroleptic malignant syndrome is a rare, life-threatening reaction to drugs that decrease dopamine. For more discussion about these problems, see Chapter 10.

Drug Interactions

Promotility drugs are contraindicated in patients who are taking phenothiazine drugs, typical and atypical antipsychotics (see Chapter 10), and levodopa/carbidopa (see Chapter 9). In addition, use of these drugs along with certain antidepressants can increase the risk for serotonin syndrome, which is discussed in greater detail in Chapter 10.

❖ Nursing Implications and Patient Teaching

◆ *Planning and implementation.* In addition to the general nursing considerations related to antiemetic drug therapy listed in Box 13.1, the following issues and actions are important. Carefully monitor the patient for symptoms of restlessness, dizziness, and fatigue. This is especially important for the older adult who may be at greater risk for confusion or falls. Also monitor the patient for any Parkinson's disease–like symptoms such as tremor, slower gait, or masklike facial appearance. If the patient experiences these side effects, notify the healthcare provider because the drug may need to be discontinued.

◆ *Patient and family teaching.* Tell the patient and family the following:

- Avoid driving, using any heavy machinery, or making important decisions while using this drug until you are aware of the effects.
- Do not drink alcohol while taking this drug, to avoid severe side effects.
- If you have any depression or thoughts of suicide, notify your healthcare provider immediately.
- Inform your healthcare provider immediately if you have any sudden increase in fever, muscle spasms, or difficulty with movement because these may be signs of a more serious health issue.
- Some men may experience erectile dysfunction or *gynecomastia* (enlargement of the breasts); some women may experience menstrual irregularities. These are generally reversible within a few weeks to a few months.

DRUGS FOR PEPTIC ULCER DISEASE AND GASTROESOPHAGEAL REFLUX DISEASE

The lining of the stomach is usually strong enough to resist the powerful digestive juices and acids that aid normal digestion. Gastric distress may be caused when stress or disease produces excess secretion of gastric acids, or when alcohol, chemicals, drugs, or disease produces destruction of the protective mucosal lining. If the protective lining is not repaired or the gastric acid level reduced, duodenal and gastric ulcers are produced. This is known as *peptic ulcer disease (PUD)*, as shown in Fig. 13.4. PUD is associated with inflammation, pain, bleeding, reduced nutrition, and reduced quality of life.

> ### 💡 Memory Jogger
> Prostaglandins maintain good blood flow to the stomach, which keeps these tissues well oxygenated and allows the immune system to help keep them healthy. This is why drugs that decrease prostaglandins, such as corticosteroids and NSAIDs, can be harmful to the stomach.

For many people, another problem is GERD, which is when the highly acidic stomach contents move backward (*reflux*) into the esophagus (Fig. 13.5). The esophagus has no protection for this acidity and thus can be damaged very easily. Drug therapies for PUD and GERD are essentially the same. Commonly used drug therapies include antacids, histamine H_2 receptor antagonists, **proton pump inhibitors** (PPIs), and cytoprotective drugs. Table 13.2

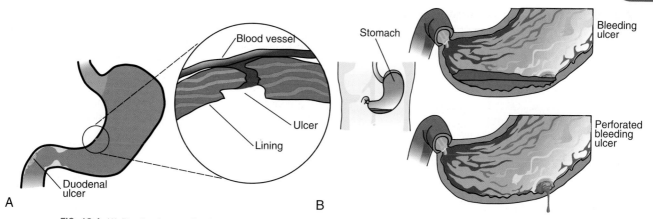

FIG. 13.4 (A) Peptic ulcer pathophysiology: The mucosa breaks down and an open sore develops. (B) A peptic ulcer may lead to bleeding, perforation, or other emergencies. (From Workman ML, LaCharity LA: *Understanding pharmacology*, ed 2, St. Louis, 2016, Elsevier.)

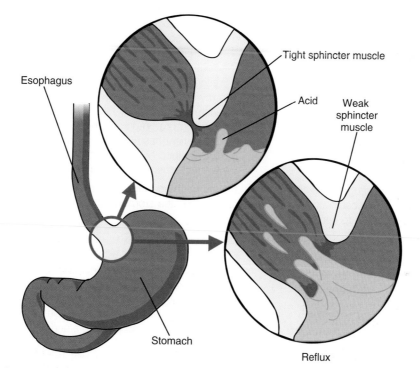

FIG. 13.5 Pathophysiology of gastroesophageal reflux disease (GERD). Acid reflux into the esophagus through the lower esophageal sphincter. (From Workman ML, LaCharity LA: *Understanding pharmacology*, ed 2, St. Louis, 2016, Elsevier.)

Table 13.2 Common Drugs for Peptic Ulcer Disease and Gastroesophageal Reflux Disease

Antacids: These drugs neutralize stomach acids to help relieve heartburn and indigestion.

DRUG/ADULT DOSAGE RANGE	NURSING IMPLICATIONS
aluminum hydroxide (Alternagel, Alu-cap) dosages vary depending on the formulation; make sure to check your drug handbook calcium carbonate (Rolaids Extra Strength, Tums, Caltrate, Maalox) dosages vary depending on the formulation; make sure to check your drug handbook magnesium hydroxide (Milk of Magnesia) regular suspension: 5–15 mL orally up to four times per day; concentrated suspension: 2.5–7.5 mL orally up to four times per day; chewable tablets: two to four tablets orally up to four times per day	• Antacids are often available as combination drugs, so make sure to review drug information carefully before giving. • Timing of antacids relating to meals and other drugs is very important. Many drugs bind with antacids and thus lose effectiveness. In general, antacids should be given 1 hour before any other drugs and 2 hours after any other drugs. • Patients with heart failure or any other cardiac diseases should avoid antacids high in sodium.

Continued

Table 13.2   Common Drugs for Peptic Ulcer Disease and Gastroesophageal Reflux Disease—cont'd

Histamine H₂ receptor antagonists: These drugs bind to the H₂ receptor in the stomach cells leading to a decrease in production of basal and nighttime gastric acid. They also decrease the amount of gastric acid that is released with meals and with substances such as caffeine.

DRUG/ADULT DOSAGE RANGE	NURSING IMPLICATIONS
famotidine (Pepcid AC) OTC 10 mg orally may repeat 1 time to maximum of 20 mg/day famotidine (Pepcid) 20 mg orally twice daily for up to 6 weeks nizatidine (Axid) 150 mg orally twice daily for up to 12 weeks ranitidine (Zantac) 150 mg orally twice daily	• Over-the-counter doses are typically about half the prescription drug doses. Patients who are taking over-the-counter histamine H₂ receptor antagonists should not take them for more than 2 weeks without seeing a healthcare provide because they may be experiencing a more significant health issue. • Monitor the patient for signs of restlessness or confusion because these side effects may increase the risk for falls.

Proton pump inhibitors: These drugs help heal gastric ulcers and reduce symptoms of GERD by stopping the acid secretory pump that is located within the gastric parietal cell membrane. This helps reduce the amount of acid secreted into the stomach.

DRUG/ADULT DOSAGE RANGE	NURSING IMPLICATIONS
esomeprazole (Nexium) 20 mg orally once daily given 60 minutes before first meal of the day for up to 8 weeks lansoprazole (Prevacid) 15–30 mg orally once daily 30–60 minutes before first meal of the day omeprazole (Prilosec) 20–40 mg orally once daily before first meal of the day for 2–8 weeks pantoprazole (Protonix) 20–40 mg orally once daily for 2–8 weeks	• Give with a full glass of water 30–60 minutes before meals for maximum benefit (read drug information carefully). • Over-the-counter proton pump inhibitors should not be taken for more than 2 weeks because failure to relieve symptoms may indicate a more severe health problem. • Prescriptions of proton pump inhibitors may vary in length from 2 to 8 weeks depending on the patient's presenting condition. • Teach patients it may take several days to experience relief once beginning proton pump inhibitors • If the patient has *H.pylori* bacteria in the stomach, the proton pump inhibitor will be combined with specific antibiotics to treat the infection so remind them to take the full prescription.

Cytoprotective drugs: These drugs protect the lining of the stomach and protect from further damage. When taken properly, some of these drugs can "stick" to the ulcerated areas in the stomach or duodenum to protect them from further damage and allow them to heal.

DRUG/ADULT DOSAGE RANGE	NURSING IMPLICATIONS

sucralfate (Carafate, Sulcrate) 1 g orally two to four times daily 1 hour before meals and at bedtime
bismuth subsalicylate (Pepto-Bismol)
  For relief of gastric distress:
  Chewable or caplets: 2 tablets orally every 30–60 minutes PRN; do not exceed eight doses per day
  Liquid regular strength: 30 mL orally every 30–60 minutes PRN; do not exceed eight doses per day
misoprostol (Cytotec) 50–200 mcg orally four times per day, with meals and at bedtime
	• Do not give antacids within 30 minutes before or 1 hour after sucralfate because they decrease the effectiveness.
	• Do not crush or chew the tablets. The tablets are scored, so they may be cut in half for easier swallowing. For patients who are unable to swallow the half or whole tablet, dissolve the tablet in 10 mL of water and allow to stand for 10–20 minutes (called a "slurry").
	• Shake the oral suspension well before giving to achieve a consistent dose of drug in solution.
	• Carefully review dosages for bismuth subsalicylate before giving because this drug can be given for several conditions besides gastric distress (e.g., treatment of diarrhea or prevention of traveler's diarrhea). It can also be used for antibiotic properties.
	• If patients do not receive relief from the recommended doses, make sure to contact the patient's healthcare provider in case there is a significant underlying condition that needs treatment.
	• Teach patients that bismuth subsalicylate can turn stools dark brown or even black while taking this drug.
	• Taking too much bismuth subsalicylate can result in symptoms of aspirin toxicity (because of the salicylate components of the drug).
	• Encourage the patient to drink at least 2–3 L of liquid unless contraindicated because this drug can cause constipation.
	• Remember that misoprostol must never be given to pregnant women because it can cause uterine contractions.

GERD, Gastroesophageal reflux disease.

lists the names, dosages, and nursing implications of common drugs for PUD and GERD. More than one drug type may be used at the same time to help in healing the initial problem.

> ### Memory Jogger
>
> Common drugs used to manage peptic ulcers and GERD are:
> - antacids
> - histamine H_2 receptor antagonists
> - PPIs
> - cytoprotective drugs

Some peptic ulcers may be caused by *Helicobacter pylori (H. pylori)*. *H. pylori* infections are typically treated by a combination of antimicrobial drugs and PPIs. Currently, patients with *H. pylori*–associated ulcers are treated for about 10 to 14 days with a standard triple therapy (consisting of a combination of a PPI and two selected antimicrobials). Alternatively, a standard quadruple therapy might be considered with a PPI and three antimicrobials. The *H. pylori* bacteria must be eradicated for successful treatment of the peptic ulcer. Chapter 5 discusses the patient teaching issues and nursing implications for antimicrobial therapy.

ANTACIDS

Action and Uses

Antacids are drugs that neutralize hydrochloric acid (HCl) and increase gastric pH (making the stomach's pH less acidic), which in turn reduces gastric irritation. Antacids are typically formulated with at least one of the following ingredients: calcium, magnesium, and aluminum. They are most often used in combination with other drugs to treat a number of GI conditions including PUD, gastritis, gastric ulcer, peptic esophagitis, hiatal hernia, gastric hyperacidity, and GERD. In most cases antacids are not used as the primary treatment for these disorders because they provide only temporary relief and do not prevent any future attacks. Table 13.2 lists the names, dosages, and nursing implications of common antacids. Be sure to consult a drug reference book for more information about specific drugs.

Expected Side Effects

Using antacids as directed rarely results in significant side effects. In general, brands with magnesium can cause diarrhea; brands with calcium or aluminum can cause constipation. Other side effects include loss of appetite, frequent burping, nausea and vomiting, fatigue, and weight loss.

Adverse Reactions

Adverse reactions are usually specific to the type of antacid. For example, if the patient is taking a magnesium-based antacid, adverse effects are usually related to hypermagnesemia, such as muscle weakness, low blood pressure, and low heart rate. Adverse effects of calcium-containing antacids include bone pain, kidney stones, and in severe cases, cardiac dysrhythmias. Aluminum-containing antacids can cause mood changes, confusion, osteoporosis, and hypercalcemia.

Drug Interactions

A major concern for all antacids is the impact on absorption of other drugs. For this reason, timing of administration of the antacids related to meals and other drugs is very important. Always consult your drug reference before you give an antacid.

❖ Nursing Implications and Patient Teaching

◆ *Planning and implementation.* In addition to the general nursing considerations related to care of the patient with PUD or GERD listed in Box 13.2, the following issues and actions are important. Antacids are available over the counter and in a variety of flavors and forms to help make them more palatable to the patient. Depending on the brand, antacids can come as liquids, chewable tablets or gummies, or as tablets that dissolve in water. The neutralizing abilities of antacids vary, so one type of antacid does not necessarily result

Box 13.2	General Nursing Considerations for the Patient With Peptic Ulcer Disease or Gastroesophageal Reflux Disease

- Teach patients to avoid eating within 3 hours of bedtime to reduce the risk of reflux while lying flat in bed.
- Recommend that the patient stop smoking because nicotine increases stomach acid.
- Recommend that the patient eat smaller portions at mealtimes.
- Tell patients to notify their healthcare provider if they have taken H_2 receptor blockers for longer than 2 weeks because these drugs can lose their effectiveness over time and the patient may need different drugs.
- GERD and peptic ulcer have similar symptoms to cancer of the stomach, and overuse of the over-the-counter drugs can mask symptoms of other health problems.
- For patients with peptic ulcer disease, make sure to monitor vital signs regularly. Make sure to notify the healthcare provider of increase in heart rate or decrease in blood pressure that may indicate internal bleeding.
- Monitor level of consciousness while patient is taking drugs for GERD and PUD because they often cause confusion or restlessness, particularly in older adult patients.
- Teach patients to avoid driving, using heavy machinery, or making important decisions while taking these drugs because they can cause drowsiness or confusion in some cases.
- Tell the patient to report any severe dizziness or changes in stool color (black) because these may be an indication of bleeding.

in the same results as another. The sodium content of various antacids must be carefully assessed before giving any antacid to patients who are on restricted sodium intake. These patients include pregnant women and patients with congestive heart failure (CHF) or other cardiac conditions, hypertension (high blood pressure), edema (fluid buildup in the body tissues), or renal failure.

◆ *Patient and family teaching.* Tell the patient and family the following:
* Antacids neutralize gastric acids and are typically most beneficial if given between meals and at bedtime.
* Take the drug exactly as prescribed. Antacids are generally taken 1 hour after meals and before bedtime.
* If you are taking other drugs, it is usually best to take them 1 hour before or 2 hours after taking the antacid. Consult your pharmacist or healthcare provider if you have any questions.
* Diarrhea or constipation are common side effects of different antacids. Contact your healthcare provider if they are severe.
* Never take more than the recommended amount, to avoid adverse effects.
* Antacids are used for short-term treatment only; they do not prevent future attacks.
* If you are taking a chewable antacid, chew it thoroughly before swallowing and with a full glass of water.
* Shake any liquid antacid well before taking to ensure the dosage is correct.

HISTAMINE H₂ RECEPTOR ANTAGONISTS

Action and Uses

Histamine H_2 receptor antagonists bind to the H_2 receptor in the stomach cells, leading to a decrease in production of *basal* (the minimum amount of acid your body needs throughout the day) and nighttime gastric acid. It also decreases the amount of gastric acid released with meals and with substances such as caffeine. They may be used intravenously before and during long, major surgical procedures to prevent ulcer formation resulting from the physiologic stress of surgery. Table 13.2 lists the names, dosages, and nursing implications of common histamine H_2 receptor antagonists. Be sure to consult a drug reference book for more information about specific drugs.

> **Memory Jogger**
>
> All the histamine H_2 receptor antagonists have the suffix *-tidine* in their generic names.

Expected Side Effects

Expected side effects include headache, nausea, diarrhea or constipation, and mild abdominal pain. Some patients may have mental status changes, including confusion, anxiety, or depression. These usually resolve when the drug is stopped.

Adverse Reactions

Severe adverse reactions to H_2 receptor blockers are rare and include severe allergic reactions, a variety of blood disorders, and cardiac dysrhythmias. Although the reason is not fully known, patients may also be at risk for pneumonia.

Drug Interactions

H_2 blockers can affect certain enzymes in the liver that metabolize drugs. This can result in changes in how certain drugs are metabolized in the body, including warfarin, beta blockers, benzodiazepines, calcium channel blockers, and alcohol. Contact the healthcare provider or pharmacist if there is any concern about interactions.

❖ **Nursing Implications and Patient Teaching**

◆ *Planning and implementation.* In addition to the general nursing considerations related to care of the patient with PUD or GERD listed in Box 13.2, the following issues and actions are important. Make sure to assess the complete blood count and check for unusual bleeding or signs of infection. Make sure to monitor patients for any changes in mental status, such as confusion or anxiety, after beginning H_2 receptor blockers. For best effects, these drugs should be given with meals and at bedtime.

◆ *Patient and family teaching.* Tell the patient and family the following:
* Once-a-day dosing of H_2 receptor blockers is best taken at bedtime to reduce symptoms of acid reflux at night.
* Avoid cigarette smoking because it increases gastric acid production and can decrease the effectiveness of H_2 blockers.
* Take H_2 blockers only for occasional episodes of heartburn because they can lose their effectiveness. If symptoms continue, contact your healthcare provider for diagnosis and treatment.
* Do not drive or operate heavy machinery until you see how the drug affects you. These drugs may cause dizziness in some people.
* Use handrails when you are using stairs in case you have any dizziness.
* Ask your family members to observe you for any changes in mental status, such as confusion or anxiety and depression.

> **Lifespan Considerations**
> **Older Adults**
>
> Older adults are more likely than younger adults to experience confusion and dizziness as side effects of H_2 blockers.

PROTON PUMP INHIBITORS

Action and Uses

PPIs help heal gastric ulcers and reduce symptoms of GERD by stopping the acid secretory pump that is located within the gastric parietal cell membrane. This helps reduce the amount of acid secreted into the stomach.

PPIs are used to reduce gastric acid in a variety of conditions including GERD or peptic ulcer, or in combination with other drugs to treat *H. pylori* infection. They also may be used in acute care settings to decrease the risk for stress ulcers in critically ill patients. Length of treatment varies according to the type of illness the patient is experiencing but typically is about 4 to 8 weeks. In some cases longer-term treatment may be indicated in patients who produce excessive amounts of gastric acid (e.g., Zollinger-Ellison syndrome). In fact, some patients may need the drug for as long as 5 years. Table 13.2 lists the names, dosages, and nursing implications of common PPIs. Be sure to consult a drug reference book for more information about specific drugs.

> **Memory Jogger**
>
> All the PPIs have the suffix -*prazole* in their generic names.

Expected Side Effects

Common side effects include headache, mild abdominal pain, nausea and vomiting, flatulence ("passing gas"), and diarrhea or constipation. Many patients experience increased sensitivity to light (*photosensitivity*). Less common side effects include dizziness, anxiety, or mild rash. Low vitamin B_{12} levels leading to anemia may develop in patients who have taken PPIs for more than 1 year.

Adverse Reactions

Possible adverse reactions include severe allergic reactions, pancreatitis, and blood abnormalities including thrombocytopenia and hemolytic anemia. There is some concern that decreased calcium absorption in the stomach may place the patient at risk for osteoporosis and bone fractures with long-term use.

Drug Interactions

PPIs also inhibit certain enzymes in the liver that are involved in metabolizing other drugs. This is important because PPIs can increase or decrease the effectiveness of other drugs. Examples include warfarin, alprazolam, drugs given to treat tuberculosis, and certain drugs used to decrease blood cholesterol.

❖ Nursing Implications and Patient Teaching

◆ *Planning and implementation.* In addition to the general nursing considerations related to care of the patient with PUD or GERD listed in Box 13.2, the following issues and actions are important. Give PPIs about 30 to 60 minutes before the first meal of the day (usually breakfast). This will help to decrease the amount of acid secreted while eating. It may take 1 to 3 days for the patient to experience any relief from symptoms. In patients at risk for or with osteoporosis, manage their

bone status according to the healthcare providers' recommendations from current clinical practice, and ensure adequate vitamin D and calcium supplementation.

◆ *Patient and family teaching.* Tell the patient and family the following:

- Avoid driving or using heavy machinery while using this drug because it may cause dizziness.
- Contact your healthcare provider for recommendations about calcium and vitamin D because this drug may increase your risk for osteoporosis.
- Do not use over-the-counter PPIs for longer than 2 weeks. If symptoms continue, contact your healthcare provider.
- If you are taking prescription PPIs, make sure to take the full prescription even if you feel better.
- These drugs do not cure ulcers, but they do reduce acid in your stomach so that the ulcer can heal.
- Wear sunscreen and protective clothing because your skin may be more sensitive to light.

CYTOPROTECTIVE DRUGS

Action and Uses

Cytoprotective drugs protect the lining of the stomach and protect from further damage. When taken properly, some of these drugs can "stick" to the ulcerated areas in the stomach or duodenum to protect them from further damage and allow them to heal.

Sucralfate aids in the healing of ulcers by forming a protective layer at the ulcer site, providing a barrier to injury from the gastric acids. Misoprostol is a synthetic prostaglandin with both an antisecretory and a mucosal protective action. Although it has other drug classifications, it is a cytoprotective drug for the GI tract. It is indicated for use in patients who have gastric distress or ulceration secondary to the use of NSAIDs. Names, usual adult dosages, and nursing implications of these drugs are listed in Table 13.2. Be sure to consult a drug reference book for more information about specific cytoprotective drugs.

DRUGS FOR CONSTIPATION AND DIARRHEA

Constipation is not considered a specific disease, but rather is a condition associated with other health problems. Normal bowel patterns vary widely, with some people having a bowel movement several times a day and others no more than three times a week. Decreased frequency of bowel movements is just one factor associated with constipation. Others include hard or dry stools, pain with having a bowel movement, feeling bloated, and/or straining with bowel movement. See Fig. 13.6 for a description of how constipation occurs.

Patients experience constipation for multiple reasons. For example, low-fiber diet, low levels of physical activity, ignoring the urge to have a bowel movement, pregnancy, or aging. Other causes include certain drugs, dehydration, certain bowel disorders, depression, or other medical problems. Most episodes of constipation

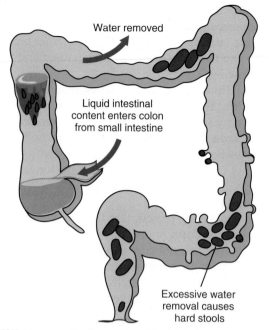

FIG. 13.6 How constipation occurs. (From Workman ML, LaCharity LA: *Understanding pharmacology*, ed 2, St. Louis, 2016, Elsevier.)

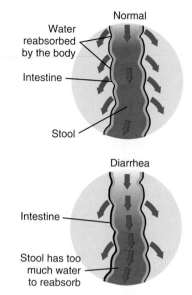

FIG. 13.7 Pathophysiology of diarrhea. (From Workman ML, LaCharity LA: *Understanding pharmacology*, ed 2, St. Louis, 2016, Elsevier.)

Box 13.3   Common Causes of Diarrhea

- Drugs (e.g., antibiotics, laxatives, chemotherapy)
- Food poisoning/traveler's diarrhea
- Gastrectomy (partial removal of the stomach)
- High-dose radiation therapy
- Medical conditions (e.g., malabsorption, inflammatory bowel diseases such as Crohn's disease or ulcerative colitis, irritable bowel syndrome, celiac disease)
- Nerve disorders (autonomic neuropathy, diabetic neuropathy)
- Other infections (bacterial, parasites)
- Viral gastroenteritis (most common cause)
- Zollinger-Ellison syndrome

From Workman ML, LaCharity L, Kruchko S: *Understanding pharmacology: Essentials for medication safety*, ed 2, St. Louis, 2010, W.B. Saunders Company, Box 19-3.

are mild and do not require drugs or input from a healthcare provider. Some are relieved with the use of an over-the-counter laxative (discussed later). However, if constipation becomes severe, a patient experiences bleeding or abdominal pain, or constipation lasts longer than a few weeks, the patient should contact his or her healthcare provider.

Memory Jogger

Signs and symptoms of constipation include:
- less than three bowel movements per week
- sudden decrease in frequency of bowel movements
- harder stools than normal
- bowels still feeling full after a bowel movement
- feeling bloated
- straining to have a bowel movement

Like constipation, diarrhea is a symptom of other health conditions. Diarrhea is caused by an increase in the amount of water in the stool. This increased water is from an imbalance between the amount of fluid secreted from the intestines and the amount of fluid absorbed back into the body. If the amount of fluid secreted is greater than the amount reabsorbed, water will remain in the colon and the stool will be loose and watery (Fig. 13.7). This may be a result of infection, drugs that change the bacteria in the colon, inflammatory bowel disorders, food poisoning, or other medical conditions (Box 13.3 lists common causes of diarrhea). Episodes of diarrhea are usually self-limiting, lasting no more than a few days. However, in certain conditions, diarrhea can be severe and long-lasting. In general, the term *acute diarrhea* is used when it lasts up to 14 days; chronic diarrhea is considered when it lasts

for more than 2 to 4 weeks. Whatever the cause or length of time, the major risks of prolonged diarrhea are dehydration and electrolyte imbalance.

Of special consideration, in cases of infection from certain bacteria or parasites, drugs to reduce diarrhea may be contraindicated. This is because the drugs would slow down or hamper the body's ability to eliminate the organism that is causing the problem. In this situation, the focus is on keeping the patient well hydrated and providing good skin care to reduce irritation to the anus and surrounding area of the skin.

DRUGS FOR CONSTIPATION

Laxatives are a class of drugs that promote bowel movements by stimulating peristalsis, increasing the bulk of the stool, or softening the stool. They are typically used to relieve constipation. Laxatives are also used to cleanse the bowel in preparation for surgery involving the GI tract, certain x-rays, or endoscopic procedures (such as colonoscopy or proctoscopy). They can also be used as part of bowel care for individuals who have lost

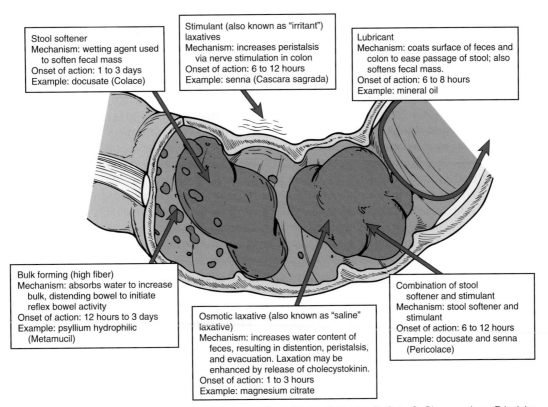

Stool softener
Mechanism: wetting agent used to soften fecal mass
Onset of action: 1 to 3 days
Example: docusate (Colace)

Stimulant (also known as "irritant") laxatives
Mechanism: increases peristalsis via nerve stimulation in colon
Onset of action: 6 to 12 hours
Example: senna (Cascara sagrada)

Lubricant
Mechanism: coats surface of feces and colon to ease passage of stool; also softens fecal mass.
Onset of action: 6 to 8 hours
Example: mineral oil

Bulk forming (high fiber)
Mechanism: absorbs water to increase bulk, distending bowel to initiate reflex bowel activity
Onset of action: 12 hours to 3 days
Example: psyllium hydrophilic (Metamucil)

Osmotic laxative (also known as "saline" laxative)
Mechanism: increases water content of feces, resulting in distention, peristalsis, and evacuation. Laxation may be enhanced by release of cholecystokinin.
Onset of action: 1 to 3 hours
Example: magnesium citrate

Combination of stool softener and stimulant
Mechanism: stool softener and stimulant
Onset of action: 6 to 12 hours
Example: docusate and senna (Pericolace)

FIG. 13.8 Sites of action for different types of laxatives. (From Fulcher E, Fulcher R, Soto C: *Pharmacology: Principles and applications,* ed 3, St. Louis, 2012, Elsevier.)

neurogenic control of the bowel. Although laxatives can be very helpful for short-term treatment of constipation, they are not a substitute for healthy diet, adequate hydration, and physical activity. There are five major categories based on their mechanism of action (Fig. 13.8): bulk-forming drugs, stool softeners, lubricants, osmotic laxatives (sometimes called *saline* laxatives), and stimulants (sometimes called *irritant* laxatives).

Action and Uses

Bulk-forming laxatives relieve constipation by absorbing water in the GI tract, altering intestinal fluid and electrolytes. The absorption of fluid expands the stool (in other words, increases the bulk). The increased bulk stimulates peristalsis, and the absorbed water softens the stool. Bulk-forming laxatives are used for the treatment and prevention of constipation. They can also be used as part of the management of irritable bowel syndrome or diverticulosis. Laxative effects can occur as soon as 12 hours after the dose to as long as 3 days later.

Stool softeners relieve constipation by reducing surface tension of the stool so water and lipids can enter the stool and soften the feces. This makes it easier to pass the stool, so they are helpful in patients after surgery or patients who should avoid straining. Softening of the stool typically takes between 1 and 3 days after starting the drug.

Lubricant laxatives relieve constipation by creating a barrier between the feces and the colon wall that prevents the colon from reabsorbing fecal fluid, thus softening the stool. The lubricant effect also eases the passage of feces through the intestine. Lubricant laxatives are used to soften stool in conditions in which straining should be avoided, such as in patients with myocardial infarction, aneurysm, stroke, or hernia or after abdominal or rectal surgery. They can help prevent pain and decrease the risk for tearing or laceration of hemorrhoids or anal fissures.

Osmotic laxatives (also known as *saline laxatives*), such as lactulose and glycerin, relieve constipation by producing an osmotic effect by drawing water into the intestinal lumen of the small intestine and colon. This increase in fluid helps soften the stool and causes distention of the stool. The distention of the stool helps stimulate peristalsis. Osmotic laxatives are typically used to cleanse the bowel in preparation for colonoscopy, x-ray studies, or GI surgery. They can work very rapidly between 30 minutes and 6 hours, and can work effectively to help empty the bowel. One of the drugs, lactulose, can also be used in patients with liver failure because it helps reduce ammonia levels by nearly 50%. It can be helpful for some patients to reduce the confusion associated with liver failure.

When rapid relief of constipation is desired, stimulant or irritant laxatives may be used. They are often used to treat acute constipation resulting from prolonged bed rest or poor dietary habits, or constipation induced by other drugs. They may be used in combination with osmotic laxatives as part of bowel preparation for surgery. *Stimulant laxatives* increase peristalsis by several mechanisms, depending on the agent. These drugs can stimulate sensitive nerve fibers in the intestine, irritate the mucosa in the intestine, and affect water and electrolyte secretion in the bowel. The result is increased peristalsis and stimulation of a bowel movement, usually within 6 to 8 hours. Some drugs may even act more rapidly, so carefully read the drug information before giving stimulant laxatives. In the past it was believed that stimulant laxatives could cause physical dependence on laxatives. More recent evidence suggests that this is not the case. Nevertheless, frequent use of stimulant laxatives should be avoided in favor of improving diet and physical activity. When constipation relief is needed long term, bulk-forming laxatives are more likely to be recommended because of the low incidence of side effects. Table 13.3 lists the names, dosages, and nursing implications of selected laxatives from each of the categories. Be sure to consult a drug reference book for more information about specific drugs.

Expected Side Effects

The most common side effects of laxatives are GI symptoms such as nausea, abdominal cramping, bloating, and diarrhea. Table 13.4 lists side effects associated with specific types of laxatives.

Adverse Effects

Bulk-forming laxatives are the safest laxatives. Nevertheless, inhaling the psyllium dust particles can cause hypersensitivity reactions. These reactions can be as severe as bronchospasm and anaphylaxis. Caution should be taken for patients with respiratory illnesses. Patients who do not take the drug with enough water (need at least 8–12 ounces of fluid) are at risk for esophageal obstruction. Swelling of the throat or choking might occur. If patients do have severe difficulty swallowing, chest pain, or difficulty breathing, they should contact their healthcare provider immediately.

Stool softeners rarely cause adverse events; however, severe allergic reactions are possible. Lubricant laxatives may produce decreased absorption of nutrients and fat-soluble vitamins. Rarely, a condition called *lipid pneumonia* can occur by inhalation of fat-containing substances like mineral oil. The risk can be reduced by avoiding giving lubricant laxatives at bedtime or before lying down. Lubricant laxatives should also be avoided in patients who are at risk for aspiration. Osmotic laxatives can produce a fluid and electrolyte disturbance if used daily or in patients with renal or cardiac impairment. Stimulant laxatives may produce muscle weakness (after excessive use of laxatives), dermatitis, pruritus, alkalosis, and electrolyte imbalance (with excessive use).

Memory Jogger

Common drugs used to manage constipation are:
- bulk-forming laxatives
- stool softeners
- lubricants
- osmotic laxatives
- stimulant laxatives

Drug Interactions

Laxatives in general may reduce absorption or bind to certain drugs because they can increase GI motility. In particular, loop diuretics, warfarin, salicylates (such as aspirin), and digoxin must be separated from administration of laxatives by at least 2 hours. Patients who take loop diuretics and digoxin are at risk for hypokalemia if they use laxatives frequently. Some laxatives given with foods that have high potassium or sodium content can increase the risk for hyperkalemia or hypernatremia.

❖ Nursing Implications and Patient Teaching

◆ *Planning and implementation.* In addition to the general nursing considerations related to care of the patient with constipation listed in Box 13.4, the following issues and actions are important. Some bulk-forming drugs are high in sugars. Suggest to patients with diabetes that "sugar-free" drugs are less likely to interfere with diabetes therapy. Even though allergic reactions are rare, certain patients may be allergic to dust particles when the drug is mixed or poured. Report any symptoms of allergy, such as rash, hives, or difficulty breathing, to the healthcare provider immediately. Bulk-forming drugs

Box 13.4	General Nursing Considerations for Drugs for Constipation

- Never give any type of laxative to a patient with severe abdominal pain, nausea and vomiting, or fever unless that patient has been thoroughly assessed by a healthcare provider or nurse practitioner. These symptoms may indicate a serious illness.
- Remember, normal bowel function will vary between individuals. Some patients may have one to three stools per day, others three times a week. Ask patients about their normal bowel history and if they have had additional symptoms of diarrhea, including difficulty passing stool, straining at bowel movement, or hard, dry stools. Also check to see if they have had mucus or blood with having a bowel movement.
- For patients who are unable to communicate clearly (e.g., after stroke or with cognitive impairment), keep accurate records of when the patient has a bowel movement.
- Ask the patient about any chronic disease (especially heart failure), allergies, edema, any other drugs being taken, and whether he or she has been prescribed a sodium-restricted diet.
- Laxatives are not a substitute for adequate hydration and nutrition to maintain adequate bowel function.
- Make sure to include a variety of fruits and vegetables per day. Recommended fruit intake for adults is between 1½ to 2 cups per day. Recommended vegetable intake is 2 to 3 cups per day.
- Assess the patient's drug list because many drugs may cause constipation, including some iron supplements, opioids, certain antacids, and anticholinergic drugs.
- Assess the patient's use of over-the-counter laxatives or herbal laxatives because some may cause electrolyte imbalances if used improperly or too often.

Table 13.3   Common Drugs for Diarrhea and Constipation

Anticholinergic drugs: These drugs reduce diarrhea and associated symptoms by selectively blocking the neurotransmitter acetylcholine from binding to its receptors in nerve cells. The nerve fibers of the parasympathetic system affect the involuntary movement of smooth muscle in the GI tract, lungs, and urinary tract.

DRUG/ADULT DOSAGE RANGE	NURSING IMPLICATIONS
dicyclomine (Bentyl) initially, 20 mg orally four times per day; after the first week, the dose may be increased as tolerated; maximum: 40 mg orally four times daily IM dosage: 10–20 mg IM four times per day for no longer than 1–2 days if the patient cannot take orally	• Do not give this drug within 2 hours of giving an antacid because it can decrease absorption. • Do not stop this drug suddenly if the patient has used this drug for a long time. Suddenly stopping the drug may cause withdrawal symptoms, including dizziness, sweating, and vomiting. • To avoid local skin reaction with local pain and edema, inject this drug into a large muscle mass.

Antispasmodic drugs: These drugs reduce muscle contraction in the GI tract. This causes decreased cramping, bloating, and diarrhea.

DRUG/ADULT DOSAGE RANGE	NURSING IMPLICATIONS
atropine, hyoscyamine, phenobarbital, scopolamine (Donnatal) 1–2 tablets orally three to four times per day; Elixir 5 to 10 mL orally three to four times per day; Extended release 1 tablet orally every 12 hours; may give 1 tablet every 8 hours if needed.	• Teach patients that they should not use contact lenses while taking these drugs because they can cause dry eyes and blurred vision. • These drugs decrease GI motility and should not be used in infectious diarrhea. • Monitor patient's vital signs carefully because these drugs can cause significant changes in heart rate (bradycardia or tachycardia). • These drugs are not recommended in older adults because they can cause confusion and other adverse effects even at low doses. • See nursing implications for anticholinergic drugs because they contain atropine, which is an anticholinergic drug.

Opioid agonists: These drugs are synthetic opioid agonists to decrease motility of the smooth muscle of the bowel. They are combined with atropine to decrease any mood-elevating effects of the opioid and reduce potential for abuse

DRUG/ADULT DOSAGE RANGE	NURSING IMPLICATIONS
loperamide (Imodium) 4 mg orally initially, followed by 2 mg orally after each unformed stool; do not exceed 16 mg/day diphenoxylate with atropine (Lomotil) initially, 5 mg (2 tablets) orally three to four times per day, reduce to 2.5 mg orally two to three times per day, if needed; discontinue as soon as possible; do not exceed 20 mg/day orally	• Remind patients to avoid sedatives, tranquilizers, and opioid pain drugs because they may increase the risk for CNS effects. • Teach patients to follow directions carefully because overuse can result in constipation. • Drugs with atropine may cause side effects such as dry mouth or blurred vision. Use caution when taking the drug. Also, patients may find that ice chips or sugar-free candy may help keep their lips and mouth moist.

Bulk-forming drugs: These act by absorbing fluids in the GI tract to form a mixture leading to softening and increased bulk of the stool. The increased bulk stimulates peristalsis leading to increased bowel mobility and more rapid transit time through the GI tract. Stools are easier to pass. In addition, these drugs can be helpful for patients with watery diarrhea by increasing the bulk and consistency of the stool.

DRUG/ADULT DOSAGE RANGE	NURSING IMPLICATIONS
methylcellulose (Citrucel) 1 rounded tablespoon orally one to three times daily with 240 mL (8 oz.) of fluid; 2 caplets orally with at least 240 mL (8 oz) of liquid, up to six times per day as needed psyllium (Fiberall, Karacil, Metamucil) 1 rounded teaspoon, tablespoon, or premeasured packet in 8 oz. of fluid orally, one to three times per day (see specific product chosen); if using wafer form, take 2 wafers orally one to three times per day with 240 mL (8 oz). of fluid	• Teach patients that these drugs typically work within 12 hours to 3 days. • Instruct patients to drink at least one full glass of water with each dose to avoid blockages in the esophagus. • These drugs can be mixed with water, fruit juices, or milk for better flavor.

Continued

Table 13.3 Common Drugs for Diarrhea and Constipation—cont'd

Emollients/Stool softeners: These drugs lower the surface tension of the stool, allowing water and lipids to permeate the stool. This results in a softer, easier to pass stool. This typically takes 1–3 days for the patient to receive the benefit.

DRUG/ADULT DOSAGE RANGE	NURSING IMPLICATIONS
docusate (Colace, Sulfolax, Surfak) capsules 50–300 mg/day orally given in single or divided doses; oral solution (containing 10 mg/mL docusate sodium) 50–200 mg/day orally given in single or divided doses	• Teach patients that they may experience a change in urine color from pinkish red to yellow-brown depending on the alkalinity or acidity of the urine. • Teach the patient that these drugs typically have an effect in 1–3 days. They are not used to treat acute constipation but to prevent constipation from occurring.

Stimulants: These drugs stimulate peristalsis by irritating the mucosal lining of the intestine, and increase the amount of fluid in the intestine, relaxing the bowel and easing the passage of stool.

DRUG/ADULT DOSAGE RANGE	NURSING IMPLICATIONS
bisacodyl (Dulcolax, Doxidan, Feen-a-Mint) 5–15 mg single oral dose; 10 mg rectally. Either a rectal suppository or oral tablet(s) may be used up to three times per week.	• These drugs are available over the counter and may be used for occasional constipation. Higher doses can be used as bowel preparation for x-rays of the colon or for colonoscopy. • Inform patients regarding the expected onset of action. Oral tablets can work within 6–12 hours; rectal suppositories can work within 15 minutes to 1 hour.

Osmotic laxatives: These drugs cause increased absorption of fluid into the stool. As a result, the stool is softer and distends the colon, leading to peristalsis and easier passage of the stool.

DRUG/ADULT DOSAGE RANGE	NURSING IMPLICATIONS
polyethylene glycol (MiraLAX) 1 heaping tablespoon of powder in 120–240 mL of fluid given orally once daily To evacuate the bowel before a colonoscopy: 238 g PEG 3350 dissolved in 64 oz. of carbohydrate-electrolyte drink (e.g., Gatorade). Note: some regimens add biscodyl tablets to bowel prep. Sodium phosphate monobasic monohydrate; sodium phosphate dibasic anhydrous (Fleet) Rectal dosage (Fleet Enema) 1 bottle (118 mL) rectally: taking more than the recommended dose in 24 hours can be harmful. NOTE: each 118-mL bottle contains 4400 mg of sodium.	• Follow directions very carefully when these drugs are used as part of bowel preparation for colonoscopy or other procedures. Protocols may vary between prescribers. The goal is to have the best visibility of the lower intestine during examination. • Instruct patients not to use these drugs more than recommended to avoid severe fluid and electrolyte imbalance. • Some preparations include high amounts of sodium, so they should be avoided in patients who require a low sodium intake. • These drugs work very quickly with onset of action within 1–3 hours. Make sure to teach patients that they should be near a place that has a bathroom or commode available.

may become dry, thick, and hardened in the throat or within the intestine if they are swallowed without sufficient water and can cause GI obstruction. The drugs should never be chewed or swallowed without one or more full glasses of water.

Laxatives high in sodium should be avoided in patients with edema, pregnancy, CHF, and sodium-restricted diets. In addition, overuse of stimulant laxatives may cause excessive fluid and electrolyte imbalance, particularly dehydration and hypokalemia. Laxatives are available without prescription; therefore it is especially important to teach the patient about risks associated with laxative use.

Top Tip for Safety

Make sure your patient has a call light available particularly after taking osmotic or stimulant laxatives because these may cause a sense of urgency to have a bowel movement.

◆ **Patient and family teaching.** Tell the patient and family the following:
- Drink a full glass of fluid with each dose of bulk-forming laxative to avoid blockage in the esophagus.
- Most laxatives are recommended for short-term use only. Contact your healthcare provider if you require laxatives on a regular basis or do not have relief with the over-the-counter drugs.
- Some laxatives are high in sodium or in sugar. Make sure to read the labels carefully if you are on a low-sodium diet or have diabetes.
- Laxatives are not a substitute for good bowel habits including regular physical activity and a diet that includes high-fiber foods, such as whole grains, fruits, and fresh vegetables.
- Many types of drugs increase the risk for constipation. If you are taking a drug that causes constipation, contact your healthcare provider to determine the best type of laxative for you.

Table 13.4 Summary of Common Side and Adverse Effects of Laxatives

DRUG	COMMON SIDE AND ADVERSE EFFECTS
Bulk-Forming Drugs (onset of action 12 hours to 3 days)	
psyllium (Metamucil)	Abdominal cramping, nausea, vomiting
Stool Softeners	
docusate (Colace, Surfak)	Mild abdominal cramping, nausea, cramps, throat irritation, rashes; urine can have a color change with some stool softeners varying from pink-red to yellow-brown depending on the acidity of the urine
Lubricants (onset of action 6–8 hours)	
glycerin suppository (Sani-Supp)	Abdominal cramping, hyperemia (increased blood flow) of rectal mucosa, rectal discomfort
Osmotic Laxatives (onset of action 1–3 hours)	
lactulose (Cephulac, Cholac, Constilac)	Abdominal distention, belching, diarrhea, flatulence, GI cramps, hypoglycemia in patient with diabetes
lubiprostone (Amitiza)	Abdominal pain and distention, diarrhea, dizziness, dry mouth, gas, headache, nausea, peripheral swelling, reflux
magnesium hydroxide (Phillips' Milk of Magnesia)	Diarrhea, flushing, sweating
polyethylene glycol (MiraLAX)	Abdominal bloating, cramping, flatulence (gas), nausea
sodium phosphate (Fleet Enema)	Abdominal bloating, abdominal pain, dizziness, electrolyte imbalances (hyperphosphatemia, hypocalcemia, hypokalemia, sodium retention), GI cramping, headache, nausea, vomiting
Stimulants (onset of action 6–12 hours)	
bisacodyl (Dulcolax)	Abdominal cramps, diarrhea, hypokalemia (low potassium), muscle weakness, nausea, rectal burning

Modified from Workman ML, LaCharity L, Kruchko S: *Understanding pharmacology: Essentials for medication safety*, ed 2, St. Louis, 2010, W.B. Saunders Company.

- Never take a laxative to treat severe abdominal pain because the drug may make conditions that cause the pain, such as appendicitis or diverticulitis, worse.
- The onset of action of laxatives varies according to the specific drug category. These drugs can work in as short of a period as an hour or as long as 2 to 3 days. Knowing the expected onset will help you plan.

DRUGS FOR DIARRHEA

Gastric motility is the spontaneous but unconscious or involuntary movement of food through the GI tract. Much of the discomfort of GI disease is caused by increased intestinal peristalsis (bowel muscle contraction) and the resulting symptoms. Abdominal cramping, bloating, and pain may be related either to acute minor illnesses associated with diarrhea and increased gas, or to chronic diseases such as ulcers or colitis. Also, many drugs have both diarrhea and increased bowel motility as common side effects or adverse reactions.

Antidiarrheals are drugs that reduce or stop loose, watery stools and help to restore normal bowel movements. Three general drug classes are used to treat these problems: anticholinergics, antispasmodics, or opioid agonists. Their actions are somewhat different, although they are often used in combination.

Action and Uses

The *anticholinergic drugs* reduce diarrhea and associated symptoms by selectively blocking the neurotransmitter acetylcholine from binding to its receptors in nerve cells. The nerve fibers of the parasympathetic system affect the involuntary movement of smooth muscle in the GI tract, lungs, and urinary tract. Anticholinergics reduce GI tract spasm and intestinal motility, acid production, and gastric motility, and thus reduce the associated pain. Gastric emptying time is slowed, and acid production is reduced. Anticholinergic drugs are rarely used alone but rather are used in combination with other drugs to reduce diarrhea.

The *antispasmodic drugs* reduce muscle contraction in the GI tract. This causes decreased cramping, bloating, and diarrhea. These drugs are typically combination drugs that affect the autonomic nervous system and the CNS. Antispasmodic drugs are used primarily to treat symptoms of irritable bowel syndrome. They can also be used to treat acute inflammation of the small bowel and colon or duodenal ulcer.

Memory Jogger

When diarrhea is caused by infection, the healthcare provider may not give antidiarrheals to allow the patient's body to get rid of the infection. In those cases, your care will be supportive to prevent dehydration and provide excellent skin care.

Some antidiarrheals are categorized as **opioid agonists.** These drugs are effective for diarrhea but do not have the analgesic or other opioid-like effects. They do, however, reduce GI motility and increase the ability of the intestine to absorb water. Feces then increase bulk and the patient loses fewer fluid and electrolytes. One more antidiarrheal, bismuth subsalicylate, is a salicylate drug. Although its action is not fully understood, bismuth subsalicylate may prevent the attachment of certain organisms to the intestinal mucosa and provide a protective coating for the intestinal mucosa. These drugs can be used to treat nonspecific diarrhea or diarrhea caused by antibiotics. Bismuth subsalicylate may be used to prevent traveler's diarrhea.

Expected Side Effects

The most common side effects of antidiarrheals include nausea, vomiting, dry mouth, and constipation. Others may be dizziness or drowsiness.

Adverse Reactions

Anticholinergics have many drug interactions (see Chapter 9 for a more specific discussion). The opioid agonists may interact with other opioid drugs to increase the opioid effect. Many of these drugs are combination drugs, so be sure to consult your nursing reference before giving them.

❖ Nursing Implications and Patient Teaching

◆ *Planning and implementation.* In addition to the general nursing considerations related to care of the patient with diarrhea discussed in Box 13.5, the following issues and actions are important. Anticholinergic drugs should not be given to patients with a history of GI obstruction, benign prostatic hypertrophy, or glaucoma because these drugs worsen these conditions. Some of the antispasmodic drugs contain phenobarbital (a sedating drug and CNS depressant). Although the dosage is very small, these drugs should be avoided in patients with a history of sensitivity to barbiturates. They should be avoided in patients with a history of substance abuse or alcoholism.

Physical dependence on opioid agonists contained in some antidiarrheal drugs is rare. Nevertheless, patients who use high doses of these drugs may experience withdrawal symptoms if they stop taking them suddenly. Table 13.3 gives a summary of anticholinergic, antispasmodic, and antidiarrheal drugs.

◆ *Patient and family teaching.* Tell the patient and family the following:

- Take this drug exactly as ordered by your healthcare provider.
- Notify your healthcare provider if any new or troublesome problems occur, especially if increased abdominal pain or fever is associated with diarrhea.
- The antidiarrheal drugs are used to relieve symptoms and to prevent dehydration until the underlying cause can be found and treated.
- Diarrhea that persists for more than 48 hours should not be self-treated. Return to your healthcare provider for further evaluation and diagnosis.
- Some antidiarrheal drugs contain habit-forming drugs; therefore they should be used only at the dosage recommended and for the length of time prescribed.

Box 13.5 | General Nursing Considerations for Drugs for Diarrhea

- Wash your hands between contact with all patients. Wear gloves when directly caring for the patients.
- Follow agency protocol to determine the need for isolation of a patient.
- Never give any type of antidiarrheal agent to a patient with severe abdominal pain, nausea and vomiting, or fever unless that patient has been thoroughly assessed by the registered nurse or healthcare provider These symptoms may indicate a serious illness.
- Assess the patient's normal bowel pattern including frequency, consistency, and regularity.
- Ask the patient about any underlying health conditions that may be causing the diarrhea.
- Check the patient's drug history because many drugs have diarrhea as a side effects (e.g., antibiotics, laxatives, statin drugs, lithium, and NSAIDs). Remind the patient to include over-the-counter and herbal drugs.
- Determine whether the patient has cramping or abdominal pain with defecation.
- Monitor stools for color, consistency, and presence of blood or mucus. If blood or mucus is present, report it to the registered nurse or healthcare provider.

- Report fever, abdominal distention, or severe pain to the registered nurse or healthcare provider.
- Track intake and output and daily weight to help prevent dehydration.
- Give oral fluids (or intravenous) to replace fluid losses from diarrhea.
- Maintain adequate nutrition including complex carbohydrates such as rice, toast, and cereal as tolerated.
- Teach patients to avoid alcohol or other CNS depressants while taking these drugs.
- Special consideration should be given to older adults or children because of their increased risk for dehydration (symptoms include orthostatic hypotension, increased heart rate, poor skin turgor, or decreased urine output).
- Monitor laboratory values for changes in electrolytes (particularly hypokalemia).

Get Ready for the NCLEX® Examination!

Key Points

- Nausea and vomiting result from a complex set of interactions that involve the brain, nervous system, inner ear, and the stomach and intestines.
- All antiemetic drugs affect the CNS and cause varying degrees of drowsiness.
- Although we tend to think of nausea and vomiting as just problems of the digestive tract, they result from a complex set of interactions that involve the brain, nervous system, inner ear, and the stomach and intestines.
- Antiemetic drugs are used to prevent and treat nausea and vomiting that occur with any problem.
- The class of antiemetic used depends on the severity of the problem and the patient's individual response. Some patients may require a combination of two or more types of antiemetic drugs for effective management of nausea and vomiting.
- The serotonin ($5-HT_3$) receptor antagonists reduce or halt nausea and vomiting by blocking ($5-HT_3$) receptors in the intestinal tract and the CTZ so serotonin cannot activate these receptors.
- The major use of serotonin ($5-HT_3$) receptor antagonists is to reduce or prevent the nausea and vomiting resulting from cancer chemotherapy, radiation therapy, and postoperative nausea and vomiting.
- Serotonin ($5HT_3$) receptor antagonists may be called *setrons* for short because they end in the suffix *-setron*.
- Common CNS side effects for serotonin ($5HT_3$) receptor antagonists include dizziness, headache, and drowsiness.
- Serotonin syndrome can occur if the patient is taking other drugs that increase serotonin (e.g., certain antidepressants and St. John's Wort) with serotonin ($5HT_3$) receptor drugs.
- Substance P/NK_1 receptor antagonists are drugs that block the substance P/NK_1 receptors in the CTZ. This prevents both substance P and neurokinin that are released from cells exposed to chemotherapy and from tissues injured during surgery from binding to and triggering the CTZ.
- Fatigue, diarrhea, headache, and dizziness are side effects of the substance P/NK_1 receptor antagonists.
- Carefully review the drug instructions for making the oral or injectable forms of substance P/NK_1 receptor antagonists to avoid foam or clumps.
- Phenothiazines are a type of antiemetic drug that reduces nausea and vomiting by blocking dopamine (D_2) receptors in the CTZ of the brain. For this reason, drugs in this class are also called *dopamine antagonists*.
- Some phenothiazines can cause urine to change to a pinkish red color. Sensitivity to sun exposure is common.
- High doses of phenothiazine drugs can cause serious EPS including tardive dyskinesia, acute dystonia, and even neuroleptic malignant syndrome.
- Patients with nausea and vomiting are at risk for dehydration, weight loss, and electrolyte imbalance.

- Monitor and report any changes in fluid balance, food intake, and laboratory value abnormalities.
- Cannabinoids reduce nausea and vomiting by binding to both cannabinoid receptors in the CTZ and by interfering with serotonin $5-HT_3$ from binding to its receptors in the CTZ. Use of cannabinoids as antiemetics is typically reserved for patients with severe nausea and vomiting that has not been relieved by other antiemetics.
- Some patients who are taking cannabinoids experience a dose-related "high" (easy laughing, elation, and increased awareness).
- Promotility drugs are used to increase contraction of the upper GI tract including the stomach and the small intestines. They may be used in patients with postoperative nausea and vomiting, chemotherapy-induced nausea and vomiting, and GERD.
- Promotility drugs should be used with caution in patients with a history of depression because they can cause depression and even suicidal ideation.
- Monitor the patient who is taking promotility drugs for any Parkinson's disease–like symptoms, such as tremor, slower gait, or masklike facial appearance. If the patient experiences these side effects, notify the healthcare provider because the drug may need to be discontinued.
- Drug therapy for both PUD and GERD are essentially the same. Commonly used drug therapies include antacids, histamine H_2 receptor antagonists, PPIs, and cytoprotective drugs.
- Some peptic ulcers may be caused by *H. pylori*. *H. pylori* infections are typically treated by a combination of antimicrobial drugs and PPIs.
- Antacids are drugs that neutralize HCl and increase gastric pH, which makes the stomach's pH less acidic and reduces gastric irritation.
- Antacids are typically formulated by at least one of the following ingredients: calcium, magnesium, and aluminum. They are most often used in combination with other drugs to treat a number of GI conditions including PUD, gastritis, gastric ulcer, esophagitis, hiatal hernia, gastric hyperacidity, and GERD.
- In most cases antacids are not used as the primary treatment for these disorders because they provide only temporary relief and do not prevent any future attacks.
- Using antacids as directed rarely results in significant side effects. In general, brands with magnesium can cause diarrhea; brands with calcium or aluminum can cause constipation.
- Antacids neutralize gastric acids and are typically most beneficial if given between meals and at bedtime.
- Histamine H_2 receptor antagonists bind to the H_2 receptor in the stomach cells, leading to a decrease in production of basal (the minimum amount of acid your body needs throughout the day) and nighttime gastric acid.
- All the histamine H_2 receptor antagonists have the suffix *-tidine* in their generic names.

Get Ready for the NCLEX® Examination!—cont'd

- Some patients who are taking H$_2$ receptor antagonists may have mental status changes, including confusion, anxiety, or depression. These usually resolve when the drug is stopped.
- Once-a-day dosing of H$_2$ receptor blockers are best taken at bedtime to reduce symptoms of acid reflux at night.
- Patients should avoid cigarette smoking because it increases gastric acid produce and can decrease the effectiveness of H$_2$ blockers.
- H$_2$ blockers should be given only for occasional episodes of heartburn because they can lose their effectiveness.
- Older adults are more likely to experience confusion and dizziness as side effects of H$_2$ receptor blockers compared with younger adults.
- PPIs help heal gastric ulcers and reduce symptoms of GERD by stopping the acid secretory pump that is located within the gastric parietal cell membrane. This helps reduce the amount of acid secreted into the stomach.
- All of the PPIs have the suffix -*prazole* in their generic names.
- Give PPIs 30 to 60 minutes before the first meal of the day (usually breakfast). This will help decrease the amount of acid secreted while eating. It may take 1 to 3 days for the patient to experience any relief from symptoms.
- Cytoprotective drugs protect the lining of the stomach from further damage. When taken properly, some of these drugs can "stick" to the ulcerated areas in the stomach or duodenum to protect them from further damage and allow them to heal.
- Signs and symptoms of constipation include less than three bowel movements a week, sudden decrease in frequency of bowel movements, harder stools than normal, bowels still feeling full after a bowel movement, feeling bloated, and straining to have a bowel movement.
- Laxatives are a class of drugs that promote bowel movements by stimulating peristalsis, increasing the bulk of the stool, or softening the stool.
- Bulk-forming laxatives absorb water in the GI tract, altering intestinal fluid and electrolytes. The increased bulk stimulates peristalsis, and the absorbed water softens the stool. They are the safest laxatives and can be used to prevent constipation.
- Stool softeners reduce surface tension of the stool so that water and lipids can enter the stool and soften the feces. This makes it easier to pass the stool, so they are helpful in postsurgical patients or patients who should avoid straining.
- Lubricant laxatives create a barrier between the feces and the colon wall that prevents the colon from reabsorbing fecal fluid, thus softening the stool.
- Osmotic laxatives (also called *saline* laxatives) work rapidly and are typically used to cleanse the bowel in preparation for colonoscopy, x-ray studies, or GI surgery.

- When rapid relief of constipation is desired, stimulant or irritant laxatives may be used.
- Frequent use of stimulant laxatives should be avoided in favor of improving diet and physical activity.
- The most common side effects of laxatives are GI symptoms such as nausea, abdominal cramping, bloating, and diarrhea.
- Laxatives in general may reduce absorption of or bind to certain drugs because they can increase GI motility.
- Bulk-forming laxatives should be given with a full glass of water to prevent obstruction in the esophagus.
- Laxatives high in sodium should be avoided in patients with edema, pregnancy, CHF, and sodium-restricted diets.
- Overuse of stimulant laxatives may cause excessive fluid and electrolyte imbalance, particularly dehydration and hypokalemia.
- Laxatives are available without a prescription; therefore it is especially important to teach the patient about risks associated with laxative use.
- Make sure your patient has a call light available particularly after taking osmotic or stimulant laxatives because these may cause a sense of urgency to have a bowel movement.
- Antidiarrheals are drugs that reduce or stop loose, watery stools and help to restore normal bowel movements.
- Anticholinergic drugs reduce GI tract spasm and intestinal motility, acid production, and gastric motility, and thus reduce the associated pain.
- Anticholinergic drugs are rarely used alone but rather are used in combination with other drugs to reduce diarrhea.
- Antispasmodic drugs reduce muscle contraction in the GI tract. This decreases cramping, bloating, and diarrhea.
- When diarrhea is caused by infection, the healthcare provider may not give antidiarrheals, to allow the patient's body to get rid of the infection.
- Opioid agonists are effective for diarrhea but do not have the analgesic or opioid-like effects. They do, however, reduce GI motility and increase the ability of the intestine to absorb water.
- Physical dependence on opioid agonists as contained in antidiarrheal drugs is rare.

Review Questions for the NCLEX® Examination

1. How do histamine (H$_2$) receptor antagonists help prevent or heal gastric ulcers?
   1. Increasing prostaglandins production of thick mucus in the stomach
   2. Neutralizing the hydrochloric acid secreted only in the stomach
   3. Blocking the activity of the proton (hydrogen ion) pumps in the stomach
   4. Reducing the stimulation of cells that produce acid in the stomach

Get Ready for the NCLEX® Examination!—cont'd

2. A patient has been given an osmotic laxative as part of bowel preparation for a colonoscopy. How long does this drug usually take to have its effect?
   1. 1 to 3 days
   2. 30 minutes to 6 hours
   3. 6 to 12 hours
   4. 13 to 24 hours

3. The patient has been taking a phenothiazine drug for nausea. The patient tells the nurse she has a pinkish red color to her urine. Which is the most appropriate response from the nurse?
   1. "This is an expected response to the drug."
   2. "This is evidence of a toxic dose of the drug."
   3. "This is an allergic response to the drug."
   4. "This response is not related to the drug."

4. The daughter of a 72-year-old man tells her neighbor (an LPN) that her father has had recent episodes of confusion. The LPN discovers that the man recently started taking over-the-counter famotidine (Pepcid) for his "heartburn." What is the best action for the LPN?
   1. Recommend that the patient's daughter increases the dosage of famotidine.
   2. Suggest that the daughter research placement of her father into a long-term care facility.
   3. Tell the daughter to contact the patient's healthcare provider because this is a common adverse effect of famotidine.
   4. Remind the daughter that her father is older and may have early signs of Alzheimer's disease.

5. A patient with liver failure has been given the drug Lactulose. What is the purpose of this drug in liver failure?
   1. Lactulose decreases constipation in patients with liver failure.
   2. Lactulose reduces the ammonia level in patients with liver failure.
   3. Lactulose increases fluid volume in the stool to reduce constipation.
   4. Lactulose also has a diuretic action that can decrease fluid in ascites.

6. Omeprazole has been prescribed for a patient with gastroesophageal reflux disease. What type of drug is omeprazole?
   1. H_2 receptor antagonist
   2. Promotility drug
   3. Cytoprotective drug
   4. Proton pump inhibitor

7. A 67-year-old patient has chemotherapy-related nausea and vomiting. She is prescribed dolasetron (Anzemet). When you are giving morning drugs, you notice that she is taking a selective serotonin reuptake inhibitor for chronic depression. What is the your best action?
   1. Give the dolasetron and tell the patient she should stop taking her antidepressant.
   2. Hold the dolasetron and contact the healthcare provider to notify him or her that the patient takes the antidepressant.
   3. Give both the dolasetron and the antidepressant and monitor the patient for signs of serotonin syndrome.
   4. Hold the dolasetron and give it later in the day so it does not interact with the antidepressant.

8. A patient with chronic constipation is prescribed psyllium (Fiberall). Which of the following statements by the patient shows a need for more teaching?
   1. "I will take this drug with a full glass of water to prevent blockage in my esophagus."
   2. "I understand that it takes a few days for this drug to work effectively."
   3. "I may feel some nausea and abdominal cramping when I start taking this drug."
   4. "This drug will replace my need for dietary fiber, so I can eat fewer fruits and vegetables."

9. Which of the following patients are most likely to require a stool softener for management of bowel movements? (Select all that apply.)
   1. An 84-year-old woman who has moved into a skilled nursing facility after having a stroke.
   2. A 64-year-old patient who states she has not had a bowel movement in a week and needs relief immediately.
   3. A 62-year-old patient who recently underwent open heart surgery to replace a heart valve.
   4. A 34-year-old pregnant woman with a prescription from her healthcare provider.
   5. A 55-year-old man who comes to the emergency room with severe abdominal pain and feels like he has to have a bowel movement.

10. A nurse is teaching a patient about the loperamide prescribed for acute diarrhea. Which of the following statements should be included in the patient teaching? (Select all that apply.)
    1. Loperamide will reduce the number of liquid stools that you are experiencing.
    2. Make sure you take 4 mg (2 tablets) initially, then 2 mg by mouth after each unformed stool. Do not exceed 8 tablets per day.
    3. This drug has an effect like opioid drugs, so you may have a "high" feeling while taking it.
    4. If your diarrhea does not stop after 48 hours, notify your healthcare provider.
    5. Loperamide helps decrease the motility of your bowel so there is more time for the body to absorb water and you will have a more formed stool.

Get Ready for the NCLEX® Examination!—cont'd

Drug Calculation Review

1. The patient is to receive famotidine (Pepcid) 40 mg orally at bedtime to treat gastric ulcer caused by *H. pylori*. The drug is available in 20-mg tablets. How many tablets should the patient receive? ____tablets

2. A patient is to receive 4 mg ondansetron (Zofran) IM as a single dose after surgery for nausea and vomiting. Ondansetron is available as 2 mg/mL. How many milliliters will the patient receive? ____mL

3. A patient is to receive sucralfate (Carafate) 1 g per gastrostomy-tube four times daily. Sucralfate is available as an oral suspension 1 g/10 mL. How many milliliters will the patient receive each day? ____mL

Case Study

Ms. McKelvey has been taking over-the-counter (OTC) famotidine for her indigestion for 2 weeks without significant relief. She decided to contact her healthcare provider because the symptoms continued to occur, particularly her heartburn symptoms. Now, however, the healthcare provider has added a proton pump inhibitor. When the healthcare provider leaves the room, Ms. McKelvey tells the nurse she is unhappy about this, because she has prided herself on keeping her "medical costs" down by using only home remedies and OTC drugs. "If they're both for ulcers," she says, "then what's the difference? Why can't I just double my dose of the antacid?"

1. What are the major differences between proton pump inhibitors and H_2 receptor antagonists?

2. What should the nurse teach Ms. McKelvey regarding the use of home remedies and OTC drugs?

3. What strategies will you use to ensure that Ms. McKelvey adheres to her new prescription?

Drugs Affecting the Hematologic System

14

Learning Outcomes

1. Describe the clotting mechanism in the human body.
2. Explain the difference between anticoagulant drugs and fibrinolytic drugs.
3. List the names, actions, possible side effects, and adverse effects of the common platelet inhibitors.
4. Explain what to teach patients and families about platelet inhibitors.
5. List the names, actions, possible side effects, and adverse effects of the common direct thrombin inhibitors.
6. Explain what to teach patients and families about direct thrombin inhibitors.
7. List the names, actions, possible side effects, and adverse effects of the common indirect thrombin inhibitors.
8. Explain what to teach patients and families about indirect thrombin inhibitors.
9. List the names, actions, possible side effects, and adverse effects of the vitamin K antagonists.
10. Explain what to teach patients and families about vitamin K antagonists.
11. List the names, actions, possible side effects, and adverse effects of fibrinolytic drugs.
12. List the names, actions, possible side effects, and adverse effects of erythropoiesis-stimulating agents.
13. Explain what to teach patients and families about erythropoiesis-stimulating agents.

Key Terms

anticoagulants (ĂN-tī-kō-Ă-gyă-lĕnts, p. 266) Drugs that interfere with one or more steps in the blood clotting process that either reduce or prevent new clots from forming, or prevents existing clots from getting larger.

clot (klŏt, p. 266) A semi-solid amount of coagulated (thickened) blood. May also be referred to as a thrombus.

deep vein thrombosis (thrăm-BŌ-sĕs, p. 270) A clot lying in a deep vein, usually in the legs.

direct thrombin inhibitor (DTI) (THRŎM-bĭn ĭn-HĬ-bă-tĕr, p. 266) Anticoagulants that delay blood clotting by directly inhibiting the enzyme thrombin.

embolism (ĔM-bĕ-lĭ-zĕm, p. 270) A blockage in an artery by a blood clot or air bubble.

erythropoiesis-stimulating agent (ESA) (ĭ-rĭth-rō-pōĭ-Ē-sĕ, p. 276) Drugs that are synthetic forms of the hormone, erythropoietin, which stimulate the bone marrow to make more red blood cells at a faster rate.

fibrin (FĬ-brĕn, p. 266) A protein formed by fibrinogen during the clotting process that assists with the formation of a clot.

fibrinogen (fĭ-BRĬ-nĕ-jĕn, p. 266) A protein found in the blood's plasma that is converted to fibrin when a blood clot is formed.

fibrinolytic drug (fĭ-brĭ-nō-LĬ-tĭk, p. 275) A drug that uses enzymes to dissolve fibrin.

indirect thrombin inhibitors (THRŎM-bĭn ĭn-HĬ-bă-tĕr, p. 266) Anticoagulant drugs that reduce clot formation by increasing the protein antithrombin III.

platelet inhibitor (PLĀT-lĕt, p. 268) Drugs that inhibit the functions of platelets, interfering with blood clotting within arteries.

thrombin (THRŎM-bĭn, p. 266) An enzyme that acts on fibrinogen (a protein found in the blood plasma) to convert it to fibrin to help clots form.

vitamin K antagonist (VĬ-tĕ-mĭn, p. 273) Anticoagulant drugs that interfere with blood clotting by reducing the amount of vitamine K available to help the liver form clotting factors.

Drugs that affect the hematologic system can work by interfering with blood clotting, reducing existing blood clots, or stimulating the production of red blood cells (RBCs). Many of these drugs are taken by patients on a daily basis, and others are given only in hospital settings. To help in fully understanding the action of these drugs, it is important to review the normal clotting mechanisms.

BLOOD CLOTTING

The ability of the blood to flow freely through blood vessels is critical in providing cells with oxygen and nutrients, and in removing waste products from tissues and organs. However, when blood vessels are damaged, clot formation is needed to prevent blood from leaving the circulatory system, causing excessive bleeding. A

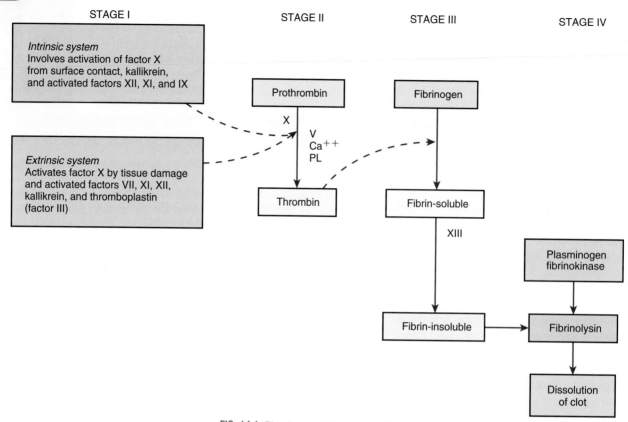

FIG. 14.1 Blood coagulation and clot lysis.

clot is a semisolid amount of coagulated (thickened) blood that blocks blood flow in a blood vessel. So at all times, the body has functions that keep circulation going, balanced along with blood functions that can start the formation of blood clots in areas of injury. In health, blood circulates to all tissues and organs continuously, and forms clots only when and where they are needed.

One of the body's protective functions is to clot blood in response to tissue injury. Any damage to the cells starts a series of reactions to protect the body (Fig. 14.1). A variety of clotting factors made by the liver are present in the blood to act quickly in an organized series of events called a *cascade* that results in the formation of a blood clot. Specifically, tissue and blood vessel damage results in the formation of *thromboplastin*, which then acts on *prothrombin* in the bloodstream to form the clotting factor thrombin. **Thrombin** is an enzyme that then acts on **fibrinogen** (a protein found in the blood plasma) to convert it to **fibrin**, a netlike substance in the blood that traps blood cells and platelets to form the matrix, or frame, of a blood clot. Vitamin K must be present to produce prothrombin and other clotting factors that are made in the liver. In addition to calcium, clotting factors, and red blood cells (RBCs), platelets and magnesium are needed in clot formation.

As part of the circulatory system, the arterial vessels carry oxygenated blood throughout the body. If these small arteries become plugged with *thrombi* (clots made of fibrin, platelets, and cholesterol), oxygen cannot get to the tissues and death may result. Abnormal blood clotting may produce a *thrombus* (a single clot) in the coronary artery, which nourishes the heart muscle. *Emboli* (small pieces of a blood clot) may break off from a site of a thrombus or a *thrombophlebitis* (inflammation and blood clot in a vein) in the lower extremities and travel through the bloodstream to block vessels in the brain or lungs. In the brain, this blockage can cause stroke or death. In the lungs, the blockage can interfere with oxygenating the blood.

ANTICOAGULANTS

Anticoagulants are drugs that interfere with one or more steps in the blood clotting process. These drugs can reduce or prevent new clots from forming and can help to prevent existing clots from getting larger (extending). They cannot dissolve formed clots. Anticoagulants are mistakenly called "blood thinners," but they do not actually thin the blood. Drugs that act as anticoagulants are classified as platelet inhibitors, **direct thrombin inhibitors (DTIs)**, indirect thrombin inhibitors (ITIs), and vitamin K antagonists. A summary of anticoagulants is provided in Table 14.1.

> 💡 **Memory Jogger**
>
> The four classes of anticoagulant drugs are:
> - platelet inhibitors
> - direct thrombin inhibitors
> - indirect thrombin inhibitors
> - vitamin K antagonists

Table 14.1   Anticoagulants

Platelet inhibitors: These drugs use a variety of mechanisms to prevent platelets from sticking together (aggregating) to form a platelet plug that starts the blood clotting cascade.

DRUGS/ADULT DOSAGE RANGE	NURSING IMPLICATIONS
aspirin (Ecotrin, low-dose aspirin, Asaphen♣, Entrophen♣) 81–325 mg orally once daily cilostazol (Pletal) 100 mg orally twice daily clopidogrel (Plavix) 75 mg once daily ticagrelor (Brilinta) 180 mg orally once as a loading dose, then begin 90 mg orally twice daily ticlopidine (Ticlid) 250 mg orally twice daily	• Avoid taking over-the-counter drugs, especially those that contain NSAIDs, because these increase the risk for bleeding. • Antacids interfere with antiplatelet drugs, so teach patients to take antiplatelet drugs 1 hour before or 2 hours after taking antacids. • Most oral antiplatelet drugs are better tolerated when given with food to prevent nausea. • Teach patients the symptoms of bleeding and to report any signs of abnormal bleeding to the healthcare provider. • Teach patients to avoid the foods, herbs, and supplements that can interfere with antiplatelet drugs. • Teach patients not to stop taking these drugs without talking to their provider. At times antiplatelet drugs may need to be held for certain surgical or dental procedures. Discuss all drugs with each healthcare provider. • Antiplatelet drugs should be avoided during the last trimester of pregnancy and should not be taken while breast-feeding.

Direct thrombin inhibitors: These drugs bind to prothrombin and prevent its conversion to thrombin, which is needed to convert fibrinogen to fibrin. With less thrombin, less fibrin is available to form the network that is the mesh forming the base of a clot.

DRUGS/ADULT DOSAGE RANGE	NURSING IMPLICATIONS
apixaban (Eliquis) 2.5–5 mg orally twice daily desirudin (Iprivask) 15 mg subcutaneously every 12 hours or 0.1 mg/kg/h continuous IV dabigatran (Pradaxa) 150 mg orally twice daily rivaroxaban (Xarelto) 20 mg daily or 15 mg orally twice daily	• Watch for signs of abnormal bleeding and teach patients to report abnormal bleeding, including heavy menses, to the healthcare provider. • Monitor patients for signs of allergy or hypersensitivity to these drugs, such as wheezing, shortness of breath, chest tightness, facial swelling, rash, or hives. • Teach patients to avoid aspirin or NSAIDs while taking thrombin inhibitors because serious hemorrhage or death could occur. • Keep the drugs in the original containers; do not place in plastic pill containers because they are sensitive to light.

Indirect thrombin inhibitors: These drugs indirectly prevent the conversion of prothrombin to thrombin by increasing the amount of active antithrombin III. This substance has the action of interfering with the conversion of prothrombin to thrombin.

DRUGS/ADULT DOSAGE RANGE	NURSING IMPLICATIONS

heparin, heparin sodium (Calcilean♣, Hepalean♣)
  IV: adult dose for bolus is based on patient weight; usually 5000–10,000 units IV bolus, followed by continuous IV infusion
  Subcutaneous injection: 8000–10,000 units every 8 hours or 5000–20,000 units every 12 hours
Low Molecular Weight Heparins
enoxaparin (Lovenox) 1 mg/kg every 12 hours or 1.5 mg/kg once daily subcutaneously
dalteparin (Fragmin) 100–200 U/kg/day once daily subcutaneously
tinzaparin (Innohep) 175 U/kg once daily subcutaneously
fondaparinux sodium (Arixtra) available in single-dose, prefilled syringe of 2.5–10 mg once daily subcutaneously
	• The IV flow rate for continuous heparin infusion is ordered by the prescriber and based on aPTT test results, so monitor aPTT results and report them to the healthcare provider.
	• Watch for signs of abnormal bleeding and teach patients to report abnormal bleeding, including heavy menses, to the healthcare provider because these may indicate overdosage.
	• Monitor patients who are receiving heparin for wheezing, shortness of breath, chest tightness, facial swelling, rash, or hives because these are indications of allergy or hypersensitivity to the drug.
	• Teach patients to avoid aspirin or NSAIDs while taking heparin preparations because excessive bleeding risks are greatly increased.
	• Assess patients who are receiving heparin for low platelet counts and indications of clot extension because these are signs of heparin-induced thrombocytopenia, a life-threatening reaction to heparin.
	• Ensure the heparin antidote, protamine sulfate, is available so that it can be given quickly in case of overdose.
	• LMWHs are given by deep subcutaneous injection. *Do not expel air bubble or aspirate before giving injection.* Do not rub the injection site. All of these actions can cause excessive bleeding, bruising, and tissue damage at the injection site.
	• Ask patients who are prescribed prefilled syringes of fondaparinux sodium (Arixtra) whether they have a latex allergy because these products contain latex rubber-tipped needle covers.

Continued

Table 14.1 Anticoagulants—cont'd

Vitamin K antagonist: Vitamin K is critical to the production of many clotting factors in the liver. These drugs reduce or prevent the formation of vitamin K in the intestinal tract. With less vitamin K, fewer clotting factors are made in the liver.

DRUGS/ADULT DOSAGE RANGE	NURSING IMPLICATIONS
warfarin (Coumadin) 2–10 mg orally daily for 2–4 days; then dose is adjusted based on INR laboratory test results	• Teach patients to limit the amount of green, leafy vegetables they eat because these vegetables are a natural source of vitamin K that can reduce the effect of warfarin. • Monitor patients' INR to determine effectiveness. • Remind patients to keep all appointments for INR laboratory tests because the dosage is changed based on the test results. • Stress the importance of not taking aspirin or NSAIDs with this drug because it can lead to excessive bleeding. • Teach patients the signs of abnormal bleeding to report to the healthcare provider. • Ensure that the warfarin antidote, vitamin K, is available so it can be given quickly in case of an overdose. • Caution women of childbearing age who are taking warfarin to avoid pregnancy, because this drug can cause birth defects and bleeding. • Many drugs and herbal supplements interfere with the action of warfarin and should be avoided.

♣ Indicates Canadian drug.

PLATELET INHIBITORS

Action

Platelet inhibitors or antiplatelet drugs act through different mechanisms to prevent platelets from sticking and clumping together (aggregating) to form a platelet plug. Platelet aggregation is an important defense mechanism when the body is injured and results in sealing the entry into the vascular system and preventing blood from going into body tissues. Platelet inhibitors work in the cardiovascular system, sometimes in specific places, to prevent clotting events in a patient who might be having reduced blood circulation to the heart before a *myocardial infarction* (heart attack). Common platelet inhibitors are aspirin, clopidogrel, dipyridamole, eptifibatide, prasugrel, ticlopidine, tirofiban, and cilostazol.

Uses

Platelet inhibitors are often the first drugs used to prevent clots in blood vessels (vascular system). These drugs are often given prophylactically (prevention) when a patient has a condition that may produce blood clots, to prevent further extension of the clot, or to prevent the further development of blood clots. Although they can prevent some clotting, they can do nothing to dissolve clots that have already developed.

Some of these drugs are used in situations where blood vessels become blocked, to keep venous and arterial grafts open and to prevent strokes. They may be given as additional drugs (adjuncts) to thrombolytic therapy in those patients who have had a heart attack to prevent them from having another one.

Acetylsalicylic acid (ASA), or aspirin, is the most commonly used antiplatelet drug. ASA reduces the risk for major blood vessel blockage that can lead to acute myocardial infarction (MI), ischemic stroke, angina, and peripheral arterial disease. Although ASA use is helpful, it also carries the risk for gastrointestinal (GI) bleeding in older patients, those with a history of peptic ulcer disease, and patients using other nonsteroidal anti-inflammatory drugs (NSAIDs) or more than one antiplatelet therapy. See Chapter 12 for information on the actions and nursing implications for aspirin.

Clopidogrel (Plavix) is a drug that is used for patients who have had an MI caused by a clot (thrombus) formed in a coronary artery. For patients who have had a stent placed into the coronary artery as a result of severe narrowing or blockage of the artery, clopidogrel prevents platelets from sticking to the stent mesh. For these patients, clopidogrel *must* be taken daily for a year or longer to prevent clots from developing and plugging up the stent. It is also used in peripheral arterial disease (PAD) to prevent blood clots in the legs, for prevention of an MI, and as additional therapy along with thrombolytic drugs to prevent further strokes after a patient has had a recent ischemic stroke.

Expected Side Effects

Most drugs that affect the blood clotting system have the potential to cause bleeding, especially when used in combination with other antiplatelet drugs. Easy bruising is common; for example, bleeding of the gums can occur when the patient brushes his or her teeth. GI effects such as diarrhea, nausea, *dyspepsia* (stomach discomfort after eating), vomiting, flatulence, and *anorexia* (lack of appetite) have been experienced. Skin effects such as rash, *pruritus* (itching), and *purpura* (bruising) have been reported.

Adverse Reactions

Excessive bleeding, including acute hemorrhage, is the most common adverse effect. Allergic reactions to aspirin and NSAIDs generally occur within a few hours of taking the drug. Symptoms of allergic reactions include itching, hives, and runny nose, with more severe reactions causing swelling of the lips, tongue, or face. Acute cardiovascular events can occur when these drugs are stopped abruptly, so they should never be discontinued without the advice of the patient's healthcare provider. Some of these drugs, including clopidogrel, can result in a decrease in platelet counts (*thrombocytopenia*) and white blood cell counts (*neutropenia*).

⚠ Safety Alert!

For any patient who is taking anticoagulants, watch for early signs of bleeding:

- easy bruising of knuckles, elbows, or any body part that experiences pressure (e.g., under watchband)
- new or excessive bleeding of gums when brushing teeth
- blood in the urine or stool, or tarry-colored stool
- tachycardia
- hypotension
- shortness of breath
- GI pain

Drug and Food Interactions

Anticoagulants have many interactions with other drugs and foods that can increase the risk for bleeding or decrease the effectiveness of the drug. Platelet inhibitors, such as aspirin and NSAIDs taken with other drugs that reduce coagulation, can cause excessive bleeding. Alcoholic beverages can also increase the risk for bleeding because of their effect on the liver, where some clotting factors are formed. Other drugs, such as vitamin K and oral contraceptives, decrease the effects of anticoagulants. Antibiotics can have a variable effect on blood clotting when taken with anticoagulants. Some drugs that protect the GI system, such as proton pump inhibitors, can interact with clopidogrel and decrease its effectiveness. Green, leafy vegetables contain vitamin K and can decrease the effectiveness of anticoagulants. Many herbal products, vitamins, and supplements can interfere with anticoagulants. For example, St. John's wort further increases the risk for bleeding when used while taking an anticoagulant. In addition, multivitamins contain vitamin K, which reduces the effectiveness of warfarin (Box 14.1). Chapter 19 describes many herbal, vitamin, and supplemental products and some of their interactions with drugs.

❖ Nursing Implications and Patient Teaching

◆ *Assessment.* Before giving the first dose of any platelet inhibitor, it is important to ask the patient what other drugs he or she has taken in the past week, including over-the-counter (OTC) drugs, vitamins, minerals, and herbal products. Many of these drugs and products can interact with platelet inhibitors and greatly increase the risk for bleeding. Ask whether he or she currently has

---

Box 14.1   Foods, Herbs, and Supplements That Affect the Clotting System

FOODS THAT MAY INTERFERE WITH ANTICOAGULANTS

Tomatoes, onions, dark, leafy greens, broccoli, garlic, bananas

Herbs and Supplements That Increase the Risk for Bleeding in Anticoagulated Patients

Angelica	Ginkgo
Cat's claw	Goldenseal
Chamomile	Grape seed extract
Chondroitin	Green leaf tea
Feverfew	Horse chestnut seed
Fish oil	Psyllium
Vitamin E	Turmeric

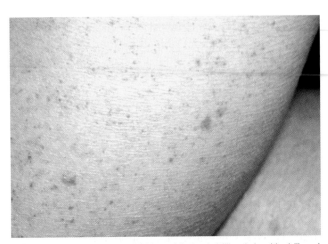

FIG. 14.2 Petechiae. (Modified from Marks J, Miller J: *Lookingbill and Marks' principles of dermatology*, ed 5, Philadelphia, 2013, Saunders.)

---

any bruising or bleeding, especially from the gums, nose, or mouth, which is a sign of low platelet count and increased bleeding risk.

Assess for signs of internal bleeding, such as:
- severe abdominal pain and tenderness
- vomiting or diarrhea that is frank red blood or coffee-colored
- cold, clammy skin

Examine the mouth and skin for any signs of bleeding, such as pale mucous membranes, bruising, or the presence of *petechiae* (tiny red/purple spots on the skin, caused by a minor bleed into the skin) (Fig. 14.2).

◆ *Planning and implementation.* Give platelet inhibitors and record the drugs given and the patient's response. Monitoring the patient's vital signs will alert you to possible adverse reactions. Tachycardia and hypotension can occur with bleeding, so monitor pulse and blood pressure at least once per shift.

Report the location and amount of bruising, or petechiae that occurs. Assist with the collection of any ordered blood work required to monitor therapy.

◆ *Evaluation.* Changes in vital signs and levels of consciousness provide important feedback about the possible risk for bleeding that can occur with these drugs. Watch for skin-related signs of bleeding, such as bruising or petechiae. Watch for signs of overdose and internal bleeding as therapy progresses. This includes bleeding gums when brushing teeth, blood in the urine, or coughing up blood.

Determine whether the patient understands why he or she is taking the drug and the symptoms of overdose. Have the patient report any signs of bruising or easy bleeding.

DIRECT THROMBIN INHIBITORS

Action

All direct thrombin inhibitors (DTIs) prevent the formation of blood clots, or thrombi, by interfering with the enzyme thrombin (factor II). This action increases the time it takes for blood to clot, preventing new clots from forming. These drugs do not dissolve clots that have already occurred. Dabigatran (Pradaxa), rivaroxaban (Xarelto), apixaban (Eliquis), and edoxaban (Savaysa) are examples of DTIs (see Table 14.1). All of these drugs act to stop the coagulation process through binding to both free thrombin in the blood and thrombin that is bound to fibrin, stopping the clotting cascade.

Uses

DTIs are used to prevent clots in both arteries and veins. They can also be used to prevent and treat **deep vein thrombosis** (DVT) or pulmonary embolism (PE), or to prevent clotting from atrial fibrillation, an abnormal heart rhythm where the upper chambers of the heart, the atria, quiver instead of beating normally to move blood out of the atria and into the ventricles. The advantage of DTIs is that they do not require the frequent laboratory blood testing as part of the monitoring process that is required by warfarin.

DTIs are used much like warfarin and other anticoagulants. They are prescribed for patients who are at risk for systemic **embolism** and stroke, especially for patients who have atrial fibrillation that is *not* caused by a heart valve problem. They are also used for prevention of blood clots after some types of surgeries.

Expected Side Effects

The DTIs can cause bleeding. Easy bruising is common, for example, bleeding gums when the patient brushes his or her teeth. Another common side effect of DTIs is gastric upset when taken on an empty stomach.

Adverse Reactions

By far, the most common adverse reactions from DTIs are excessive bleeding and thrombocytopenia. Early signs of overdose or internal bleeding include bleeding from the gums while brushing teeth, excessive bleeding or oozing from cuts, unexplained bruising or nosebleeds, and unusually heavy or unexpected menses in women. These are the "must know" symptoms that suggest the patient needs prompt attention.

Drug Interactions

DTIs can interact with many commonly prescribed drugs and some supplements, such as atorvastatin, azithromycin, carvedilol, clarithromycin, cyclosporine, diltiazem, and St. John's wort, to name a few. When taken together, the concentration of DTIs increases, which greatly increases the risk for excessive bleeding. When taken with carbamazepine, dexamethasone, phenobarbital, phenytoin, or rifampin, the concentration and action of DTIs is reduced, decreasing their effectiveness. Antacids may also reduce the action of DTIs.

> **! Drug Interaction Alert**
>
> - Common drugs that increase the activity and bleeding risks with DTIs are atorvastatin, azithromycin, carvedilol, clarithromycin, cyclosporine, and diltiazem.
> - Drugs that decrease the effectiveness of DTIs are carbamazepine, dexamethasone, phenobarbital, phenytoin, rifampin, and antacids.

❖ Nursing Implications and Patient Teaching

◆ *Assessment.* Assess patients for any of the following, which may be a sign or symptom of serious bleeding:
- unusual bruising
- blood in the urine, stool, or vomitus
- coughing up blood
- headaches, dizziness, or weakness
- recurring nosebleeds
- unusual bleeding from gums
- menstrual bleeding that is heavier than normal

◆ *Planning and implementation.* Teach the patient and family members to take DTIs on time. When a dose is missed, the scheduled dose should be taken as soon as possible on the same day. However, if there will be *less than* 6 hours between scheduled doses, the missed dose should not be taken. Accidental overdose may lead to excessive bleeding. If needed, the reversal agent (idarucizumab) can be prescribed by the healthcare provider.

Teach patients and family members not to discontinue DTIs without talking to the healthcare provider who prescribed it because the risk for serious clotting events increases.

Instruct patients to keep DTIs in the original bottle to protect the drug from moisture and light. Teach them not to put DTIs in pill boxes or pill organizers.

Teach patients not to chew or break the capsules before swallowing them because the drug may be absorbed too rapidly or destroyed by stomach acid. Instruct patients to take DTIs with a full glass of water to prevent stomach irritation and improve absorption.

◆ *Evaluation.* Watch for signs of overdose and internal bleeding. These include bleeding gums when brushing teeth, blood in the urine, or coughing up or vomiting of blood.

Have the patient or family explain to you the purpose of taking this drug and the symptoms of overdose.

Note any signs of bruising or easy bleeding, and document your findings according to agency policy.

INDIRECT THROMBIN INHIBITORS

Actions

Indirect thrombin inhibitors (ITIs) are anticoagulant drugs that decrease clot formation by increasing the amount and action of a protein called antithrombin III. This protein inhibits thrombin from doing its job in the blood clotting cascade, and clot formation is reduced. Commonly used ITIs are heparin sodium (Calcilean✦, Hepalean✦); low-molecular-weight heparin (LMWH), dalteparin (Fragmin), enoxaparin (Lovenox), tinzaparin (Innohep), and fondaparinux (Arixtra). Heparin is given only by injection because it cannot be absorbed orally.

LMWH is a special formulation with a more steady anticoagulation effect than unfractionated heparin sodium. LMWH works by binding to antithrombin and inhibiting factor Xa, which disrupts part of the clotting cascade. The half-life of LMWH is longer than heparin sodium, ranging from 2 to 4 hours after intravenous injection to 3 to 6 hours after subcutaneous injection.

Therapy with heparin sodium must be monitored for its anticoagulation effect by a blood test known as the activated partial thromboplastin time (aPTT). The prescriber maintains or adjusts dosages according to this test result. The LMWH formulation does not require testing.

Uses

Anticoagulant therapy with heparin is used to prevent new clot formation or to stop existing clots from growing in size. Heparin therapy is used *prophylactically* (as a preventative) during and after many types of surgery, especially surgery involving the heart or circulatory system. It is also used in patients with heart valve disease, in patients with some *dysrhythmias* (irregular heartbeats), and in patients receiving hemodialysis. Any patient on bed rest for a long time is at risk for the development of blood clots, especially patients with a history of clotting problems or recent orthopedic, thoracic, or abdominal surgery. LMWH is used especially in the prevention of venous thromboembolism and may often be used when pulmonary embolism is present.

Expected Side Effects

Heparin sodium can cause easy bleeding and bruising, pain, redness, warmth, irritation, or skin changes where the drug was injected. Other side effects may include foot itching or bluish-colored skin.

Adverse Reactions

A number of other adverse reactions may occur, including hemorrhage, thrombocytopenia, shortness of breath, wheezing, chills, fever, alopecia, and *hypersensitivity* (allergic) reaction. In cases of heparin overdose, protamine sulfate is given to counteract the effect of heparin. Serious adverse reactions include *heparin-induced thrombocytopenia* (HIT) and *heparin-induced thrombocytopenia and thrombosis* (HITT). In HIT, antibodies against heparin are formed and activate platelets, which then clump together and cause small clots in the bloodstream, and the platelet count falls. If major clots develop and block vessels, the condition is even more serious and is called HITT.

Drug Interactions

Heparin can interact with aspirin, NSAIDs, glucocorticoids, and other anticoagulants (warfarin) to increase the risk for GI bleeding. Antihistamines, digoxin, nicotine, and tetracycline decrease the anticoagulant effect of heparin.

❖ Nursing Implications and Patient Teaching

◆ *Assessment.* Heparin is derived from animal tissue and is more likely to cause an allergic reaction than other anticoagulants. When giving it to patients who have a history of allergy, observe them closely.

This drug should be used cautiously in patients with liver or kidney disease or hypertension, during menses, after delivery, or in patients with indwelling catheters. A higher incidence of bleeding may be seen in older patients.

◆ *Planning and implementation.* Dosages for heparin are given in heparin units. Heparin is given only by IV injection, IV infusion, or subcutaneous injection. Heparin is not given by IM injection because these injections produce hematomas, irritation, and pain at the injection site.

Do not shake the bottle containing the heparin; only roll it carefully between your hands before inserting the needle. If the heparin solution is discolored or contains a precipitate or particles at the bottom of the bottle, do not use it. Heparin is strongly acidic and is incompatible with many other drugs in solution, so it must not be piggybacked with other drugs into an infusion line. Never mix any drug with heparin in a syringe when bolus therapy is given.

> **❗ Drug Alert**
>
> **Administration Alert**
>
> Roll the heparin bottle between your hands rather than shaking it. Do not give heparin in the same IV line or same syringe with any other drug.

Use a small (25-gauge) needle and a tuberculin syringe for the subcutaneous injection (often given in the abdomen around the umbilicus). Subcutaneous heparin is usually given every 12 hours. There are several things to remember about heparin injection. First, once the needle has been inserted into the patient, do not attempt to pull back on the plunger or aspirate blood before injection. Second, do not move the needle while the heparin is being injected. Third, do not massage injection

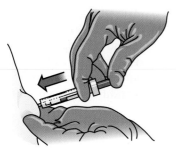

FIG. 14.3 Deep subcutaneous injection for low-molecular-weight heparin. (From Workman ML, LaCharity LA: *Understanding pharmacology*, ed 2, St. Louis, 2016, Elsevier.)

sites before or after injection. Doing any of these things increases tissue damage from the heparin. Avoid giving IM injections of other drugs while the patient is receiving heparin, because hematomas and bleeding into nearby areas may occur. LMWH preparations are given by deep subcutaneous injection (Fig. 14.3).

> ### ⊕ Top Tip for Safety
>
> When injecting subcutaneous heparin, do not pull back on the syringe to aspirate for blood or move the needle in the tissue during the injection. Do not massage the injection site. All of these actions increase the risk for bleeding, bruising, and tissue damage at the injection site.

Rotate the sites of subcutaneous injections of heparin to avoid formation of hematomas (see Chapter 4 and Fig. 4.14 for recommended rotation sites). In the hospital setting, once the heparin is drawn into the syringe, double-check the dose drawn up with another nurse, because of the adverse effects if inaccurate doses are given.

If intermittent IV therapy is prescribed, blood for partial thromboplastin time (PT) determination should be drawn an hour before the next scheduled heparin dose. Blood for partial thromboplastin times can be drawn any time after 8 hours of continuous IV heparin therapy. However, blood should *not* be drawn from the tubing of the heparin infusion line or from the vein being used for infusion. Blood should always be drawn from the arm *not* being used for heparin infusion.

Continuous intravenous therapy with heparin is first started by a bolus of heparin that is based on the weight of the patient (usually 5000 to 10,000 units). Obtaining an accurate weight is important before initiating heparin therapy. Check intravenous heparin infusions frequently, even if pumps are in good working order, to ensure the proper dose is being given.

If heparin is being given at the same time as warfarin, blood should not be drawn for PT within 5 hours of IV heparin administration, or within 24 hours if heparin is given subcutaneously.

Patients who require rapid anticoagulation are commonly hospitalized. Heparin is usually started for

an immediate effect and gradually replaced by oral anticoagulants.

The most commonly used blood test for determining the therapeutic range for heparin is the activated partial thromboplastin time (aPTT). The dosage of heparin is considered adequate when the aPTT is about 1.5 to 2.5 times the laboratory control value. PT and international normalized ratio (INR) tests are ordered when the patient is started on oral anticoagulants and at regular intervals thereafter. The normal range for the INR is 0.8 to 1.2, with a therapeutic target range of 2.0 to 3.0. For patients with mechanical heart valves, this therapeutic range is slightly higher at 2.5 to 3.5, because of the high risk for clots forming within the valve itself. When the oral anticoagulant shows proper effect, and the prothrombin activity is in the therapeutic range, heparin therapy may be stopped and the oral anticoagulant therapy continued.

It is important for you to be sure that the heparin antidote, protamine sulfate, is available for use whenever patients are on heparin therapy while hospitalized, in the event of accidental overdosage or an acute bleeding event. You will need to urgently contact the appropriate healthcare provider for an order before giving protamine sulfate.

◆ *Evaluation.* If heparin is given by continuous IV infusion, the coagulation time should usually be determined every 4 hours in the early stages of treatment. Many medical centers have adopted protocols that indicate heparin dosing based on previous aPTT results, and determine when the next aPTT should be drawn.

Watch for signs of allergy, such as difficulty breathing, wheezing, swelling around the eyes, itching, rash, or hives. Watch for signs of overdose and internal bleeding as therapy progresses. Check with the patient and/or family to ensure they understand the dosage schedule, side effects, adverse effects, and which signs of adverse effects to report to the healthcare provider. These include bleeding gums when brushing teeth, blood in the urine, or coughing up blood. Teach patients to report all drugs and supplements taken.

> ### ⊕ Top Tip for Safety
>
> - Teach women of childbearing age to notify the healthcare provider if they are pregnant or plan to become pregnant while using heparin. There is a risk for birth defects and bleeding in the last trimester that is associated with heparin use in pregnancy.
> - If anticoagulation is needed for an expectant mother, heparin is the anticoagulant that will be used.
> - Breast-feeding is safe during heparin therapy because the drug is not found in breast milk.
> - The heparin antidote protamine sulfate should be available in the event of accidental overdose or hemorrhage.
> - Monitor the patient's platelet counts for declines that can be associated with HIT or HITT.

VITAMIN K ANTAGONISTS

Vitamin K is necessary for the production of specific proteins that are needed in the clotting process. **Vitamin K antagonists,** which are anticoagulant drugs that interfere with blood clotting by reducing the amount of vitamin K that is available to help the liver form clotting factors, are from the coumarin category of drugs. The most common drug in this class is warfarin (Coumadin).

Actions

Vitamin K antagonists inhibit the enzyme needed for final activation of vitamin K. Without adequate amounts of vitamin K, the liver cannot make blood coagulation factors II, VII, IX, and X. Blood clotting requires the actions of all of the clotting factors, so limiting any clotting factor reduces blood clot formation.

Uses

For long-term therapy in chronic conditions that might involve problems with clot formation (such as coronary artery disease, atrial fibrillation, knee and hip replacement surgery, and immobility), warfarin (Coumadin, Jantoven, Warfilone♣) is the drug of choice. Warfarin is given orally for the prevention of blood clots and emboli. Patients typically begin warfarin while on heparin. Heparin is then discontinued when the INR blood clotting test reaches the therapeutic range.

Expected Side Effects

The potential for easy bruising and bleeding is common. For example, bleeding gums may occur when the patient brushes his or her teeth; blood in the stool or urine is also common. Warfarin may produce GI upset (e.g., diarrhea or nausea), headache, and skin rash.

Adverse Reactions

Adverse reactions of warfarin include excessive bleeding, or hemorrhage that can be seen with very heavy menstrual bleeding, frank blood or dark, tarry stools, or coffee-colored vomitus with excessive dosage. Warfarin can cause skin necrosis (death) that can occur within the first 10 days of therapy, and is associated with larger dosages (Fig. 14.4). Obese, menopausal women are at greatest risk for this rare adverse reaction. Warfarin can also cause birth defects or death to the fetus. It is not given during pregnancy.

In response to some bleeding disorders or warfarin overdosage, vitamin K (phytonadione [AquaMEPHYTON]) may be given either orally or parenterally to help stimulate the liver to resume manufacture of prothrombin and serve as an anticoagulant antagonist. However, this clotting activity may not return for 48 to 72 hours. Blood products that contain clotting factors may have to be given to stop severe bleeding. Even in

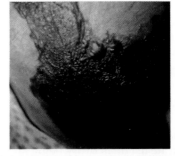

FIG. 14.4 Warfarin-induced skin necrosis. (From Hoffman R, Benz EJ Jr, Shattil SJ, Furie B, Silberstein LE, McGlave P, Heslop H: *Hematology: Basic principles and practice,* ed 5, Philadelphia, 2008, Churchill Livingstone.)

urgent situations, giving phytonadione requires an order from the healthcare provider.

⌂ Top Tip for Safety

Signs that suggest internal bleeding include:
- abdominal pain or swelling, back pain, or constipation (resulting from paralytic ileus or intestinal obstruction);
- bloody or tarry stools, bloody or dark-colored urine, coughing up or vomiting blood or "coffee-ground" substance;
- dizziness or cold, clammy skin;
- severe or continuous headache; and
- tachycardia (fast pulse), hypotension (low blood pressure), and tachypnea (rapid breathing).

Drug and Food Interactions

Vitamin K antagonists, such as warfarin, interact with many other drugs. Use a drug reference or consult with the healthcare provider or pharmacist as needed for patient care or teaching, because the list of drugs that interact with vitamin K antagonists is very long. In general, many antibiotics, anti-inflammatory drugs, antidysrhythmics, GI drugs, statins, and steroids can lengthen bleeding time effects of warfarin, whereas antacids, antihistamines, barbiturates, large doses of vitamin C, and oral contraceptives can shorten it. Lengthening the bleeding time greatly increases the risk for hemorrhage and death. It is critically important for the patient and family to accurately report all current drugs before beginning therapy with warfarin. Vitamin K antagonists also interact with many herbal preparations and supplements, so patients should consult with the healthcare provider before beginning any of these while taking these drugs.

Anticoagulant effects may be increased with acute alcohol intoxication, but decreased with chronic alcohol abuse. Some antidiabetic drugs taken with anticoagulants may increase the effect of either the diabetes drug or the anticoagulant, so close patient monitoring is needed. Eating excessive amounts of green, leafy vegetables (i.e., spinach, broccoli) can interfere with the purpose of vitamin K antagonist therapy, decrease bleeding time, and reduce effectiveness of the treatment, leading to new blood clot formation.

❖ Nursing Implications and Patient Teaching

◆ *Assessment.* Obtain a complete health history from the patient, including the current health problem, medical and surgical histories, and any drug and food allergies or hypersensitivity reactions. Ask the patient for a current, accurate list of all drugs being taken, including herbal products, supplements, or OTC drugs.

Ask about any conditions that would prevent the use of some anticoagulants, such as alcoholism, blood diseases and conditions associated with bleeding, or uncontrolled hypertension. Patients with heart failure may be more sensitive to vitamin K antagonists.

Make absolutely sure that female patients who are taking a vitamin K antagonist are not pregnant or breast-feeding. A pregnancy test may be performed for women of childbearing age before beginning these drugs. Teach sexually active women who are taking warfarin to use two reliable methods of birth control.

◆ *Planning and implementation.* Warfarin can have an unpredictable and variable effect in some patients, especially in older adult (>65 years) patients and those of Asian descent. Warfarin has a very narrow range (therapeutic index) that produces the anticoagulant effects without also producing bleeding in the patient. Frequent blood tests for PT/INR are done to monitor bleeding risk while still providing the anticoagulation needed. To avoid variation in testing methods, a system called the INR is used to standardize PT reporting. In a person who is not receiving anticoagulation therapy, the normal INR is 0.9 to 1.1. The typical INR goal for a patient who needs anticoagulation therapy is 2 to 3, except in mechanical cardiac valve replacement, in which a higher INR is necessary to prevent clot formation. The INR goal may be different for specific disorders that require anticoagulation.

Initially, the PT/INR may be done daily, but after stabilization, tests are performed at 1-week to 4-week intervals, depending on patient response. For hospitalized patients and those in long-term care facilities, be sure to obtain the blood tests on time, and report abnormal findings to the healthcare provider as soon as they are received.

The antidote for warfarin overdosage (vitamin K) should be available at all times.

Caution patients to wear a MedicAlert bracelet or carry an identification card indicating the use of an anticoagulant.

Teach patients and family members about warfarin, the expected side effects, and adverse effects that should be reported immediately.

Teach patients and family members to avoid adding any drugs, herbs, and supplements without the express permission of the healthcare provider, because these agents can interfere with the actions of warfarin.

Teach patients to swallow the tablets whole, without cutting, crushing, or chewing them, to ensure proper drug absorption.

Protect the drug from humidity and light exposure (they are dispensed in an opaque plastic container or a dark-colored glass container) because the drug's activity is reduced by exposure to light and moisture. Do not transfer the drug to another storage container.

Teach patients and family members to avoid increasing the intake of green leafy vegetables, because these contain vitamin K and can decrease the effectiveness of warfarin. Instruct patients to avoid alcohol while taking warfarin because alcohol ingestion changes the drug's activity.

Teach patients to keep all appointments for laboratory tests and visits to the healthcare provider because blood clotting can change and dosage changes may be needed based on test results.

Teach patients to use caution when brushing teeth, trimming nails, and shaving. (An electric shaver should be used when possible.)

Teach patients to apply pressure to stop bleeding from accidental cuts or scrapes. If bleeding persists after 10 minutes, tell the patients to contact their healthcare provider.

Tell patients not to suddenly stop taking any of the oral anticoagulants because this may trigger severe cardiovascular problems and clotting.

Instruct patients to avoid contact sports or other activities that could lead to injuries.

The effects of anticoagulants usually require at least 2 days to recover blood clotting ability once anticoagulation is stopped.

> ### 🍃 Lifespan Considerations
> **Older Adults**
>
> Older adults may be more sensitive to the effects of anticoagulants, and a lower maintenance dose is usually recommended for the older adult patient, along with very close supervision and monitoring. This is particularly true for patients who receive warfarin and may be vitamin K deficient because of low intake of green, leafy vegetables.

◆ *Evaluation.* Warfarin takes up to 72 hours before it reaches an effective level for anticoagulation. Heparin is given when an immediate anticoagulant effect is required; so often the hospitalized patient will be receiving both heparin and warfarin at the same time. Thus monitoring of the PT/INR is especially critical during this period.

> ### 💡 Memory Jogger
> Heparin and warfarin can be taken at the same time, whereas most other anticoagulants cannot.

Watch for signs of overdose and internal bleeding as therapy progresses. Indications include bleeding gums when brushing teeth, blood in the urine or stool, and coughing up or vomiting blood.

Assess whether the patient understands why he or she is taking the drug, as well as the symptoms of overdose. Have the patient explain to you the actions he or she would take when signs of bruising or easy bleeding are noted.

Remind patients to always consult the prescriber before starting any new drug (including OTC drugs and vitamins), changing a drug dose, or discontinuing any drug. Many drugs can change the effects of an anticoagulant in the body.

Determine whether the patient and family members understand the dietary instructions regarding the intake of green, leafy vegetables (e.g., broccoli, cabbage, collard greens, lettuce, and spinach). See Box 14.1 for a list of herbs that increase the risk for bleeding or interfere with anticoagulant action.

Top Tips for Clinical Care

- Teach patients to tell their dentist and all their healthcare providers that they are taking anticoagulants.
- Patients who are taking anticoagulants and who require dental or surgical procedures may need to discontinue the drug before surgery to avoid problems with bleeding. Surgical procedures may be a particular risk if patients have a traumatic injury or require emergency surgery.
- Drugs such as clopidogrel (Plavix), used after stent placement, should never be abruptly stopped without consultation with a cardiologist. Abruptly stopped clopidogrel in this case might prompt the stent to become blocked with a clot.

FIBRINOLYTIC DRUGS

Action

Fibrinolytic drugs (formerly called *thrombolytic* drugs) actually do dissolve and break down existing blood clots. For this reason they are sometimes referred to as "clot busters." Fibrinolytic drugs work by converting plasminogen to the enzyme plasmin, which degrades or breaks down fibrin clots, fibrinogen, and other plasma proteins. These products are used especially for *lysis* (dissolving) of thrombi and are used only in a critical care setting. A summary of fibrinolytics is provided in Table 14.2.

Uses

Fibrinolytic drugs are used in the acute care setting such as the emergency department or intensive care unit. These drugs are given for a variety of reasons, including acute MI, acute pulmonary emboli, acute ischemic stroke, and acute arterial occlusion. These drugs dissolve clots and emboli, ultimately reducing the extent of cellular damage from arterial blockage. Timing is a critical factor for using these drugs. If fibrinolytics are begun within 12 hours of a heart attack or 3 hours of the onset of a stroke, the blood clot blocking the artery can be dissolved and blood flow restored. The most commonly used fibrinolytic drugs are alteplase (Activase, tPA), reteplase (Retavase), and tenecteplase (TNKase). Be careful not to confuse tPA and TNKinase. Although both are fibrinolytics, the dosages and administration are different. These drugs are high-alert drugs and are given through an IV line.

Table 14.2 Fibrinolytics

Fibrinolytics: These drugs dissolve clots by activating plasminogen to plasmin, which is an enzyme that breaks down the fibrin fiber network that is the mesh holding a clot together.

DRUGS/ADULT DOSAGE RANGE	NURSING IMPLICATIONS
alteplase (Activase, tPA; Activase, rtPA♣): adult dose is based upon condition being treated	• Before therapy, ensure the patient has no history of active internal bleeding, recent stroke, spinal surgery, blood pressure >200/120 mm Hg, bleeding disorders, pregnancy or delivery, head trauma, prolonged cardiopulmonary resuscitation, or pending aortic dissection because these conditions are absolute contraindications for fibrinolytic therapy.
Myocardial Infarction	
15 mg IV bolus, then 50 mg IV over 30 min, then 35 mg IV over 60 min; followed by heparin therapy	• Watch for signs of hemorrhage, especially bleeding into the brain, because these drugs greatly increase the risk for bleeding anywhere.
Pulmonary Embolism	
100 mg IV over 2 hours; followed by heparin therapy	• Monitor patients who are taking heparin for wheezing, shortness of breath, chest tightness, facial swelling, and rash or hives because this drug is made from animal products and has a higher risk for causing allergy and hypersensitivity.
Stroke	
0.9 mg/kg IV over 1 hour (limit total dose to 90 mg, with 10% of the dose given as a bolus) reteplase (Retavase) adult dose: 10 units IV bolus, then another 10 units IV bolus 30 min later tenecteplase (TNKase) adult dose is based on weight: 30–50 mg IV push[a]	• Monitor coagulation laboratory tests because drug dosages are based on the results of these tests. • Monitor for the presence of severe headache or changes in alertness because these may signal stroke from bleeding in the brain. • Avoid giving IM drugs because of the risk for bleeding. If IV line is removed, apply pressure for 30 minutes.

[a]Not given by LPN/VN.
♣ Indicates Canadian drug.

Expected Side Effects

Bleeding is the most obvious side effect of fibrinolytic drugs. Bleeding of the gums or injection or IV sites can occur. Low blood pressure (hypotension) can also occur.

Adverse Reactions

Allergic reactions and hypersensitivity can occur with symptoms of shortness of breath, wheezing, chest tightness, facial swelling, skin rash, or hives. Hemorrhage is the most critical adverse reaction that can occur. In addition, because these drugs break up clots, there is a risk for stroke, especially in older adult patients with hypertension. There are contraindications for receiving fibrinolytic drugs, in which case they cannot be given. These contraindications include known bleeding disorders, pregnancy or recent delivery (<24 hours), history of stroke within the past 2 months, hypertension with a blood pressure >200/120 mm Hg, head trauma, and aortic dissection.

Drug Interactions

Giving fibrinolytic drugs together with other anticoagulants increases the potential for bleeding and hemorrhage.

❖ Nursing Implications and Patient Teaching

◆ *Assessment.* Fibrinolytic drugs are given by the healthcare provider or advanced practitioners in life-threatening situations of MI or stroke. They are most helpful when given within the first hour after the onset of symptoms from the thrombosis. Ask the patient or family when chest pain (for MI) or stroke symptoms first began to determine the exact time sequence of events and what happened before the patient was brought to the hospital. Ask whether the patient has a history of prior stroke or bleeding disorder.

Ask whether any other drugs, such as aspirin, have been taken. Aspirin helps reduce platelet adhesion; for patients suspected of having an MI, the standard protocol is to have the patient chew a 325-mg aspirin (ASA) tablet. The aspirin may have been taken at home or given by paramedics before arrival at the hospital.

Ask the patient or family whether he or she has had surgery or given birth within the past 48 hours.

◆ *Planning and implementation.* Fibrinolytic drugs come as a powder that requires reconstitution. Have all of the equipment and materials assembled and ready for infusion.

Carefully monitor and record the vital signs of the patient who is receiving thrombolytic therapy. Report these findings to the healthcare provider. Once the fibrinolytic drug has been given, do not remove IV lines or give IM injections because of the risk for severe bleeding. If an IV line must be removed, apply pressure to the area for 30 minutes.

◆ *Evaluation.* Monitor the patient carefully for bleeding. Bleeding may be superficial, coming from the infusion site. Other more significant bleeding indicates overdose and is shown by *hematuria* (blood in the urine), *hematemesis* (blood in the vomitus), abdominal pain and swelling, tachycardia, tachypnea, and hypotension that can indicate internal bleeding.

◆ *Patient and family teaching.* Ensure that the patient and family understand the purpose, risks, and benefits of fibrinolytic therapy. Teach the patient to report any unusual symptoms, signs of allergic reaction to the drug, and any unusual bleeding that occurs.

ERYTHROPOIESIS-STIMULATING AGENTS

Action

Erythropoiesis-stimulating agents (ESAs) are synthetic forms of the hormone *erythropoietin*, which is naturally produced by the kidneys when red blood cell (RBC) counts decline because of anemia. The decrease in RBCs results in poor tissue oxygenation, because the hemoglobin in the RBC carries oxygen to the body organs and tissues. So anemia signals the kidneys to secrete erythropoietin, which then travels to the bone marrow, stimulating the marrow to increase production of RBCs. This process is known as *erythropoiesis*. The synthetic forms of erythropoietin work just like the natural hormone. ESAs come in vials or in prefilled syringes, and are given by IV or subcutaneous routes. A summary of ESAs is provided in Table 14.3.

Uses

ESAs are usually given to patients with a condition that causes anemia, and who need to increase the production of RBCs. Patients with chronic kidney disease cannot make enough erythropoietin to provide adequate oxygen to tissues. Patients who are anemic from the effects of chemotherapy on the bone marrow or who may be anemic before surgery are often prescribed ESAs. These drugs reduce the need for transfusions and reduce the complications of transfusions, such as fluid overload.

Expected Side Effects

Pain at the injection site is the most common side effect of ESAs. Generalized body aches and pain, skin rash, redness, or warmth at the injection site can occur.

Adverse Reactions

The use of ESAs is not without significant risks. As RBC production increases, the blood itself becomes thicker. This can result in a higher risk for hypertension, blood clots, stroke, and MI (heart attack). In some advanced cancers, increased tumor growth occurred when ESAs were given. There is a risk for severe allergic reactions to ESAs.

Table 14.3   Erythropoiesis-Stimulating Agents

Erythropoiesis-stimulating agents: These drugs induce the bone marrow to increase the production of red blood cells and some other blood cells.

DRUGS/ADULT DOSAGE RANGE	NURSING IMPLICATIONS
darbepoetin alfa (Aranesp) 0.45 mcg/kg IV or subcutaneously each week; can be given in divided doses epoetin alfa (Epogen, Procrit, Eprex♣) 50–100 U/kg IV or subcutaneously three times weekly to maintain hemoglobin level at prescribed range	• Monitor blood pressure for increases due to increased blood viscosity (thickness), headaches, body aches, fever, or chills. • Monitor blood counts, especially hemoglobin, to help determine drug effectiveness. • Follow directions for drug mixing and preparation because these vary by product and drug effectiveness depends on correct administration. • Check for signs or symptoms of allergic reactions, which are possible adverse effects of these drugs. • Teach patients to immediately report chest pain or shortness of breath, drooping face, or numbness in face or extremities, calling an ambulance to the emergency department; these are signs of heart attack or stroke, and ESAs increase the risk for these health problems.

♣ Indicates Canadian drug.

❖ Nursing Implications and Patient Teaching

◆ *Assessment.* Assess the patient's vital signs and weight. Report the presence of hypertension, which may need to be controlled before beginning ESAs.

Obtain a complete health history, especially for a history of stroke, blood clots, MI, other blood clotting disorders, or sickle cell disease.

Ask about symptoms of allergic reactions if the patient received ESAs in the past. Ask about the presence of latex allergy because the covers of prefilled syringes contain latex.

Assess the result of the patient's complete blood count. Notify the healthcare provider if the hemoglobin is 12 g/dL (or higher) before giving ESAs. Monitor the patient's iron status (transferrin, serum ferritin) levels and notify the healthcare provider of results before beginning ESAs.

◆ *Planning and implementation.* Give supplemental iron as ordered by the healthcare provider.

Do not expose the ESA vial to light and do not shake the vial. After giving the drug, discard any unused or leftover drug in the vial or in the prefilled syringes.

Do not give intravenous (IV) ESAs with any other drugs.

Give subcutaneous injections in the outer area of the upper arms, the abdomen (except for the 2-inch area around the umbilicus), the front middle of the thigh, or the outer area of the buttocks.

Teach the patient and family the following:
• Weigh yourself daily and report a weight gain of 2 lb in 24 hours or 4 lb in a week to your healthcare provider because these drugs can cause water retention.
• Go immediately to the nearest hospital if you have chest pain because these drugs increase blood thickness and raise blood pressure, which can increase your risk for having a heart attack.
• Inform your healthcare provider if you are pregnant, breast-feeding, or plan to become pregnant.

◆ *Evaluation.* Report signs of an allergic reaction, such as rash, wheezing, facial swelling, difficulty breathing, or hypotension. Report signs of stroke, or the presence of chest pain or shortness of breath, or increases in the patient's blood pressure.

Get Ready for the NCLEX® Examination!

Key Points

• Anticoagulants are used to prevent new clots from forming and existing clots from getting larger.
• Fibrinolytics dissolve existing clots and reduce the formation of new clots.
• All anticoagulants and fibrinolytics greatly increase the risk for excessive bleeding.
• Before starting anticoagulation therapy, ask the patient which other drugs (prescribed or OTC), vitamins, or herbal supplements he or she takes, and check with the pharmacist to determine whether any of them affect blood clotting.
• When injecting subcutaneous heparin, do not pull back on the syringe to aspirate for blood or move the needle in the tissue during the injection.
• Do not massage the subcutaneous heparin injection site.
• The antidote for a heparin overdose is protamine sulfate.
• The risk for allergic reactions is higher with heparin than with other anticoagulants because heparin is made from animal products.

Get Ready for the NCLEX® Examination!—cont'd

- Warfarin is teratogenic (can cause birth defects) and should never be used during pregnancy.
- The antidote for warfarin overdose is vitamin K injection (AquaMEPHYTON).
- DTIs are light sensitive and must be stored in their original opaque bottles, not in daily pill organizers.
- A patient may receive warfarin at the same time he or she is receiving heparin.
- The anticoagulation effect for patients who are taking warfarin daily is usually measured weekly by INR.
- The "must know" signs that require prompt attention for patients who are taking anticoagulant drugs are excessive gum bleeding, continuous bleeding or oozing from cuts, unexplained nosebleeds, and unusually heavy menstrual flow.
- All fibrinolytic drugs are given intravenously and are high-alert drugs.
- ESAs are used to increase hemoglobin levels to improve oxygen transport to vital organs and tissues.
- Patient and family teaching is especially important for the patient who is undergoing long-term therapy.

Review Questions for the NCLEX® Examination

1. You are caring for a patient who has just begun anticoagulant therapy with heparin for the treatment of a pulmonary embolus. Which response from the patient confirms that the patient understands the purpose of this therapy?
   1. "This drug will heal the scarring in my lung."
   2. "This drug will not cause any additional bleeding."
   3. "This drug will break up the clot that is in my lung."
   4. "This drug will prevent new clots from forming in my body."

2. A female patient who is being treated with subcutaneous heparin reports having an unusually heavy menstrual period. What is the most appropriate response to this patient's concern?
   1. "This is only concerning if you develop a fever."
   2. "I will be sure to notify the prescriber right away of this issue."
   3. "This shows that the heparin is working correctly in your body."
   4. "Please keep a chart of your periods so that we can note any unusual trends developing."

3. You are caring for a patient who is taking an NSAID for the treatment of arthritis and will also be treated with heparin. Based on this report, what may you expect that the patient will experience?
   1. A decrease in arthritis pain
   2. An increase in arthritis pain
   3. A decreased effect of the heparin
   4. An increased effect of the heparin

4. Which of the following menu selections would demonstrate understanding of the dietary teaching for a patient treated with an anticoagulant?
   1. Bacon, lettuce, and tomato sandwich and iced tea
   2. Chef salad, whole grain crackers, and orange juice
   3. Baked chicken, macaroni and cheese, and low-fat milk
   4. Pork chops, broccoli and cheese, and iced tea

5. What is the most important action to take as you give heparin to a patient?
   1. Heparin can be mixed with other drugs, preventing the need for multiple injections.
   2. Always pull back on the plunger to aspirate before giving the injection.
   3. Keep the needle firmly in place while injecting the drug.
   4. Massage the injection site after giving the injection.

6. Which drugs belong to the direct thrombin inhibitor class of anticoagulants? (Select all that apply.)
   1. Acetylsalicylic acid
   2. Apixaban
   3. Clopidogrel
   4. Dabigatran
   5. Heparin
   6. Protamine sulfate
   7. Rivaroxaban
   8. Warfarin

7. You are caring for a patient who will be receiving warfarin sodium (Coumadin) 10 mg by mouth daily. You have warfarin 5 mg tablets available to give. What is your best action?
   1. Give the patient two (2) tablets.
   2. Skip this dose until you obtain 10 mg tablets.
   3. Break the tablet in half and give ½ a tablet.
   4. Give 2½ tablets.

8. A patient is prescribed 2000 U/mL heparin subcutaneously. The drug on hand is heparin 5000 U/mL. How many milliliters is the correct dose? _____ mL

Case Study

Mr. Dooley, a 75-year-old male patient, was hospitalized for new-onset atrial fibrillation. During his hospital stay he was receiving IV heparin. He will be discharged tomorrow after being started on warfarin 5 mg daily. He has been following a vegetarian diet for the past 30 years and states that he has a health regimen that includes his vegetarian diet and several supplements and herbal products.

1. While Mr. Dooley receives heparin in the hospital, what blood test should you monitor to determine whether he is at risk for heparin-induced thrombocytopenia?

2. What blood test is useful in determining how much heparin should be given?

3. What information should be included in the dietary teaching for Mr. Dooley?

4. What should you tell Mr. Dooley about taking supplements and herbs while taking warfarin?

5. What drug is the antidote for warfarin overdosage?

6. You are completing the drug teaching about warfarin before Mr. Dooley's discharge home. What should you teach him about the adverse effects of warfarin?

Drugs for Immunization and Immunomodulation

15

Learning Outcomes

1. Explain the differences between innate immunity and acquired immunity.
2. Describe the role of antibodies in providing true immunity.
3. Explain how vaccination affects acquired immunity.
4. Describe the proper technique for giving drugs for routine immunization.
5. Describe the recommended schedules for vaccination for children, adults, and older adults.
6. List issues for vaccination during pregnancy.
7. List the names, actions, possible side effects, and adverse effects of selective immunosuppressant drugs.
8. Explain what to teach patients and families about selective immunosuppressant drugs.

Key Terms

acquired immunity (ă-KWĪRD ĭ-MYŪ-nĭ-tē, p. 281) A long-acting and "learned" protective response by lymphocyte production of antibodies that are directed against specific microorganisms.

active immunity (ĂK-tĭv ĭ-MYŪ-nĭ-tē, p. 281) Acquired immunity in which your body makes specific antibodies to antigens. Can be natural or artificial.

antibody (ĂN-tĭ-bŏ-dē, p. 281) A blood protein that is produced in response to and binds with any substance that the body's WBCs consider foreign such as bacteria, viruses, and foreign substances in the blood.

antibody titer (TĪ-těr, p. 284) A test that detects and measures the amount of antibodies in the blood to help determine the strength of a person's immunity against a specific microorganism.

antigen (ĂN-tĭ-jĕn, p. 281) Any substance your body's WBCs recognize as foreign that will cause lymphocytes to produce an antibody against it.

antiproliferative drugs (ĂN-tĭ-prō-LĬF-ĕ-rāt-ĭv, p. 287) Drugs that slow the growth of those lymphocytes most responsible for autoimmune diseases and for transplant rejection.

antirejection drugs (ĂN-tĭ-rĭ-JĔK-shĕn, p. 287) Drugs that suppress the cells and factors of the immune system responsible for the receiving patient's rejection of transplanted tissues and organs.

artificial acquired active immunity (ahr-tĭ-FĬ-shĕl ă-KWĪRD ĂK-tĭv ĭ-MYŪ-nĭ-tē, p. 282) The type of immunity that a person develops against a specific microorganism when a form of it is deliberately injected into his or her body as a "vaccination" or "immunization."

artificial acquired passive immunity (ahr-tĭ-FĬ-shĕl ă-KWĪRD PĂ-sĭv ĭ-MYŪ-nĭ-tē, p. 282) The type of immunity that is transferred as "premade" antibodies from one person or persons and even from animals into another person to provide immediate protection against a specific dangerous infection.

attenuated vaccine (ĕ-TĔN-yu-wāt-ĕd văk-SĒN, p. 283) A vaccine containing live organisms that have been weakened and rendered harmless so that they are not capable of causing disease but are still able to produce an immune response.

biosynthetic vaccine (BĪ-ō-sĭn-THĔ-tĭk văk-SĒN, p. 283) A vaccine composed of man-made substances that are very similar to the parts of a virus or bacterium that cause disease.

calcineurin inhibitors (KĂL-sē-NYŪR-ĭn, p. 287) A class of drugs that works by forming a complex around the normal calcineurin present inside T-lymphocytes preventing the calcineurin from activating those cells.

immunity (ĭ-MYŪ-nĭ-tē, p. 280) The body's physical resistance to becoming ill every time it comes into contact with pathogenic (disease-causing) microorganisms.

immunization (Ĭ-myū-nī-ZĀ-shŭn, p. 282) The result of successful vaccination that causes a person to develop his or her own antibodies for immunity against the substance in the vaccine. Often used in the same way as the term vaccination.

immunosuppressant drugs (Ĭ-myū-nō-sĕ-PRĔ-sănt, p. 287) Drugs that subdue or decrease the strength of the body's immune system.

inactivated vaccine (ĭ-NĂK-tĕ-vāt-ĕd, p. 283) A vaccine in which the organisms have been killed or inactivated by heat, radiation, or chemicals to prevent them from reproducing and causing disease but that can still trigger antibody production and immunity. Also called a "killed" vaccine.

279

innate immunity (ĭ-NĀT ĭ-MYŪ-nĭ-tē, p. 280) The body's intact protective barriers and the cellular responses of inflammation.

natural acquired active immunity (NĂ-chĕ-rĕl ă-KWĪRD ĂK-tĭv ĭ-MYŪ-nĭ-tē, p. 281) The type of immunity a person develops to a microorganism that invades his or her body, usually making him or her sick, and triggering his or her immune system to make antibodies against it.

natural acquired passive immunity (NĂ-chĕ-rĕl ă-KWĪRD PĂ-sĭv ĭ-MYŪ-nĭ-tē, p. 282) The immunity provided by the antibodies that a woman transfers to her fetus during pregnancy and to her infant during breastfeeding.

passive immunity (PĂ-sĭv ĭ-MYŪ-nĭ-tē, p. 281) Acquired immunity in which antibodies made in another person or animal are given to you and your body had no part in making them. Can be natural or artificial.

toxoid (TŎK-sōĭd, p. 283) A pathogenic microorganism that is modified chemically so it is no longer toxic and can be used as a vaccine.

vaccination (văk-sĭ-NĀ-shĕn, p. 282) An injection or ingestion of a harmless form of bacteria or virus to stimulate antibody production against a certain disease.

vaccine (văk-SĒN, p. 282) A preparation of a synthetic, killed, or weakened form of a bacteria or virus that can be injected or ingested in order to stimulate antibody production against certain diseases.

OVERVIEW OF IMMUNITY

Immunity is your body's physical resistance to becoming ill every time you come into contact with pathogenic (disease-causing) microorganisms. It is provided by the immune system working together with the protective barriers of intact skin and mucous membranes along with the body's normal flora. The immune system has two main divisions, innate immunity (also known as nonspecific or general immunity), and acquired immunity (also known as specific or adaptive immunity). When all these protections are working well, we are healthy and well more often than we are sick, even when exposed to invading bacteria, viruses, and other organisms. Think of all the times someone in your family caught a cold, influenza, or some other contagious illness, but not everyone in the family got sick.

INNATE IMMUNITY

Innate immunity is the body's intact protective barriers and the cellular responses of inflammation. *Inflammation* is a predictable set of tissue and blood vessel actions caused by white blood cells (WBCs) and their products whenever the body is injured or invaded by microorganisms. Whenever microorganisms enter the body, many WBCs recognize them as "foreign" and take nonspecific actions against them to kill, neutralize, or eliminate them to prevent illness. WBCs can recognize invading organisms as foreign because all of your cells have a unique code on the surface that works like a universal product code for you (Fig. 15.1). Invaders have a different "code" on their cell surfaces than your cells do, and your WBCs recognize the difference (Fig. 15.2) and take actions against only the invader, not your own cells. These inflammatory responses and actions are general and can be overwhelmed, such as when you are heavily exposed to thousands of one type of streptococcal bacteria and develop a strep throat infection. If innate immunity were the only type of immunity you had, you would probably get another strep throat the next time the same type of streptococcal bacteria heavily invaded your body. This general part of innate immunity helps keep you well from day to day, but it does not provide you with the true immunity that acquired immunity does.

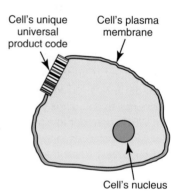

FIG. 15.1 Human cell with unique universal product code. (From Workman ML, LaCharity LA: *Medical-surgical nursing: Patient-centered collaborative care,* ed 2, St. Louis, 2016, Elsevier.)

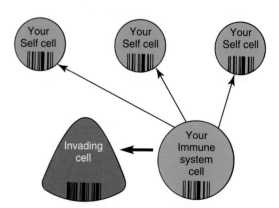

FIG. 15.2 Immune system cell recognizing an invading or foreign cell by differences in its universal product code. (Modified from Ignatavicius DD, Workman ML: *Medical-surgical nursing: Patient-centered collaborative care,* ed 8, St. Louis, 2016, Elsevier; and Workman ML, LaCharity LA: *Medical-surgical nursing: Patient-centered collaborative care,* ed 2, St. Louis, 2016, Elsevier.)

Acquired Immunity

Acquired immunity is a long-acting and "learned" protective response by lymphocyte production of antibodies that are directed against specific microorganisms, which are considered foreign substances known as antigens. Exposure to antigens is the trigger for lymphocytes to begin producing antibodies. (Thus an **antigen** is anything your WBCs recognize as foreign that will cause lymphocytes to produce an **antibody** against it.) These antibodies can be made in such high amounts that, when you are reinfected by the same microorganism, they attack and destroy it or rid the body of it before it can make you sick again. For example, if you are overwhelmingly infected with thousands of the 234 type of streptococcus (this is a made-up type) and developed a strep throat from the infection, at the same time your lymphocytes would be learning how to make antibodies to streptococcus-234. Then the next time you were heavily exposed to streptococcus-234, you would make so many anti-streptococcus-234 antibodies that they would be killed or eliminated before you could get sick from them again. You would then be immune to streptococcus-234. (Unfortunately there are many different types of streptococcus and until you have had them all, you will not have antibodies to all of them.)

Acquired immunity is specific, which means that antibodies to streptococcus-234 probably will not recognize and attack streptococcus-422. So until your body is exposed to type 422 and learns to make anti-streptococcus-422 antibodies, you could get sick from being infected with streptococcus-422.

Acquired immunity has two major forms, *natural* and *artificial,* each of which can be active or passive. Both types involve the production of specific antibodies in response to exposure to an antigen. One difference between these two types is in *how* you are exposed to the antigen. Remember, your immune system cannot make an antibody against a specific antigen unless the antigen actually enters the body and the immune system is exposed to the antigen. Whether immunity is active or passive depends on who made the antibodies. When your body makes the antibodies, immunity is **active**. When the antibodies are made by another person or an animal, immunity is **passive** (because your body was not actively involved in making the antibody). Fig. 15.3 shows how the four different types of acquired immunity develop.

Natural Acquired Active Immunity

Natural acquired active immunity is the type of immunity you develop to a microorganism that invades your body naturally, usually making you sick and triggering your

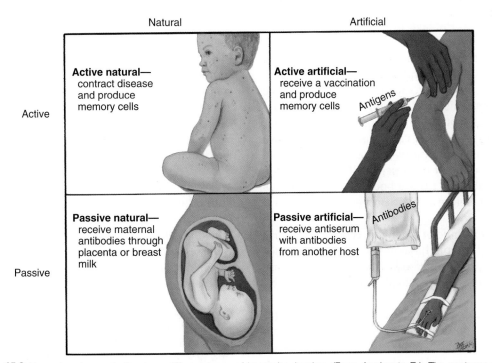

FIG. 15.3 Examples demonstrating how different types of immunity develop. (From Applegate EJ: *The anatomy and physiology learning system,* ed 4, St. Louis, 2011, Saunders.)

immune system to make antibodies against it. After your immune system learns to make these specific antibodies, every time you are reexposed to the micro-organism, you make more and more antibodies against it. So you continually "self-boost" your immunity to it. This self-boosting part of natural acquired active immunity makes it the most long-lasting type of immunity to a specific microorganism. Therefore natural acquired active immunity is *true immunity*.

Natural Acquired Passive Immunity

Natural acquired passive immunity is composed of the antibodies that a woman transfers to her fetus during pregnancy and to her infant during breast-feeding. This immunity is short term but critically important in preventing young infants from developing illnesses during the first 6 months after birth.

Artificial Acquired Active Immunity

Artificial acquired active immunity is the type of immunity that you develop against a specific microorganism when a form of it is deliberately injected into you as a vaccination or immunization. It is still active immunity because your body has to work to learn how to make the antibodies, and it is artificial because you did not just "catch" the microorganisms, you were deliberately injected with them (or deliberately ingested them). Although this is a common type of immunity and usually works well, it wears off faster than natural acquired active immunity because you are injected with fewer microorganisms than the amount that entered your body naturally to make you sick. As a result, you will need periodic booster shots to help your immune system remember how to make the antibodies to these specific microorganisms.

Artificial Acquired Passive Immunity

Artificial acquired passive immunity is the type of immunity that is transferred as premade antibodies from one person or persons and even from animals to you. It is called *passive* because your body did not actively make these antibodies. This type of immunity is used only when a person is exposed to and highly likely infected with a microorganism that can cause serious disease and he or she has no immunity against it. The purpose of giving a person a lot of these specific antibodies is to have the antibodies rid the body of the dangerous microorganisms before the person becomes sick with the disease.

Rabies is an example of when this type of immunity is needed. Most people have never received a rabies vaccination and have no antibodies to it. Once the disease occurs, it is almost always fatal. If a person is bitten by an animal with rabies, immediate passive immunity can help prevent him or her from developing rabies and dying. As soon as possible the exposed person is given a series of injections of rabies antibodies that were made by other people or animals. These injected antibodies then attack and destroy the rabies virus before the disease

can develop. This immunity is immediate but only temporary. Within a few weeks, the person's immune system will then destroy the "foreign" antibodies. Some other highly dangerous infections and disorders that can be managed with artificial acquired passive immunity include poisonous snakebites, tetanus, and Ebola.

> **Memory Jogger**
>
> Artificially acquired passive immunity through the transfer of premade antibodies from another person or animal provides only very short-term protection against a specific infectious disease.

VACCINATION

Vaccinations work to prevent possible life-threatening infections. If a person acquires an infection naturally, he or she becomes immune to that microorganism; however, death or complications of the disease can occur. For instance, polio can cause paralysis, and measles can cause blindness. The first vaccine was for smallpox; it was created in 1796 by Dr. Edward Jenner. Today, more than 20 infectious diseases can be prevented with available vaccines.

Vaccination is an injection or ingestion of a harmless form of bacteria or virus to stimulate antibody production by B lymphocytes (B cells) against a certain disease. (The B cells are the only type of WBC that can form antibodies in response to exposure to a specific antigen.) These antibodies provide immunity to the disease caused by the antigen. Although some vaccines, such as for polio, can be taken orally, most are injected. A **vaccine** is a preparation of a synthetic, killed, or a weakened form of a bacteria or virus that can be injected or ingested to stimulate antibody production against certain diseases. As a result of vaccination, the person's B cells start making the desired antibodies. However, vaccination is not as efficient in stimulating antibody-mediated immunity compared with when a person develops naturally acquired active immunity by actually becoming sick with the disease first. So for full immunity to develop from vaccination, more than one injection vaccination with the same vaccine over time may be needed. In addition, this immunity wears off eventually and the person requires a periodic booster shot with revaccination to ensure continued production of enough antibodies to maintain immune resistance against the organism. Many people use the terms *vaccination* and *immunization* interchangeably; however, **immunization** is the result of successful vaccination that causes a person to develop his or her own antibodies for immunity against the substance in the vaccine.

> **Memory Jogger**
>
> Successful vaccination causes immunization to develop with the production of antibodies against the organisms in the vaccine, leading to immunity.

Types of Vaccines

Vaccines are prepared in different ways for different organisms. Often inactivated viruses or bacteria are used. **Inactivated vaccines** are composed of organisms that could cause diseases but have been killed or inactivated by heat, radiation, or chemicals that prevent the organisms from reproducing and causing disease. Diseases for which inactivated vaccines are commonly used include influenza, cholera, hepatitis A, and rabies.

Attenuated vaccines (also called *live virus vaccines*) contain live organisms that have been weakened and rendered harmless so that they are not capable of causing disease but are still able to produce an immune response. Usually modifying the organisms through attenuation makes them noncontagious to people who have normal immune systems. Diseases for which attenuated vaccines are commonly used include measles, mumps, rubella, polio, and chickenpox.

Toxoids are pathogenic microorganisms that are modified chemically so that they are no longer toxic and can be used as a vaccine. Disease for which toxoid vaccines are commonly used include tetanus, diphtheria, pertussis (whooping cough), human papilloma virus (HPV), and hepatitis B virus (HVB).

Biosynthetic vaccines are those made by genetic engineering that contain a synthetic or natural extract of the virus or bacterium that causes disease. Many modern vaccines are produced this way.

> ### Memory Jogger
>
> The four types of vaccines that are currently available are:
> - inactivated vaccines
> - attenuated vaccines
> - toxoids
> - biosynthetic vaccines

Vaccination and Boosting Schedules

Vaccinations for artificial acquired active immunity usually require more than one injection to ensure that enough B cells are sufficient to the specific antigen and can begin making antibodies. As stated earlier, additional vaccinations (boosters) that contain smaller doses of the original antigens are needed to continue immunity. For example, "baby shots," which are vaccinations that contain antigens for diphtheria, tetanus, and pertussis (DTaP) mixed into one injection, are given to infants three separate times, usually at ages 2, 4, and 6 months. Boosters of this vaccination are repeated once between the ages of 15 and 18 months, and once again between the ages of 4 and 6 years. Another booster with a different formulation of these same three antigens (known as Tdap [tetanus, diphtheria, acellular pertussis]) should be given once to children between the ages of 11 and 12 years and to women during each pregnancy. It is also recommended that all adults older than 19 years receive this booster vaccination every 10 years. Other common vaccinations recommended during childhood

to prevent severe complications of contagious diseases include HVB, *Haemophilus influenza* type B (Hib), pneumonia, polio, measles, mumps, rubella, hepatitis virus A (HVA), varicella, rotavirus, HPV, meningitis, and seasonal influenza.

In addition to immunizing to prevent disease and complications of disease in individual persons, it is necessary to immunize to protect the population. When a significant portion of the public is immunized against a specific contagious disease, most people within that population are protected against that disease because an outbreak has little chance of occurring. People who cannot receive certain vaccines, such as pregnant women or those who are immunocompromised, are still protected because exposure to the disease is either limited or nonexistent. This is known as *herd immunity* and is the principle used to promote vaccination yearly for seasonal influenza. It is also the reason polio has been eradicated in the United States since 1979.

The Centers for Disease Control and Prevention (CDC) website has free printable schedules for both regular and catch-up versions of immunizations to download so healthcare professionals can easily keep up to date and safely give vaccinations for both children and adults. You can access these schedules, as well as educational tools, at the CDC website. The website is published every year based on recommendations of the American Academy of Pediatrics, the CDC Advisory Committee, and the American Academy of Family Physicians. This website also features a phone app that is free to download and is available for both Android and iPhones for quick access to this information.

> ### Bookmark This!
>
> To access up-to-date immunization schedules for children: https://www.cdc.gov/vaccines/schedules/index.html.

Fig. 15.4 shows a sample of what is available on the website. It is meant to simply be a sample and although current for the year 2017, it is not entirely complete. The CDC site includes a schedule for those who fall behind on vaccinations or who start late. There are also separate schedules for those who are immunosuppressed. Footnotes are included to provide further guidance on the use of all the vaccines that are available.

> ### Top Tip for Safety
>
> Tdap and DTaP have similar names but are used in different patients and different circumstances: DTaP is used for active immunization in infants and children, and Tdap is used as a booster vaccine for older children and adults.

Vaccination and immunization are needed in adulthood, not just in childhood. Vaccines are recommended to stimulate protection for adults against common infectious diseases, especially for older adults and those

Vaccine	Birth	1mo-2mos	2mos	4mos	6mos	9mos	12mos-15mos	15mos-18mos	18mos	19-23mos	2-3yrs	4-6yrs	7-10yrs	11-12yrs	13-15yrs	16-18yrs
Hepatitis B (HepB)	1st dose	2nd dose			3rd dose											
Rotavirus 2 dose (RV1)			1st dose	2nd dose												
Diptheria, tetanus, & acellular pertussis (DTaP)			1st dose	2nd dose	3rd dose			4th dose				5th dose		(Tdap dose)		
Haemophilus influenza (Hib)			1st dose	2nd dose	3rd dose											
Pneumococcal conjugate (PCV13)			1st dose	2nd dose	3rd dose		4th dose									
Poliovirus (IPV)			1st dose	2nd dose	3rd dose							4th dose				
Measles, mumps, rubella (MMR)							1st dose					2nd dose				
Varicella (VAR)							1st dose					2nd dose				
Hepatitis A (HepA)							2 dose series									
Human papillomavirus (HPV)														3 dose series		
Meningococcal conjugate vaccines														1st dose		Booster

FIG. 15.4 Sample immunization schedule for children aged 0 to 18 years.

who have chronic health problems. For these people, even less serious contagious disease, especially pneumonia and influenza, can have fatal consequences. Additional recommended vaccinations include those to prevent shingles (varicella), HVA, HVB, and pertussis. Recommendations for adults against other childhood disorders vary, depending on whether the person actually had these diseases as a child. See the CDC website for adult vaccination schedules.

Bookmark This!

To access immunizations schedules for adults: https://www.cdc.gov/vaccines/schedules/index.html.

Additional vaccinations may be recommended for adults depending on the person's history, job, or travel. For example, the rabies vaccine is not part of a recommended set of vaccinations. However, for veterinarians and other animal handlers, the vaccine is readily available. Military personnel and others who travel to areas of the world where contagious diseases are common may be vaccinated against diseases such as yellow fever, cholera, typhoid, malaria, anthrax, and many others, depending on which area of the world they enter. Many of these less common vaccinations require more than one injection on a specific schedule to ensure effective immunity. Vaccine guidelines and schedules for these contagious diseases can be found on the CDC website.

Bookmark This!

For vaccination guidelines and schedules for contagious diseases:
https://www.cdc.gov/vaccines/hcp/acip-recs/index.html

It is important to properly store, handle, and give vaccines so that potency and safety are maintained. Box 15.1 has important nursing responsibilities and actions for vaccine handling, storage, and administration.

Antibody Titer

Does vaccination always result in successful immunization? A person's immunity to a specific organism can be assessed by performing a blood titer for that antibody. An **antibody titer** is a test that detects and measures the amount of specific antibody in the blood to help determine the strength of a person's immunity against a specific organism. This titer can be used to determine the effectiveness of vaccination, as well as to determine whether a person has retained immunity to a disease he or she once had. For example, a person who has a 0 titer for anti–chickenpox antibody (anti–varicella zoster virus [anti-VZV] or varicella) has no antibodies to the chickenpox virus and is highly likely to develop the

Box 15.1   Nursing Responsibilities and Actions for Vaccine Administration

STORAGE
- Immediately unpack vaccines as soon as received from the manufacturer and store in a designated area with a designated refrigerator that is separate from other drugs or food.
- Ensure the refrigerator is labeled "DO NOT UNPLUG" and is plugged into an outlet that has emergency power.
- Keep all opened and unopened vials in their original boxes.
- Do not place vaccine vials on the door of the refrigerator or in the freezer.
- Check the vials weekly for expiration dates, and discard those that are expired.

BEFORE ADMINISTRATION
- Check the recommended schedule for whether the vaccination is appropriate for the patient.
- Check the expiration date on the vaccine vial and, if a diluent is to be used, check the expiration date on the diluent's vial.
- Read the package insert to determine all vaccine components (i.e., preservatives); the recommended dosage, techniques, and solutions for dilution; and any special instructions for administration.
- Ask the patient (or parent) whether he or she has ever had a reaction to the vaccine or its components.
- Ask the patient (or parent) when he or she last received this or any other vaccine.

- Ask the patient (or parent) about any known allergies.
- Ask whether the patient is ill or has been ill within the previous 24 hours (some vaccines should *not* be given to a patient who has a fever or any type of infection).
- Using aseptic technique and the recommended type of syringe, draw up the appropriate dose. Use an appropriate needle for the patient size and vaccine type.
- Inject the drug using the recommended technique and site.

AFTER ADMINISTRATION
- Document the following information in the patient's medical record or permanent vaccination log:
  - Name and age of the patient
  - Name of the vaccine
  - Manufacturer, lot number, and expiration date of the vaccine
  - Dosage of the vaccine
  - Site of vaccination
  - Condition of the site
- Give the patient or parent a copy of the specific vaccine's Vaccine Information Statement (VIS).
- Document which VIS was given to the patient or parent.
- Observe the patient as recommended by the manufacturer for any immediate reaction.
- Tell the patient what side effects to expect and which ones require immediate attention.

---

disease if he or she is heavily exposed to the organism. A person who has a positive antibody titer of 32 has so much antibody that it is still detectable even when the blood has been diluted to a ratio of 1 part blood to 31 parts diluent. This result indicates good immunity to the chickenpox virus. Overall, this test can indicate whether you have ever had a specific infectious disease (or have been vaccinated against it) and how much immunity you had to it at the time the test was performed. The interpretation of antibody titers is guided by laboratory reference values that are specific to the antibody of the disease.

Seasonal Influenza Vaccination

Many people wonder why adults and children are recommended to receive seasonal influenza vaccination every year. Doesn't the protection from an influenza vaccination last longer than a year? There are many strains of influenza. Each strain is somewhat different and has a different unique code. If you get sick with one specific strain this year, you will develop active immunity to it. However, each year different strains may come to your community. Last year's antibodies do not provide immunity to this year's strain and, if sufficiently infected, you will get sick with the new strain of influenza. The case with flu shots is the same. When you receive this year's seasonal flu shot, the vaccination contains antigens for the three or four viruses that are predicted by the CDC to be the most common

ones prevalent this year. Receiving the vaccination helps you develop active immunity only to these three or four influenza strains, which then protects you against those strains for a long time. However, next year the predicted most common strains may not be the ones you were vaccinated against this year. So if you skip next year's vaccination, you may not have any immunity to the different strains of influenza and could become sick if you are heavily exposed to one or all of them. It is advisable for healthcare workers to receive the flu shot every year not only to prevent individual sickness, but also to prevent giving the flu to an already sick population, which could make them sicker and even lead to untimely death. It takes about 2 weeks to develop antibodies after being vaccinated.

Memory Jogger

Some infectious organisms have many strains with different codes. Immunity to each requires either becoming sick with each strain or being vaccinated against each strain.

Lifespan Considerations

Pediatric Vaccination

For best effect, the recommended pediatric vaccination schedules must be followed closely. Most vaccinations given before 6 months of age require multiple doses over time because more time is needed for the infant's immature immune system to learn to make antibodies.

Vaccination and Pregnancy

Some, but not all, vaccinations can be safely given during pregnancy. Live virus vaccinations, such as for chickenpox, polio, measles, mumps, and rubella, are *not* recommended during pregnancy. Vaccinations that are recommended during pregnancy include seasonal influenza and Tdap.

Vaccinations and Older Adults

As a person ages, previously acquired immunity slowly declines. As a result, older adults gradually lose immunologic protection, even natural active immunity. They need to receive scheduled booster shots to immunizations they have already received and need new immunizations to other organisms such as influenza, pneumonia, and the VZV (the same virus that causes chickenpox). Many older adults are not aware of their loss of immunologic protection and the need for additional vaccination. Urge all older adults to follow the recommended schedules for vaccination and revaccination.

Expected Side Effects

All vaccines can cause side effects, but they are generally minor. A sore arm and minor swelling and redness at the injection site or low-grade fever are common and go away within a few days. Fever can be relieved by keeping the child cool or with age-appropriate doses of acetaminophen or ibuprofen. Cool compresses to the injection area will relieve minor swelling and discomfort. Fever over 101°F should be reported to the healthcare provider because this may indicate an infection.

Adverse Reactions

Vaccines are constantly monitored for safety, but just like all other drugs they can cause adverse effects. The risk for rare complications from vaccines outweighs the risk for the serious problems that disease can cause for both the child and all others who come in contact with the child. The CDC lists all vaccines licensed in the United States. Expected side effects and any adverse reactions associated with each of them can be found on the CDC website.

Bookmark This!

For adverse side effects of individual vaccinations: https://www.cdc.gov/vaccines/vac-gen/side-effects.htm

❖ Nursing Implications and Patient Teaching

◆ *Assessment.* Obtain a medical history, in particular a history of any immune deficiency disease such as HIV, any specific congenital immunodeficiency disease, pregnancy, or plan to become pregnant that will prohibit vaccination with a live virus. Some vaccines can be given during pregnancy, but other vaccines, such as the measles, mumps, rubella (MMR) vaccine, must be given a month or more before pregnancy occurs.

Obtain a drug history, including immunosuppressant drugs, immune globulins, or blood products. Some drugs may interfere with the antibody response of vaccines. Intervals between live vaccines and blood product transfusions are recommended because live vaccines must replicate to initiate an immune response. Antibodies against injected live vaccine antigen in transfused blood may interfere with that replication. People who are immunocompromised are at increased risk for an adverse reaction after administration of live attenuated vaccines because they have less of an ability to build up an effective immune response. Ask if there is an immunocompromised person living with the person who is to be vaccinated. Before receiving a vaccination with a live vaccine, the household member's healthcare provider should be consulted because the patient with reduced immunity may be at increased risk for contracting the virus the vaccine is designed to prevent.

A complete allergy history that includes drugs, foods, vaccines, and environmental allergens should be taken. An updated CDC recommendation for people with egg allergy can be found at https://www.cdc.gov/flu/protect/vaccine/egg-allergies.htm. Recent studies examining the use of injectable influenza vaccine in egg-allergic persons indicate that severe allergic reactions are highly unlikely. The only contraindication for allergic individuals is a previous severe allergic reaction to flu vaccine for any reason.

Assess the patient for symptoms of illness with or without fever that may require a delay in giving the vaccination until symptoms have subsided. Take a complete immunization history so current vaccination needs can be determined. In addition, ask about family and household members who are immunocompromised or unvaccinated so their health and safety also can be assessed.

◆ *Planning and implementation.* Adhere to the vaccination storage (see Box 15.1 for nursing responsibilities and actions) to ensure the vaccination will be effective. *Never mix vaccines in the same syringe.* Keep epinephrine or an anaphylactic kit readily available for immediate use in case of an anaphylactic reaction.

◆ *Evaluation.* Observe the patient for any signs and symptoms of adverse reactions and provide the patient with a record of the vaccinations (see Box 15.1).

◆ *Patient and family teaching*

- Teach the parent or patient that localized reactions to the injection can occur. The discomfort can be relieved with cool compresses to the site and age-appropriate acetaminophen or ibuprofen as directed by the healthcare provider.
- Advise the parents or patient to notify the healthcare provider of fever greater than 101°F, rash, itching, or shortness of breath.
- Tell the parent or patient to keep a current record of the immunizations. It is advisable to keep two copies in case of loss.

- Teach the parent or patient the risks of contracting the disease that the vaccine is preventing.
- Tell female patients that they should not become pregnant for at least 1 month after receiving the MMR vaccine.
- Remind the parent or patient to bring the immunization record with them to all visits.
- Give the parent or patient information and an appointment date to return for the next vaccination.

IMMUNOMODULATING THERAPY

SELECTIVE IMMUNOSUPPRESSANTS FOR AUTOIMMUNE DISEASES

Although the immune system is protective most of the time, for some people it can overreact in certain tissues as a result of autoimmune disorders, such as rheumatoid arthritis or psoriasis. In such disorders the immune system sees normal body tissue as "foreign" and attacks it. These problems can be chronic and destructive, requiring that the immune responses be selectively modified or suppressed. In addition, immune modification is needed after organ transplantation to prevent destruction of the transplanted organ by an immune system that sees this new organ as "foreign." In both cases, management involves suppression of the immune response.

Some **immunosuppressant drugs** are nonselective and cause such general immune suppression that the patient is at high risk for life-threatening infections. These general immunosuppressive drugs include corticosteroid anti-inflammatories and some types of cancer chemotherapy, such as methotrexate. Their use has decreased and, even when they are used today, the dosages are lower because they are used along with more selective immunosuppressants. The actions, effects, nursing implications, and other information specific for corticosteroids are detailed in Chapter 11.

More recent drug therapy for autoimmune disorders uses selective immunosuppressants that confine their effects to those cells and products of the immune system most directly involved in tissue-damaging actions. The most common drug category of selective immunosuppressants for this use is the disease-modifying antirheumatic drugs (DMARDs). The actions, effects, nursing implications, and other information specific for DMARDs are detailed in Chapter 11.

SELECTIVE IMMUNOSUPPRESSANTS TO PREVENT TRANSPLANT REJECTION

The immune system of a person who receives a transplanted organ (from anyone who is not an identical sibling) recognizes the transplanted organ as "foreign" and tries to attack it. For a transplanted organ to remain healthy in the recipient, the parts of his or her immune system that usually attack it must be suppressed forever.

Drug therapy to prevent solid-organ rejection is lifelong and uses combination drug therapy. **Antirejection drugs** suppress the cells and factors of the immune system responsible for the receiving patient's rejection of transplanted tissues and organs. The dosages must be adjusted to the immune response of each patient because these drugs do cause some degree of general immunosuppression. In addition to corticosteroids and some DMARDs, the selective immunosuppressant drugs for this purpose are the antiproliferative drugs and calcineurin inhibitors.

Action

Antiproliferative drugs slow the growth of those lymphocytes most responsible for autoimmune diseases and for transplant rejection. A less selective drug in this class is azathioprine. It inhibits the metabolism of purines, which are important in DNA synthesis and cell division. This inhibition suppresses the actions of T lymphocytes that are toxic to transplanted organs and also are responsible for causing tissue damage in some autoimmune diseases. The names, usual adult dosages, and nursing implications of the antiproliferative drugs are listed in Table 15.1.

Mycophenolate is more selective in suppressing T and B lymphocyte activity by inhibiting an enzyme needed for lymphocyte reproduction. It also prevents T cell activation. As a result, the immune responses most associated with autoimmune tissue destruction and transplant rejection are selectively suppressed.

Sirolimus selectively inhibits T cell activation and reproduction by blocking the mammalian target or rapamycin (mTOR) signal pathways that promote completion of cell division for T cells. If fewer T cells are present, then there is less tumor necrosis factor and other substances present to attack normal tissues and transplanted organs. Sirolimus also suppresses B cell growth and maturation (which makes antibodies against normal tissue and against transplanted organs), so there are fewer antibody attacks on these tissues.

Everolimus is a drug that acts very similarly to sirolimus. It also inhibits the mTOR pathway, so lymphocyte cell division and growth are reduced. It is more specific against those immune system cells that attack normal self-cells and transplanted organs than are the general antiproliferative drugs.

Calcineurin inhibitors work by forming a complex around the normal calcineurin present inside T lymphocytes preventing the calcineurin from activating those cells. With less ability to be activated, the T cells have less power to attack and damage transplanted tissues and organs. The two main calcineurin inhibitors are cyclosporine and tacrolimus. The names, usual adult dosages, and nursing implications of the antiproliferatives are listed in Table 15.1.

Expected Side Effects

All selective immunosuppressants reduce immunity to some extent and increase the patient's risk for infection. So these drugs are not to be used when a patient

Table 15.1   Examples of Selective Immunosuppressants for Transplant Rejection

Antiproliferative drugs: reduce transplant rejection by slowing the growth of many immune system cells that are responsible for transplant rejection

DRUG/ADULT DOSAGE RANGE	NURSING IMPLICATIONS
azathioprine (Azasan, Imuran) 1–5 mg/kg orally once daily or 1–1.5 g IV mycophenolate (CellCept, Myfortic) 1.5 g orally twice daily or 1.5 g IV twice daily sirolimus (Rapamune) 6 mg orally loading dose, followed by 2 mg orally once daily for maintenance everolimus (Zortress) 0.75 mg orally every 12 hours initially; dosages adjust according to patient responses	• Teach patients to look for signs of bleeding, such as bleeding gums, easy bruising, and nosebleeds, because these drugs can decrease platelet counts as well as WBC counts. • All patients should have BUN and creatinine levels checked as ordered and notify the healthcare provider for signs of renal failure such as decreased urine output, fatigue, swelling, or shortness of breath. • Antiproliferative drugs commonly cause nausea and vomiting. Warn patients that if these symptoms are accompanied by fever and diarrhea, they should notify their healthcare provider. • Teach patients not to take these drugs with grapefruit juice because it can cause increased toxicity. • Allopurinol use with azathioprine can cause increased toxicity of the drug, leading to an extreme decrease in WBCs and bone marrow suppression, which can be life-threatening. • Mycophenolate is associated with congenital abnormalities if used in pregnancy. Remind female patients who are sexually active to use two forms of birth control while on this or any of these antiproliferative drugs. • Mycophenolate can cause hyperglycemia. Caution diabetic patients that it may be difficult to control sugar levels. • Sirolimus and cyclosporine doses must be separated by at least 4 hours to ensure the best effect. • Oral solutions of sirolimus must be mixed in a glass container with milk, orange, or apple juice and *not* water.

Calcineurin drugs: reduce transplant rejection from T cell activation by binding to protein and forming a complex that inhibits calcineurin present in some immune system cells that is needed to allow these cells to function and reproduce

DRUG/ADULT DOSAGE RANGE	NURSING IMPLICATIONS

cyclosporine (Neoral, Gengraf, Sandimmune) 4–8 mg/kg orally twice daily initially
tacrolimus (Astagraf XL, HECORIA, Prograf)
  Immediate-release capsules, 0.1 mg/kg orally every 12 hours
  Extended-release capsules, 0.2 mg/kg orally once daily
	• Both of these drugs can cause significant kidney and liver toxicity. Monitor serum electrolyte, BUN, and creatinine levels closely along with liver enzymes.
	• All patients should have BUN and creatinine levels checked as ordered. Notify the healthcare provider for signs of renal failure such as decreased urine output, fatigue, swelling, or shortness of breath.
	• Teach patients who are taking cyclosporine to monitor their blood pressure daily because this drug causes hypertension.
	• Teach patients who are taking cyclosporine to practice good oral hygiene because it can cause gingival hyperplasia.
	• Neoral and Gengraf cannot be used interchangeably with Sandimmune because the absorption is different between them.
	• These drugs should not be given with grapefruit juice because it can lead to toxicity.
	• Many drug interactions can occur, most commonly with St. John's wort and NSAIDs. Remind the patient to never take any over-the-counter drugs before checking first with the pharmacist or healthcare provider.
	• Do not crush or split the tablets or capsules because they are extended release and could cause toxicity.
	• Oral solutions of cyclosporine must be mixed in a glass container with milk, orange, or apple juice and *not* water.

has a systemic infection. With reduced immunity and inflammation, the symptoms of infection may not be present even when the patient has a significant infection.

Side effects of the selective immunosuppressants vary depending on the exact mechanism of action. All of these drugs cause GI problems and many skin rashes.

Tacrolimus can cause diabetes mellitus. Sirolimus and everolimus increase blood cholesterol levels.

The calcineurin inhibitors increase blood cholesterol levels, which leads to hypertension. They also increase blood glucose levels (hyperglycemia), making diabetes more difficult to control. Many patients who are taking cyclosporine develop gingival (gum) hyperplasia.

Adverse Effects

All selective immunosuppressants increase the risk for cancer development, especially skin cancers, because they reduce immunity. This problem is thought to be related to reduced immunosurveillance by loss of immune system early recognition of when normal cells transform into cancer cells. The risk is higher for the drugs that are taken long term, including the antiproliferatives and the calcineurin inhibitors.

Antiproliferative drugs given intravenously can cause phlebitis and thrombosis at the administration site. Liver toxicity and liver failure have occurred with all of the antiproliferative drugs and the calcineurin inhibitors. The risk is increased if the patient has other liver problems or is exposed to other substances that are liver toxic, such as alcohol and acetaminophen. Other adverse effects vary by the drug's mechanism of action. Most of these drugs can cause imbalances of potassium, phosphorus, and magnesium. Patients who are taking selective immunosuppressant drugs are advised to avoid vaccinations with live vaccines because their reduced immunity increases their risk for getting the disease the vaccine is designed to prevent.

Drug Interactions

All the selective immunosuppressants interact with numerous other drugs. Transplant patients usually need other drugs in addition to their lifetime immunosuppressant therapy, which increases their risk for drug interactions. Be sure to consult a drug reference book or pharmacist for more information about specific drug interactions with the antiproliferative drugs and the calcineurin inhibitors.

❖ Nursing Implications and Patient Teaching

◆ *Assessment.* A healthcare provider completes a detailed history and physical for each patient who will receive a transplant. Transplantation is a multifaceted medical and ethical issue, and the many healthcare team members include specialty healthcare providers, nurses, nurse practitioners, social services, psychologists, and a variety of other professionals involved in the care of a transplant patient and the patient's family. Your continued assessment after transplantation will be guided by the individual medical needs of the patient and are covered in the following subsection.

◆ *Planning and implementation.* The antiproliferative drugs can be absorbed through skin and mucous membranes, and they exert effects on whoever prepares them. So using personal protective equipment (PPE) of gowns, gloves, and masks is critical when preparing and giving these drugs to prevent accidental exposure of these drug to yourself.

Be sure to obtain a list of all other drugs (prescribed and over-the-counter drugs) that the patient takes because most selective immunosuppressant drugs interact with many other agents. Be sure to consult a drug reference book or pharmacist for more information about specific drug interactions. If needed, consult with the prescriber about dosage or changing the patient's other drugs.

All patients who are taking or receiving any selective immunosuppressant have baseline laboratory tests that include complete blood cell counts, electrolyte studies, platelet counts, kidney function tests, liver function tests, bilirubin levels, and ECGs. These tests, as well as assessment and documentation of signs and symptoms of infection and bleeding, are done at regular intervals throughout the patient's lifetime to prevent drug toxicities. Review the results of laboratory tests and notify the healthcare provider for any abnormal results.

For best effects, intravenous (IV) formulations of these drugs *must* be mixed with the manufacturer-recommended diluent. Do not mix or give selective immunosuppressants with other IV drugs, and do not give other drugs through the same IV line used for immunosuppressant therapy. Assess the site for irritation, phlebitis, and thrombosis. Monitor patients closely during infusions of any immunosuppressant drugs for signs of allergic (hypersensitivity) reactions and anaphylaxis. If these occur, stop the infusion immediately and follow your institution's protocol for an emergency situation. If you are in a clinic, make sure the crash cart or emergency drug box is close by. Be sure to document the reaction to the drug, flag the chart, and alert the patient that the drug should not be taken again.

Assess the functioning of all patient organ systems. Assess vital signs and report abnormalities. Ask the patient about fever, chills, fatigue, lethargy, cough, or difficult breathing that may indicate infection. Look in the mouth for signs of gum hyperplasia (can be caused by cyclosporine) or evidence of fungal infection. Assess the patient for yellowing of the skin or whites of the eyes that may indicate liver dysfunction. Kidney function can be affected, especially with tacrolimus, so weigh the patient to assess for changes in fluid balance. A weight gain of 1 kg is equal to 1 L of fluid. In addition, check the blood urea nitrogen (BUN), creatinine, and electrolyte studies, and ask the patient about color, amount, and consistency of urine. Small amounts of dark yellow concentrated urine can indicate dehydration, infection, or a problem with the kidneys caused by drug toxicity.

◆ *Patient and family teaching.* Tell the patient and family the following:

- Take your temperature daily and watch for the common signs and symptoms of infection because these drugs reduce your ability to fight infection. Common indications of infection include fever, foul-smelling drainage, pain or burning on urination, sore throat, and cough.
- Immediately report any indication of infection to your healthcare provider.
- Check with your healthcare provider for what types of vaccinations you should receive while on immunosuppressive therapy.

- Keep all appointments for monitoring of blood counts and other laboratory tests.
- Take your drugs exactly as prescribed to maintain the effectiveness in preventing transplant rejection. Even a few missed doses can lead to tissue-damaging responses and transplant rejection episodes.
- Notify your healthcare provider if you develop yellowing of the skin or eyes, darkening of the urine, or lightening of the stools. These problems are signs of liver toxicity, a serious adverse effect of these drugs.
- Avoid drinking alcohol or using acetaminophen while taking these drugs because these substances also can cause liver damage.
- If you are taking the oral suspensions of sirolimus or cyclosporine, mix the drug exactly as directed, using the recommended solution (e.g., milk, orange juice, or apple juice); *do not mix with water.* After drinking the suspension, rinse the container with the same solution and drink the rinse for better drug effectiveness. Remember that cyclosporine must be mixed in a glass container, not a plastic one.

- If you are taking both sirolimus and cyclosporine, separate the drug dosages by at least 4 hours to ensure the best effect.
- Do not take sirolimus or tacrolimus with grapefruit juice because it decreases the effectiveness of the enzyme that metabolizes these drugs, and their blood levels could become dangerously high, leading to toxic side effects.
- Do not take other drugs or supplements without checking with your healthcare provider because the antiproliferatives and calcineurin inhibitors interact with so many other drugs.

Lifespan Considerations

Pregnancy and Selective Immunosuppressants

Pregnancy is an absolute contraindication for the use of antiproliferative drugs because these drugs are associated with birth defects and other severe problems. Tell sexually active women of childbearing age to use two reliable methods of contraception during this therapy and for at least 12 weeks after the therapy is discontinued. These drugs also enter breast milk and can have an adverse effect on the infant.

Get Ready for the NCLEX® Examination!

Key Points

- Innate immunity helps protect a person from infection but does not provide true immunity to any specific infectious microorganism.
- The immune system cannot make an antibody against a specific antigen unless it is exposed to that antigen.
- Antibodies made by one person or animal can be transferred to another person for short-term passive immunity.
- The four types of vaccines currently available are inactivated ("killed") vaccines, attenuated ("live") vaccines, toxoids, and biosynthetic vaccines.
- Vaccinations usually require more than one dose and often must be "boosted" for best long-term immunity to a specific organism.
- For some infectious microorganisms there are many different strains of the microorganisms, each of which requires vaccination for immunity. One example is seasonal influenza.
- Pregnant women should receive seasonal influenza vaccination and the Tdap vaccination during every pregnancy. Most other vaccinations are avoided during pregnancy.
- Vaccinations are used to help people develop immunity to a dangerous disease without the risk for becoming sick first.
- Immunizing the majority of a community produces herd immunity, which prevents disease transmission to those persons who are unable to become vaccinated.
- The immune systems of patients who receive transplanted organs (unless from an identical sibling) can attack and reject the new organ. They need to take immunosuppressive drugs daily to prevent transplant rejection.

- All patients who are taking immunosuppressive drugs are at increased risk for infection and cancer development.
- Ask patients about all other drugs or supplements they take before giving any selective immunosuppressant drug because these drugs have many interactions.
- Use PPE when preparing or giving selective immunosuppressants to prevent accidental exposure of the drug to you.
- The antiproliferative drugs are associated with poor pregnancy outcomes; therefore teach sexually active women of childbearing age who are taking these drugs to use two reliable methods of contraception during therapy and for 12 weeks after antiproliferative drugs are discontinued.

Review Questions for the NCLEX® Examination

1. Which condition is a contraindication for receiving a measles, mumps, rubella (MMR) vaccine?
   1. Cold symptoms
   2. Pregnancy
   3. Urinary tract infection
   4. Anemia
2. Which of the following symptoms are considered expected side effects of IM vaccinations? (Select all that apply.)
   1. Rash
   2. Fever less than 101°F
   3. Redness and soreness of injection site
   4. Shortness of breath
   5. Earache
   6. Sore throat

Get Ready for the NCLEX® Examination!—cont'd

3. A patient asks what all the adverse reactions of a yellow fever vaccination are before consenting to the injection. Which response by the nurse is the most appropriate?
   1. "There are side effects to every drug, but the side effects far outweigh getting yellow fever."
   2. "The expected side effects are redness and soreness at the injection site. A warm compress and some acetaminophen will take care of those symptoms."
   3. "You should ask the pharmacist or healthcare provider that question."
   4. "The CDC regularly monitors adverse side effects of all vaccinations. Let's pull up the CDC website so we can look up the adverse effects of the vaccine, as well as the dangers of getting yellow fever."

4. Which type of immunity does an injection with rabies antibodies represent?
   1. Natural acquired active immunity
   2. Natural acquired passive immunity
   3. Artificial acquired active immunity
   4. Artificial acquired passive immunity

5. A mother brings her 9-month-old child to the clinic for his scheduled immunizations. Which statement by the mother would cause the nurse to question giving the child his immunization at this visit?
   1. "Ethan's nose has been stuffy for a week."
   2. "Ethan's thigh was really sore and red the last time he was vaccinated."
   3. "Ethan was cranky, crying, and wouldn't eat his dinner the last time he was vaccinated."
   4. "Ethan had a fever last night, but it is back to normal since I gave him ibuprofen."

6. A 45-year-old female patient is receiving cyclosporine (Neoral, Sandimmune) after a kidney transplant. The patient has a sore throat, fatigue, and a fever of 99°F. What should the nurse suspect at this time?
   1. The patient's kidney has begun to fail.
   2. The patient is rejecting the kidney.
   3. The patient may have an infection.
   4. The patient is beginning to have an adverse reaction to the cyclosporine.

7. Which laboratory test on a transplant patient is most important to monitor closely for an adverse effect of tacrolimus?
   1. Liver enzymes
   2. Electrolytes
   3. Platelet count
   4. Serum creatinine

8. Which of the following fruits should be avoided when a patient is taking cyclosporine?
   1. Apples
   2. Grapefruit
   3. Apricots
   4. Oranges

9. A patient on long-term immunosuppressants should adhere to which of the following behaviors? (Select all that apply.)
   1. Staying away from persons who are sick
   2. Using acetaminophen for minor discomfort
   3. Routinely have a healthcare professional check for skin lesions
   4. Receiving only inactivated or dead vaccines
   5. Washing fruits and vegetables well before eating
   6. Not straining while bearing down for a bowel movement

10. Order: cyclosporine (Sandimmune) 15 mg/kg orally as a single dose for a child who weighs 77 lb. Cyclosporine (Sandimmune) is available in a 100 mg/1 mL oral solution.
    A. How many mg of cyclosporine should be given? (35 kg × 15 mg = 525 mg)
    B. How many mL of oral solution will you give the child? (5.25 mL of oral solution)

Case Study

Jennifer Walden is a 32-year-old mother who presents to the clinic for vaccinations. She desires a hepatitis B vaccine for herself because she will be returning to work as a healthcare worker in the jail infirmary and must have the vaccinations up to date before she begins employment. She also requests immunizations for her 4-year-old son, Joey, who will be starting kindergarten in the fall. He is so far up to date on all of his immunizations. Using the CDC website, answer the following questions.

1. How long will it take for Jennifer to complete the vaccination series?

2. What appointment schedule will you give Jennifer assuming her first dose will be given today?

3. Jennifer tells you she had a booster tetanus shot when she was in high school. Should she receive another booster of DTaP or Tdap? How often should Jennifer receive this booster?

4. Which vaccinations will Joey need to receive before beginning school in the fall?

5. Jennifer asks you if it is wise for her and Joey to receive a seasonal flu shot. What will you tell her and why?

6. Using the CDC website (https://www.cdc.gov/vaccines/schedules/hcp/imz/adult.html), determine what other immunizations Jennifer might receive.

Learning Outcomes

1. Explain the role of hormone replacement therapy for general health and endocrine problems.
2. List the names, actions, possible side effects, and adverse effects of drugs for thyroid problems.
3. Explain what to teach patients and families about drugs for thyroid problems.
4. List the names, actions, possible side effects, and adverse effects of drugs for adrenal gland problems.
5. Explain what to teach patients and families about drugs for adrenal gland problems.
6. List the names, actions, possible side effects, and adverse effects of drugs for sex hormone replacement and contraception.
7. Explain what to teach patients and families about drugs for sex hormone replacement and contraception.
8. List the names, actions, possible side effects, and adverse effects of drugs for osteoporosis.
9. Explain what to teach patients and families about drugs for osteoporosis.

Key Terms

aldosterone (ăl-dō-STĔR-ōn, p. 297) A hormone secreted by the adrenal cortex that regulates sodium and water balance.

anabolic steroids (ă-nă-BŎL-ĭk STĔR-ōĭd, p. 304) Synthetic drugs with the same use and actions as androgens.

androgens (ĂN-drĕ-jĕns, p. 304) Synthetic or natural hormones that help to develop and maintain the male sex organs at puberty and develop secondary sex characteristics in men (facial hair, deep voice, body hair, body fat distribution, and muscle development).

antithyroid drugs (ĂN-tĭ-THĪ-rōĭd, p. 296) Thyroid-suppressing drugs that work directly in the thyroid gland to stop production of new hormones by preventing an enzyme from connecting iodine (iodide) with tyrosine to make active thyroid hormones.

bisphosphonates (bĭs-FŎS-fĕ-nāts, p. 306) Calcium-modifying drugs that both prevent bones from losing calcium and increase bone density by moving blood calcium into the bone, binding to calcium in the bone, and preventing osteoclasts from destroying bone cells and resorbing calcium.

corticosteroid (kōr-tĭ-kō-'STĔR-oid, p. 297) Drug similar to natural cortisol, a hormone secreted by the adrenal cortex that is essential for life.

estrogen agonist/antagonist (Ĕ-strĕ-jĕn Ă-gă-nĭst/ăn-TĂ-gĕ-nĭst, p. 307) Drug for osteoporosis that activates (agonizes) estrogen receptors in the bone to promote calcium retention in the bone and blocks (antagonizes) estrogen receptors in breast tissue and uterine tissue.

hormonal contraception (hōr-MŌ-năl, p. 302) The use of hormones to suppress ovulation for the intentional prevention of pregnancy.

hormone (HŌR-mōn, p. 292) A protein secreted by an endocrine gland that changes the action of another gland or tissue, known as its target tissue.

hormone replacement therapy (HRT) (HŌR-mōn rĭ-PLĀS-mĕnt THĔR-ĕ-pē, p. 293) Temporary or permanent therapy with drugs that perform the function of natural endocrine hormones.

osteoporosis (Ŏ-stē-ō-pĕ-RŌ-sĭs, p. 305) The gradual loss of bone density and strength, which leads to spinal shortening and increased risk for bone fractures.

thyroid hormone agonist (THĪ-rōĭd HŌR-mōn Ă-gă-nĭst, p. 294) Drug that mimics the effect of thyroid hormones, T_3 and T_4, helping to regulate metabolism.

OVERVIEW OF THE ENDOCRINE SYSTEM

The endocrine system involves many glands that secrete hormones (Fig. 16.1). A **hormone** is a protein secreted by an endocrine gland that changes the action of another gland or tissue, known as its *target tissue*. Unlike some glandular secretions, such as from the salivary glands in which a secretion moves through a duct directly to its site of action, hormones do not require a duct to reach their target tissues. For this reason endocrine glands are known as "ductless" glands. Instead, hormones are released into the bloodstream, where they circulate throughout the body. When a specific hormone, such as insulin, reaches a tissue or organ that has insulin

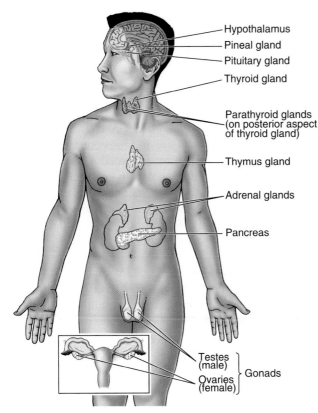

FIG. 16.1 The endocrine system. (Modified from Herlihy B: *The human body in health and illness,* ed 5, Philadelphia, 2014, Elsevier.)

Labels:
- Hypothalamus
- Pineal gland
- Pituitary gland
- Thyroid gland
- Parathyroid glands (on posterior aspect of thyroid gland)
- Thymus gland
- Adrenal glands
- Pancreas
- Testes (male) / Ovaries (female) } Gonads

Symptoms Associated With Thyroid Problems

HYPOTHYROIDISM

- Tired, with no energy, sleeps a lot
- Gains weight while eating minimal amounts
- Heart rate, blood pressure, and respiratory rate low for age and size
- Always feels cold when others are comfortable
- Body temperature below normal
- Constipation
- Increased facial and body hair, decreased scalp hair
- Is less interested in surroundings and appears to think more slowly
- Tongue seems thicker, making speech more difficult
- Skin dry and flakey
- Decreased sex drive
- Decreased or absent menstruation
- Erectile dysfunction

HYPERTHYROIDISM

- Lots of energy, difficulty sleeping
- Weight loss even when appetite and eating are increased
- Heart rate and blood pressure elevated
- Always feels too warm when others are comfortable
- Body temperature above normal
- Multiple bowel movements daily, diarrhea
- Thinning scalp hair
- Skin moist, sweaty
- Difficulty concentrating, may be irritable
- Hand tremors
- Menstrual cycle irregular

receptors, insulin recognizes its target tissue and binds to the receptors, causing a change in the target tissue activity.

Many hormones are necessary for life. Some, such as estrogen, are useful at different times during a person's life but are not essential for maintaining critical physiologic functions. At times endocrine glands develop problems and are no longer able to produce adequate amounts of specific hormones. For example, pancreatic beta cells can stop producing insulin, which causes the person to have diabetes. At other times, an endocrine gland may be surgically removed for a specific problem and the person then would be deficient for that hormone. Depending on how important the function of the hormone is to a patient's health and well-being, **hormone replacement therapy (HRT)** with drugs that perform the function of natural hormones may be needed. HRT may be used for a short time, such as for relief of menopause symptoms, or permanently, such as replacement of thyroid hormones after removal of the thyroid gland.

Common uses of hormone replacement therapy include drugs for thyroid problems, adrenal gland problems, sex hormone replacement, contraception, and diabetes. The issues for diabetes management are complex and are discussed separately in Chapter 17.

DRUGS FOR THYROID PROBLEMS

The thyroid gland in the neck (see Fig. 16.1) produces two thyroid hormones that are critical for life: thyroxine (T_4) and triiodothyronine (T_3). These hormones enter all cells in the body, where they bind to receptors inside the cell and activate the genes for metabolism. T_4 and T_3 increase the rate of metabolism, which is the energy use and work performed in the body. These hormones are critical for the following body actions:

- brain development and function, including the ability to think, remember, and learn
- heart and skeletal muscle contraction and strength
- endocrine system production of other hormones
- breathing and oxygen use in all cells

HYPOTHYROIDISM

Hypothyroidism, also known as underactive thyroid, is a common problem in which the thyroid gland produces little or no thyroid hormones, slowing all aspects of metabolism. Other symptoms such as weakness, fatigue, weight gain, or depression also occur. If left untreated, serious problems of the cardiovascular, pulmonary, and nervous systems and brain result. Children may have such poor brain development that they are cognitively impaired. Adult metabolism can slow to the point that death from cardiac or respiratory failure can occur. These problems can be prevented using HRT with thyroid hormone agonists. Usually this therapy is needed for the rest of the person's life. Box 16.1 lists the symptoms associated with hypothyroidism.

THYROID HORMONE AGONISTS

Action and Uses

Thyroid hormone agonists are drugs that mimic the effect of the thyroid hormones T_3 and T_4, helping to regulate metabolism. These drugs work just like natural thyroid hormones by moving through the blood and entering all cells. The drugs then enter the nucleus and bind to receptors on the DNA, which then activates the genes for metabolism. As a result of turning on these genes, thyroid hormone agonists increase the cells' rate of metabolism, which speeds up both the energy use and the work of each cell. Table 16.1 lists the names, dosages, and nursing implications for the most commonly prescribed thyroid hormone agonists. Consult a drug reference or pharmacist for information about other thyroid hormone agonists.

Expected Side Effects

Thyroid hormone agonist drugs have few side effects because they mimic normal hormones. As cell metabolism increases, the patient may experience symptoms of hyperthyroidism. The symptoms most easily noticed are diarrhea, rapid pulse, high blood pressure (*hypertension*), difficulty sleeping (*insomnia*), excessive sweating, and heat intolerance.

Adverse Effects

The most serious adverse effects of thyroid hormone agonists occur in the cardiac and nervous systems. The activity of both systems increase, sometimes to dangerous levels. Increased cardiac activity can lead to *angina* (chest pain), *myocardial infarction* (heart attack), or heart failure.

Increased nervous system activity can lead to seizures, although this is more likely to occur in patients who already have a seizure disorder.

Drug Interactions

When thyroid hormone agonists are taken with drugs that reduce blood clotting (anticoagulants), especially warfarin (Coumadin), their actions are increased. This response can cause excessive bleeding and bruising.

Table 16.1   Examples of Common Drugs for Thyroid Problems

Thyroid hormone agonists: These synthetic drugs have the same structure as thyroid hormones and work in the same way to activate the gene for metabolism, speeding up the energy use and work output of each cell.

DRUG/ADULT DOSAGE RANGE	NURSING IMPLICATIONS
levothyroxine sodium [synthetic] (Estre, Eltroxin ♣, Levo-T, Levothroid, Levoxyl, Synthroid, Unithroid) Oral: 25–250 mcg once daily IV: 12.5–150 mcg once daily liothyronine sodium [synthetic] (Cytomel, Triostat) 25–100 mcg orally once daily.	• Check the patient's heart rate and blood pressure before giving this drug because increased heart rate and blood pressure can result. • Check the patient's entire prescription and over-the-counter drug list for potential interactions with thyroid hormone agonist drugs. • Report the use of anticoagulants or NSAIDs because these drugs can interact with levothyroxine and cause excessive bruising and bleeding. • Pregnant women may need a higher dose, and women who are taking thyroid hormone agonists are advised not to breast-feed, because the drug can be found in the mother's breast milk. • Check the dose and the specific drug name carefully. Thyroid hormone agonists are *not* interchangeable because the strength of each drug varies. • Levothyroxine may affect the blood sugar of diabetic patients. Check blood sugar levels closely.

Antithyroid drugs: These drugs reduce thyroid hormone levels by entering the thyroid gland and combining with the enzyme responsible for connecting iodine (iodide) with tyrosine. Without this iodide–tyrosine connection, thyroid hormone production is suppressed.

DRUG/ADULT DOSAGE RANGE	NURSING IMPLICATIONS
methimazole (Northyx, Tapazole) Usual maintenance dosage: 5–30 mg orally every 8 hours propylthiouracil (Propacil, Propyl-Thyracil ♣, PTU) Usual maintenance dosage: 100–150 mg orally every 8 hours	• Check the patient's complete blood cell count for signs of bone marrow suppression such as a low white blood cell count, anemia, or thrombocytopenia. • Assess the patient for signs of infection. • Assess the patient's skin for signs of bruising or bleeding such as ecchymosis or petechiae. • Check the patient's drug list for drugs that have antiplatelet actions, such as warfarin. • Check the patient's liver function tests before giving these drugs. Both thyroid-suppressing drugs are hepatotoxic. Check the patient daily for yellowing of the skin or sclera that indicates jaundice. • Check the dose and the specific drug name and prescribed dosage carefully. These drugs are not interchangeable because the strength of each drug varies. • Notify the healthcare provider if adverse effects, such as bone marrow suppression or altered liver function, occur.

♣ Indicates Canadian drug.

❖ Nursing Implications and Patient Teaching

◆ *Assessment.* Before giving the first dose of a thyroid hormone agonist drug, check the patient's heart rate and blood pressure because these drugs can increase metabolic rate and cardiac activity.

Check the patient's entire drug list, including prescription drugs, vitamins, minerals, and supplements for potential interactions with thyroid hormone agonist drugs. Report the use of anticoagulants or NSAIDs to the healthcare provider because these drugs can interact with thyroid hormone agonists and cause excessive bruising and bleeding.

Assess women of childbearing age for possible pregnancy before beginning thyroid hormone agonists. Pregnant women may need a higher dose, and women who are taking thyroid hormone agonists are advised not to breast-feed because the drug can be found in the mother's breast milk.

Carefully check the drug name and dose because thyroid hormone agonists drugs are *not* interchangeable. Although the actions are similar, the strength of each drug varies.

> 🔒 **Top Tip for Safety**
>
> Do not give one brand of thyroid hormone in place of another. The strength of different brands and types vary, and so can patient responses. Liothyronine is four times as potent as levothyroxine.

◆ *Planning and implementation.* When hypothyroidism is first diagnosed, the thyroid hormone drug dose is kept low for the first several weeks. The drug dose is then increased slowly every 2 to 3 weeks until the patient has normal blood levels of thyroid hormone and signs of normal metabolism.

The absorption of thyroid hormone agonists in the GI tract is greatly reduced by food and fiber. Give the drug 2 hours before a meal or fiber supplement or at least 3 hours after a meal or a fiber supplement has been taken.

◆ *Evaluation.* The effects of the drug may not be apparent for several weeks. Check the patient's heart rate and blood pressure to determine whether the drug is working and to check for any side effects because hypothyroid symptoms may be most notable in the cardiac system. The following changes indicate that the drug is effective and the dose is appropriate:

- The patient's vital signs (i.e., body temperature, heart rate, blood pressure, and respiratory rate) are within normal limits.
- The patient's activity level and mental status are normal for him or her.
- The patient's body weight is consistent with the amount of calories he or she eats and his or her activity level.
- The patient's bowel habits are what they were before the thyroid problem occurred.

Assess the patient for indications of adverse effects on the cardiac system. The first indications may be chest pain or discomfort and hypertension.

For patients who are also taking drugs that affect blood clotting, especially warfarin (Coumadin), assess the patient at least once per shift for any sign of increased bleeding. Indications are bleeding from the gums; the presence of unusual or excessive bruising anywhere on the skin; bleeding around intravenous (IV) sites; bleeding for more than 5 minutes after an IM injection or discontinuing an IV; and visible blood in urine, stool, or vomit.

◆ *Patient and family teaching.* Teach the patient and family the following:

- Take only the dose that is prescribed for you, because increasing the drug too quickly can lead to adverse effects such as a heart attack or seizures.
- Do not skip doses, and you must take the drug daily to maintain normal body function.
- Take a missed dose as soon as you remember it. However, if it is almost time for the next dose, skip the missed dose and continue your regular dosing schedule. Do not take a double dose to make up for a missed one.
- Do not stop the drug suddenly or change the dose (up or down) without contacting your healthcare provider, to prevent underdosing or overdosing.
- Take the drug 2 to 3 hours before a meal or before taking a fiber supplement or at least 3 hours after a meal or after taking a supplement because food and fiber greatly decrease absorption of the drug.
- Check your pulse each morning before taking the drug and again each evening before going to bed. If the pulse rate becomes 20 beats higher than the normal rate for 1 week or if it becomes consistently irregular, notify your healthcare provider.
- Go to the emergency department immediately if you start to have chest pain.
- If you are ill and cannot take the drug orally, contact your healthcare provider to get an injection dose of the drug.
- If you also take warfarin (Coumadin), keep all follow-up appointments and appointments for blood-clotting tests because these drugs increase the effectiveness of warfarin.
- Avoid situations that can lead to bleeding and other drugs (such as aspirin) that can make bleeding worse.

> 🍃 **Lifespan Considerations**
>
> **Pediatric**
>
> Hypothyroidism can occur in children and some are born with it. Any child with the disorder must take thyroid hormone replacement drugs for his or her entire life. Infants and children going through periods of rapid growth need higher dosages of thyroid agonist drugs.

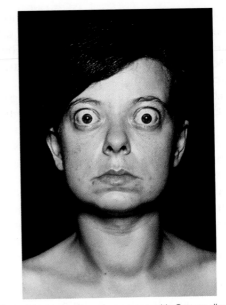

FIG. 16.2 Facial appearance of a woman with Graves disease. (From Ignatavicius DD, Workman ML: *Medical-surgical nursing: Patient-centered collaborative care*, ed 8, St. Louis, 2016, Saunders.)

HYPERTHYROIDISM

Hyperthyroidism, also called an *overactive thyroid* or *thyrotoxicosis*, is a condition in which the thyroid gland secretes excessive amounts of thyroid hormones (T_3 and T_4). This hormone excess causes general body metabolism to be greatly increased. Although there are different causes of hypothyroidism, the most common type is Grave's disease. Box 16.1 lists the symptoms associated with hypothyroidism. Some types of hyperthyroidism cause the patient to have a *goiter*, which is a swelling in the neck caused by an enlarged thyroid gland. The effects of continued excessive amounts of thyroid hormones can cause toxic side effects to some organs, especially the heart and nervous system. When hyperthyroidism is caused by Grave's disease, bulging or protruding eyes (exophthalmos) (Fig. 16.2) and blurred vision may occur.

Severe hyperthyroidism that causes life-threatening hypertension, heart failure, and seizures is called *thyroid crisis* or *thyroid storm*. Often a fever is the first indication of a problem. This condition is an emergency and can lead to death if the thyroid hormone levels are not decreased immediately.

ANTITHYROID DRUGS

Actions and Uses

Without treatment, hyperthyroidism has serious consequences. For some people, treatment consists of surgical removal of all or part of the thyroid gland. Radiation therapy with radioactive iodine can also reduce thyroid gland function and production of thyroid hormones. Therapy with antithyroid drugs can be used short-term before surgery or long-term to prevent thyroid hormone production and control of the disease. Antithyroid drugs are methimazole and propylthiouracil, which belong to the thionamide class of drugs. Table 16.1 lists the names, dosages, and nursing implications for common

antithyroid drugs. These drugs are not interchangeable because methimazole is 10 times stronger than propylthiouracil.

Antithyroid drugs work directly in the thyroid gland to stop production of the hormones. They serve as a decoy for the enzyme that normally connects iodine (iodide) with tyrosine to make active thyroid hormones. So the enzyme works on the drug instead of connecting these two substances. As a result, new hormones are not made, but the ones already made and stored in the thyroid gland are not affected by the drug. The drugs do not affect stored hormones, so it may take several weeks before the effects of all of the stored thyroid hormones are gone.

Expected Side Effects

Most common side effects of antithyroid drugs are minor. Some of these include taste changes, headache, itchiness, rash, muscle and joint aches, drowsiness, nausea, vomiting, enlarged lymph nodes, and swelling of the lower extremities.

Adverse Effects

Bone marrow suppression can occur and make the patient anemic and more at risk for infection. These drugs often induce hypothyroidism in patients who take them. Propylthiouracil can be hepatotoxic (liver damage). Methimazole is preferred over propylthiouracil. In some patients these drugs can also damage the kidneys.

Drug Interactions

Both methimazole and propylthiouracil drugs increase the effectiveness of anticlotting drugs, especially warfarin (Coumadin). As a result, patients who are taking these drugs with any anticlotting drug are at greater risk for excessive bleeding and bruising.

❖ Nursing Implications and Patient Teaching

◆ *Assessment.* Assess the patient's vital signs, especially for elevated temperature that may be associated with infection.

Check the patient's blood counts for signs of bone marrow suppression, such as a low white blood cell count, anemia, or thrombocytopenia.

Check the patient's drug list for drugs that have antiplatelet actions, such as warfarin. Assess the patient's skin for signs of bruising or bleeding, such as ecchymosis or petechiae. Notify the healthcare provider if these appear.

Before giving these drugs, check the patient's liver function tests because both are toxic to the liver *(hepatotoxic)*, especially propylthiouracil. For patients who already have liver problems, the effects of antithyroid drugs on the liver are more severe and occur at lower doses.

◆ *Planning and implementation.* Carefully check the dose and the specific drug name and prescribed dosage. These drugs are not interchangeable because methimazole is 10 times stronger than propylthiouracil.

Notify the healthcare provider if adverse effects such as bone marrow suppression or altered liver function occur.

◆ *Evaluation.* Check the patient's complete blood cell count (CBC) whenever it is drawn because these drugs cause some degree of bone marrow suppression. When white blood cells are reduced, the patient's risk for infection increases. Report changes in blood cell counts to the healthcare provider.

Bone marrow suppression can increase the risk for bleeding. Also, these drugs increase the action of anticlotting drugs. For patients who also take anticlotting drugs, look for bleeding from the gums; unusual or excessive bruising anywhere on the skin; bleeding around IV sites or for more than 5 minutes after discontinuing an IV; and the presence of blood in urine, stool, or vomit.

Both drugs are hepatotoxic, especially propylthiouracil, so check the patient daily for yellowing of the skin or sclera (jaundice), coffee-colored urine, and clay-colored stools. These are all symptoms of liver problems.

◆ *Patient and family teaching.* Tell the patient and family the following:

- Even if you do not notice a reduction of your symptoms in the first 1 to 2 weeks, do not increase the dosage on your own. These drugs take several weeks to be effective.
- Keep all follow-up appointments and appointments for blood-clotting tests because these drugs increase the effectiveness of warfarin.
- Avoid situations that can lead to bleeding and other drugs that can make bleeding worse.
- Avoid crowds and people who are ill because these drugs can reduce your immunity and resistance to infection.
- Check the color of the roof of the mouth and the whites of your eyes daily for a yellow tinge that may indicate a liver problem. If this appears, notify your healthcare provider as soon as possible.

🍃 Lifespan Considerations
Pregnancy and Breast-Feeding

Antithyroid drugs increase the risk for birth defects, fetal damage, and miscarriages. They should not be taken during pregnancy unless the benefits of treatment outweigh the risks. Women who are taking antithyroid drugs should not breast-feed because these drugs enter breast milk and would suppress the infant's thyroid function.

🍃 Lifespan Considerations
Older Adults

Older adults who are taking antithyroid drugs are more likely to have more severe adverse effects. The older patient's immune system is already lower than that of a younger person, which increases the older person's risk for infection. Bone marrow suppression from these drugs increases the risk for severe infection. For older adults who also take warfarin (Coumadin), the risks for bleeding are even greater while taking an antithyroid.

DRUGS FOR ADRENAL GLAND PROBLEMS

ADRENAL GLAND HYPOFUNCTION

The adrenal glands are a pair of small endocrine glands located on top of the kidneys, although they are not part of kidney function (Fig. 16.3). They have an outer layer known as the cortex and an inner layer known as the medulla. The cortex secretes aldosterone and cortisol. Both are steroid hormones, also called **corticosteroids**, which means their main structure is composed of the steroid cholesterol. **Aldosterone** controls sodium and water balance. It is also known as a *mineralocorticoid* because it regulates sodium. Cortisol, of which there are many types, has many more functions that are essential for life. Cortisol helps maintain critical blood glucose levels, the stress response, excitability of cardiac muscle, immunity, and blood sodium levels.

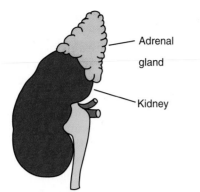

FIG. 16.3 Location of adrenal gland on top of the kidney. (From Workman ML, LaCharity LA: *Understanding pharmacology*, ed 2, St. Louis, 2016, Elsevier.)

Because cortisol was first discovered to affect blood glucose levels, it is also known as a *glucocorticoid*.

Adrenal gland hypofunction is a disorder in which the adrenal gland produces little or no cortisol and aldosterone. Conditions that cause it include autoimmune disease attacking and destroying the adrenal glands, adrenalectomy, abdominal radiation therapy, and reduced function of the anterior pituitary gland. Major problems from adrenal gland hypofunction are *hypoglycemia* (low blood glucose levels), salt wasting, hypotension, weakness, and high blood potassium levels. Without replacement of cortisol and aldosterone, this endocrine problem eventually leads to death. Corticosteroid replacement therapy involves the glucocorticoids, especially prednisone. If further help is needed to replace aldosterone action, fludrocortisone (Florinef) may be used.

Action and Uses
Although glucocorticoids (corticosteroids) are used for HRT, their most common use is as powerful antiinflammatory drugs. See Chapter 12 for a detailed discussion of corticosteroid drug therapy, including specific drugs, side effects, adverse effects, and nursing implications.

Glucocorticoid drugs act just like natural cortisol. Because glucocorticoids have some mineralocorticoid action, many people with adrenal gland hypofunction only need HRT with glucocorticoids. When this replacement is not enough to manage blood sodium levels, fludrocortisone may be added to correct the deficiency.

Fludrocortisone (Florinef) is a synthetic drug that acts like natural aldosterone. With the use of this drug more sodium is retained to prevent excessive sodium wasting and more potassium is excreted to prevent dangerously high blood potassium levels. So fludrocortisone helps prevent hyponatremia, hyperkalemia, and hypotension. The usual adult dosage is 0.1 to 0.2 mg orally once daily.

Expected Side Effects
Side effects of fludrocortisone therapy include hypertension, edema formation, low blood potassium levels, and high blood sodium levels. The cause of these problems is the drug's action on fluid and electrolyte balance.

Adverse Effects
Congestive heart failure is a serious adverse effect of fludrocortisone. It requires that the drug dose be either reduced or stopped.

❖ Nursing Implications and Patient Teaching
◆ *Patient and family teaching.* Tell patients and families the following:
- Take fludrocortisone at the same time daily with food to prevent GI problems.
- Weigh yourself daily and keep a record because the drug can cause fluid retention with weight gain, edema, and heart failure.
- Report a weight gain of 2 lb in a day or 3 lb in a week to the healthcare provider immediately.

ADRENAL GLAND HYPERFUNCTION
Most of the time when adrenal gland hyperfunction occurs, only one hormone is oversecreted. Excessive secretion of cortisol is known as hypercortisolism or *Cushing's disease.* Excessive secretion of aldosterone is hyperaldosteronism. The most common cause of adrenal gland hyperfunction is an adrenal gland tumor. Sometimes a problem in the pituitary gland produces excessive amounts of hormones that stimulate the adrenal gland to produce adrenal hormones in excess.

Action and Uses
Surgery is the most common treatment for adrenal gland hyperfunction that is caused by a problem in the adrenal gland. Drug therapy can help manage the problems caused by adrenal gland hyperfunction before surgery or for those patients unable to have surgery. Table 16.2 lists the names, dosages, and nursing implications of the most common drugs used to manage adrenal gland hyperfunction. Some drugs reduce cortisol production, whereas others help control the problems caused by hyperaldosteronism.

Mitotane (Lysodren) is a steroid production inhibitor that works by directly preventing adrenal gland production of cortisol and other adrenal cortex hormones. A specialized drug for hypercortisolism is Mifepristone (Korlym). This drug works by blocking corticosteroid receptors. Although this does not reduce cortisol levels, it does inhibit cortisol responses in different tissues. It is approved for use *only* in people who have type 2 diabetes and hypercortisolism.

Drug therapy for hyperaldosteronism focuses on reducing potassium levels and relies on spironolactone (Aldactone, Spironol, Novo-Spiroton), a potassium-sparing diuretic. See Chapter 8 for more information on spironolactone therapy.

Table 16.2 Examples of Common Drugs to Treat Adrenal Gland Hyperfunction

Corticosteroid receptor blocker: reduces symptoms and problems of hypercortisolism by interfering with the binding of cortisol with its receptor, acting as an antagonist

DRUG/ADULT DOSAGE RANGE	NURSING IMPLICATIONS
mifepristone (Korlym) 300 mg orally once daily; can be increased to 1200 mg orally daily	• This drug is to be given *only* for use in people who have type 2 diabetes and hyperglycemia along with hypercortisolism. • Instruct sexually active woman of childbearing age to use two reliable forms of birth control while taking mifepristone because this drug can cause a pregnancy loss.

Steroid production inhibitors: reduce symptoms and problems of hypercortisolism by preventing the adrenal cortex from producing cortisol and other adrenal cortex hormones

DRUG/ADULT DOSAGE RANGE	NURSING IMPLICATIONS
mitotane (Lysodren) 1–2 g orally every 6–8 hours	• Teach patients the signs and symptoms of adrenal insufficiency: hypoglycemia, salt craving, muscle weakness, hypotension, and fatigue. • Teach patients the importance of laboratory blood work because these drugs affect levels of sodium and potassium. • Teach patients to take these drugs with food because they can cause nausea, vomiting, and other GI upsets.

Expected Side Effects

Common side effects for drugs that suppress adrenal hormone production are likely to cause nausea, vomiting, skin rashes, and dizziness. Mitotane can also cause bloody urine (hematuria). Mifepristone causes many side effects, including menstrual irregularities.

Adverse Effects

Any drug that suppresses adrenal production of cortisol can lead to problems of adrenal insufficiency. Allergic reaction to mifepristone can occur. Emergency help is needed for hives, difficult breathing, and swelling of the face, lips, tongue, or throat. Mifepristone is also used to induce abortion and can cause pregnancy loss.

Patient Teaching

Teach patients who are taking any drug that suppresses adrenal hormone production the signs and symptoms of adrenal insufficiency. Common indicators are salt craving, muscle weakness, hypotension, hypoglycemia (with headache, difficulty concentrating, shakiness), and fatigue.

Tell the patient and family the following:

• Keep all appointments for laboratory blood work because these drugs alter blood levels of sodium and potassium.
• Report symptoms of adrenal insufficiency to your healthcare provider immediately. These include salt craving, muscle weakness, hypotension, low blood glucose levels, headache, difficulty concentrating, shakiness, and fatigue.
• Take these drugs with food because they all can cause nausea, vomiting, and other GI upsets.
• If you are a sexually active woman in your childbearing years, use two reliable forms of birth control while taking mifepristone because this drug can cause a pregnancy loss.

Lifespan Considerations

Pregnancy and Pediatric

The drugs used for suppressing adrenal hormone production are not approved for use in children or in women who are pregnant or breast-feeding.

FEMALE SEX HORMONES

OVERVIEW

Hormones secreted throughout a woman's menstruating years promote conception and pregnancy. The beginning of menstruation is menarche, usually occurring during adolescence. Menstruation occurs as a result of the secretion of *gonadotropin-releasing hormone* (GnRH) in the brain. Secretion of this hormone begins with the start of puberty in both females and males to initiate sex hormone secretion and start the physical changes leading to interest in sexual activity (libido) and the ability to perform sexual intercourse. During menstruation, shedding of the uterine lining occurs resulting from changes in hormone levels in females during their menstrual cycles. Estrogen is the main female sex hormone secreted by the ovaries and adrenal glands.

In females the secretion of GnRH from the hypothalamus stimulates the release of two hormones from the pituitary gland: *follicle-stimulating hormone* (FSH) and *luteinizing hormone* (LH) (Fig. 16.4). FSH triggers the ovary to make and secrete estrogen, along with maturing one ovum (egg) each month. Rising estrogen levels allow the uterine lining to grow and thicken (see Fig. 16.4). After about 14 days (midcycle), the uterine lining is thick enough to allow a fertilized egg to implant. At this time, GnRH triggers the release of LH, which, in turn, causes secretion of progesterone by the ovary

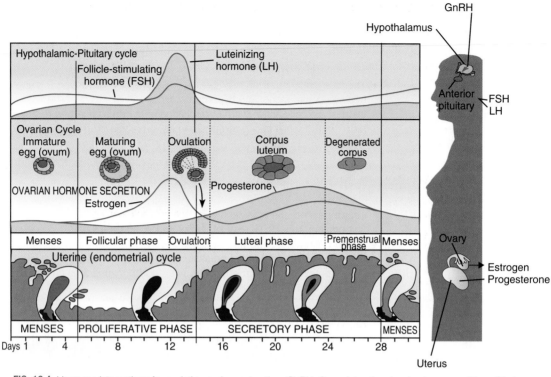

FIG. 16.4 Hormone interactions for ovulation and menstruation. *GnRH,* Gonadotropin-releasing hormone. (From Workman ML, LaCharity LA: *Understanding pharmacology,* ed 2, St. Louis, 2016, Elsevier.)

and allows the release of the mature ovum or egg *(ovulation).*

When the ovulated egg is fertilized by a sperm, the egg's outer covering grows and secretes both estrogen and progesterone. It is these two hormones that keep the uterine lining intact and able to support a pregnancy until the placenta forms and maintains the pregnancy. Therefore functional pregnancy resulting in birth requires conception, continued secretion of estrogen and progesterone, successful implantation 5 to 8 days after conception, and placental development.

If, after ovulation, conception and pregnancy do not occur, the outer covering from the released ovum degenerates, and circulating levels of estrogen and progesterone decline in about 12 days. Low levels of these hormones cause the uterine lining to shed as menstruation. Fig. 16.5 shows the feedback loops controlling the secretion of estrogen and progesterone.

MENOPAUSE

Menopause is the life period of women when menstruation and ovulation no longer occur. This occurs because of age-related changes that make the ovary stop functioning. Estrogen secretion and ovulation stop. *Perimenopause* is when a woman transitions from having regular menstrual periods from hormone cycles to when menstrual periods have stopped for a full year as a result of reduced hormone levels. The reduction of hormone levels causes a variety of uncomfortable symptoms.

As a result of negative feedback, decreased blood levels of estrogen trigger the brain to secrete GnRH, which then forces the pituitary gland to oversecrete FSH (see Fig. 16.5). The FSH has no effect on the ovary because these cells are no longer functional and blood levels of estrogen remain low. Continuing low blood estrogen levels constantly stimulate the brain to secrete GnRH in large amounts for a time, resulting in the secretion of even more FSH (Fig. 16.6). This extra FSH does not have any effect on the ovary but does cause responses in other body tissues. Box 16.2 lists the symptoms associated with decreased estrogen levels and increased FSH levels.

Memory Jogger

- Symptoms of menopause are caused by low levels of estrogen and high levels of FSH.
- Hot flashes (hot flushes) with facial redness and feelings of overheating are caused by high levels of FSH acting on blood vessels to make them dilate suddenly.
- At night, hot flashes or hot flushes may be followed by excessive sweating that leaves nightclothes and bedding wet.

DRUGS FOR MENOPAUSE RELIEF

Action and Uses

Menopausal HRT during the perimenopausal period is the replacement of naturally secreted estrogen and progesterone with hormones given in the form of a

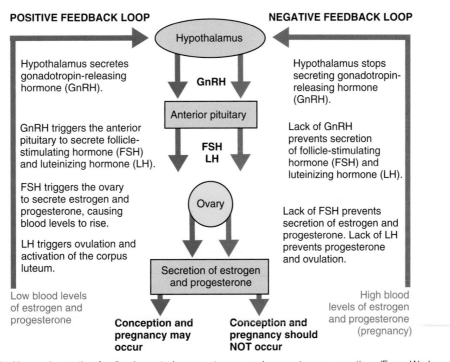

POSITIVE FEEDBACK LOOP   **NEGATIVE FEEDBACK LOOP**

Hypothalamus secretes gonadotropin-releasing hormone (GnRH).

GnRH triggers the anterior pituitary to secrete follicle-stimulating hormone (FSH) and luteinizing hormone (LH).

FSH triggers the ovary to secrete estrogen and progesterone, causing blood levels to rise.

LH triggers ovulation and activation of the corpus luteum.

Low blood levels of estrogen and progesterone

Hypothalamus stops secreting gonadotropin-releasing hormone (GnRH).

Lack of GnRH prevents secretion of follicle-stimulating hormone (FSH) and luteinizing hormone (LH).

Lack of FSH prevents secretion of estrogen and progesterone. Lack of LH prevents progesterone and ovulation.

High blood levels of estrogen and progesterone (pregnancy)

FIG. 16.5 Positive and negative feedback control over estrogen and progesterone secretion. (From Workman ML, LaCharity LA: *Understanding pharmacology,* ed 2, St. Louis, 2016, Elsevier.)

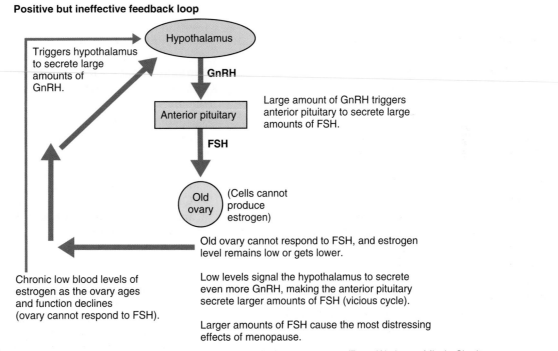

FIG. 16.6 Mechanism for hot flushes and night sweats associated with menopause. (From Workman ML, LaCharity LA: *Understanding pharmacology,* ed 2, St. Louis, 2016, Elsevier.)

drug. Giving a woman low doses of estrogen increases blood estrogen levels. The mildly increased estrogen levels help reduce perimenopausal symptoms by relieving the problems from low estrogen levels (see Box 16.2) and by inhibiting the feedback system to lower the FSH levels. This action reduces hot flashes, night sweats, and difficulty sleeping. Table 16.3 lists the names, dosages, and nursing implications for common drugs used for relief of menopausal symptoms. Be sure to consult a drug handbook or drug reference source for information about additional drugs for relief of menopausal symptoms.

Table 16.3 Examples of Common Drugs for Relief of Menopausal Symptoms

Conjugated female sex hormones: reduce menopausal symptoms by providing enough estrogen or estrogen and progesterone to disrupt the feedback loop and lower follicle-stimulating hormone levels

DRUG/ADULT DOSAGE RANGE	NURSING IMPLICATIONS
conjugated estrogens (Cenestin, C.E.S. ♣, Enjuvia, Premarin) 0.3, 0.45, or 0.625 mg orally once daily, given cyclically or continuously, alone in women without a uterus, in combination with a progestin in women with a uterus conjugated estrogens: medroxyprogesterone (Premphase) 0.625 mg conjugated estrogens orally once daily on days 1–14, then 1 light-blue tablet (0.625 mg conjugated estrogens, 5 mg acetate) orally once daily on days 15–28 medroxyprogesterone (Prempro) 0.3 or 0.45 mg along with medroxyprogesterone acetate 1.5 mg/day, or 0.625 mg along with medroxyprogesterone 2.5 mg, and the 0.625 mg along with 5 mg medroxyprogesterone	• Teach the patient to take drugs for perimenopausal hormone replacement therapy exactly as prescribed to reduce the risk for excessive uterine bleeding. • Advise the patient to quit or reduce smoking to reduce the risk for blood clots, heart attacks, and strokes. • Teach the patient to assess the color of the roof of the mouth and the sclera of the eyes weekly for the presence of jaundice. • Instruct the patient to call 911 immediately for chest pain, difficulty breathing, swelling in one leg, or symptoms of stroke. • Teach the patient that taking hormone replacement therapy for long periods increases the risk for cancers of the cervix, breast, ovary, and uterus.

♣ Indicates Canadian drug.

Box 16.2 Symptoms Associated With the Low Estrogen Levels and High FSH Levels of Menopause

SYMPTOMS CAUSED BY REDUCED ESTROGEN LEVELS
• Irregular and absent menses
• Dry skin and vaginal mucous membranes
• Painful intercourse
• Increased rate of osteoporosis

SYMPTOMS CAUSED BY INCREASED FSH LEVELS
• Hot flushes/flashes
• Night sweats
• Sleep difficulty
• Difficulty concentrating on cognitive tasks

Expected Side Effects

The most common side effects of perimenopausal HRT are breast tenderness, breakthrough bleeding, fluid retention, weight gain, and acne. These occur with estrogen alone and when estrogen is combined with progesterone.

Adverse Effects

Women who are taking estrogen-based HRT have been found to have a slightly higher incidence of myocardial infarction (heart attack). For this reason perimenopausal HRT is not recommended for long-term therapy.

Estrogen and progesterone drugs increase the risk for blood clotting and inappropriate development of thrombi and emboli. These risks increase with age and are greatly increased with cigarette smoking. Potential health problems associated with increased clot formation include heart attack, stroke, pulmonary embolism, and deep vein thrombosis.

The uterine lining in women who have a uterus and who take perimenopausal HRT can become very thick and bleed excessively. In addition, perimenopausal HRT promotes the growth of hormone-sensitive cancers of the cervix, uterus, ovary, and breast. These hormones should not be used by women who have a history of or are at high risk for these types of cancer. Perimenopausal HRT also is associated with liver impairment, gallbladder disease, and pancreatitis.

❖ **Nursing Implications and Patient Teaching**
◆ *Patient and family teaching.* Tell the patient and family the following:
• Take drugs for perimenopausal HRT exactly as prescribed with regard to dosage and timing. Taking perimenopausal HRT drugs more often than prescribed or not following instructions for timing increases the risk for excessive uterine bleeding.
• Quit or reduce smoking during the time you take these drugs to reduce your risk for blood clots, heart attacks, and strokes.
• Check the color of the roof of your mouth and the whites of your eyes weekly for the presence of a yellow tinge because these drugs can impair the liver. If you see this yellowing, report it to your healthcare provider as soon as possible.
• Go to the emergency department or call 911 immediately if you have chest pain or difficulty breathing, swelling in one leg, or symptoms of stroke.
• Taking HRT for long periods of time increases the risk for cancers of the cervix, breast, ovary, and uterus. Discuss the optimum length of time for taking these drugs with your healthcare provider.

DRUGS FOR HORMONAL CONTRACEPTION

Hormonal contraception is the use of hormones to suppress ovulation for the intentional prevention of pregnancy. When used correctly, hormonal contraception

Table 16.4	Common Hormonal Contraceptives
GENERIC NAMES	**TRADE NAMES**
Combination Oral Contraceptives	
drospirenone; ethinyl estradiol	Yasmin
ethinyl estradiol; desogestrel	Apri, Azurette, CAZIANT, Cyclessa, Desogen, Kariva, Mircette, Ortho-Cept, Pimtrea, Reclipsen, Solia, Velivet
ethinyl estradiol; ethynodiol diacetate	Demulen, Kelnor, Zovia
ethinyl estradiol; levonorgestrel	Aviane, Enpresse, Jolessa, Lessina, Levlen, Levlite, Levora, Lutera, Portia, Quasense, Seasonale, Seasonique, Sronyx, Tri-Levlen, Triphasil, Trivora
ethinyl estradiol; norethindrone	Aranelle, Balziva, Brevicon, Femcon, Genora, Jenest, Leena, Modicon, Necon, Norinyl, Nortrel, Ortho-Novum, Ovcon, Tri-Norinyl, Zenchent
ethinyl estradiol; norethindrone acetate	Estrostep, Femhrt, Junel, Loestrin, Microgestin, Pirmella, Tilia, Tri-Legest
ethinyl estradiol; norgestimate	MonoNessa, Ortho Tri-Cyclen, Previfem, Sprintec-28, Tri-Previfem, Tri-Sprintec, TriNessa
ethinyl estradiol; norgestrel	Cryselle, Low-Ogestrel, Ogestrel, Ovral
mestranol; norethindrone	Genora, Necon, Necon, Norinyl, Ortho-Novum
Combination Topical Contraceptives	
Vaginal Rings ethinyl estradiol; etonogestrel	NuvaRing
Patches ethinyl estradiol; norelgestromin	Ortho Evra
Progestin-Only Oral Contraceptives norethindrone	Aygestin, Camila, Errin, Jolivette, Nor-QD, Nora-BE, Ortho Micronor
norgestrel	Ovrette
Intrauterine Contraceptives (Progestin Only) levonorgestrel	Mirena
Subcutaneous Implants (Progestin Only) etonogestrel	Implanon
levonorgestrel	Norplant

is highly effective. These hormones can be taken orally; used as topical applications in the form of transdermal patches, uterine rings, or released by a device directly in the uterus; implanted under the skin; and injected parenterally as a slow-absorbing drug form (Table 16.4). *Oral contraceptives* (*OCs*; often called *birth control pills* or *BCPs*) are the most commonly used form of hormonal contraceptive. The mechanism of action and side effects of hormonal contraception are the same for all forms.

Action and Uses

As described earlier, the control of natural estrogen and progesterone secretion is through a "feedback" system involving the hypothalamus, the pituitary gland, and the ovary (see Fig. 16.5). In a manner similar to perimenopausal hormone replacement therapy, OCs provide enough estrogen and/or progesterone to interfere with feedback and decrease the body's natural production of estrogen and progesterone. As a result, ovulation stops and the cervical mucous thickens, making fertilization difficult (see Fig. 16.5). The most effective OCs contain two synthetic hormones, a synthetic estrogen and progestin, a synthetic progesterone. When taken

consistently, this hormone combination keeps the blood levels of estrogen and progesterone high, signaling the hypothalamus that further secretion of these hormones is not needed. With this influence, GnRH, FSH, and LH secretion are stopped and the ovary has no stimulation to produce estrogen or progesterone. Ovulation does not occur and the lining of the uterus is too thin to support pregnancy. So OCs make the endocrine system act as though the woman is pregnant and further hormone production by the ovary is not needed. The specific drugs in combination and their dosages vary, as does the dosing schedule. Be sure to consult a drug handbook for specific dosages and scheduling.

Mini-pills are OCs that contain only progestin rather than a combination of estrogen and progestin. They increase blood levels of progesterone, turning off the hormone pathway with positive feedback, which prevents ovulation. Mini-pills are not as effective as combination OCs and most must be taken daily continuously.

Expected Side Effects

The most common side effects of OCs include breast enlargement and tenderness, nausea, fluid retention, and weight gain. Depending on dosage and whether the OCs contain estrogen and progestin or only progestin, breakthrough vaginal bleeding can occur. Acne can become worse for some women or clear up for others while taking OCs.

Adverse Effects

Just as for other types of sex hormones, OCs increase the risk for blood clot formation. This problem can lead to deep vein thrombosis, pulmonary embolism, myocardial infection, and stroke. The risk increases among women who smoke and in those older than 35 years.

Most hormonal contraceptives cause fluid and sodium retention, which can lead to hypertension. Hormonal contraception is not recommended for women with moderate-to-severe hypertension.

The estrogen and progestin in OCs can cause liver toxicity. Indications of liver toxicity include elevated liver enzymes, yellowing of the skin and whites of the eyes, tiredness, coffee-colored urine, clay-colored stools, and nausea. Hormonal contraceptives are not recommended for women who have known liver problems.

The estrogen and/or progestin of OCs promote the growth of hormone-sensitive cancers of the cervix, uterus, ovary, and breast. Hormonal contraceptive should not be used by women who have a history of or are at high risk for these types of cancer.

OCs that use drospirenone as the progestin (Ocella, Yasmin, YAZ28) can increase the serum potassium level, which can lead to heart block and other irregular heart rhythms. Women who have kidney, liver, or adrenal disease and those who are taking other drugs that increase potassium levels (e.g., angiotensin-converting enzyme inhibitors for hypertension and potassium-sparing diuretics) are not recommended to use contraceptives that contain drospirenone.

Drug Interactions

Many drugs and herbal supplements interact with OCs. Be sure to ask women prescribed to take OCs about all other drugs and supplements. Check with the pharmacist to avoid a possible drug interaction.

❖ Nursing Implications and Patient Teaching

◆ *Patient and family teaching.* Tell the patient and family the following:

- Use an additional method of contraception during the first cycle because OCs require a full cycle before they are effective.
- Take the drug as prescribed or an unplanned pregnancy may result because scheduling is important for best effectiveness.
- Remember that OCs are only effective at preventing pregnancy when taken *exactly* as prescribed.
- Take the OC with food once daily at the same time each day for best effect and remember to take it.
- Do not smoke or use nicotine in any form to reduce your risk for blood clots, heart attacks, and strokes.

- If you miss one dose within the cycle, the drug should still be effective in preventing pregnancy. However, if you miss more than one dose within a cycle, especially two doses in a row, continue to use it for the rest of the cycle but also use another method of contraception for the rest of the cycle.
- Be sure to tell any other healthcare provider that you are taking this drug, because of the potential for drug interactions.
- Do not take any over-the-counter drug without checking with your healthcare provider who prescribed the contraceptive, to prevent possible interactions.
- Notify your healthcare provider if you develop yellowing of the skin or eyes, darkening of the urine, or lightening of the stools. These problems are signs of liver toxicity, a serious adverse effect of hormonal contraceptives.

⚘ Lifespan Considerations
Pregnancy and Lactation

- Hormonal contraceptives should not be used during pregnancy because they can interrupt the pregnancy and can cause birth defects. Women should know for certain that they are not pregnant before starting hormonal contraceptives. Instruct women to immediately notify their healthcare provider if a pregnancy is suspected.
- Hormonal contraceptives interfere with lactation. They are also present in breast milk and may harm the infant. These drugs should not be used by lactating women.

MALE SEX HORMONES

OVERVIEW

Male sex hormones are produced under the influence of the anterior pituitary gland. The male hormone testosterone and its related hormones are called *androgens*. **Androgens** help to develop and maintain the male sex organs at puberty and develop secondary sex characteristics in men (e.g., facial hair, deep voice, body hair, body fat distribution, and muscle development). They promote the anabolic or tissue-building processes in the body. **Anabolic steroids** are synthetic drugs with the same use and actions as androgens. These drugs may be given as replacement therapy for testosterone deficiency.

ANDROGENS

Action and Uses

Androgens are steroid hormones synthesized from cholesterol, and they work to stimulate or control the development and maintenance of male characteristics. This includes the activity of the male sex organs and the development of male secondary sex characteristics. Androgens are primarily used in the treatment of hypogonadism, hypopituitarism, *eunuchism* (absence of testes or undeveloped gonads in a male), *cryptorchidism* (undescended testes), *oligospermia* (lack of sperm in the semen), and general androgen deficiency in males. The most commonly used androgen is testosterone. Androgens also help in the development of skeletal muscle cells exerting action on several cell types in skeletal muscle tissue.

Expected Side Effects

Common side effects of androgens include edema caused by sodium retention (usually with larger doses), acne, *hirsutism* (excessive body hair), male pattern baldness, mouth irritation, diarrhea, nausea, and vomiting.

Adverse Reactions

Tumors of the liver, liver cancer, or hepatitis have occurred with long-term, high-dose therapy with androgens. Adverse reactions to androgens also include jaundice, a decreased sperm count, *gynecomastia* (enlargement of the breasts), impotence, and urinary retention. In children, use of androgens may result in early puberty and short stature because of premature closing of the bone growth plates.

Drug Interactions

Anabolic steroids may increase the effects of anticoagulants, antidiabetic agents, and other drugs. Corticosteroids given at the same time as androgens increase the possibility of edema. Barbiturates decrease the therapeutic effects of androgens because of increased breakdown in the liver.

❖ **Nursing Implications and Patient Teaching**

◆ *Patient and family teaching.* Tell the patient and family the following:

- Take this drug as instructed by your healthcare provider.
- Do not increase the dose without consulting your healthcare provider if you do not see the expected effects within the first 1 to 2 months because response to the drug may take several months.
- Report any new or troublesome symptoms that may develop, including fluid retention, especially in the feet and hands, breast enlargement, shortness of breath, excessive physical or sexual stimulation, prolonged or painful penile erection of the penis, impotence, urinary retention, and jaundice.
- If you are taking the drug under the tongue (*sublingually*) or putting the drug in your cheek (*buccally*), do not eat, drink, smoke, or chew tobacco until the drug is dissolved for best absorption.
- If you are using a topical gel form of the drug, do not let women or children come into contact with the areas where you have applied it, to prevent them from absorbing the drug.

DRUGS FOR OSTEOPOROSIS

Good health and mobility require that bones remain strong enough to support mobility. Normal bone

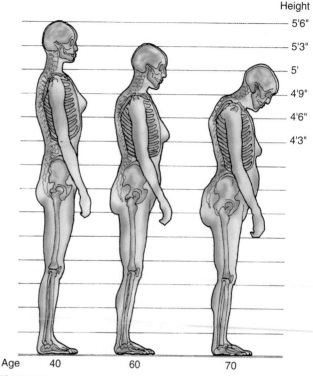

FIG. 16.7 A normal spine at age 40 years and osteoporotic changes at age 60 and 70 years. (From Ignatavicius DD, Workman ML: *Medical-surgical nursing: Patient-centered collaborative care*, ed 8, St. Louis, 2016, Saunders.)

formation and maintenance continue throughout the lifespan, not just during childhood growth. Even after bones have achieved their final length, old bone cells are continually removed by a process known as *osteoclastic* activity, and new bone cells are continually added by a process known as *osteoblastic* activity. For bones to remain strong and dense, these two processes must be balanced.

Osteoporosis is the gradual loss of bone density and strength, which leads to spinal shortening and increased risk for bone fractures (Fig. 16.7). This results when osteoclastic activity occurs at a faster rate than osteoblastic activity. When excessive osteoclastic activity occurs, minerals (especially calcium) are lost from the bones, making them thinner and weaker. Osteoporosis is commonly more severe in women after menopause, but it does occur in people of both genders at any age. The rate and degree of bone density loss varies from person to person but does occur to some degree in everyone during the aging process. For some people, severe osteoporosis is present as early as age 40 years. For other people, bone density loss may not be obvious until 75 years or older. Factors that influence at what age a person develops this bone-thinning problem and how severe it is include a genetic predisposition, nutritional status, amount of weight-bearing activity, cigarette smoking, presence of sex hormones, and drug use. Osteoporosis occurs earlier and at faster rates in

Table 16.5   Examples of Common Drugs for Osteoporosis

Bisphosphonates: reduce the rate of osteoporosis by moving blood calcium into the bone, binding to calcium in the bone, and preventing osteoclasts from destroying bone cells and resorbing calcium

DRUG/ADULT DOSAGE RANGE	NURSING IMPLICATIONS
alendronate (Fosamax) 10 mg orally daily ibandronate (Boniva) 2.5 mg orally daily or 150 mg orally once per month, or 3 mg IV bolus once every 3 months risedronate (Actonel, Atelvia) 5 mg orally daily, or 35 mg orally once weekly, or 75 mg orally twice per month, or 150 mg orally once per month zoledronic acid (Reclast) 5 mg IV infusion over 15–30 minutes once yearly	• Teach patients to take drug first thing in the morning before breakfast and before taking other drugs for best absorption and to prevent drug interactions. • Tell patients to remain upright (sitting or standing) for 30 minutes after taking the drug to help prevent esophageal irritation or reflux. • Remind patients to have a dental examination every 6 months and to tell the dental professional about taking a bisphosphonate because it can cause jaw bone osteonecrosis. • Infuse the IV form of the drug slowly over 15–30 minutes to reduce the risk for cardiac complications.

Estrogen agonists/antagonists: slow the rate of osteoporosis by activating estrogen receptors in the bone, which leads to reduced calcium resorption and increased bone density

DRUG/ADULT DOSAGE RANGE	NURSING IMPLICATIONS
estrogen/bazedoxifene (Duavee) 1 tablet orally daily (contains 0.45 mg conjugated estrogen and 20 mg bazedoxifene) raloxifene (Evista) 60 mg orally once daily	• Urge patients not to smoke while taking these drugs to reduce the risk for blood clots, heart attacks, and strokes.

Osteoclast monoclonal antibodies: work by binding to a receptor on immature osteoclasts and on certain white blood cells, preventing them from becoming mature and attacking bone tissue; the result is decreased bone loss and increased bone density and strength

DRUG/ADULT DOSAGE RANGE	NURSING IMPLICATIONS
denosumab (Prolia) 60 mg subcutaneously once every 6 months	• Remind patients to have a dental examination every 6 months and to tell the dental professional about taking this drug because it can cause jaw bone osteonecrosis.

people who have a strong family history for the problem; smoke; have a diet poor in calcium, other minerals, vitamin D, and protein; have lower than normal levels of estrogen (women) or testosterone (men); and who take corticosteroids daily.

Although osteoporosis cannot be cured or completely prevented, its progress can be delayed with drug therapy. Drugs and supplements that are used to manage the disorder include calcium, activated vitamin D, bisphosphonates, estrogen agonists/antagonists, and osteoclast monoclonal antibodies. The names, dosages, and nursing implications for common examples of these drugs are summarized in Table 16.5.

Bone density requires a constant supply of calcium, and dietary calcium requires activated vitamin D for absorption from the intestinal tract, so these supplements are needed for osteoporosis management. These nutritional supplements are discussed in Chapter 19.

BISPHOSPHONATES

Action and Uses
Bisphosphonates are calcium-modifying drugs that prevent bones from losing calcium by moving blood calcium into the bone, binding to calcium in the bone, and by preventing osteoclasts from destroying bone cells and resorbing calcium. They also prevent certain white blood cells from damaging or destroying bone.

Exactly how the bisphosphonates increase bone production is not yet known.

Bisphosphonates are used mainly in women to prevent and manage osteoporosis. Reducing bone density loss reduces the risk for bone fractures. Additional uses are the prevention of skeletal fractures in patients with bone metastases and multiple myeloma, Paget's disease, and the treatment of cancer-induced hypercalcemia.

Bisphosphonates contain nitrogen, and their effectiveness requires that patients have an adequate intake of both calcium and vitamin D.

Expected Side Effects and Adverse Effects
Common side effects of the bisphosphonates are headache, esophageal reflux, and nausea. Jawbone necrosis (osteonecrosis) can develop with tooth extraction or other invasive dental procedures in which the jawbone is damaged. This adverse reaction is more common in patients who are taking higher doses or the IV form of the drug.

❖ **Nursing Implications and Patient Teaching**
◆ *Patient and family teaching.* Tell the patient and family the following:
• Take the drug early in the morning, right after breakfast, and drink a full glass of water.

- Remain in the upright position (sitting, standing, or walking) for at least 30 minutes after taking these drugs to prevent esophageal irritation and reflux.
- Be sure to inform your dentist or oral surgeon that you are taking a bisphosphonate before you have any tooth extraction or invasive dental procedure involving the jawbone.

ESTROGEN AGONISTS/ANTAGONISTS

Action and Uses

Estrogen agonists/antagonists are drugs that activate (agonize) estrogen receptors in the bone to promote calcium retention in the bone and block (antagonize) estrogen receptors in breast tissue and uterine tissue. These opposing responses increase bone density and prevent excessive growth of breast tissue (that may promote breast cancer cell growth) and overgrowth of uterine endometrial tissues that can lead to excessive uterine bleeding.

Expected Side Effects and Adverse Effects

Common side effects of these drugs are muscle spasms, nausea, and indigestion. Some people have hot flashes, sodium retention, and edema formation. These drugs agonize some estrogen receptors; therefore a possible adverse effect is the increased risk for thrombotic events, which include deep vein thrombosis, stroke, myocardial infarction, and pulmonary embolism. Estrogen agonists/antagonists should not be used by patients who have had a previous thrombotic event or who smoke.

❖ Nursing Implications and Patient Teaching

◆ *Patient and family teaching.* Tell patients and families the following:
- Do not smoke while taking this drug, to prevent forming dangerous blood clots that could cause a stroke or heart attack.

- Avoid excessive salt and sodium intake to prevent edema.

OSTEOCLAST MONOCLONAL ANTIBODIES

Action and Uses

Osteoclast monoclonal antibodies are antibodies directed against immature osteoclasts. Binding of the antibodies to these cells prevents them from maturing and reducing bone density. This drug has some dangerous side effects and is recommended only to treat severe osteoporosis in patients who have tried other treatments that were not effective.

Expected Side Effects and Adverse Effects

Skin rashes and muscle and joint pain are the most common side effects of osteoclast monoclonal antibodies. This drug can cause allergic reactions and possible anaphylaxis. The risk increases with repeated dosage of the drug. Jaw osteonecrosis also can occur with the use of osteoclast monoclonal antibodies.

❖ Nursing Implications and Patient Teaching

◆ *Planning and implementation.* Assess the patient for an allergic reaction during and after subcutaneous injection of denosumab (Prolia). Keep emergency equipment in the room with the patient.

◆ *Patient and family teaching.* Tell patients and families the following:
- Be sure to inform your dentist or oral surgeon that you are taking denosumab (Prolia) before you have any tooth extraction or invasive dental procedure involving the jawbone.
- If you start having chest pain, shortness of breath, dizziness, or just do not feel right when you are receiving this drug, call for help immediately.

Get Ready for the NCLEX® Examination!

Key Points

- Hormones exert their actions only on target tissues that have receptors for that specific hormone.
- Common uses of HRT include drugs for thyroid problems, adrenal gland problems, sex hormone replacement, contraception, and diabetes.
- Teach patients who are taking oral bisphosphonates to remain upright (sitting or standing) for at least 30 minutes after taking the drug to reduce the risk for esophageal irritation and reflux.
- Overdoses of thyroid replacement hormones have the same symptoms as hyperthyroidism.
- Older adults with hypothyroidism are very sensitive to the drugs and are started on lower initial doses than are younger adults.
- Thyroid crisis (or thyroid storm) is an emergency that can lead to death without prompt treatment.

- The effects of antithyroid drugs usually are not until 2 to 4 weeks after therapy has started because these drugs do not affect the levels of stored thyroid hormones.
- HRT to relieve menopausal symptoms increase the risk for blood clot formation, increasing the risk for heart attack, stroke, pulmonary embolism, and deep vein thrombosis.
- Osteoporosis occurs to some degree in all older adults, but the rate and severity are related to genetic predisposition and risk factors such as smoking, sedentary lifestyle, and long-term use of corticosteroids.
- Teach patients using the topical gel form of testosterone to avoid letting women or children come into contact with the areas where drug has been applied, to prevent their accidental absorption of the drug.

Get Ready for the NCLEX® Examination!—cont'd

Review Questions for the NCLEX® Examination

1. Which drug therapy for an endocrine problem drug can cause pregnancy loss?
   1. liothyronine sodium (Cytomel)
   2. spironolactone (Aldactone)
   3. mifepristone (Korlym)
   4. mitotane (Lysodren)

2. Which precaution is most important to teach a patient who is taking hormone replacement therapy for hypothyroidism?
   1. Take the drug at least 3 hours before or 3 hours after taking an oral fiber supplement.
   2. Avoid aspirin and aspirin-containing products while on this therapy.
   3. You can stop taking the drug as soon as you feel normal again.
   4. Use reliable birth control methods while on this therapy.

3. You are preparing to give instructions to an older adult patient who is starting treatment with thyroid hormone. Which symptom reported by the patient indicates an adverse effect of the drug?
   1. Difficulty swallowing
   2. Sleep apnea
   3. Chest pain
   4. Increased temperature

4. Which food or beverage will you advise a patient who is taking methimazole to avoid?
   1. Alcohol
   2. Aged cheese
   3. Dairy products
   4. Leafy green vegetables

5. What should a woman who takes a combination oral contraceptive do if she misses two consecutive doses?
   1. Finish the package as prescribed for the rest of the cycle and start the next cycle's package without taking any time off.
   2. Finish the package as prescribed for the rest of the cycle and use an additional method of contraception.
   3. Take two tablets daily for the next 2 consecutive days and then finish the package as prescribed.
   4. Take two tablets daily for the rest of the current cycle.

6. What would indicate that a patient understands his androgen therapy regimen? (Select all that apply.)
   1. The patient understands that the effects of the drug may not be seen for several months.
   2. The patient understands to report the presence of jaundice.
   3. The patient understands that these drugs can only be delivered by injection.
   4. The patient understands to report the presence of lower extremity edema.
   5. The patient understands that the gel should not be applied to children or females.
   6. The patient understands that these drugs can cause regression of the testes.

7. Which precaution is most important to teach a patient newly prescribed to take a bisphosphonate?
   1. Avoid calcium-containing foods and vitamin supplements.
   2. Do not have any dental work while taking this drug.
   3. Immediately report any muscle pain while taking this drug.
   4. Be sure to sit or stand for 30 minutes after taking this drug.

8. A 26-year-old woman has begun an initial course of oral contraceptives (OCs). Which of the following is a serious side effect of OCs?
   1. Blood clots
   2. Risk for infection
   3. Fracture of the jaw
   4. Bone marrow suppression

9. A patient is prescribed levothyroxine 30 mcg by IV push. The drug on hand is levothyroxine sodium 100 mcg/mL. How many mL should be given?
   1. 30 mL
   2. 0.3 mL
   3. 5 mL
   4. 0.5 mL

10. A patient is prescribed to receive Synthroid 100 mcg orally daily. The drug on hand is Synthroid 25 mcg per tablet. How many tablets should be given?
    1. 2 tablets
    2. 2½ tablets
    3. 4 tablets
    4. ¼ tablet

Drug Therapy for Diabetes

http://evolve.elsevier.com/Visovsky/LPNpharmacology/

Learning Outcomes

1. Describe the differences between diabetes mellitus type 1 and type 2, and explain why most drugs used for diabetes type 2 are not useful for diabetes type 1.
2. List the names, actions, possible side effects, and adverse effects of the insulin stimulators and the biguanides.
3. Explain what to teach patients and families about the insulin stimulators and the biguanides.
4. List the names, actions, possible side effects, and adverse effects of the insulin sensitizers and the alpha-glucosidase inhibitors.
5. Explain what to teach patients and families about the insulin sensitizers and the alpha-glucosidase inhibitors.
6. List the names, actions, possible side effects, and adverse effects of the incretin mimetics and the amylin analogs.
7. Explain what to teach patients and families about the incretin mimetics and the amylin analogs.
8. List the names, actions, possible side effects, and adverse effects of the DPP-4 inhibitors and the sodium-glucose cotransport inhibitors.
9. Explain what to teach patients and families about the DPP-4 inhibitors and the sodium-glucose cotransport inhibitors.
10. List the names, actions, possible side effects, and adverse effects of insulin preparations.
11. Explain what to teach patients and families about insulin preparations.

Key Terms

alpha-glucosidase inhibitor (ĂL-fah glū-KŌ-sě-dās ĭn-HĬ-bă-těr, p. 315) A category of oral non-insulin antidiabetic drugs that lowers blood glucose levels by preventing enzymes in the intestinal tract from breaking down starches and more complex sugars into glucose.

amylin analog (Ă-mě-lěn Ă-ně-lŏg, p. 317) A category of injectable non-insulin antidiabetic drugs similar to natural amylin, which is a hormone produced by pancreatic beta cells that works with and is co-secreted with insulin in response to blood glucose elevation. It prevents hyperglycemia by delaying gastric emptying and making the patient feel full so he or she eats less.

biguanides (bī-GWŎN-īd, p. 314) A category of oral non-insulin antidiabetic drugs that lowers blood glucose levels by reducing the amount of glucose the liver releases and by reducing how much and how fast the intestines absorb the glucose in food.

diabetes mellitus (DM) (dī-ě-BĒ-těz MĚ-lě-těs, p. 310) A common chronic endocrine problem in which either the lack of insulin or poor function of insulin impairs glucose metabolism, which then leads to problems in fat metabolism and protein metabolism.

DPP-4 (dipeptidyl peptidase-4) inhibitors (p. 318) A category of non-insulin antidiabetic drugs that helps prevent hyperglycemia by reducing the amount of the enzyme (DPP-4), which inactivates the normal incretins, GLP and GIP. This actions allow the naturally produced incretins to be present and work with insulin to control blood glucose levels.

glucagon (p. 310) A hormone produced by alpha cells of the pancreas that works to raise the concentration of glucose and fat in the bloodstream.

glucose (GLŪ-kōs, p. 310) A sugar-based nutrient critically important for energy production in cells and organs.

hyperglycemia (hī-pěr-glī-SĒ-mē-ě, p. 311) A condition of higher-than-normal blood glucose levels.

hypoglycemia (hī-pō-glī-SĒ-mē-ě, p. 310) A condition of lower-than-normal blood glucose levels.

incretin mimetics (ĭn-KRĒ-tĭn mĭ-MĚ-tĭks, p. 316) A category of non-insulin antidiabetic drugs that acts like the natural gut hormones (e.g., GLP-1) that are secreted in response to food in the stomach. They work with insulin to prevent blood glucose levels from becoming too high after meals by slowing the rate of gastric emptying.

insulin (ĬN-sŭ-lĭn, p. 310) A protein hormone produced by the pancreas or injected as a drug that binds to insulin receptors on many cells, which then promotes the movement of glucose from the blood into the cells.

insulin sensitizer (ĬN-sŭ-lĭn SĚN-sĭ-tīz-ěr, p. 314) A category of oral non-insulin antidiabetic drugs that lowers blood glucose levels by making insulin receptors more sensitive to insulin, which increases cellular uptake and use of glucose.

insulin stimulator (ĬN-sŭ-lĭn STĬM-ū-lā-těrs, p. 312) A category of oral non-insulin antidiabetic drugs that lowers blood glucose levels by triggering the release of insulin stored in the beta cells of the pancreas. The sulfonylureas and the meglitinides are the two classes of drugs in this category.

non-insulin antidiabetic drugs (p. 312) Oral and injectable drugs that use a variety of mechanisms other than binding to insulin receptors to help lower blood glucose levels back to the normal range.

sodium-glucose cotransport inhibitor (SŌ-dē-em GLŪ-kōs kō-TRĂNS-pōrt ĭn-HĬ-bă-tĕrz, p. 320) A category of non-insulin antidiabetic drug that lowers blood glucose levels by preventing the kidney from reabsorbing glucose that was filtered from the blood into the urine. This glucose then remains in the urine and is excreted rather than moved back into the blood.

DIABETES

BLOOD GLUCOSE CONTROL

Glucose is a sugar-based nutrient that is critical for energy production in cells and organs. **Insulin** is a protein hormone produced by the pancreas that binds to insulin receptors on many cells. Like other hormones, insulin is a "key" that binds to its receptors (the "locks"). When insulin binds to its receptors, the "doors" on cell membranes open for glucose to enter cells, which lowers the blood glucose level. Glucose in the cells undergoes metabolism to generate the cellular energy needed to perform all functions, particularly organ physiologic functions.

When blood glucose levels are lower than normal (**hypoglycemia**), glucose is not available for cells and organs to metabolize it into energy substances, and cellular function can be greatly reduced. However, too much glucose leads to the many serious complications of **diabetes mellitus (DM)**. So good glucose control, sometimes called *glycemic control,* requires balancing blood glucose so levels are constantly in the normal range. Table 17.1 lists the desired laboratory values that indicate good blood glucose control for the two most common tests (fasting blood glucose levels and hemoglobin A1c).

The healthy pancreas controls blood glucose levels through the actions of insulin and another hormone, glucagon. Insulin prevents hyperglycemia by allowing body cells to take up, use, and store carbohydrate, fat, and protein. It is known as the "hormone of plenty" because its release is triggered by a high blood glucose level. **Glucagon** is a hormone that has actions opposite those of insulin. It prevents low blood glucose levels by triggering the release of glucose from storage sites in the liver and skeletal muscle. Glucagon is known as the "hormone of starvation" because the trigger for its release is a lower-than-normal blood glucose lever. When these two hormones are released appropriately, blood glucose levels remain in the normal range.

> 💡 **Memory Jogger**
>
> *Insulin* is the hormone of plenty, which is released when blood glucose levels are above normal. Its function is to lower blood glucose levels and prevent hyperglycemia.
>
> *Glucagon* is the hormone of starvation, which is released when blood glucose levels are lower than normal. Its function is to raise blood glucose levels and prevent hypoglycemia.

In addition to insulin and glucagon, other organs and hormones help maintain normal blood glucose levels by balancing glucose uptake by cells and glucose production by the liver. Blood glucose levels after a meal are controlled by the emptying rate of the stomach and delivery of nutrients to the small intestine, where they are absorbed into circulation. Incretin hormones (e.g., glucagon-like peptide-1 [GLP-1]), secreted in response to food in the stomach, work with insulin to prevent blood glucose levels from becoming too high after meals. The actions of incretins increase insulin secretion, inhibit glucagon secretion, and slow the rate of gastric emptying. All of these actions help prevent high blood glucose levels.

The neurons and the brain require a continuous supply of glucose from the blood because the brain cannot store it. Other organs can use fats, as well as glucose, to generate energy. In the liver and muscles, glucose is stored as glycogen. Fats are stored as triglyceride in fat cells. During a prolonged fast or after illness, proteins are broken down and some of the amino acids are converted into glucose. Insulin not only keeps blood glucose levels from becoming too high, it also helps keep blood lipid levels in the normal range and prevents muscle protein breakdown.

LOSS OF GLUCOSE CONTROL

Diabetes mellitus is a common chronic endocrine problem in which either the *lack of insulin* or *poor function of insulin* impairs glucose metabolism. When glucose metabolism is poor, problems in fat metabolism and protein metabolism also occur. When there is not enough insulin or when insulin does not bind well to its receptor,

Table 17.1	Goals for Blood Glucose Control
LABORATORY TEST	**INDICATIONS OF GOOD BLOOD GLUCOSE CONTROL**
Fasting blood glucose	Less than 100 mg/dL or 5.6 mmol/L Controlled levels for older adults usually increase by about 1.0 mg/dL or 0.05 mmol/L for every decade of life
Glycosylated hemoglobin (A1c), also known as hemoglobin A1c	4%–6%

glucose does not enter cells and circulates unused and at high levels in the blood. So the main feature of DM is chronic high blood glucose levels (**hyperglycemia**) because glucose movement from the blood into cells and organs is impaired.

> ### Memory Jogger
>
> The main feature of DM is chronic high blood glucose levels (hyperglycemia) because glucose movement from the blood into cells and organs is impaired.

About 29 million people in the United States and 2 million people in Canada are living with DM. Nearly one-third of people with diabetes have not been diagnosed and are not being treated. Another 90 million have *prediabetes,* which is abnormal glucose metabolism that has a high risk for developing into actual DM.

DM that is not well controlled can reduce the function of all organs and tissues. Complications of uncontrolled or poorly controlled DM include hypertension, high blood lipid levels, early-onset cardiovascular disease, kidney failure, strokes, and blindness, to name only the more serious ones. The complications of DM can be delayed or reduced with good blood glucose (*glycemic*) control, along with keeping blood pressure and blood cholesterol levels as close to normal as possible.

The lack of insulin production or a problem with insulin binding to its cell receptors prevents some cells from using glucose for energy. The body then breaks down fat and protein in an attempt to provide energy and increases the production of glucose from other sources. Muscle protein is reduced, and the body uses fats in the blood in place of glucose for cellular energy. When this stored fat is used for energy, ketoacids are formed and collect in the blood, resulting in a dangerous and potentially fatal condition known as *ketoacidosis.* The classic symptoms of DM are *polydipsia* (increased fluid intake), *polyuria* (excessive urination), and *polyphagia* (hunger with excessive eating). The person with untreated DM remains in metabolic starvation until insulin is available to move glucose into the cells.

> ### Memory Jogger
>
> **Hyperglycemia**
>
> | EARLY SIGNS | LATE SIGNS |
> | --- | --- |
> | • Frequent urination | • Fruity-smelling breath |
> | • Increased thirst | • Abdominal pain |
> | • Dry mouth | • Nausea and vomiting |
> | • Blurred vision | • Shortness of breath |
> | • Fatigue | • Weakness |
> | • Headache | • Confusion |
> | | • Coma |

CLASSIFICATION OF DIABETES MELLITUS

In addition to the diabetes that can occur with pregnancy (*gestational diabetes*), there are two main types of DM.

Diabetes mellitus (DM type 1) is an autoimmune disorder in which the beta cells of the pancreas that store and release insulin are destroyed when a person's own immune system takes destructive actions and produces antibodies against the insulin-secreting cells in the pancreas. This immune attack can be caused by a genetic predisposition or exposure to certain viruses. This most commonly begins after a viral infection such as mumps and coxsackievirus infection. Often DM type 1 is diagnosed in childhood, sometimes even before the child is a year old. Older names for DM type 1 are *insulin-dependent diabetes mellitus (IDDM)* or *juvenile diabetes.* With DM type 1, the pancreas produces no insulin. The patient must take insulin daily for life unless a pancreas transplant is received.

Diabetes mellitus type 2 (DM type 2) is a disorder in which the person continues to make some insulin, but it does not bind well to its receptors so there is a reduced response of the body to insulin, known as *insulin resistance.* Eventually, the pancreas makes less and less insulin. Insulin resistance develops from obesity and decreased physical activity in people who are genetically predisposed. Obesity is a common finding in many, but not all, patients with DM type 2. Usually DM type 2 develops in adulthood, although with childhood obesity on the rise, some children are also being diagnosed with it. Older names for DM type 2 are *non-insulin-dependent diabetes mellitus (NIDDM)* or *adult-onset diabetes.*

About 90% of people with DM have diabetes type 2. The pancreas still makes some insulin, so the symptoms occur over a long time and many people are not aware they have the disease until long-term complications begin. So far fewer people have DM type 1, although it is usually diagnosed more quickly because the initial symptoms are so sudden and severe. It is important to remember that whether a person has DM type 1 or type 2, the long-term complications are the same and often shorten the person's lifespan.

> ### Bookmark This!
>
> The American Diabetes Association: http://www.diabetes.org

DRUG THERAPY FOR DIABETES MELLITUS

NON-INSULIN ANTIDIABETIC DRUGS

Patients with DM type 2 usually have a pancreas that functions a little and can be stimulated by drugs to produce more insulin. Drug therapy can also improve how well insulin interacts with its receptors. Insulin may also be necessary for some people with DM type 2, although diet, weight reduction, and non-insulin antidiabetic drugs are often effective in maintaining good blood glucose control.

Non-insulin antidiabetic drugs are *oral* and *injectable* drugs that use a variety of mechanisms other than binding to insulin receptors to help lower blood glucose levels back to the normal range. At one time some of these drugs were called *oral hypoglycemic agents,* although this term was never correct. The goal of drug therapy for DM type 2 is to help keep blood glucose levels within the normal target range for each person, not to make the person hypoglycemic. In fact hypoglycemia is a serious adverse effect of some of these drugs, not the desired effect.

Non-insulin antidiabetic drugs are prescribed when diet and exercise alone are not enough for a patient with DM type 2 to maintain the blood glucose target range identified for him or her. These drugs are not a substitute for diet and exercise for blood glucose control, but are used in addition to them. Usually one drug is started at the lowest effective dose and increased every 1 to 2 weeks until the patient either reaches his or her target blood glucose levels or the maximum drug dose is reached without the desired blood glucose control. If the first drug does not adequately control blood glucose levels, a second non-insulin antidiabetic drug that works differently may be added to the first or used alone. Insulin therapy is used only when blood glucose target ranges cannot be met with the use of two or three different types of non-insulin antidiabetic agents.

The non-insulin antidiabetic drugs are divided into eight categories. These categories are the *insulin stimulators* (secretogogues, which include the sulfonylureas and the meglitinide analogs), the *biguanides*, the *insulin sensitizers*, the *alpha-glucosidase inhibitors*, the *incretin mimetics*, the *DPP-4 (dipeptidyl peptidase-4) inhibitors*, the *amylin analogs*, and the *sodium-glucose cotransport inhibitors*. Some are oral agents and others are taken by subcutaneous injection. The drug tables in this chapter list the mechanisms of action, usual adult dosages, nursing implications, and common drugs for each class.

> ### 💡 Memory Jogger
>
> The eight categories of non-insulin antidiabetic drugs are:
> * insulin stimulators (secretogogues)
> * biguanides
> * insulin sensitizers
> * alpha-glucosidase inhibitors
> * incretin mimetics
> * amylin analogs
> * DPP-4 inhibitors
> * sodium-glucose cotransport inhibitors

INSULIN STIMULATORS (SECRETOGOGUES)

Action and Uses

Insulin stimulators are oral drugs that lower blood glucose levels by stimulating the release of insulin stored in the beta cells of the pancreas. Therefore the patient must have some functioning beta cells if these drugs are to work. In addition, they improve the movement of glucose into cells by either *increasing the number* of insulin receptors present on the cells or by *enhancing the actions* of activated insulin receptors. They are used only for DM type 2 and are often used with other non-insulin antidiabetic drugs for best blood glucose control. They also can be used with insulin. The sulfonylureas and the meglitinides are the two classes of drugs in this category. Names, usual adult dosages, and nursing implications of the insulin stimulators are listed in Table 17.2. Be sure to consult a drug reference book for more information about specific insulin stimulators.

The sulfonylureas were the first type of non-insulin antidiabetic drugs available to help manage DM type 2. These early drugs, known as *first-generation* sulfonylureas, are rarely used today because of the extensive number of drug interactions associated with them. The second-generation sulfonylureas are much more potent than first-generation drugs and have fewer interactions with other drugs.

The meglitinide analogs are newer insulin stimulators. They work in the same way as sulfonylureas but are more likely to increase insulin release just after a meal, when it is most needed.

Expected Side Effects

Some common side effects of sulfonylureas are heartburn, nausea, vomiting, abdominal pain, and diarrhea caused by increased gastric acid secretion. In addition, they increase sun sensitivity (*photosensitivity*), which increases the risk for severe sunburns.

Common side effects of meglitinides are upper respiratory infections, back and joint pain, and dizziness.

Adverse Effects

All of the insulin stimulators can cause hypoglycemia because they force the pancreas to secrete insulin even when blood glucose levels are normal or low. A serious problem with insulin stimulators is that over long periods of use they eventually cause the beta cells of the pancreas to stop producing insulin, a condition known as secondary beta cell failure. In addition, all of these drugs can affect the liver and increase liver enzyme levels.

> ### 💡 Memory Jogger
>
> #### Indications of Hypoglycemia
>
> * Headache
> * Hunger sensation
> * Difficulty concentrating
> * Nervousness
> * Tremors
> * Increased sweating
> * Pale, clammy skin
> * Rapid heart rate
> * Anxiety, confusion

Table 17.2 Examples of Insulin Stimulators and Biguanides

Insulin stimulators: drugs that lower blood glucose levels by triggering the release of preformed insulin from beta cells

DRUG/ADULT DOSAGE RANGE	NURSING IMPLICATIONS

Second-Generation Sulfonylurea Agents
 	
glimepiride (Amaryl, Apo-Glimepiride ❦)
  1–4 mg orally once daily with breakfast
glipizide (Glucotrol) 10–15 mg orally once
  daily before breakfast
glyburide (DiaBeta, Micronase) 0.75–12 mg
  orally daily
 	
Meglitinide Analogs
 	
nateglinide (Starlix) 120 mg orally three
  times daily with meals
repaglinide (Prandin) 0.5–4 mg orally with
  meals up to four times daily
	• Assess patients for indications of hypoglycemia before giving an insulin stimulator, to prevent increasing the risk for hypoglycemia.
	• Avoid giving the drug until the patient has his or her food tray, to prevent hypoglycemia.
	• If a patient is NPO or is not eating a meal, do not give that dose of the insulin stimulator, to prevent hypoglycemia.
	• Teach patients the indications of hypoglycemia (i.e., hunger, headache, tremors, sweating, and confusion) because all insulin stimulators lower blood glucose levels even when hyperglycemia is not present.
	• Instruct patients to take these drugs with or just before meals to prevent hypoglycemia.
	• Instruct patients taking a sulfonylurea to check with his or her healthcare provider or a pharmacist before taking any supplements, over-the-counter drugs, or prescribed drugs because sulfonylureas interact with many other drugs.
	• Warn patients about the common side effects of sulfonylureas (i.e., nausea, headache, and weight gain) to ensure they are prepared for these effects and are not anxious.

Biguanides: drugs that lower blood glucose levels by reducing the amount of glucose the liver releases and by reducing how much and how fast the intestines absorb the glucose in food

DRUG/ADULT DOSAGE RANGE	NURSING IMPLICATIONS

metformin (Glucophage, Glumetza)
  Immediate release: 500–850 mg orally
    twice daily with meals
  Extended release: 500–2000 mg orally
    once daily with evening meal
	• Check with the healthcare provider about stopping the drug 24 hours before and for 48 hours after a test using a radioactive dye is scheduled, to reduce the risk for an interaction that can cause kidney damage.
	• Teach patients not to cut, crush, or chew the extended-release capsule, to prevent rapid absorption of the drug that could lead to adverse effects.

❦ Indicates Canadian drug.

Drug Interactions

Sulfonylureas and the meglitinides interact with many other drugs. Some drugs or drug groups enhance the *hypoglycemic effect* of insulin stimulators. These include aspirin and other nonsteroidal anti-inflammatory drugs (NSAIDs), angiotensin II receptor antagonists (ARBs), angiotensin converting enzyme inhibitors (ACEIs), beta blockers, warfarin, azole antifungal drugs, and many antibiotics. Other common drugs, such as corticosteroids, furosemide, isoniazid, pseudoephedrine, antiretroviral protease inhibitors, and thiazide diuretics, increase the *hyperglycemia risk* by reducing the effectiveness of insulin stimulators. Be sure to consult a drug reference book or pharmacist for more information about specific drug interactions with sulfonylureas and the meglitinides.

⌂ Top Tip for Safety

Drug Interactions

Sulfonylureas may decrease the effectiveness of certain contraceptive drugs. Women of childbearing years who are taking this antidiabetic drug will need an alternative contraceptive method to avoid an unplanned pregnancy.

❖ Nursing Implications and Patient Teaching

◆ *Planning and implementation.* Assess patients for any signs or symptoms of hypoglycemia before giving an insulin stimulator to avoid making hypoglycemia worse. Signs of hypoglycemia include tremors, sweating, confusion, rapid heart rate, hunger, headache, nervousness, and inability to concentrate. If any indications are present, check the patient's blood glucose level.

Do not give an insulin stimulator at the same time as other drugs known to increase the hypoglycemic effect. When in doubt, consult a drug reference book or pharmacist for which other drugs increase hypoglycemic effects.

Ensure that these drugs are given with a meal *or* no more than 15 minutes before a meal to prevent hypoglycemia. It is a good idea to wait until the patient's tray is actually in his or her room before giving the drug. If the patient is NPO or is not eating a meal for some other reason, do not give the drug.

⌂ Top Tip for Safety

Do not give an insulin stimulator drug to a patient who is NPO or who is skipping a meal.

◆ *Patient and family teaching.* Tell the patient and family the following:
• Take these drugs with or just before meals to prevent hypoglycemia. If you must skip a meal, also skip the drug dose.

- Signs and symptoms of hypoglycemia, which include feelings of hunger, nervousness, confusion, sweating, and tremors.
- Check with your healthcare provider or a pharmacist before taking any supplements, over-the-counter drugs, or other prescribed drugs because these drugs interact with many other drugs that can change your blood glucose levels.
- Common but expected side effects of these drugs are nausea, headache, and weight gain.

BIGUANIDES

Action and Uses

Biguanides are oral, non-insulin antidiabetic drugs that lower blood glucose levels by reducing the amount of glucose the liver releases and by reducing how much and how fast the intestines absorb the glucose in food. In addition, biguanides also increase how well insulin binds to its cellular receptor site. Unlike the insulin stimulators, biguanides do not force the pancreas to release insulin from its beta cells. The only drug in this class is metformin. The dosages and nursing implications for this drug are presented in Table 17.2.

Expected Side Effects

The most common side effects of metformin are related to the gastrointestinal (GI) system and include nausea, diarrhea, flatulence, and weight loss. These side effects usually decrease over time.

Adverse Effects

Metformin use is associated with a risk for lactic acidosis, an unusually high concentrate of lactate in the body. Signs of lactic acidosis include nausea, vomiting, rapid, deep breathing, and weakness. When used without other antidiabetic drugs, metformin alone does not cause hypoglycemia.

Drug Interactions

Metformin interacts with the dye (contrast medium) used in some diagnostic tests and can lead to kidney failure. For this reason, metformin is to be stopped at least 24 hours before radioactive dye is used and not started again until 48 hours after the test is completed.

❖ Nursing Implications and Patient Teaching

◆ *Planning and implementation.* Assess the patient's kidney function. Metformin should not be given to patients with kidney disease because it can cause kidney failure. Assess the patient for signs of lactic acidosis and report any concerning findings to the healthcare provider.

Check the patient's blood sugar as ordered, and assess the patient for signs of hypoglycemia.

Metformin is safe in pregnancy for the treatment of gestational diabetes.

◆ *Patient and family teaching.* Tell the patient and family the following:

- Avoid drinking alcohol while taking metformin because this can increase the chance of developing lactic acidosis.
- The common side effects of metformin are mostly GI upset; nausea, vomiting, and diarrhea may occur, especially when the drug is first started or the dose is increased.
- Check with your healthcare provider about stopping metformin at least 24 hours before radiopaque dye is used, and not restarting it again until 48 hours after the test is completed.
- Keep all appointments for laboratory tests to check homocysteine and vitamin B$_{12}$ levels because metformin increases homocysteine levels (and increases the risk factor for cardiovascular disease) and may cause vitamin B$_{12}$ deficiency.

> ⊕ **Top Tip for Safety**
>
> Metformin should be stopped 24 hours before any diagnostic tests that use radiopaque dye. Metformin should not be restarted until 48 hours after the test is completed.

INSULIN SENSITIZERS

Action and Uses

Insulin sensitizers are a category of oral non-insulin antidiabetic drugs that lower blood glucose levels by making insulin receptors more sensitive to insulin, which increases cellular uptake and use of glucose. The drugs in this class are the thiazolidinediones, also called the "glitazones" or TZDs. They are used only for DM type 2 and are often used together with other non-insulin antidiabetic drugs for best blood glucose control. They also can be used with insulin. The names, usual adult dosages, and nursing implications of the glitazones are listed in Table 17.3.

Expected Side Effects

Hypoglycemia is a potential side effect of rosiglitazone, as well as all agents to treat diabetes, and can be more frequent and severe if combined with the use of insulin as part of the diabetes treatment plan. Headache, sneezing, and sore throat can also occur.

Adverse Effects

Thiazolidinediones have been associated with severe cardiovascular side effects and must be used with care. Currently, rosiglitazone is a drug only available to selected patients, but pioglitazone is still generally available, although closely monitored. Rosiglitazone can also cause fluid retention, liver problems, and macular edema.

Drug Interactions

Rosiglitazone has many drug interactions. Gemfibrozil, rifampin, and drugs to treat hypertension can all interact with rosiglitazone. Check your drug reference guide or ask a pharmacist about specific drug interactions.

❖ Nursing Implications and Patient Teaching

◆ *Planning and implementation.* Assess the patient for signs of allergic reaction (e.g., hives, facial swelling, and itching).

Assess the patient for signs of heart failure, which include weight gain, shortness of breath, tachycardia, and edema.

Assess for symptoms of hypoglycemia (e.g., hunger, sweating, pale skin, irritability, dizziness, feeling shaky, or trouble concentrating).

◆ *Patient and family teaching.* Tell the patient and family the following:

- Take the drug as prescribed. If you miss a dose, take it as soon as possible. Do not double up on the drug to make up for missed doses.
- Report itching, hives, or swelling of the face or hands to your healthcare provider immediately should any of these symptoms of allergic reaction occur.
- Report any changes in vision or blurred vision to your healthcare provider.
- Report swelling of the feet or ankles, or rapid weight gain to your healthcare provider.
- Avoid alcohol because this can affect blood glucose levels, causing both hypoglycemia and hyperglycemia depending on how much alcohol is ingested.
- When signs and symptoms of hypoglycemia are present (e.g., hunger, sweating, pale skin, irritability, dizziness, feeling shaky, or trouble concentrating), eat or drink something that contains real sugar, as your healthcare provider directed.

- When signs or symptoms of hyperglycemia such as headache, increased thirst, dry mouth, blurred vision, fatigue, abdominal pain, or weakness are present and persist, notify your healthcare provider.
- Check your blood sugar frequently, especially during times of stress or illness, because these problems can affect blood glucose levels.

ALPHA-GLUCOSIDASE INHIBITORS

Action and Uses

Alpha-glucosidase inhibitors are a category of oral non-insulin antidiabetic drugs that lower blood glucose levels by preventing enzymes in the intestinal tract from breaking down starches and more complex sugars into glucose. This action slows glucose absorption. These drugs are primarily prescribed for patients who have high blood sugars following meals.

Alpha-glucosidase inhibitors were first approved to help manage DM type 2 but can also be used for DM type 1 (along with insulin) because they work in the GI tract independently from insulin. Used alone they cannot cause hypoglycemia. Alpha-glucosidase inhibitors can be used with sulfonylureas, insulin, or metformin. The names, usual adult dosages, and nursing implications of the alpha-glucosidase inhibitors are listed in Table 17.3.

Expected Side Effects

Because alpha-glucosidase inhibitors prevent the breakdown of complex carbohydrates (starches such

---

Table 17.3   Examples of Insulin Sensitizers and Alpha-Glucosidase Inhibitors

Insulin sensitizers: drugs that lower blood glucose levels by making insulin receptors more sensitive to insulin, which increases cellular uptake and use of glucose

DRUG/ADULT DOSAGE RANGE	NURSING IMPLICATIONS
pioglitazone (Actos) Initial dosage: 15–30 mg orally daily with meal; may increase up to 45 mg daily maximum rosiglitazone (Avandia) Initial dosage: 4 mg orally once daily or divided into 2 mg every 12 hours; may increase to 8 mg orally once daily, or divided and given every 12 hours	• Teach patients to report indications of allergic reactions (itching, hives, facial swelling) immediately to the healthcare provider. • Monitor patients carefully for signs and symptoms of heart failure (e.g., excessive, rapid weight gain, dyspnea, and/or edema) because these drugs have been known to cause or worsen heart failure symptoms. • Monitor for symptoms of hypoglycemia (i.e., hunger, sweating, pale skin, irritability, dizziness, feeling shaky, or trouble concentrating).

Alpha-glucosidase inhibitors: non-insulin antidiabetic drugs that lower blood glucose levels by preventing enzymes in the intestinal tract from breaking down starches and more complex sugars into glucose

DRUG/ADULT DOSAGE RANGE	NURSING IMPLICATIONS
acarbose (Prandase, Precose) Initial dosage: 25 mg orally three times daily at meals, with a maximum dosage of 100 mg orally three times daily miglitol (Glyset) Initial dosage: 25 mg orally every 8 hours at meals; maintenance dosage: 50 mg orally every 8 hours, with a maximum dosage of 100 mg orally every 8 hours	• Assess the patient for signs of an allergic reaction to the drug. • Monitor the patient for hypoglycemia especially when combined with insulin or other diabetic drugs. • Monitor the patient for GI discomfort or diarrhea, and report findings to the healthcare provider. GI side effects are common because the intestinal tract is the site of action for these drugs. • Take these drugs at the start of a meal because their antidiabetic action is to reduce the conversion of the ingested complex carbohydrates into glucose.

as bread, cereals, corn, and potatoes) into glucose, the carbohydrates remain in the intestine, causing gas formation (*flatulence*), feeling bloated, and diarrhea. These side effects usually go away as the body adjusts to the drug and dose.

Adverse Effects

Alpha-glucosidase inhibitors can cause the worsening of conditions associated with inflammation of the bowel, such as colitis, Crohn's disease, or intestinal obstruction. There is the potential for hypoglycemia when alpha-glucosidase inhibitors are given with insulin or other drugs for the treatment of diabetes. These drugs can cause liver impairment with elevated liver enzyme levels.

Drug Interactions

There is a risk for hypoglycemia when alpha-glucosidase inhibitors are combined with other diabetes drugs such as sulfonylureas, insulin, and meglitinides.

❖ Nursing Implications and Patient Teaching

◆ *Planning and implementation.* Assess the patient for signs of allergic reaction to the drug (e.g., hives, itching, and facial swelling). Monitor the patient for any signs or symptoms associated with hypoglycemia when combined with insulin or other diabetic drugs. Monitor the patient for GI discomfort or diarrhea, and report findings to the healthcare provider because a dose adjustment may be needed.

◆ *Patient and family teaching.* Tell the patient and family the following:
- These drugs work best when they are used in conjunction with diet and exercise.
- Alpha-glucosidase inhibitors must be taken at the start of meals to get the most benefit because these drugs work by interfering with digestive enzymes.
- The drug effect on blood sugar levels after meals will depend on the amount of complex carbohydrates in the meal.
- Avoid alcohol because it can increase the risk for liver impairment while taking these drugs.
- Report any signs of allergic reaction to the healthcare provider immediately.

INCRETIN MIMETICS

Action and Uses

Incretin mimetics are injectable drugs that act like the natural gut hormones (e.g., glucagon-like peptide-1 [GLP-1]) that are secreted in response to food in the stomach. Just like the gut hormone, these drugs work with insulin to prevent blood glucose levels from becoming too high after meals. This results in an increase in insulin secretion, a decrease in glucagon secretion, and a slower rate of gastric emptying. All of these actions help prevent high blood glucose levels. In addition, these drugs make the person feel full (have *satiety*), which may help them to eat less. These injected drugs work with naturally secreted insulin, so they are only approved for use in patients who have DM type 2 that has not been controlled with oral drugs. These drugs are given by the subcutaneous route, and some are long-acting, needing only weekly dosing. The names, usual adult dosages, and nursing implications of the incretin mimetics are listed in Table 17.4.

Expected Side Effects

Common side effects of the incretin mimetics include nausea, vomiting, diarrhea, and upper respiratory tract symptoms. Many patients lose weight when taking this drug.

Adverse Effects

Incretin mimetics can cause allergic reactions (hives, facial swelling, and trouble breathing). There are several long-term potential adverse effects. Pancreatitis can occur in people with DM who are obese. These drugs also appear to increase the risk for thyroid cancer.

Drug Interactions

Many herbal products or drugs interact with incretin mimetics. Ask the healthcare provider or pharmacist about potential interactions. Sulfonylureas increase the risk for hypoglycemia. Incretin mimetics slow the absorption of other drugs, including antibiotics and contraceptive drugs. Take other drugs 1 hour before incretin mimetics.

❖ Nursing Implications and Patient Teaching

◆ *Planning and implementation.* Assess the patient for signs of allergic reaction to the drug. Assess the patient for signs of abdominal pain, bloating, and nausea. Assess the patient's blood sugar level, especially after beginning this drug.

Ensure that the patient and family understand and can demonstrate cleansing the skin, injecting the drug, rotation of injection sites, and proper disposal of the needles and syringes.

Assess the patient for signs of thyroid cancer such as a lump in the throat or difficulty swallowing.

◆ *Patient and family teaching.* Tell the patient and family the following:
- Report any signs or symptoms of allergic reaction to your healthcare provider. If you have difficulty breathing, a "lump" in your throat, or swelling of the mouth and tongue, call 911 or go to the nearest emergency department immediately.
- Avoid alcohol intake because it makes the risk for pancreatic inflammation worse when you are taking these drugs.
- Monitor your blood sugar regularly, especially if you are taking more than one drug for your diabetes.
- Seek immediate help for severe abdominal pain and nausea that can signal pancreatitis.
- If a dose is accidentally missed, do not double up injections; simply take the missed dose as soon as possible.

Table 17.4 Examples of the Amylin Analogs and Incretin Mimetics

Incretin mimetics: Non-insulin antidiabetic drugs that act like the natural gut hormones (e.g., GLP-1) secreted in response to food in the stomach. They work with insulin to prevent blood glucose levels from becoming too high after meals. This results in an increase in insulin secretion, a decrease in glucagon secretion, and a slower rate of gastric emptying.

DRUG/ADULT DOSAGE RANGE	NURSING IMPLICATIONS
albiglutide (Tanzeum) 30–50 mg subcutaneously once weekly (prefilled pen) dulaglutide (Trulicity) 0.75–1.5 mg subcutaneously once a week exenatide (Byetta) 5–10 mcg subcutaneously every 12 hours within 60 minutes before meals exenatide extended-release (Bydureon) 2 mg subcutaneously once every 7 days liraglutide (Victoza) 0.6 mg subcutaneously once daily for 7 days, then 1.2–1.8 mg once daily subcutaneously lixisenatide (Adlyxin) Initial dose: (green pen 50 mcg/mL) 10 mcg subcutaneously before first meal of the day; maintenance dose: (burgundy pen 100 mcg/mL in 3 mL) 20 mcg subcutaneously 1 hour before the first meal of the day	• Assess for signs of an allergic reaction to the drug. • Assess the patient for pancreatitis (i.e., abdominal pain, bloating, and nausea) because this is a possible adverse effect of incretin mimetics. • Assess the patient's blood sugar level before injecting the drug to prevent hypoglycemia. • Teach the patient and family the correct procedure for preparing the skin, injecting the drug with the pen injector, and proper disposal of needles and syringes to ensure best action and prevent complications. • Assess the patient for signs of thyroid cancer (i.e., lump in the throat or difficulty swallowing) because these drugs are associated with an increased risk for the disease. • Instruct the patient to avoid alcohol because together alcohol and the incretin mimetics increase the risk for pancreatitis.

Amylin analogs: Injectable non-insulin antidiabetic drugs that are similar to natural amylin, which is a hormone produced by pancreatic beta cells that works with and is co-secreted with insulin in response to blood glucose elevation. They prevent hyperglycemia by delaying gastric emptying and making the patient feel full so he or she eats less.

DRUG/ADULT DOSAGE RANGE	NURSING IMPLICATIONS
pramlintide (Symlin) Initial dose: 15 mcg subcutaneously immediately before meals; maintenance: 30–60 mcg subcutaneously immediately before meals	• Assess for signs of an allergic reaction to pramlintide. • Check blood sugar levels after meals because this is the drug's time of action and when hypoglycemia is most likely to occur. • Monitor for symptoms of hypoglycemia. • Monitor the patient for the presence of dizziness, which is a possible side effect of this drug. • Teach the patient/family proper skin preparation and how to correctly inject the drug using the pen injector because drug effectiveness is related to correct administration of the drug. • Teach the patient/family to rotate the injection sites and proper disposal of the needles and syringes to prevent complications. • Instruct the patient to avoid alcohol because together alcohol and pramlintide increase the risk for pancreatitis.

GLP-1, Glucagon-like peptide-1.

• Give the subcutaneous injection in the thigh, upper arm, or abdomen, rotating injection sites regularly.
• Inject the drug 60 minutes *before* meals, not after meals.
• Refrigerate unused injectable pens until they are used or expired. Dispose of them in a regulation sharps container.

Memory Jogger

Symptoms of Acute Pancreatitis

• Severe upper abdominal pain that radiates to the back
• Indigestion
• Nausea and vomiting
• Bloating with distended abdomen
• Rapid heart rate

AMYLIN ANALOGS

Action and Uses

Amylin analogs are a category of injectable non-insulin antidiabetic drugs that are similar to natural amylin, which is a hormone produced by pancreatic beta cells that works with and is secreted along with insulin in response to blood glucose elevation. The only drug currently in this class is pramlintide, which prevents hyperglycemia by delaying gastric emptying and making the patient feel full so he or she eats less. It is used for patients with DM type 1 and type 2. Patients with DM type 1 take this drug because people who do not secrete insulin are usually deficient in amylin. The usual adult dosages and nursing implications for pramlintide are listed in Table 17.4.

Expected Side Effects

Nausea, vomiting, headache, abdominal pain, weight loss, and fatigue can occur with pramlintide. This drug can cause dizziness.

Adverse Effects

This drug can cause severe hypoglycemia, especially if used with insulin to treat diabetes. If it occurs, severe hypoglycemia will develop within 3 hours of injecting the drug. The drug is associated with pancreatitis.

Drug Interactions

Some drugs that can affect how pramlintide works include aspirin, atropine, disopyramide, fluoxetine, pentoxifylline, certain blood pressure and cholesterol drugs, and monoamine oxidase (MAO) inhibitors. Pramlintide interferes with the absorption of antibiotics and birth control pills, which should be taken at least 1 hour *before* pramlintide.

📭 Top Tip for Safety

Teach patients to take prescribed antibiotics and oral contraceptives at least 1 hour *before* taking pramlintide because it interferes with the absorption of these other drugs.

❖ Nursing Implications and Patient Teaching

◆ *Planning and implementation.* Assess for signs of allergic reaction to pramlintide.

Check blood sugar after meals to assess effectiveness of the drug and to screen for hypoglycemia.

Monitor the patient for dizziness; if present, notify the healthcare provider because the dose may need adjustment.

Ensure the patient and family understand and can demonstrate the process for drawing up the drug, cleansing the skin, injecting the drug, rotation of injection sites, and proper disposal of the needles and syringes.

◆ *Patient and family teaching.* Tell the patient and family the following:

- This drug is injected into the thigh or stomach area, rotating the injection site regularly.
- Opened vials and injectable pens should be kept refrigerated. If not refrigerated, they must be used within 28 days, then discarded.
- Allow the drug to warm to room temperature before injecting it.
- Give this injectable drug right before your meal.
- Never mix pramlintide with insulin in the same syringe.
- Dispose of all used syringes and needles into a regulation sharps container.
- If you miss a dose, and cannot take it within a reasonable time period, skip the dose. Do not double up on doses to make up for a missed dose.
- Do not drink alcohol while taking pramlintide because the risk for pancreatitis increases if you drink alcohol while taking this drug.

- Check your blood sugar regularly. Do not take pramlintide if your blood sugar is too low.
- This drug can cause dizziness. Do not drive or operate machinery until you know how this drug affects you.
- Report signs and symptoms of hypoglycemia to your healthcare provider.

DPP-4 INHIBITORS

Action and Uses

DPP-4 (dipeptidyl peptidase-4) inhibitors are a category of non-insulin antidiabetic drugs that help prevent hyperglycemia by reducing the amount of the enzyme DPP-4, which inactivates the normal gut hormones (incretins), such as GLP (glucagon-like peptide) and GIP (gastric inhibitory polypeptide). These actions allow the naturally produced incretins to be present and work with insulin to control blood glucose levels. These drugs are approved for use only in patients who have DM type 2. The names, usual adult dosages, and nursing implications of the DPP-4 inhibitors are listed in Table 17.5.

Expected Side Effects

Nasopharyngitis, with cold-like symptoms of sneezing, runny nose, cough, and swelling of the nasal passages, can occur. Diarrhea has also been reported with the use of DPP-4 inhibitors.

Adverse Effects

Hypoglycemia can occur when given in combination with insulin or a sulfonylurea. Allergic reactions with symptoms of hives, facial swelling, and itching can occur. Reports of acute and even fatal pancreatitis have occurred with these drugs. It is unknown whether persons with a history of pancreatitis are at increased risk.

Severe arthralgia (joint pain) has been reported in patients who are taking DPP-4 inhibitors. Bullous pemphigoid, a rare skin condition that results in large, fluid-filled blisters that most often occur in the lower abdomen, upper thighs, or armpits, has also been reported (Fig. 17.1).

Drug Interactions

The effectiveness of DPP-4 inhibitors may be reduced when taken with erythromycin, ketoconazole, and other drugs that change the activity of metabolizing enzymes. Consult a drug reference or a pharmacist to determine whether other drugs the patient is prescribed change the effectiveness of DPP-4 inhibitors.

❖ Nursing Implications and Patient Teaching

◆ *Planning and implementation.* Assess for signs of allergic reaction or angioedema (swelling of the face, mouth, tongue, or larynx, often accompanied by hives; see Fig. 8.10). If any of these indications appear, notify the healthcare provider immediately.

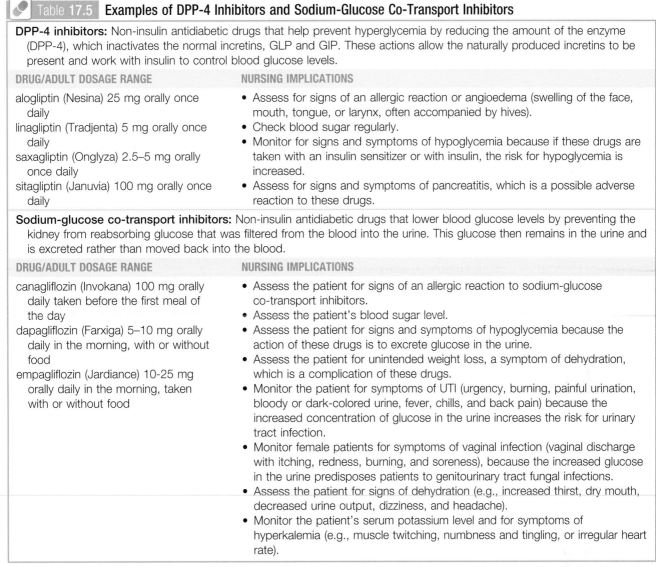

Table 17.5 Examples of DPP-4 Inhibitors and Sodium-Glucose Co-Transport Inhibitors

DPP-4 inhibitors: Non-insulin antidiabetic drugs that help prevent hyperglycemia by reducing the amount of the enzyme (DPP-4), which inactivates the normal incretins, GLP and GIP. These actions allow the naturally produced incretins to be present and work with insulin to control blood glucose levels.

DRUG/ADULT DOSAGE RANGE	NURSING IMPLICATIONS
alogliptin (Nesina) 25 mg orally once daily linagliptin (Tradjenta) 5 mg orally once daily saxagliptin (Onglyza) 2.5–5 mg orally once daily sitagliptin (Januvia) 100 mg orally once daily	• Assess for signs of an allergic reaction or angioedema (swelling of the face, mouth, tongue, or larynx, often accompanied by hives). • Check blood sugar regularly. • Monitor for signs and symptoms of hypoglycemia because if these drugs are taken with an insulin sensitizer or with insulin, the risk for hypoglycemia is increased. • Assess for signs and symptoms of pancreatitis, which is a possible adverse reaction to these drugs.

Sodium-glucose co-transport inhibitors: Non-insulin antidiabetic drugs that lower blood glucose levels by preventing the kidney from reabsorbing glucose that was filtered from the blood into the urine. This glucose then remains in the urine and is excreted rather than moved back into the blood.

DRUG/ADULT DOSAGE RANGE	NURSING IMPLICATIONS
canagliflozin (Invokana) 100 mg orally daily taken before the first meal of the day dapagliflozin (Farxiga) 5–10 mg orally daily in the morning, with or without food empagliflozin (Jardiance) 10-25 mg orally daily in the morning, taken with or without food	• Assess the patient for signs of an allergic reaction to sodium-glucose co-transport inhibitors. • Assess the patient's blood sugar level. • Assess the patient for signs and symptoms of hypoglycemia because the action of these drugs is to excrete glucose in the urine. • Assess the patient for unintended weight loss, a symptom of dehydration, which is a complication of these drugs. • Monitor the patient for symptoms of UTI (urgency, burning, painful urination, bloody or dark-colored urine, fever, chills, and back pain) because the increased concentration of glucose in the urine increases the risk for urinary tract infection. • Monitor female patients for symptoms of vaginal infection (vaginal discharge with itching, redness, burning, and soreness), because the increased glucose in the urine predisposes patients to genitourinary tract fungal infections. • Assess the patient for signs of dehydration (e.g., increased thirst, dry mouth, decreased urine output, dizziness, and headache). • Monitor the patient's serum potassium level and for symptoms of hyperkalemia (e.g., muscle twitching, numbness and tingling, or irregular heart rate).

GIP, Gastric inhibitory polypeptide; *GLP-1,* glucagon-like peptide-1; *UTI,* urinary tract infection.

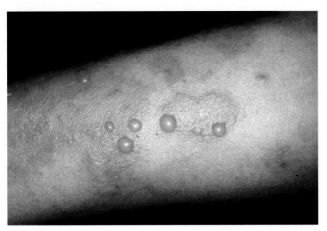

FIG. 17.1 Bullous pemphigoid. (From Habif TP: *Clinical dermatology,* ed 6, St. Louis, 2016, Elsevier.)

Check blood sugar to assess the effectiveness of the drug and to screen for hypoglycemia, especially if the patient is taking insulin or a sulfonylurea.

◆*Patient and family teaching.* Tell the patient and family the following:

- Take the drug as ordered. If a dose is accidentally missed and cannot be taken within a reasonable time, do not double up on the drug dose. Take the next dose as scheduled.
- Check your blood sugar regularly, report any hypoglycemia incidents to your healthcare provider.
- Report symptoms of allergic reaction or angioedema associated with the drug to your healthcare provider.
- Report symptoms of acute pancreatitis (e.g., upper abdominal pain radiating to the back, nausea and vomiting, fever, or rapid pulse) to your healthcare provider immediately.
- Inform your healthcare provider if you become pregnant, because it is unknown whether these

drugs are safe for use during pregnancy or when breast-feeding.

- Tell your healthcare provider all of the drugs you are taking, because many drugs can interfere with the effectiveness of DPP-4 inhibitors.

⚠ Safety Alert!

Drug Interactions

- Many drugs used to treat diabetes interact with other drugs the patient may be taking.
- Obtain a complete list of all drugs and supplements that the patient is taking.
- Oral contraceptives and antibiotics can interact with drugs for diabetes, reducing their effectiveness.

SODIUM-GLUCOSE CO-TRANSPORT INHIBITORS

Action and Uses

Sodium-glucose co-transport inhibitors are a new category of non-insulin antidiabetic drugs that lower blood glucose levels by preventing the kidney from reabsorbing glucose that was filtered from the blood into the urine. This glucose then remains in the urine and is excreted rather than moved back into the blood. These drugs are approved for use only in patients who have DM type 2. The names, usual adult dosages, and nursing implications of sodium-glucose co-transport inhibitors are listed in Table 17.5.

Expected Side Effects

An increased need to urinate has been reported in patients who are taking sodium-glucose co-transport inhibitors. Patients who are using glucose strips to check for glucose in the urine will see a positive result most of the time because glucose is excreted in the urine. Weight loss initially through the loss of fluid followed by loss of fat mass can occur.

Adverse Effects

Vaginal yeast infections and urinary tract infections (UTIs) are the most commonly reported problems, with the greatest risk being in female patients and uncircumcised men. Kidney failure, *hyperkalemia* (high level of potassium in the blood), ketoacidosis, increased risk for bladder cancer, and *hypotension* (low blood pressure) are other potential serious adverse effects. Also allergic reactions, hypoglycemia, and dehydration can occur.

Drug Interactions

Combining sodium-glucose co-transport inhibitors with insulin increases the likelihood for hypoglycemia. When these drugs are given with diuretics, the frequency of urination increases and can result in dehydration. Some drugs such as rifampin, phenytoin, ritonavir, and phenobarbital decrease the efficacy of sodium-glucose co-transport inhibitors, requiring an increased dose.

❖ Nursing Implications and Patient Teaching

◆ *Planning and implementation.* Assess the patient for signs of allergic reaction to sodium-glucose co-transport inhibitors.

Assess the patient's blood sugar level to check for hypoglycemia.

Check the patient's weight at the start of therapy, and at regular intervals, as these drugs can cause weight loss.

Monitor the patient for symptoms of urinary tract infection (UTI): urgency, burning, painful urination, bloody or dark-colored urine, fever, chills, and back pain.

Monitor female patients for symptoms of vaginal infection (vaginal discharge with itching, redness, burning, and soreness).

Assess the patient for signs of dehydration (increased thirst, dry mouth, decreased urine output, dizziness, and headache).

Monitor the patient's serum potassium level and for symptoms of hyperkalemia (muscle twitching, numbness and tingling, and irregular heart rate).

◆ *Patient and family teaching.* Tell the patient and family the following:

- Notify your healthcare provider if you have any symptoms of an allergic reaction to the drug.
- Check your blood sugar at regular intervals.
- Weigh yourself at least once a week and report any undue or unexpected weight loss.
- Report any signs of a UTI or vaginal infection to your healthcare provider.
- Make sure you are drinking enough fluids throughout the day to prevent dehydration.
- You will see the presence of glucose in your urine if you test your urine with a glucose test strip. This is to be expected because the drug works by excreting glucose into the urine for elimination.

INSULIN

Action and Uses

The pancreas is responsible for making insulin and glucagon, both of which work to maintain blood glucose levels. Insulin is made by the beta cells of the pancreas. When levels of glucose are abnormally elevated in the blood, this is known as *hyperglycemia*. When blood sugar levels become elevated, insulin is released from the beta cells of the pancreas to help restore normal blood sugar levels by moving insulin into cells and allowing insulin to bind to insulin receptors on the cell membrane (Fig. 17.2). A fasting glucose level of 70 to 90 mg/dL is considered normal.

Once insulin binds to the insulin receptor, a series of reactions take place in the cell, making it easier for glucose to pass into the cell. In addition to its role in glucose control, insulin is also very important in fat metabolism. Adequate amounts of insulin inhibit the release of fatty acids into the blood, thus preventing high blood lipid levels. Insulin is an *anabolic* hormone

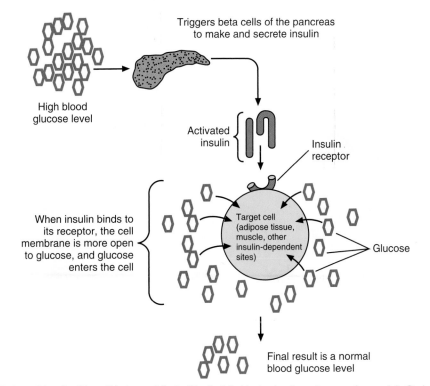

High blood
glucose level

Triggers beta cells of the pancreas
to make and secrete insulin

Activated
insulin

Insulin
receptor

When insulin binds to
its receptor, the cell
membrane is more open
to glucose, and glucose
enters the cell

Target cell
(adipose tissue,
muscle, other
insulin-dependent
sites)

Glucose

Final result is a normal
blood glucose level

FIG. 17.2 Action of insulin. (From Workman ML, LaCharity LA: *Understanding pharmacology*, ed 2, St. Louis, 2016, Elsevier.)

(one that converts simple substances into more complex compounds) that helps maintain stores of fatty acids, glycogen, and protein. Insulin is considered a *high-alert drug*.

🔔 Top Tip for Safety

High-Alert Drug

- Insulin is a high-alert drug that can cause great harm when given at too high a dose, too low a dose, not given to a patient for whom it was prescribed, or given to someone who does not have diabetes.
- If insulin is given to a patient without diabetes, or if given at a high dose, the patient can become severely hypoglycemic, which can result in death.
- If insulin is given at too low a dose, a patient's blood glucose level is poorly controlled, increasing the risk for severe hyperglycemia, ketoacidosis, and even death.
- Older patients with poor vision may benefit from prefilled insulin syringes, cartridges, or pens to prevent dosing errors.

Recent recommendations for glucose control in DM type 1 consist of multiple-dose insulin injections (three to four injections per day), known as *intensive insulin therapy*, or by continuous subcutaneous insulin infusion via an insulin pump (Fig. 17.3). Insulin must be given by the parenteral route because it is destroyed by stomach acids and intestinal enzymes. At present, most patients use specific insulin syringes with a small, thin needle designed specifically for insulin dosage (in units)

and subcutaneous injection into the thigh, upper arm, or abdomen (Fig. 17.4). Various injection devices have also been developed to simplify insulin injection. Some of these look like a pen, and patients just have to dial the insulin dosage needed and touch the tip to their skin where the insulin is automatically injected (Figs. 17.5 and 17.6). These products do not need to be refrigerated, so they can easily be carried by the patient. Internal or external insulin pumps are computer driven and can be programmed to release small doses of insulin continuously as needed, or hourly.

Each patient with DM who needs insulin therapy will be placed on an *insulin regimen*, which is the schedule of insulin aimed at preventing hyperglycemia. The dose of insulin and how often it is to be given or taken varies between patients. Generally, patients are scheduled to receive a long-acting insulin in the morning, with short-acting insulin given to cover meals and snacks. Whenever short-acting insulin is given before a meal, the patient will need to eat the meal within 15 minutes of receiving the injection to prevent hypoglycemia.

🔔 Top Tip for Safety

Whenever short-acting insulin is given before a meal, the patient will need to eat the meal within 15 minutes of receiving the injection to prevent hypoglycemia.

The insulin regimen is determined by the patient's blood glucose levels, age, activity level, and eating habits. Some insulin regimens require the patient to self-inject

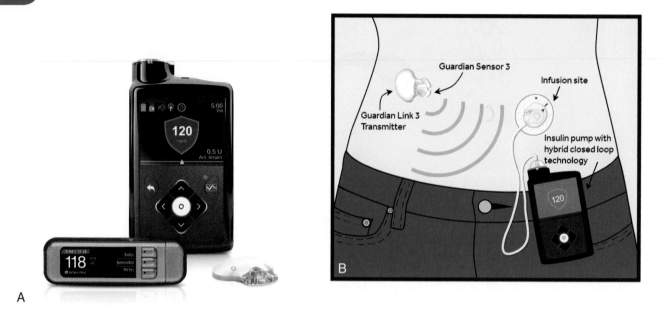

FIG. 17.3 Insulin pump. (A) MiniMed 670G System. (B) MiniMed system in use on a patient. (Courtesy Medtronic MiniMed, Inc.)

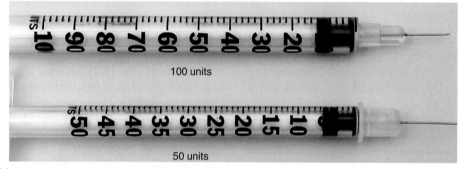

FIG. 17.4 U-100 and U-50 syringes. (From Workman ML, LaCharity LA: *Understanding pharmacology*, ed 2, St. Louis, 2016, Elsevier.)

two different types of insulin once daily. Patients need to be taught home glucose testing and to maintain a written or electronic record of their test results. This information, along with hemoglobin A1c testing, is used by the healthcare provider to adjust the insulin regimen.

Patients with diabetes type 2 may require insulin, because over time diabetes type 2 tends to worsen and the pancreas no longer makes enough insulin. The addition of insulin also increases the glucose-lowering effect when oral drugs alone are not adequate. Insulin is also used in patients with diabetes type 2 if the patient has allergies to other antidiabetic drugs, has liver or renal dysfunction, or is pregnant or contemplating pregnancy.

Types of Insulin

Many types of insulin are available for use. Insulin is available in rapid, short-acting, intermediate-acting, and long-acting formulas. So the amount of insulin available in the blood to prevent hyperglycemia varies mostly by the duration of action. Almost all insulin used today is synthetic. In the past, insulin was obtained from pork and beef pancreatic sources, but the development of antibodies to these types of insulin led to the development of human synthetic insulin, which is used today. All types of insulin are regarded as *high-alert drugs* because of the severity of effects that can occur if insulin is given in the wrong dose or to the wrong patient. Table 17.6 lists commonly used types of insulin and their durations of action.

Expected Side Effects

Expected side effects of insulin include mild allergic reactions, such as swelling, itching, or redness around the injection site, and changes to the skin at injection sites (lipodystrophy).

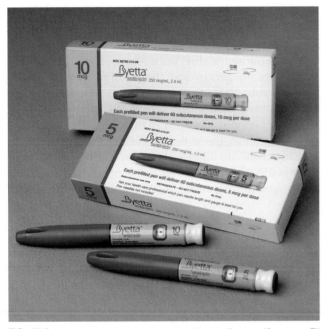

FIG. 17.5 Injection pen for the incretin mimetic Byetta. (Courtesy Eli Lilly & Company, Indianapolis, IN, and Amylin Pharmaceuticals, San Diego, CA.)

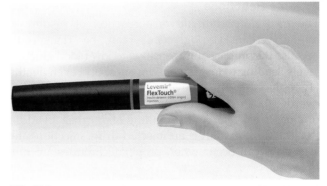

FIG. 17.6 Example of an insulin pen injector. (Courtesy Novo Nordisk Inc.)

Table 17.6   Examples of Commonly Used Types of Insulin

PREPARATION	BRAND	ONSET (HOURS)	PEAK (HOURS)	DURATION (HOURS)
Rapid-Acting Insulin Analogs				
Insulin aspart injection	NovoLog	0.25	1–3	3–5
Insulin glulisine injection	Apidra	0.3	0.5–1.5	3–4
Human lispro injection	Humalog	0.25	0.5–1.5	5
Human lispro injection U-200	Humalog U-200	0.25	0.5–1.5	5
Insulin human inhalation powder	Afrezza	0.25	1–1.25	2.5
Short-Acting Insulin				
Regular human insulin injection	Humulin R	0.5	2–4	5–7
	Novolin R	0.5	2.5–5	8
	ReliOn R	0.5	2.5–5	8–12
Humulin R (Concentrated U-500)	Humulin R (U-500)	1.5	4–12	24
Intermediate-Acting Insulin				
Isophane insulin NPH injection	Humulin N	1.5	4–12	16–24+
	Novolin N	1–4	4–14	10–24+
	ReliOn N	1–4	4–14	10–24+
70% human insulin isophane suspension/30% human insulin injection	Humulin 70/30 Novolin 70/30 ReliOn 70/30	0.5	2–12	24
70% insulin aspart protamine suspension/30% insulin aspart injection	NovoLog Mix 70/30	0.25	1–4	24
75% insulin lispro protamine suspension/25% insulin lispro injection	Humalog Mix 75/25	0.25	1–2	24
Long-Acting Insulin Analogs				
Insulin glargine injection	Lantus	2–4	None	24
Insulin glargine injection U-300	Toujeo	2–4	12	24
Insulin detemir injection	Levemir	1	6–8	5.7–24
Insulin degludec injection U-100, U-200	Tresiba U-100 Tresiba U-200	1 1	9 9	42 42

Adverse Reactions

The most important adverse reaction of insulin is hypoglycemia. Hypoglycemia can be dangerous because the brain is quite sensitive to low blood glucose levels, leading to loss of consciousness and even death. Hypoglycemia may develop because of an insulin overdose, increased work or exercise, skipping a meal, or illness associated with vomiting or diarrhea. In addition, because insulin is an injected drug, injection-site infections can occur when proper techniques are not followed.

Drug Interactions

Insulin needs may be increased by insulin antagonists such as oral contraceptives, corticosteroids, epinephrine, and thiazide diuretics. Alcohol, warfarin, and anabolic steroids may increase the hypoglycemic effects of insulin. Beta blockers can mask the signs and symptoms of hypoglycemia.

❖ Nursing Implications and Patient Teaching

◆ *Planning and implementation.* Test the patient's blood sugar each time before giving insulin. Carefully check the order for the time, type, and amount of insulin to be given. Ensure you are giving the right insulin concentration (U-50, U-100, or U-500), with the correct syringe designed for the insulin concentration (Fig. 17.7).

⬆ Top Tip for Safety

Before giving any insulin dose, carefully check the order for the time, type, and amount of insulin to be given. Ensure you are giving the right insulin concentration (U-50, U-100, or U-500), with the correct syringe designed for the insulin concentration.

Check insulin vial for color and clarity. Some insulins are clear (rapid-acting, short-acting, insulin glargine [Lantus], and insulin detemir [Levemir]). All other types of insulin have a cloudy appearance (Fig. 17.8).

When drawing up two different types of prescribed insulin, check to be sure they are compatible for mixing. Insulin glargine (Lantus) and insulin detemir (Levemir) cannot be mixed with any other type of insulin. Inject the air into the shorter-acting insulin first and then inject air into the longer-acting insulin. Draw up the longer-acting insulin first, followed by the short-acting insulin. Follow the directions shown in Fig. 17.8.

Be sure to gently roll the insulin vial or device between your hands to gently mix and warm the insulin.

Select the injection site (Fig. 17.9), then cleanse the site with alcohol. Grasp a skin fold with your nondominant hand, insert the needle at a 90-degree angle, and inject the insulin (without aspirating). Withdraw the needle and place mild pressure on the injection site without massaging it. Make sure to document the injection site and note rotation of sites to prevent lipodystrophy.

Make sure the patient has a meal ready to eat before giving insulin. Check the patient at hourly intervals for signs and symptoms of hypoglycemia.

◆ *Patient and family teaching.* Teach patients and family members the correct procedures to store, draw up, and inject insulin, rotating injection sites, as described in Box 17.1. Use a return demonstration to ensure the effectiveness of the teaching plan. In addition tell the patient and family the following:

- When signs and symptoms of hypoglycemia are present (hunger, sweating, pale skin, irritability, dizziness, feeling shaky, or trouble concentrating), eat or drink something that contains real sugar, as your healthcare provider directed.
- When signs or symptoms of hyperglycemia, such as headache, increased thirst, dry mouth, blurred vision, fatigue, abdominal pain, or weakness, are present and persist, notify your healthcare provider.
- Seek emergency treatment for symptoms of ketoacidosis, which include nausea, vomiting, and changes in level of consciousness.
- Test your blood glucose levels at home as you were taught, and maintain a chart of the results to show your healthcare provider.
- An insulin vial in use may be stored in the refrigerator, or for 1 month at room temperature.
- Allow insulin to warm to room temperature for use because the injection of cold insulin may irritate the tissues.
- Check the expiration date of the insulin vial to make sure the insulin is not out of date.
- Gently roll the insulin vial before drawing the insulin up. Vigorous shaking may result in air bubbles and breaks down protein molecules in the insulin.
- Avoid drinking alcohol because it can intensify the hypoglycemia produced by insulin, causing blood glucose levels to fall too low.
- Insulin requirements increase when you are under stress or are ill with an infection. Check your blood sugar frequently and report abnormal results to your healthcare provider.
- Carry a readily available source of sugar at all times, in case you suddenly develop symptoms of hypoglycemia.

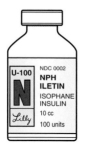

FIG. 17.7 NPH insulin vial.

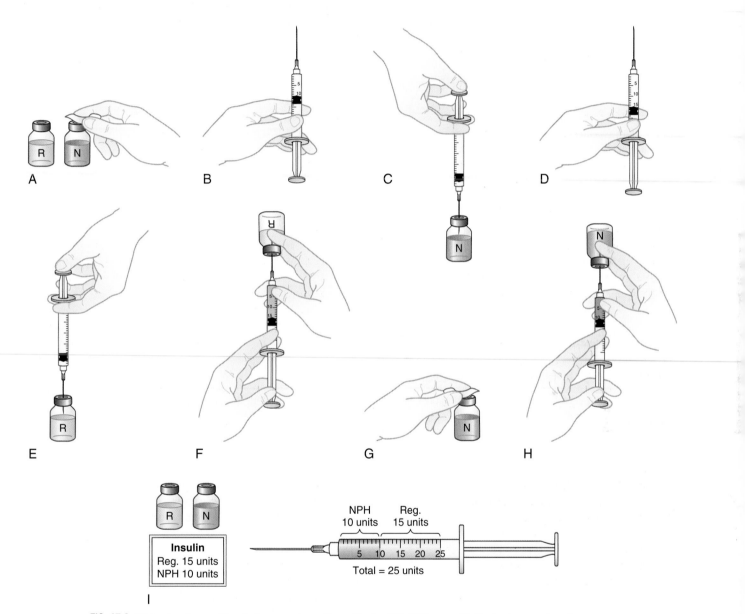

FIG. 17.8 Mixing two types of insulin in one syringe. (From Clayton BD, Willihnganz M: *Basic pharmacology for nurses,* ed 17, St. Louis, 2017, Mosby.)

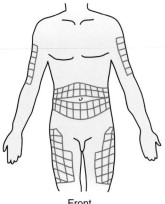

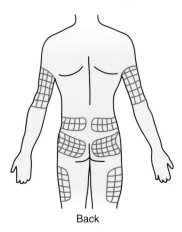

Front

Back

FIG. 17.9 Injection sites for insulin. (From Workman ML, LaCharity LA: *Understanding pharmacology,* ed 2, St. Louis, 2016, Elsevier.)

Box 17.1   **Steps to Teach Patients How to Self-Inject Insulin**

- Always wash your hands before preparing and injecting your insulin dose.
- Look at the insulin bottle and examine it carefully for the type of insulin it contains and the expiration date. If the expiration date has passed, open a new bottle.
- Make sure that the bottle of rapid-acting insulin, short-acting insulin, insulin glargine, or insulin detemir is clear and has no particles. If particles are in the insulin or if it is cloudy, do not use this bottle. Open a new bottle.
- For any other type of insulin, gently roll the bottle, pen, or cartridge between your hands to mix the insulin.
- If using an insulin bottle, clean the stopper with an alcohol sponge (not needed for prefilled pens or cartridges).
- Uncap the needle and pull back the plunger to draw in the same amount of air into the syringe as the amount of insulin you will be withdrawing from the bottle.
- Push the needle through the rubber stopper and inject the air into the insulin bottle with the bottle in the upright position (do not let the air bubble into the insulin).
- With the needle still in the bottle stopper, turn the bottle upside down and withdraw the same amount of insulin from the bottle as the amount of air you put into the bottle.

- Make sure that the tip of the plunger is on the line of the syringe for your insulin dose.
- If air bubbles are present, tap the syringe while holding it upside down, letting the bubbles come to the top of the syringe where the needle is attached. Push out any air bubbles and recheck to ensure that the tip of the plunger is on the same line as your insulin dose.
- Remove the needle from the bottle stopper and recap the needle until you are ready to inject the insulin.
- Select an area within your usual injection site that has not been injected within the past 2 weeks.
- Cleanse the skin area with an alcohol swab.
- Remove the cap from the needle on the insulin syringe.
- Pinch up a fold of skin in the area you cleaned and push the needle in at a 90-degree angle.
- Push the plunger all the way down to ensure that the entire insulin dose is injected.
- Release the fold of skin and remove the needle straight out quickly.
- Do not rub or massage the spot where you injected the insulin.
- Place the syringe with the needle (without recapping it) into a puncture-proof container.

Modified from Workman ML, LaCharity LA: *Understanding Pharmacology,* ed 2, St. Louis, 2016, Elsevier.

Get Ready for the NCLEX® Examination!

Key Points

- Insulin is the hormone of plenty, which is released when blood glucose levels are *above* normal. Its function is to lower blood glucose levels and prevent hyperglycemia.
- Glucagon is the hormone of starvation, which is released when blood glucose levels are *lower* than normal. Its function is to raise blood glucose levels and prevent hypoglycemia.
- Most people with DM have type 2 and many are not aware they have the disease.
- Regardless of whether a person has DM type 1 or type 2, the serious long-term complications are the same and often shorten the person's lifespan.
- Good management of DM that maintains blood glucose levels within the normal range most of the time can delay or prevent serious complications.
- People who have DM type 1 must use insulin to control blood glucose levels for the rest of their lives because their bodies produce no insulin.
- All insulin stimulator drugs can cause hypoglycemia when given or taken alone.
- Assess patients for any signs or symptoms of hypoglycemia (i.e., tremors, sweating, confusion, rapid heart rate, hunger, headache, nervousness, and inability to concentrate) before giving an insulin stimulator, to avoid making hypoglycemia worse. When a patient with diabetes has any of these symptoms, immediately check his or her blood glucose level.
- Do not give an insulin stimulator drug (i.e., sulfonylurea or meglitinide) to a patient who is NPO or who is skipping a meal.
- Sulfonylureas may decrease the effectiveness of certain contraceptive drugs. Women of childbearing years who are taking this antidiabetic drug will need an alternative contraceptive method to avoid an unplanned pregnancy.
- Metformin increases the risk for development of lactic acidosis.
- Metformin should be stopped 24 hours before any diagnostic tests that use radiopaque dye and not restarted until 48 hours after the test is completed.
- Alpha-glucosidase inhibitors work by interfering with digestive enzymes, so these drugs must be taken at the start of meals to get the most benefit.
- Teach patients to take prescribed antibiotics and oral contraceptives at least 1 hour *before* taking pramlintide because it interferes with the absorption of these other drugs.
- Never mix pramlintide with insulin in the same syringe.
- The sodium-glucose co-transport inhibitors increase the glucose concentration in the urine and have been associated with a risk for kidney failure.
- Insulin is a high-alert drug that can cause great harm when given at too high a dose, too low a dose, or to someone who does not have diabetes.
- Before giving any insulin dose, carefully check the order for the time, type, and amount of insulin to be given. Ensure you are giving the right insulin concentration (U-50, U-100, or U-500) and with the correct syringe designed for the insulin concentration.
- Whenever short-acting insulin is given before a meal, the patient will need to eat the meal within 15 minutes of receiving the injection to prevent hypoglycemia.
- When drawing up two different types of prescribed insulin, check to be sure they are compatible for mixing before placing them in the same syringe.
- Remind patients who use insulin or who take antidiabetic drugs that can cause hypoglycemia to always carry a readily available source of sugar at all times, in case they suddenly develop symptoms of hypoglycemia.

Review Questions for the NCLEX® Examination

1. You are preparing an injection of Lantus insulin for a diabetic patient and you note that it appears cloudy. What action should you prepare to take?
   1. Notify the pharmacy of the cloudy appearance.
   2. Vigorously shake the vial to disperse the drug.
   3. Give the insulin to the patient as scheduled.
   4. Give a rapid-acting insulin instead because they are interchangeable.
2. Which symptoms would indicate to you that a diabetic patient in your care is experiencing hypoglycemia? (Select all that apply.)
   1. Coma
   2. Tremors
   3. Confusion
   4. Pinpoint pupils
   5. Hunger sensation
   6. Fruity odor to the breath
3. A patient with newly diagnosed DM type 2 is scheduled to begin treatment with metformin. Which of the following should be part of the patient teaching plan?
   1. Metformin should be stopped 24 hours before diagnostic tests that use radiopaque dye.
   2. Metformin works by excreting glucose in the urine, which will be present on test strips.
   3. Metformin is one of the drugs injected subcutaneously to treat DM type 2.
   4. Metformin does not cause hypoglycemia when used with insulin.
4. A patient with diabetes requests to be given the oral form of insulin instead of an insulin injection. What is your best response?
   1. "Most health insurance plans will not cover this type of insulin."
   2. "Insulin is destroyed by gastric secretions and cannot be taken orally."
   3. "Insulin given by injection causes less hypoglycemia as compared with oral insulin."
   4. "Oral insulin must be taken up to four times daily; injectable insulin is taken once daily."

Get Ready for the NCLEX® Examination!—cont'd

5. A diabetic patient has been prescribed a sodium-glucose co-transport inhibitor. What adverse effect should you alert this patient to report?
   1. Signs or symptoms of a urinary tract infection
   2. Signs or symptoms of hypokalemia
   3. Redness at the injection site
   4. Abdominal pain or bloating

6. A patient with DM type 2 has been prescribed sitagliptin 100 mg daily. You have 50-mg tablets available. How many tablets should you give this patient?
   1. 3 tablets
   2. 1.5 tablets
   3. 2 tablets
   4. 0.5 tablets

7. Which problem is an adverse effect of insulin therapy?
   1. Increased blood clotting
   2. Decreased blood clotting
   3. Injection-site infection
   4. Foot ulcer formation

8. Which patient taking insulin do you need to check most frequently for hypoglycemia?
   1. 32-year-old who is pregnant with twins and allergic to avocados
   2. 40-year-old who drinks 6 to 8 cups of coffee daily and has a sedentary lifestyle
   3. 55-year-old who takes hormone replacement therapy for menopausal symptoms
   4. 70-year-old who also takes warfarin (Coumadin) daily for atrial fibrillation

9. When preparing to give a subcutaneous insulin injection to a very thin patient, which adjustment in injection technique will you make to reduce the risk for complications?
   1. Selecting a 30-gauge needle rather than a 28-gauge needle
   2. Switching the injection site to the thigh rather than the abdomen
   3. Applying pressure for at least 5 minutes after removing the needle
   4. Placing the needle at a 45-degree angle rather than at a 90-degree angle

10. A patient who received 20 units of regular insulin an hour ago is now pale, sweaty, and has trembling hands, but is alert and able to talk. What is your best first action?
    1. Prepare to give 100 mg of glucose intravenously immediately.
    2. Check the patient's blood glucose level immediately.
    3. Notify the healthcare provider immediately.
    4. Give the patient a high-protein snack immediately.

Case Study: Critical Thinking Activity

An obese 72-year-old woman with DM type 2 has been prescribed the amylin analog pramlintide. In addition to diabetes, her medical history includes high cholesterol levels and hypertension.

1. What would you tell Mrs. F. about the drug she is going to start taking?
2. What potential drug interactions should be considered?
3. What side effects may occur with this class of drug?
4. What potential adverse effects should Mrs. F. be aware of?
5. What additional teaching should be part of the care plan for an obese woman with DM type 2?

Drugs for Ear and Eye Problems

18

Learning Outcomes

1. Explain what types of drugs are used topically to manage ear problems.
2. Describe the proper technique to give drugs to the ear.
3. Explain what types of drugs are used topically to manage eye problems.
4. Describe the proper technique to give eye drops and eye ointments.
5. List the names, actions, possible side effects, and adverse effects of drugs for glaucoma.
6. Explain what to teach patients and families about different drug categories to manage glaucoma.
7. Describe lifespan considerations for drugs for glaucoma.

Key Terms

alpha-adrenergic agonists (ăd-rĕn-ĔRJ-ĭk ĂG-ō-nĭsts, p. 340) These drugs bind to receptor sites in the eye and reduce the amount of aqueous humor produced.

beta-adrenergic antagonists (BĔ-tă ăd-rĕn-ĔRJ-ĭk, p. 336) Drugs that inhibit adrenergic receptor sites in the eye and decrease production of aqueous humor.

carbonic anhydrase inhibitors (CAIs) (kăr-BŎN-ĭk ăn-HĪ-drāz ĭn-HĬB-ĭ-tŏr, p. 342) A type of diuretic that also can lower intraocular pressure by decreasing production of aqueous humor by 50-60%.

cerumenolytics (sĕ-RŪ-mĭ-nō-LĬ-tĭk, p. 331) Drugs that soften earwax.

cholinergic drugs (kō-lĭn-ĔRJ-ĭk, p. 341) Drugs that increase the availability of acetylcholine to activate specific receptors. This leads to decreased production of aqueous humor and improving outflow of aqueous humor to decrease intraocular pressure.

ophthalmic drugs (ŏf-THĂL-mĭk, p. 331) Liquid or ointment drugs prepared to place on the eye or the conjunctiva.

otic drugs (Ō-tĭk, p. 330) Drugs prepared for delivery into the external ear canal.

prostaglandin agonists (prŏ-stă-GLĂN-dĭn ĂG-ō-nĭsts, p. 335) Drugs that bind to specific prostaglandin receptor sites in the eye causing an increase outflow of aqueous humor.

EAR PROBLEMS

EAR STRUCTURE AND FUNCTION

The ear, along with the brain, is the organ that allows hearing. It has three parts that are important to hearing: the external ear, the middle ear, and the inner ear.

The external ear is known as the pinna (Fig. 18.1). It is made of cartilage covered by skin and attached to the side of the head. The external ear extends from the pinna through the external ear canal to the *tympanic membrane* (eardrum) (Fig. 18.2). The *ear canal* is an S-shaped tube open to the outside that ends at the eardrum. This canal is lined with hair cells and cells that produce *cerumen* (also called "earwax") and oil. Cerumen helps protect and lubricate the ear canal. In adults, the ear canal tilts downward and is slightly curved in an S-shape that is about 1 to 1½ inches (2.5–3.75 cm) long. In children the canal is shorter and straighter.

The middle ear is a small compartment that extends from the eardrum to the oval and round windows of the wall separating it from the inner ear. It contains the top opening of the *eustachian tube* and three small bones known as the *bony ossicles*, which are the *malleus* (hammer), the *incus* (anvil), and the *stapes* (stirrup) (see Fig. 18.2). The bony ossicles are joined loosely, which allows them to move and "jiggle" with vibrations created when sound waves hit the eardrum. The eustachian tube extends from the floor of the middle ear to the back of the throat. This allows pressure on both sides of the eardrum to equalize. (You may have felt this as a "popping" sensation when you swallow or yawn, especially when traveling in a car up and down steep hills.) The eustachian tube normally allows secretions to drain from the middle ear into the throat. This opening from the throat to the middle ear also allows organisms in the throat to move upward (ascend) into the middle ear and cause *otitis media* (middle ear infection).

The inner ear is on the other side of the oval window and contains the semicircular canals, the cochlea, the vestibule, and the end of the eighth cranial nerve (see Fig. 18.2). The *semicircular canals* are tubes that contain fluid and hair cells and are connected to the eighth cranial nerve. The fluid and hair cells within the canals help maintain the sense of balance. The *cochlea* is the fluid-filled organ with hair cells that detect vibration from sound and stimulate the eighth cranial nerve.

Hearing is the main function of the ear and occurs when sound waves are moved through the air to the external ear canal. These waves then hit the movable eardrum, creating vibrations that are transferred to the bones (ossicles) of the middle ear. The vibrations move the three small, loose bones in the middle ear, which then allows the vibrations to be transmitted to the cochlea of the inner ear. In the cochlea, the vibrations stimulate the nerve of hearing (the eighth cranial nerve), which carries the impulse to the areas of the brain that allow the nerve impulses to be "heard" and interpreted as sounds.

DRUGS TO MANAGE EAR PROBLEMS

The most common ear problems are infection and inflammation that occur in the external ear and in the middle ear. When these problems occur in the middle ear, antimicrobials and anti-inflammatories are given systemically, most often by the oral route. The actions, side effects, and nursing implications of systemic antimicrobials are discussed in Chapter 5. The actions, side effects, and nursing implications of systemic anti-inflammatories are discussed in Chapter 12.

Infections and inflammation of the pinna and the ear canal are most often managed by topical drug application because the external ear can be reached from the outside. The actions of topical antimicrobial drugs and anti-inflammatories are the same as those given systemically and are discussed in Chapters 5 and 12. Drugs that are prepared to apply into the external ear canal are **otic drugs**. Box 18.1 presents the techniques involved in giving *(instilling)* eardrops into the ear canal. Fig. 18.3 shows the correct techniques for instilling eardrops into adults (see Fig. 18.3A) and children younger than 3 years (see Fig. 18.3B).

> ⌂ **Top Tip for Safety**
>
> Apply only drugs and liquids labeled "for otic use" into the ear canal.

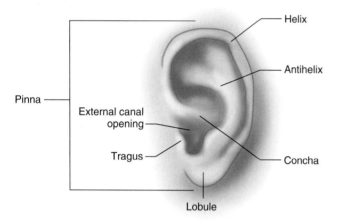

FIG. 18.1 The external ear (pinna). (From Ignatavicius D, Workman ML, Rebar C: *Medical-surgical nursing,* ed 9, St. Louis, 2018, Saunders.)

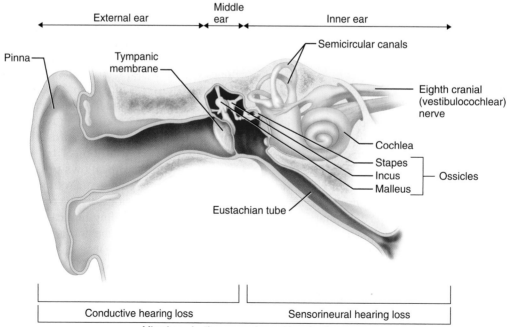

FIG. 18.2 Anatomy of the middle and inner ear. (From Ignatavicius D, Workman ML, Rebar C: *Medical-surgical nursing,* ed 9, St. Louis, 2018, Saunders.)

The length and angle of ear canals differ between young children and adults. In adults the ear canal tilts downward, is longer, and is slightly curved in an S-shape. In children the canal is shorter and straighter. These differences require differences in technique when instilling drugs into the ear canal.

- When instilling eardrops into an adult's ear, gently pull the external ear up and back (see Fig. 18.3A).
- When instilling eardrops into a child's ear, gently pull the external ear down and back (see Fig. 18.3B).

Box 18.1	Technique for Instilling Eardrops Into a Patient's Ear

- Make sure that the patient's eardrum is intact. This may require assessment by the RN or other healthcare provider. Never give an ear drug if there is damage to the eardrum.
- Read the label of the drug carefully to ensure that it is "for otic use." Never put any solution in the ear that is not labeled specifically for use in ears.
- Verify the drug using the 9 Rights of Drug Administration.
- Wash your hands and don a pair of clean gloves.
- Warm the eardrops to room temperature.
- Ask the patient to lie down with the head turned so that the affected ear is turned upward; if the patient is sitting in a chair, tilt the patient's head so the affected ear is up.
- For a young child (younger than 3 years), gently pull the pinna down and back.
- For an older child or adult, pull the pinna up and back.
- Using the applicator, place only the prescribed number of drops into the patient's ear. Aim the drops onto the side of the ear canal and let them run into the ear.
- Insert a cotton ball into the opening of the ear canal to keep the drops from rolling out of the ear.
- Remind the patient to keep his or her head in this position for 2 to 5 minutes as directed to allow the drops to flow.
- Remove your gloves and wash your hands.

Another problem that can occur in the external ear canal is an excessive buildup of cerumen to such an extent that sound waves are blocked, hearing is reduced, and the patient has ear pain. For this problem, instillation of **cerumenolytic** drugs (that soften earwax) may be used before irrigation of the ear. (Review ear irrigation in your fundamentals or medical-surgical nursing textbook.) These drugs are available over the counter and most often contain a carbamide peroxide combination (Table 18.1). An important issue to remember and to teach patients about the use of such a product is to *never* use it in an ear that has drainage or discharge because the eardrum may not be intact and the solution could enter the middle ear, causing an infection. Also, do not instill a cerumenolytic or irrigate an ear canal in a person who is dizzy, because these actions will increase the dizziness. Recent literature suggests that distilled water or saline may be just as effective as oil- or peroxide-based solutions. Carefully review the order and do not hesitate to ask the healthcare provider if you have questions.

Never place a drug into the ear canal or irrigate the ear canal if there is drainage present because it could enter the middle ear and cause an infection.

EYE PROBLEMS

Together the eye and the brain allow sight (vision). Although many problems can affect the eye and vision, those that can be managed with drug therapy are inflammation, infection, and glaucoma. Drugs for these problems are **ophthalmic drugs**, which come in liquid drops or ointment form. Chapter 12 discusses various types of anti-inflammatory drugs, nearly all of which have an ophthalmic form. Chapter 5 discusses antimicrobial drug therapy. Many antimicrobial and anti-inflammatory drugs have an ophthalmic form, and their

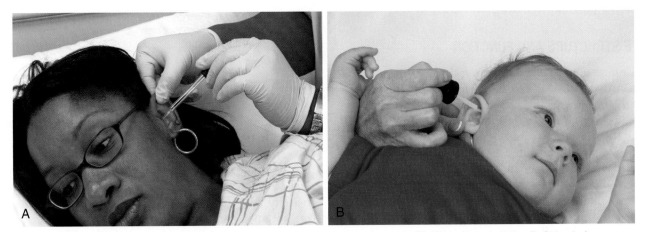

FIG. 18.3 Correct techniques for giving eardrops to an adult (A) and to a child (B). (From Perry A, Potter P, Ostendorf W: *Clinical nursing skills & techniques*, ed 8, St. Louis, 2014, Mosby.)

Table 18.1 **Example of Cerumenolytic**

Cerumenolytics: These agents are typically solvents used to break up or soften earwax so that it can be easily removed.

DRUG/ADULT DOSAGE RANGE	NURSING IMPLICATIONS
Carbamide peroxide (Debrox, Murine Ear Wax removal Adults, adolescents, and children 12 years and older: Instill 5–10 drops twice daily in the affected ear(s) for up to 4 days. Keep drops in ear for 5 minutes by keeping head tilted or placing cotton in ear. Do not use for more than 4 days. The kit comes with an ear syringe for flushing.	• Teach patients that side effects are rare and include redness, itching, or rash. • Do not give drug if patient has any symptoms of infection or any discharge from the ear because this may cause damage to the middle or inner ear. • To avoid dizziness, give the drug while the patient is lying down and the affected ear is turned upward. • Do not insert the tip of the applicator into the ear canal to avoid contamination of the tip or damage to the ear. • Remind the patient to remain lying down for at least 5 minutes after giving the drops for maximum effectiveness. • Make sure that the drug is room temperature. Drugs that are too cold or too warm can cause dizziness, nausea, and even burns to the ear. • To avoid infection, do not share the drug with other patients. • Gently flush the ear with warm water after application of drug with a bulb syringe or the syringe provided by the manufacturer. • Remind patient that they may hear a bubbling sound after they instill the eardrops.

actions are the same as the systemic form. Follow directions carefully when giving the ophthalmic form to avoid underdosing or overdosing.

This chapter focuses on drug therapy to manage the chronic eye disorder of glaucoma, which cannot be cured but can be controlled. Although the actions and uses for these drugs differ, some nursing implications are the same for all of them. In addition, many of the points to teach patients and families about these drugs are the same. Box 18.2 describes these common nursing considerations for ophthalmic drugs, and Box 18.3 describes general patient teaching points. Nursing considerations and patient teaching issues specific to any single drug type are listed with the individual drug categories.

Drug therapy for any eye problem requires that the drops or ointment be instilled using correct technique to ensure the drug is in contact with the eye and that no harm or infection occurs. Box 18.4 describes the correct technique for instilling opthalmic drugs to a patient, and Box 18.5 describes the correct technique to teach patients how to place drugs into their own eyes.

EYE STRUCTURE AND FUNCTION

Vision results from light moving through the eye and meeting the optic nerve, where images are interpreted by the brain. Fig. 18.4 shows the basic anatomy of the eye, as well as the *lacrimal gland* (tear gland), *lacrimal sack* (tear sac), and *nasolacrimal* duct. Fig. 18.5 shows much greater detail of the eye itself. From the side view, you can see the eye is divided into the *anterior segment* and the *posterior segment*. Then the anterior segment divides into the *anterior chamber* and the *posterior chamber*. The space between the cornea and the lens is filled with a watery fluid called *aqueous humor*. Aqueous humor is produced by the *ciliary body* and flows from the

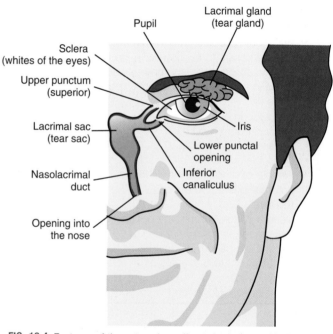

FIG. 18.4 Features of the external eye (front view) along with the tear gland and duct system. (From Workman ML, LaCharity LA: *Understanding pharmacology*, ed 2, St. Louis, 2016, Elsevier.)

posterior chamber to the anterior chamber, where it drains through the trabecular network and is reabsorbed by the body. Normal circulation of the fluid through this space is important in maintaining a normal *intraocular pressure* (IOP). Normal IOP is between 10 and 20 mm Hg. Maintenance of a normal IOP keeps the eye healthy and helps prevent blindness. This will be important when you learn later in this chapter how drugs work to treat glaucoma. From the side view (Fig. 18.5), you can see that the cornea covers the eye. The

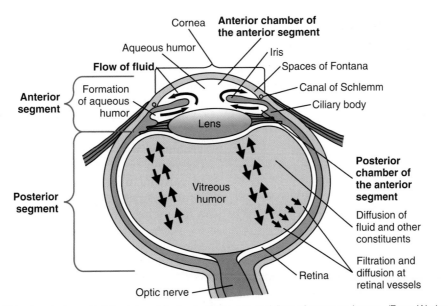

FIG. 18.5 Side view (cutaway) of the internal features of the eye and flow of aqueous humor. (From Workman ML, LaCharity LA: *Understanding pharmacology,* ed 2, St. Louis, 2016, Elsevier.)

clarity of the cornea is important because the cornea allows light to enter the eye.

The iris is the muscular ring around the eye (see Figs. 18.4 and 18.5). Pigments in the iris give you the color of your eyes (as determined by your genetic makeup). The muscular iris helps adjust the pupil size to determine how much light enters the eye at any given time. Impulses from the autonomic nervous system cause the muscle to make the adjustment. Constriction of the pupil reduces the amount of light into the eye, and dilation of the pupil increases the light let into the eye (Fig. 18.6). Constriction of the pupil is called *miosis*; dilation of the pupil is called *mydriasis*. An easy way to remember this is: "miosis—small word, small pupil; mydriasis—large word, large pupil."

Constriction and dilation of the pupil occur continually as we adjust to varying amounts of light in our environment. For example, when you walk from a dark room into the sunlight, your pupil constricts to reduce the amount of light that gets to the retina (too much light can be very uncomfortable). When you come from the daylight into a dark movie theater, your pupils dilate to let more light in so you can get to your seat (see Fig. 18.6).

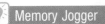

> **Memory Jogger**
>
> Pupil constriction is *miosis* (small word, small pupil size). Pupil dilation is *mydriasis* (larger word, larger pupil size).

The *posterior segment* of the eye contains the retina and the optic nerve (see Fig. 18.5). The *retina* is the lining on the back of the eye. The retina is light sensitive and contains special cells involved in helping to turn light into electrical impulses. The posterior segment is

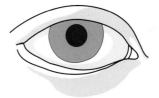

A Normal pupil slightly dilated for moderate light.

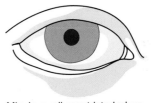

B Miosis–pupil constricted when exposed to increased light or close work, such as reading. (Smaller word, smaller opening.)

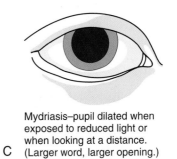

C Mydriasis–pupil dilated when exposed to reduced light or when looking at a distance. (Larger word, larger opening.)

FIG. 18.6 Comparison of pupil size: normal (A), miosis (B), and mydriasis (C). (From Workman ML, LaCharity LA: *Understanding pharmacology,* ed 2, St. Louis, 2016, Elsevier.)

filled with a jelly-like fluid called *vitreous humor*. The optic nerve in the back of the eye carries messages from the special cells in the retina to the brain, where we then "see" the images. Any increase in pressure in the eye can damage blood vessels in the retina, which then damages the specialized cells in the retina and the optic nerve that carries messages to the brain.

Memory Jogger

Normal IOP is between 10 and 20 mm Hg. Maintenance of a normal IOP keeps the eye healthy and helps prevent blindness in patients with glaucoma.

Bookmark This!

The National Eye Institute (https://nei.nih.gov/) has fantastic resources for healthcare professionals, patients, and their families about a wide range of eye disorders. In particular, the National Eye Institute has a great bank of photographs and videos that will help explain what happens in these disorders. Resources are available in English and in Spanish.

GLAUCOMA

Glaucoma is a chronic eye disease of increased IOP that causes damage to the optic nerve (Fig. 18.7). If untreated, glaucoma causes loss of peripheral vision and even blindness (Fig. 18.8). The disease is described as a "thief of the night" because the patient typically has no symptoms other than a gradual loss of *peripheral* side vision. By the time the patient realizes that vision is decreased, he or she has already experienced a degree of permanent vision loss. Those at great risk include African Americans older than 40 years, patients with a family history of glaucoma, and patients older than 60 years, especially Mexican Americans. Although glaucoma typically occurs in adults, eye trauma can cause glaucoma in children.

Glaucoma is an eye disorder that results from too much aqueous humor. As mentioned earlier, aqueous humor is a fluid, similar to plasma, produced by the ciliary body in the eye (see Fig. 18.5). This fluid provides oxygen and nutrients to the cornea, trabecular meshwork, and the lens of the eye. Normally aqueous humor flows freely in the eye, providing nutrition and removing waste products. In the most common type of glaucoma,

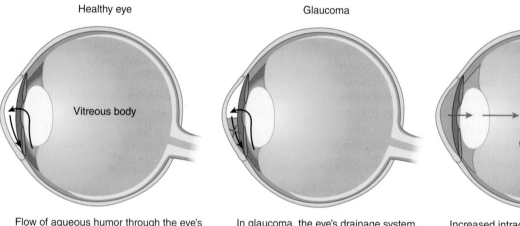

Healthy eye

Vitreous body

Glaucoma

Flow of aqueous humor through the eye's drainage system (trabecular network)

In glaucoma, the eye's drainage system does not work properly so fluid builds up and intraocular pressure increases

Increased intraocular pressure damages the optic nerve in the back of the eye leading to blindness

FIG. 18.7 Increased intraocular pressure from too much aqueous humor causing damage to the optic nerve in glaucoma.

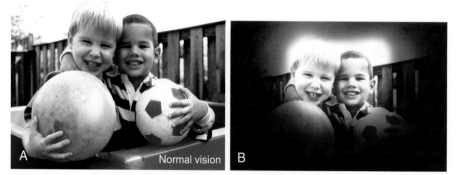

A   Normal vision   B

FIG. 18.8 (A) Scene as viewed by a person with normal vision. (B) Scene as viewed by a person with glaucoma. (Courtesy National Eye Institute, National Institutes of Health.)

primary open-angle closure glaucoma, aqueous humor does not drain through the normal pathways. This results in a buildup of fluid and increased IOP in the anterior chamber of the eye (see Fig. 18.7). The fluid increases pressure in the eye leading to damage of the retina and the optic nerve.

In rare situations a condition called *acute angle closure glaucoma* causes a sudden increase in IOP. This leads to severe eye pain, nausea and vomiting, and the patient may report seeing halos around lights. Acute angle closure glaucoma is a medical emergency. Any patient with symptoms of acute angle closure glaucoma should receive emergency treatment to avoid blindness.

> **Memory Jogger**
>
> Glaucoma is a chronic disease with no cure. Drug therapy can prevent further damage and blindness, and must continue for rest of the patient's life.

Drug therapy for patients with glaucoma involves reducing the amount of aqueous humor produced by the ciliary body or improving drainage and reabsorption of the aqueous humor. This decreases fluid pressure in the eye and relieves pressure on the retina and the optic nerve. Drugs for glaucoma are typically given as eye drops to the affected eye(s). In emergency cases of acute angle closure glaucoma, drugs may be given orally or intravenously to rapidly reduce IOP. Healthcare providers may recommend select drugs from five classes to manage glaucoma: prostaglandin agonists (sometimes called *prostaglandin analogs*), beta-adrenergic antagonists (blockers), alpha-adrenergic agonists, cholinergic drugs, and carbonic anhydrase inhibitors (CAIs).

> **Memory Jogger**
>
> The five classes of drugs to treat glaucoma are:
> - prostaglandin agonists (sometimes called *prostaglandin analogs*)
> - beta-adrenergic antagonists (blockers)
> - alpha-adrenergic agonists
> - cholinergic drugs
> - CAIs

PROSTAGLANDIN AGONISTS

Action and Uses

Prostaglandin agonists help to control glaucoma by binding to prostaglandin receptor sites in the eye and relaxing eye blood vessel smooth muscles, which allows these blood vessels to dilate and absorb aqueous humor. As a result, more aqueous fluid enters the blood and less is present in the eye, lowering the IOP. For many people, the prostaglandin agonists are very effective at controlling IOP. They are used only once a day and have fewer systemic side effects than other drugs. Names, usual adult dosages, and nursing implications of these drugs are listed in Table 18.2. Be sure to consult a drug reference book for more information about specific prostaglandin agonists.

Expected Side Effects

The most common side effects of prostaglandin agonists are eye itching and eye redness when they are first applied. In some cases, patients have a foreign body sensation (feels like something is in their eye).

Over time patients who take prostaglandin agonists may develop changes in the color of the iris from lighter colors to brown (Fig. 18.9). This is a gradual change

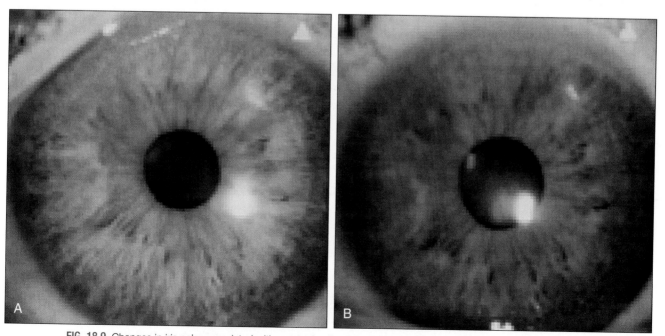

FIG. 18.9 Changes in iris color associated with prostaglandin agonist drug therapy for glaucoma. (A) Before treatment. (B) After treatment. (From Yanoff M, Duker J: *Ophthalmology*, ed 4, St. Louis, 2014, Mosby.)

and is permanent. The color change is most common in people who have brown pigment in their eyes. The drug also causes thickening and lengthening of the eyelashes and darkening of the skin on the eyelids.

Adverse Effects

In rare cases patients who are taking prostaglandin agonists can experience systemic effects including infection, asthma, and corneal erosion (damage to the cornea).

❖ Nursing Implications and Patient Teaching

◆ *Assessment.* In addition to the general nursing considerations related to eye drug therapy listed in Box 18.2, make sure to assess the patient's understanding that glaucoma is a chronic disease and will require adherence to drug therapy to prevent decreased vision and even blindness. For all patients who are taking prostaglandin agonists, it is important to check the affected eye for any scratches (corneal abrasion) or other signs of trauma. Never give these drugs if there is any damage to the eye surface.

> #### ⬦ Top Tip for Safety
>
> Never instill prostaglandin agonists into an eye that has been scratched or has an infection. Contact the healthcare provider for instructions about continuing glaucoma therapy and managing the corneal problem.

◆ *Patient and family teaching.* In addition to the general teaching points listed in Box 18.3, tell the patient and the family the following:

- Avoid using higher than prescribed doses because higher doses can reduce the effectiveness of the drug in controlling glaucoma.
- If you have lighter eyes, your eye and eyelid color can change over time, and the lashes can become thicker and longer. If only one eye has glaucoma, the color and lash changes will occur only in that eye.
- If you have glaucoma only in one eye, do not place the drops in the unaffected eye even though the colors of your eyes may now be different.

BETA-ADRENERGIC ANTAGONISTS

Actions

Beta-adrenergic antagonists (also called *beta blockers*) reduce the amount of aqueous humor produced from the ciliary body of the eye. They do this by binding to beta-adrenergic receptors in the ciliary body of the eye. Normally cells in the ciliary body produce aqueous humor, so blocking the action of these cells reduces the production of aqueous humor. Common beta blockers for glaucoma, dosages, and nursing implications are listed in Table 18.2. Be sure to consult a drug reference book for more information about specific beta-blocking agents to control glaucoma.

Expected Side Effects

Expected side effects for beta-adrenergic antagonists often occur within a few minutes of instilling the drops in the eye. These include temporary blurring of vision, slight burning or stinging, and tearing of the eye. Later the patient may notice less tear production and dry, itchy, or red eyes. Beta blockers constrict the pupil (i.e., cause miosis). It is important for patients to understand that their pupils do not dilate as easily when they go into a dark room.

> #### 💡 Memory Jogger
>
> To determine whether a drug is a beta blocker, look for the suffix (word ending) *-olol.*

Adverse Effects

The greatest risk of problems from beta-blocker ophthalmic drugs occurs when they are unintentionally absorbed systemically. This can occur if drops are absorbed through the conjunctiva, the tear ducts, the nose, or other eye tissues. If absorbed systemically, beta blockers can cause the same effects you would see if you gave them orally, as discussed in Chapter 8. Patients could experience decreased heart rate, decreased blood pressure, and even heart failure. Systemic absorption of beta blockers can also cause bronchoconstriction and asthma symptoms.

❖ Nursing Implications and Patient Teaching

◆ *Assessment.* In addition to the general nursing considerations related to eye drug therapy listed in Box 18.2, determine the patient's baseline vital signs. Watch for changes in heart rate and blood pressure. If the patient has any respiratory problems such as asthma or chronic obstructive pulmonary disease (COPD), make sure to monitor for any shortness of breath or changes in pulse oximetry. Assess carefully to determine whether the patient is also taking oral beta blockers (see Chapter 8) to control blood pressure or other heart dysrhythmia. If so, notify the healthcare provider to make sure he or she is aware of the oral drug before giving the eye drops. Ophthalmic beta blockers may increase the risk for expected side effects and adverse effects of the oral beta blocker.

◆ *Planning and intervention.* Never touch the tip of the eye dropper or touch the tip directly to the patient's eye, to avoid contaminating the tip. To decrease systemic absorption of eye drops, use only the prescribed amount of the eye drops. After giving the drops, ask the patient to close his or her eyes for 2 minutes. Closing the eyes for 2 minutes reduces the amount of drug absorbed systemically. Another option to reduce systemic absorption of the drug is *digital nasolacrimal occlusion* (this technique has also been called *punctal occlusion*). Simply speaking, this means putting gentle pressure with the index finger over the tear duct in the inner corner of the eye for about 3 minutes after giving the eye drops.

Box 18.2   General Nursing Considerations for Ophthalmic Drug Therapy

- Always wash your hands before and after giving eye drops (use gloves if available).
- Assess the patient's eye for redness, drainage, or open areas. In some cases redness is a side effect of the eye drugs but could also be a sign of infection. If there is any new redness, drainage, or open areas, notify the RN or healthcare provider before giving the eye drugs.
- Never touch the tip of the applicator/dropper or the inside of the cap to avoid contamination and reduce the risk for infection.
- Always check to make sure that you are giving the correct concentration of the drug and correct number of drops in the correct eye.
- Only use drugs that are specifically labeled for ophthalmic use.
- Remove contact lenses before giving eye drops and read the drug inserts carefully to see if the patient is able to use his or her contact lenses over the course of the therapy.
- If giving more than one type of eye drop, wait at least 5 minutes between instillations to avoid drug interaction.
- Teach the patient that his or her vision may be slightly blurry for a few minutes after giving eye drops and slightly longer for eye ointment. Avoid any significant activity until the blurred vision passes to reduce risk for falls.
- Always report any sudden eye pain or sudden changes in vision to the healthcare provider immediately because these symptoms may indicate potential for eye injury and even blindness.
- Follow the directions in Box 18.4 for instilling eye drops or ointments into a patient's eye.
- Fig. 18.10 shows the correct technique for applying eye drops.
- After giving eye drops, ask the patient to close his or her eyes for 2 minutes; this reduces the amount of drug absorbed systemically. A second option to reduce systemic absorption of the drug is to apply gentle pressure with the index finger over the tear duct in the inner corner of the eye for about 3 minutes after giving the eye drops (Fig. 18.11).
- Fig. 18.12 shows the correct technique for applying eye ointments.

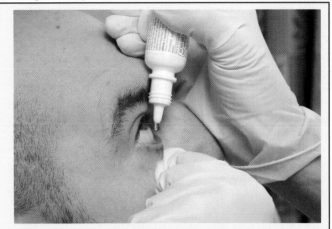

FIG. 18.10 Correct technique for instilling eye drops. (From Perry A, Potter P, Ostendorf W: *Clinical nursing skills & techniques,* ed 9, St. Louis, 2017, Mosby.)

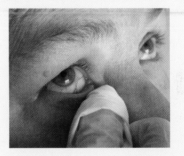

FIG. 18.11 Applying digital nasolacrimal occlusion (also called *punctal occlusion*) to prevent systemic absorption. (From Workman ML, LaCharity LA: *Understanding pharmacology,* ed 2, St. Louis, 2016, Elsevier.)

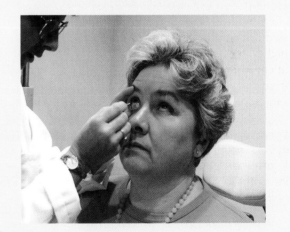

FIG. 18.12 Correct technique for instilling ointment into the eye. (From Ignatavicius D, Workman ML, Rebar C: *Medical-surgical nursing,* ed 9, St. Louis, 2018, Saunders.)

Box 18.3 **General Teaching Points for Patients and Families During Topical Eye Drug Therapy**

- Use only drugs that are labeled "for ophthalmic use only." Never place any solution in the eye that is not properly labeled.
- Eye drops are typically clear, thin, liquid drugs that are supplied in a bottle specifically labeled "for ophthalmic use only."
- Eye ointments are thick, often appear "greasy," and come in a squeezable tube. The ointment remains in contact with the eye for a longer period than the eye drops.
- The concentration of the drugs is on the label and must be carefully compared with the drug order.
- Use only the prescribed number of eye drops into the eye because too much of the drug can lead to adverse effects.
- Never share eye drops or ointments with another person to avoid eye injury and decrease risk for infection.
- Wash your hands thoroughly and, if available, put on clean gloves.
- Ask the patient to remove glasses or contact lenses before giving the eye drugs (contact lenses can absorb the eye drugs so they must be removed).
- Remove the cap of the eye drug and place it upside down on the table to avoid contamination.
- Never touch the tip of the eye dropper/applicator with your finger or to the patient's eye. The tip should remain sterile.

- Ask the patient to tilt his or her head back slightly to look at the ceiling. With a tissue, gently retract the lower lid to expose the conjunctival sac.
- Teach the patient (or family) the proper technique for giving eye drops. Over-the-counter saline drops can be used to practice the technique and avoid waste of the eye drugs.
- The patient should never drive or use heavy machinery if having blurred vision after taking the eye drugs.
- After giving eye drops, ask the patient to close his or her eyes for 2 minutes; this reduces the amount of drug absorbed systemically. A second option to reduce systemic absorption of the drug is to apply gentle pressure with the index finger over the tear duct in the inner corner of the eye for about 3 minutes after giving the eye drops.
- Always report any sudden eye pain or sudden changes in vision to the healthcare provider immediately because these symptoms may indicate potential for eye injury and even blindness.
- Teach patients that if there are any new symptoms while taking the drug (whether relating to the eye or general symptoms) to let their healthcare provider know right away.
- Should there be any sudden decrease or loss of vision, teach the patient to go to the emergency department or call 911.

Box 18.4 **Technique for Giving Eye Drops or Ointments to a Patient**

1. Check the name, strength, expiration date, color, and clarity of the eye drops to be instilled. If the drug is an ointment, be sure that it is an ophthalmic (eye) preparation and not a general topical ointment.
2. Check to see whether only one eye is to have the drug or whether both eyes are to receive the drug.
3. If both eyes are to receive the same drug and one eye is infected, use two separate bottles or tubes and carefully label each with "right" or "left" for the correct eye.
4. Wash your hands and put on gloves.
5. Explain the procedure to the patient.
6. Make sure the patient is not wearing contact lenses; if the patient is, ask him or her to remove them.
7. Have the patient sit in a chair while you stand behind the patient (or alternatively stand in front of the patient who is sitting in a chair or over the patient who is lying in bed).
8. Ask the patient to tilt his or her head backward, with the back of the head resting against you (or the back of the chair), and look up at the ceiling.
9. Gently pull the lower lid down against the patient's cheek, forming a small pocket.
10. Hold the eye-drop bottle or ointment tube (with the cap off) like a pencil, with the tip pointing down.
11. For ointment, squeeze a small amount out onto a tissue (without touching the tip to the tissue) and discard this ointment.

12. For eye drops, gently squeeze the bottle and release the prescribed number of drops into the pocket that you have made with the patient's lower eyelid. Do not touch any part of the eye or lid with the tip of the bottle. For ointment, gently squeeze the tube and release a small amount of ointment into the pocket that you have made with the patient's lower eyelid. Do not touch any part of the eye or lid with the tip of the tube.
13. Gently release the lower eyelid.
14. Ask the patient to close his or her eye gently, without squeezing the lids tightly, and roll the eye under the lid to spread the drug across the eye for about 2 minutes.
15. As an alternative to closing the eyes after giving eye drops, with a gloved finger, gently press and hold the corner of the eye nearest the nose to close off the tear duct for about 3 minutes to prevent the drug from being absorbed systemically.
16. Without pressing on the eyelid, gently blot or wipe away any excess drug or tears with a tissue.
17. Gently release the lower lid.
18. Remove your gloves.
19. Recap the tube or bottle.
20. Wash your hands again.
21. Replace contact lenses as appropriate.
22. Remind patients that their vision will be blurry and not to drive until their vision clears.

Adapted from Workman ML, LaCharity LA: *Understanding pharmacology*, ed 2, St. Louis, 2016, Elsevier.

Table 18.2 Examples of Prostaglandin Agonist and Beta-Adrenergic Antagonist Drugs

Prostaglandins agonists: help control glaucoma by binding to prostaglandin receptor sites in the eye and relax eye blood vessel smooth muscles, which allows these blood vessels to dilate and absorb aqueous humor

DRUG/ADULT DOSAGE RANGE	NURSING IMPLICATIONS
bimatoprost (Lumigan) 1 drop of a 0.01% solution in the affected eye or eyes daily in the evening latanoprost (Xalatan 0.005%) 1 drop (1.5 mcg) in affected eye or eyes daily in the evening travoprost (Travatan 0.004%, Travatan Z 0.004%) 1 drop in affected eye or eyes daily in the evening	• Check the eye carefully for any scratches or signs of trauma. If so, hold the drug and contact the registered nurse or healthcare provider because these drugs should not be given if there are any breaks in the tissue. • Teach patients that they may notice changes in the color of the affected eye (usually becomes darker). Patients may notice a slightly darker color on the eyelid. These color changes may be permanent. • Eyelashes on the affected eye may grow longer and thicker. Do not attempt to use the drops in the unaffected eye to make the eyelashes match because the drug may be dangerous if used inappropriately.

Beta-adrenergic antagonists: reduce the amount of aqueous humor by binding to beta-adrenergic receptors in the ciliary body of the eye

DRUG/ADULT DOSAGE RANGE	NURSING IMPLICATIONS
betaxolol hydrochloride (Betoptic, Kerlone) 1–2 drops (0.5% solution) in affected eye every 12 hours carteolol (Cartrol, Ocupress) 1 drop (1% solution) in affected eye every 12 hours levobunolol (Ak-Beta, Betagan) 1–2 drops (0.25% solution) in affected eye every 12 hours; 1–2 drops (0.5% solution) in affected eye once daily metipranolol (OptiPranolol) 1 drop (0.3% solution) in affected eye every 12 hours timolol (Betimol, Istalol, Timoptic) 1 drop (0.25% solution or 0.5% solution) in affected eye once or twice daily timolol GFS (gel-forming solution) (Timoptic-XE) 1 drop (0.25% solution or 0.5% solution) in affected eye once or twice daily	• To reduce the risk for systemic absorption, perform digital nasolacrimal occlusion on the affected eye or remind the patient to keep the eye closed for 2–3 minutes. • Check vital signs every 4–8 hours while the patient is receiving these drugs to assess for any decreases in heart rate or blood pressure, or note any increased respiratory effects because these can be signs of systemic absorption. • Recheck the blood sugar in patients with diabetes regularly because beta blockers can mask the symptoms of hypoglycemia.

Box 18.5 Technique for Self-Administration of Eye Drugs

1. Check the name, strength, expiration date, color, and clarity of the eye drops to be instilled. If the drug is an ointment, be sure that it is an ophthalmic (eye) preparation and not a general topical ointment.
2. Check to see whether only one eye is to have the drug or if both of your eyes are to receive the drug.
3. If both eyes are to receive the same drug and one eye is infected, use two separate bottles or tubes and carefully label each with "right" or "left" for the correct eye.
4. Wash your hands.
5. Remove the cap from the bottle or tube, keeping the cap upright to prevent contaminating it.
6. Remove contact lenses if present.
7. Tilt your head backward, open your eyes, and look up at the ceiling.
8. Using your nondominant hand, gently pull the lower lid down against your cheek, forming a small pocket.
9. Hold the eye-drop bottle or ointment tube (with the cap off) like a pencil with the tip pointing down with your dominant hand.
10. For ointment, squeeze a small amount out onto a tissue (without touching the tip to the tissue) and discard this ointment.
11. Rest your wrist that is holding the bottle or tube against your mouth or upper lip.
12. For eye drops, gently squeeze the bottle and release the prescribed number of drops into the pocket that you have made with your lower lid. Do not touch any part of the eye or lid with the tip of the bottle. For ointment, gently squeeze the tube and release a small amount of ointment into the pocket that you have made with your lower eyelid. Do not touch any part of the eye or lid with the tip of the tube.
13. Gently release your lower eyelid.
14. Close your eye gently (without squeezing the lids tight) and roll your eye under the eyelid to spread the drug across the eye.
15. Keep your eye closed for about 2 minutes.
16. As an alternative to keeping your eye closed for two minutes, gently press and hold the corner of the eye nearest to your nose to close off the punctum for about 3 minutes and prevent the drug from being absorbed systemically.
17. Without pressing on your eyelid, gently blot or wipe away any excess drug or tears with a tissue.
18. Gently release your lower eyelid.
19. Recap the bottle or tube.
20. Replace contact lenses as appropriate.
21. Wash your hands again.
22. Do not drive or operate heavy machinery while your vision is blurry.

Adapted from Workman ML, LaCharity LA: *Understanding pharmacology*, ed 2, St. Louis, 2016, Elsevier.

A word of caution: Even with the techniques to decrease systemic absorption of the eye drops, you will still need to carefully monitor for adverse effects of the drug.

⬆ Top Tip for Safety

To reduce systemic absorption of eye drops, give only the prescribed number of eye drops; then ask the patient to close his or her eyes for 2 minutes or place a gloved finger over the tear duct and apply gentle pressure for about 3 minutes.

◆ *Evaluation.* Monitor the patient for expected side effects and adverse effects. Report any significant change in vital signs, particularly blood pressure below 90/60 mm Hg or heart rate less than 60. Watch for any changes in respiratory status including shortness of breath or wheezing, or decreased pulse oximetry below 92%.

⬆ Top Tip for Safety

To avoid contamination, never touch the tip of the applicator with your finger or directly on the patient's eye.

◆ *Patient and family teaching.* In addition to the general teaching points listed in Box 18.3, tell the patient and family the following:

- Do not increase the dose or use the drug more often because excessive use increases the risk for heart and breathing problems, especially if you have asthma, COPD, or other respiratory problems.
- Use good lighting when reading and use caution in darker rooms because the eye pupil will not dilate to let in more light, and it may be harder to see objects in dim light. This problem can increase your risk for falls.
- Avoid driving at night as your vision will be reduced.
- If you have diabetes, check your blood glucose more often because these drugs can mask the symptoms of hypoglycemia if the drug is absorbed systemically.

🍃 Lifespan Considerations

Beta-Adrenergic Blocking Agents for Older Adults

Before giving beta-blocker eye drops to patients, make sure they are not taking any oral beta-blocker drugs for a cardiac condition. If so, notify the healthcare provider. Older adults are more likely to have cardiac and respiratory problems from systemic absorption of eye drops.

ALPHA-ADRENERGIC AGONISTS

Action and Uses

In patients with glaucoma, **alpha-adrenergic agonists** act to reduce the amount of aqueous humor produced in the eye. In addition, alpha-adrenergic agonists improve the flow of aqueous humor out of the anterior chamber of the eye. These actions reduce the IOP in the eye. Common alpha-adrenergic agonists for glaucoma, dosages, and nursing implications are listed in Table 18.3. Be sure to consult a drug reference book for more information about specific alpha-adrenergic agonists to control glaucoma.

Expected Side Effects

Side effects commonly experienced by patients who are taking alpha-adrenergic agonists for their glaucoma include tearing, redness, blurring of vision, and burning or stinging after giving the eye drops. Some patients may experience a sensation of a foreign body being in their eye.

Adverse Effects

Adverse effects of adrenergic agonists include bradycardia or tachycardia and a drop in blood pressure. These can result from giving too many drops of the drug, causing systemic absorption. Other adverse effects include allergic reaction, fatigue, and respiratory symptoms.

❖ Nursing Implications and Patient Teaching

◆ *Assessment.* In addition to the general nursing considerations related to eye drug therapy listed in Box 18.2, make sure to assess the patient's vital signs, especially heart rate, because the drug can cause either tachycardia or bradycardia. Patients may also experience a drop in blood pressure and/or orthostatic hypotension. Let the prescriber know if the patient is taking antianxiety agents (particularly benzodiazepines), antidepressants, or sedatives because these may increase central nervous system (CNS) effects.

◆ *Planning and implementation.* Carefully monitor the patient's heart rate and blood pressure for changes after giving the eye drops. Make sure to read the label carefully to confirm that you are giving the correct concentration of the drug. Give the exact number of eye drops prescribed by the healthcare provider to the patient to decrease the risk for adverse effects. Make sure to ask the patient to close his or her eyes for 2 minutes or place a gloved finger over the tear duct and apply gentle pressure for about 3 minutes. Always wipe any excess drug that spills on the eyelid or face to avoid systemic absorption.

◆ *Patient and family teaching.* In addition to the general teaching points listed in Box 18.3, tell the patient and family the following:

- Make sure to read packaging carefully because some drugs may need to be stored in the refrigerator and protected from light to maintain potency.
- Wear dark glasses when you are in the sunlight or other bright light conditions because your pupil will be dilated and your eye will be sensitive to light.
- If you have been prescribed to use the drug for a limited time such as 1 week, do not continue the

| Table 18.3 | Examples of Common Alpha-Adrenergic Agonists and Cholinergic Drugs for Glaucoma |

Alpha-adrenergic agonists: These drugs act to reduce the amount of aqueous humor produced in the eye. In addition, alpha-adrenergic agonists improve the flow of aqueous humor out of the anterior chamber of the eye. These actions reduce the intraocular pressure in the eye.

DRUG/ADULT DOSAGE RANGE	NURSING IMPLICATIONS
apraclonidine (Iopidine) 1–2 drops (0.5% solution) in affected eye every 8 hours dipivefrin hydrochloride (AK-Pro, Propine) 1 drop (0.1% solution) in affected eye every 12 hours	• Remind patients that these drops can sometimes make them feel they have something in their eye, so do not rub the eyelid. • Monitor vital signs regularly because these drugs can cause increased or decreased blood pressure if absorbed systemically. • Report upper respiratory symptoms such as cough, shortness of breath, sore throat, or runny nose because these can be adverse effects of the alpha-adrenergic agonists. • These drugs may be used for short-term reduction of intraocular pressure or in addition to other types of drugs for patients who do not respond to other drugs. • Wait at least 5 minutes before using other types of eye drops.

Cholinergic drugs: These drugs increase availability of acetylcholine to activate specific receptors. This leads to decreased production of aqueous humor and improving outflow of aqueous humor to decrease intraocular pressure.

DRUG/ADULT DOSAGE RANGE	NURSING IMPLICATIONS
carbachol (Isopto Carbachol) 2 drops (1.5% solution or 3% solution) in affected eye every 8 hours pilocarpine (Isopto Carpine, Pilopine) 1–2 drops (1% solution or 2% solution) in affected eye every 6–8 hours, depending on strength of solution and patient response to the drug. Also available as gel and as an ocular insert, follow administration directions carefully.	• Remind patients that vision may be decreased at night, so patients may need to avoid night driving. • Teach patients to wear protective sunglasses in bright lights because these drugs can cause photophobia. • Report symptoms such as sweating, bradycardia, drop in blood pressure, diarrhea, nausea, and vomiting because these may indicate systemic absorption.

drug beyond that time period. These drugs not only lower elevated IOP, they can also lower normal IOP, which can cause problems.

CHOLINERGIC DRUGS

Action and Uses

Cholinergic drugs decrease IOP by reducing the amount of aqueous humor produced and improving its flow. By increasing the amount of acetylcholine, the pupil becomes smaller (miosis). This in turn increases the amount of space between the lens and the iris, allowing the aqueous fluid to flow freely and decreasing IOP. Common cholinergic drugs for glaucoma, dosages, and nursing implications are listed in Table 18.3. Be sure to consult a drug reference book for more information about specific cholinergic drugs to control glaucoma.

Expected Side Effects

Expected side effects of cholinergic drugs include tearing, stinging, redness of the eye, and blurred vision. Cholinergic drugs cause miosis, so patients may experience difficulty with vision at night and even night blindness. Like other eye drugs we have discussed, systemic side effects are possible and include headache, increased saliva, increased urination, and sweating. Side effects are intensified if patients are prescribed an oral form of cholinergic drugs.

Adverse Effects

Adverse effects are more common with systemic absorption of the drug. Examples include changes in blood pressure and abnormal heart rhythms. Other adverse effects include double vision and retinal detachment.

❖ Nursing Implications and Patient Teaching

◆ *Assessment.* In addition to the general nursing considerations related to eye drug therapy listed in Box 18.2, carefully monitor the patient's vital signs. You will be assessing blood pressure, heart rate, and respiratory rate because they may all be sensitive to changes from cholinergic drugs. Assess the patient for the side effects you might expect from any drug that increases acetylcholine including increased saliva, increased urination, and sweating.

💡 Memory Jogger
Patients who are taking eye drugs for glaucoma may have unequal pupil size. If there is any question about neurologic status, make sure to contact the registered nurse (RN) or healthcare provider for assessment.

Cholinergic drugs should be avoided in people who have breathing problems such as asthma or chronic bronchitis. These drugs should be avoided in patients with gallbladder or liver disease. Always use the right dose and wipe any excess drug off of the patient's skin because it can be absorbed and cause systemic effects. Use digital nasolacrimal occlusion technique or ask the patient to close his or her eyes for at least 2 minutes after giving the drug.

> **Top Tip for Safety**
>
> To decrease the risk for side effects and adverse effects, make sure to wipe off any excess drug from the skin rather than let it absorb. Never give more drops than are prescribed.

◆ *Evaluation.* Report significant changes in the patient's vital signs including decreased heart rate less than 60 beats per minute or any trouble breathing. Symptoms such as drooling, severe sweating, respiratory failure, and severe neuromuscular weakness indicate cholinergic toxicity.

> **Top Tip for Safety**
>
> A sudden change in blood pressure, heart rate, or difficulty breathing may be related to cholinergic eye drugs. Notify the healthcare provider immediately.

◆ *Patient and family teaching.* In addition to the general teaching points listed in Box 18.3, tell the patient and family the following:
- Use caution in moving from light to dark rooms. Your pupils will not dilate normally so it may be difficult to see. Make sure to use good lighting for reading and other daily activities.
- Make sure to remove any excess drug if it spills on skin to avoid absorption.
- Report any increase of drooling or sweating, or any difficulty breathing to your healthcare provider immediately because those symptoms may indicate a toxic level of the drug.

CARBONIC ANHYDRASE INHIBITORS

Action and Uses

Carbonic anhydrase inhibitors (CAIs) lower IOP by reducing aqueous humor in the anterior chamber of the eye. CAIs are a type of diuretic. They are available in oral forms, as eye drops, and intravenously (for patients who need a rapid decrease in IOP to prevent serious optic nerve damage). Common CAIs for glaucoma, dosages, and nursing implications are listed in Table 18.4. Be sure to consult a drug reference book for more information about specific cholinergic drugs to control glaucoma.

Expected Side Effects

Eye drops can cause slight burning or stinging with administration. Some patients may experience a bitter or sour taste in the mouth. In rare cases, redness of the conjunctiva can occur. CAIs can cause CNS effects and must be used with caution. Patients may experience drowsiness, fatigue, and headache with oral and intravenous forms. Blood sugar levels may fluctuate when the patient is taking oral CAIs.

Adverse Effects

Some CAIs are related to sulfonamide drugs and may cause an allergic reaction in patients who are allergic to any sulfa drug. The allergic response can happen even in the eye drops, so make sure to notify the healthcare provider before giving a CAI to a patient with a sulfa allergy.

When CAIs are taken orally or intravenously, the patient can experience a wide range of adverse effects, including neurologic effects (i.e., confusion, dizziness, numbness of the hands and feet, and even paralysis), severe skin infections, severe electrolyte imbalances, and liver failure.

❖ Nursing Implications and Patient Teaching

◆ *Assessment.* In addition to the general nursing considerations related to eye drug therapy listed in Box 18.2,

Table 18.4 Examples of Carbonic Anhydrase Inhibitors

Carbonic anhydrase inhibitors: lower intraocular pressure by reducing aqueous humor in the anterior chamber of the eye

DRUG/ADULT DOSAGE RANGE	NURSING IMPLICATIONS

acetazolamide (Diamox)
   sustained-release capsules: 250 mg orally one to four times daily
   extended-release capsules: 500 mg by mouth twice daily
 brinzolamide (Azopt) 1 drop (1% solution) in affected eye every 8 hours
 dorzolamide (Trusopt) 1 drop (2% solution) in affected eye every 8 hours
 methazolamide (Neptazane, Glauctabs) 50–100 mg orally every 8–12 hours
	• Double-check allergies before giving these drugs because some may have cross-sensitivity with sulfonamide antibiotics.
	 • Report any GI side effects to the healthcare provider because these may be side effects of carbonic anhydrase inhibitors.
	 • Monitor electrolytes (particularly sodium and potassium) because these drugs are also categorized as diuretics.
	 • Monitor for CNS side effects such as drowsiness, fatigue, depression, and irritability. These may require a change in drugs.
	 • Notify the healthcare provider if the patient has a history of gout because these drugs may increase uric acid level.

monitor the patient for side and adverse effects, particularly CNS effects that are more likely with the oral or intravenous drugs. Ask about and report any sulfa allergy to the healthcare provider before giving any CAI.

> ### ⬆ Top Tip for Safety
> Never give a CAI to a patient who has a sulfa allergy because these drugs are a type of sulfonamide.

◆ *Evaluation.* Assess the patient's response to the drug. Report any severe side effects or adverse effects to the healthcare provider. One side effect, bitter or sour taste in the mouth, may affect the patient's dietary intake,

so monitor for this problem carefully. Shortness of breath, dizziness, hives, or itching may be symptoms of an allergic response.

> ### ✦ Lifespan Considerations
> #### Carbonic Anhydrase Inhibitors
> **Pediatric Considerations**
> CAIs should not be given to children because they can slow growth if used long term.
> **Considerations for Pregnancy and Breast-Feeding**
> CAIs should be avoided during pregnancy and breast-feeding.

Get Ready for the NCLEX® Examination!

Key Points

- Apply only drugs and liquids labeled "for otic use" into the ear canal.
- When instilling eardrops into an adult's ear, gently pull the external ear up and back. When instilling eardrops into a young child's ear, gently pull the external ear down and back.
- Place eardrops or solutions only in the affected ear.
- Never give a drug to the ear canal or irrigate the ear canal if there is drainage present, to avoid causing a middle ear infection.
- Glaucoma is a chronic disease with no cure; drug therapy can prevent blindness and must continue for the patient's life.
- Pupil constriction is *miosis* (small word, small pupil size). Pupil dilation is *mydriasis* (larger word, larger pupil size).
- Normal IOP is between 10 and 20 mm Hg. Maintenance of a normal IOP keeps the eye healthy and helps prevent blindness in patients with glaucoma.
- Never instill prostaglandin agonists into an eye that has been scratched or has an infection. Contact the healthcare provider for instructions about continuing glaucoma therapy and managing the corneal problem.
- Prostaglandin agonists can cause a change in the color of the iris of the eye and increase the length of eyelashes.
- Before giving beta-blocker eye drops to a patient, make sure he or she is not also taking any oral beta-blocker drugs for any cardiac conditions.
- Use digital nasolacrimal occlusion (also called *punctal occlusion*) to reduce systemic absorption of eye drops. Give only a prescribed number of eye drops; then ask the patient to close his or her eyes for 2 minutes or place a gloved finger over the tear duct and apply gentle pressure for about 3 minutes.
- All opthalmic drugs must be labeled specifically for "ophthalmic use."
- Give eye drops or eye ointment in the affected eye only.
- Never touch the tip of the bottle or tube to your fingers or directly on the patient's eye to avoid contamination.
- Gently pull the lower lid down on the affected eye so that you can place the eye drops or ointment into the conjunctival sac.
- Glaucoma drugs are typically available in varying strengths. Make sure to read the label carefully and only give the strength prescribed for the patient.
- Adrenergic agonists cause mydriasis. The patient's pupils are dilated, so the eyes are more sensitive to bright lights. Patients may need to wear protective sunglasses in bright conditions.
- Beta blockers and cholinergic drugs cause miosis. Patients may have difficulty adjusting to dim lighting because their pupils are smaller. Patients will need to use caution to avoid falls.
- Teach patients to report any dizziness or shortness of breath to the healthcare provider because these indicate side effects of the glaucoma drugs.
- Advise patients with diabetes that beta blockers can mask the symptoms of low blood sugar. Regular checking of blood sugar will be very important.
- Symptoms of too much cholinergic drug include increased saliva, increased urination, and sweating.
- Patients who are taking eye drugs for glaucoma may have unequal pupil size. If there is any question about neurologic status, make sure to contact the RN or healthcare provider for assessment.
- Cholinergic drugs should be avoided in people who have breathing problems such as asthma or chronic bronchitis.
- To decrease the risk for side and adverse effects of any spilled ophthalmic drug, make sure to wipe any excess drug from the skin rather than let it absorb.
- CAIs can cause severe neurologic or electrolyte imbalances and must be given with caution.
- CAIs are not approved for children because they slow growth. They are not used during pregnancy or breast-feeding because these drugs are known to cause birth defects in animals.

Get Ready for the NCLEX® Examination!—cont'd

Review Questions for the NCLEX® Examination

1. A 78-year-old woman is prescribed 1 drop of 0.25% timolol (Timoptic ophthalmic) to her left eye every day for glaucoma. How does the LPN/VN teach the patient to perform digital nasolacrimal occlusion?
   1. Teach the patient to gently press her index finger over the inner corner of her eye over her tear duct for 3 minutes after putting in the eye drop.
   2. Teach the patient to press her index finger over the outer portion of her eye (between her eye and her cheek) for 3 minutes after putting in the eye drop.
   3. Teach the patient to press her index finger over the inner part of her eye over her tear duct for 10 to 20 seconds after putting in the eye drop.
   4. Teach the patient to press her index finger over the outer portion of her eye (between her eye and her cheek) for 10 to 20 seconds after putting in the eye drop.

2. A patient reports slight stinging after applying her eye drops for glaucoma. What is the nurse's best action?
   1. Culture the patient's eye for bacteria and send it to the laboratory.
   2. Report the stinging to the healthcare provider and ask for a change in the prescription.
   3. Reassure the patient that it is normal to have slight stinging after applying her eye drops.
   4. Document the comments as the only action.

3. A patient is taking an ophthalmic drug that causes mydriasis. Which of the following effects are associated with mydriasis?
   1. The patient's pupil remains constricted even in dark rooms.
   2. The patient's pupil remains dilated even in bright lights.
   3. The patient's pupil remains dilated even in dark rooms.
   4. The patient's pupil remains constricted in bright lights.

4. A patient is prescribed an ophthalmic beta blocker for his glaucoma. Which of the following adverse effects is possible if the drug is absorbed into the blood system?
   1. Heart rate less than 60
   2. Increased tearing
   3. Increased blood pressure
   4. Redness of eyes

5. Which of the following are common side effects of prostaglandin agonists? (Select all that apply.)
   1. Changes in color of the affected eye
   2. Increased length of eyelashes
   3. Dilation of the pupil
   4. Foreign body sensation
   5. Increased heart rate

6. A patient who is taking latanoprost for glaucoma was accidentally poked in the eye by a grandchild and thinks the cornea is scratched. What is the nurse's best action?
   1. Tell the patient to continue the eye drops and apply cool compresses.
   2. Teach the patient to give the eye drops to the unaffected eye so that he or she does not miss the dose.
   3. Tell the patient to hold the eye drops and wait until the pain from the scratch goes away before putting in the drops.
   4. Tell the patient to hold the eye drops and contact the healthcare provider immediately.

7. The patient is taking metoprolol for his high blood pressure. The healthcare provider orders timolol eye drops for the patient's glaucoma. Which of the following actions will the nurse do first?
   1. Monitor the patient's blood pressure four times a day while the patient is taking the drugs.
   2. Give the eye drops and apply digital nasolacrimal occlusion to prevent systemic absorption.
   3. Increase fluid intake to 2000 to 3000 mL/day to avoid dehydration.
   4. Contact the healthcare provider to clarify the order to avoid a potential adverse drug effect.

8. An elderly woman with cognitive impairment accidentally takes three times the prescribed number of pilocarpine eye drops for her glaucoma. Which of the following symptoms would suggest cholinergic toxicity? (Select all that apply.)
   1. Increased sweating
   2. Constipation
   3. Neuromuscular weakness
   4. Drooling
   5. Diarrhea
   6. Dilated pupils

9. The patient is prescribed latanoprost (Xalatan) 0.005% ophthalmic solution, 1 drop (1.5 mcg) to the left eye every evening for glaucoma. The bottle holds 2.5 mL. In latanoprost, 1 mL is equal to 33 drops. How many days will the drug last if the patient uses the drug exactly as prescribed?

10. A patient is prescribed the carbonic anhydrase inhibitor acetazolamide 250 mg by mouth three times a day for glaucoma. How many milligrams will the patient take each day?

11. A patient comes to the outpatient clinic and states that hearing is decreased in the left ear. The nurse practitioner checks the patient's ear and notices a large amount of earwax obstructing the eardrum. The LPN carefully reads the label of the drug to ensure that it is "for otic use." Place the nurse's next actions in the correct order.

1. Ask the patient to lie down with the head turned so that the affected ear is turned upward; if the patient is sitting in a chair, tilt the patient's head so the affected ear is up.

2. Using the applicator, place only the prescribed number of drops into the patient's ear. Aim the drops onto the side of the ear canal and let them run into the ear.

3. Insert a cotton ball into the opening of the ear canal to keep the drops from rolling out of the ear.

4. Wash your hands and don a pair of clean gloves.

5. For an older child or adult, pull the pinna up and back.

6. Remove your gloves and wash your hands.

Case Study

Mr. Brown is a 43-year-old African American who was diagnosed with glaucoma after a screening event sponsored by his church. His healthcare provider prescribed latanoprost (Xalatan) 1 drop (1.5 mcg) in both eyes once daily. As he was leaving the office, he mentioned that he just could not believe he had glaucoma because "only old people get glaucoma." You are concerned about his willingness to adhere to his treatment plan.

1. What are the risk factors for glaucoma?

2. Latanoprost belongs to which class of glaucoma drugs?

3. What are some common side effects of latanoprost?

4. What information will you give to Mr. Brown to encourage adherence to his treatment plan?

19

Over-the-Counter Drugs, Herbal and Alternative Drugs, and Vitamins and Minerals

Learning Outcomes

1. Explain what to teach patients and families about over-the-counter drugs.
2. List side effects and precautions needed for herbal preparations and those used for complementary and alternative medicine.
3. List the actions, side effects, and precautions to take when giving the most common vitamins prescribed for supplementation.
4. Explain what to teach patients and families about supplemental vitamins.
5. List the actions, side effects, and precautions to take when giving the most common minerals prescribed for supplementation.
6. Explain what to teach patients and families about supplemental minerals.

Key Terms

alternative medicine (ăl-TĔR-nă-tĭv, p. 347) Medical therapies such as herbalism, homeopathy, and acupuncture that are not considered mainstream.

ascorbic acid (ăs-KŎR-bĭk, p. 354) Vitamin C.

complementary medicine (kŏm-plĕ-MĔN-tă-rē, p. 347) Alternative medicine therapies used in conjunction with a conventional or mainstream approach.

herbal (ĔR-băl, p. 349) Plants used in cooking and medicine.

hypervitaminosis (hī-pĕr-VĪ-tĕ-mĭ-NŌ-sĭs, p. 351) A high storage level of vitamins (notably ADEK) which can lead to toxic symptoms.

integrative practices (ĬN-tĕ-grā-tĭv, p. 347) Complementary and conventional approaches to healthcare that mainly focus on health and wellness.

minerals (MĬN-ĕr-ălz, p. 356) Substances found in food that are necessary for normal body function.

niacin (NĪ-ă-sĭn, p. 352) Vitamin B$_3$ or nicotinic acid helpful in lowering triglycerides and preventing pellagra.

over-the-counter (OTC) drugs (p. 346) Actual drugs approved by the US Food and Drug Administration that do not require a prescription to purchase.

vitamins (VĪ-tă-minz, p. 350) Substances found in food that are necessary for body functions.

OVERVIEW

We often forget that many of the drugs patients use are bought in stores without a prescription or are recommendations from a healthcare provider. In the late 2000s, Americans spent about $18 billion annually on nonprescription remedies. That number has more than doubled. **Over-the-counter (OTC) drugs** are actual drugs approved by the US Food and Drug Administration (FDA) that do not require a prescription to purchase.

Patients, neighbors, and family members will likely seek your knowledge when purchasing OTC products. Will you know how to advise them in a well-informed way that will answer all of their questions?

DOCUMENTING PATIENT HEALTHCARE PRACTICES

It is important for you to be familiar with the many nonprescription products now available to patients. Many of these products contain chemicals that are useful in treating common health problems but carry with them safety concerns as well. Dangerous interactions can occur. You must become familiar with these products to help patients choose the safest product for their current health concerns, problem, or illness.

Patients do not always think to mention herbals because they may regard them as natural and harmless, and not drugs at all. Many Americans consider OTC products to be safe because they are available without prescription. Herbals and OTC drugs may not be safe without keeping in mind the particular disease process and all other drugs, legal or otherwise, that the patient may be taking. When taking a drug history, always ask patients if they are taking OTC or herbal drugs and document the answers. Questionable products need to be brought to the attention of the healthcare provider.

Ask patients to bring in all herbs or drug remedies they are using so they may be accurately recorded. Sometimes patients do not know the active ingredients that are in the products. Products in their original bottles or boxes give you more information that may help determine whether the products are safe and whether drug interactions or complications are possible.

Patients who rely on **complementary and alternative medicine (CAM)** may take herbs, supplements, or other drugs instead of prescription drugs because of the cost, or they may use such products in addition to prescription drugs. Some of the reasons patients use these OTC, herbal, or complementary products include:

- Patients seek products they hope will keep them in good health, prevent disease, or provide treatment for health problems they now have.
- They have tried traditional drugs and treatments without success.
- The traditional prescribed drugs had undesirable side effects.
- There is no known drug therapy that will cure their problem, but CAM products provide them with some relief.
- Trusted people in their family or community have told them about the product.
- They are seeking a cheaper drug to replace a prescription drug.
- Traditional drugs or treatment violates their religious or spiritual beliefs.
- They seek a more **integrative medicinal** approach to their health care.

OVER-THE-COUNTER DRUGS

The role of OTC agents in healthcare today is growing. The Nonprescription Drug Manufacturers Association estimates that more than 100,000 products are now available OTC. These products contain 1 or more of about 800 active chemicals and come in a variety of dosage forms, sizes, and strengths. The sales of OTC products are currently estimated at $38 billion a year.

Nonprescription drugs, or OTC products, are drugs that are considered to be safe and effective for people to use without instructions from a healthcare provider about how they are to be taken. OTC products differ from prescription drugs in the following ways:

- The label information is more complete than prescription drug labels. Be aware, however, that because they are so complete, the print can be difficult for some patients to read.
- OTC drugs have a wider margin of safety because of the substantial testing they have undergone before advertising. In addition, the formulation of many OTC products has been changed by the manufacturer based on information gathered after years of usage by consumers.
- OTC drugs are widely available and advertised.
- The dose is often lower than the same drugs available with a prescription.
- These products are usually not covered by insurance.

The most common categories of OTC drugs are similar to those available by prescription. Laxatives, peptic acid disorder products (antacids and H_2 receptor antagonists),

analgesics, cough and cold products (antihistamines, decongestants, expectorants, and antitussives), vaginal antifungals, smoking cessation products, and topical steroids are all available OTC. Drugs that were once available only by prescription are given OTC status on a regular basis. Frequently they are available in lower dosages. Ibuprofen is such an example. Ibuprofen is available as an OTC drug sold in 200-mg tablets but is available by prescription in 800-mg tablets.

OTC drugs are sold in pharmacies, grocery stores, gas stations, and department stores. It is important to learn the generic drug name instead of just the product (trade) name because there are so many different names and versions of these products. Many of these products have multiple ingredients. The cost of the combination products can be more than buying all of the ingredients singly, so it is important to check out commonly used products for price comparisons. An example of this is the OTC drug Tylenol (acetaminophen) PM, which contains both acetaminophen (Tylenol) and diphenhydramine (Benadryl).

PRODUCT LABELING

The FDA requires that OTC product labels contain important information in a manner that a typical person can read and understand. Drug companies are required to use a standard labeling format for all OTCs sold in the United States. Key information begins with active ingredients and is followed by purposes, uses, warnings, and directions. The labeling is placed in the same order on all OTC packages in an easy-to-read format.

Surveys show that women are the family members most likely to buy OTC products, and they are also more likely than men to read labels before taking drugs.

One of the most important things to look for on the OTC label is the presence of other chemicals in a product that might pose a risk. These "hidden" chemicals are used for different purposes: to help make the drug taste better, to help preserve the drug, to give color, and to help deliver the product or make it more stable. Consumers who have an allergy or intolerance to even small amounts of any of these hidden chemicals may not be aware of the risk unless they read the label. Table 19.1 lists a number of common hidden chemicals in OTC products.

PATIENT TEACHING

There are some basic facts that healthcare providers should tell patients about OTC products. Sometimes this information is printed and given to the patient because it is so important for patients to know. Whether they are given verbally or in writing, following are some of the key facts patients should learn:

- Always read the instructions on the label.
- Do not take OTC drugs in higher dosages or for a longer time than the label states.
- If you do not get well within 2 weeks, stop treating yourself and talk with a healthcare professional.

Table 19.1	Common Active Ingredients in Over-the-Counter Products	
HIDDEN DRUG	**OTC CLASS**	**PERSONS AT RISK**
Alcohol	Cough syrups, cold medications, mouthwash	Recovering alcoholics
Phenylephrine, pseudoephedrine	Antihistamines, analgesics, antiemetic, asthma products, cold and allergy products, menstrual products, motion sickness, sleep aids, decongestants	Difficult urination in enlarged prostate, can worsen diabetes, interact with antihypertensive and cardiac drugs, antihistamines complicate glaucoma, interact with ADHD drugs, hyperthyroidism
Calcium, carbonate, magnesium, sodium	Antacids	Kidney or heart disease, sodium and magnesium salts negatively affect disease process
Bismuth subsalicylate	Kaopectate, Pepto-Bismol	Hard to excrete in kidney disease
Ibuprofen, Naproxen	Ibuprofen	Kidney and liver disease, stomach ulcers, bleeding disorders
Acetaminophen	Analgesics, antidiarrheal, cold, allergy and sleep products	Liver disease or alcoholism; it is easy for anyone to overdose with acetaminophen because it is hidden in many products
Caffeine	Analgesics, cold, migraine, allergy, diuretics, menstrual products, stimulants, weight control	Can worsen heart disease, hypertension, sleep disorders
Sugar	Cough syrups or other syrup-based OTC drugs	Diabetes
Salicylate (aspirin)		Bleeding disorders, ulcers, children with flu symptoms because it can cause Reye's syndrome
Diphenhydramine	Antihistamines, sleep aids, cough and cold products	Confusion, falls, disorientation especially in older adults

ADHD, Attention deficit/hyperactivity disorder; *OTC,* over-the-counter.
Modified from Katzung BG: *Basic and clinical pharmacology,* ed 10, New York, 2006, McGraw-Hill Medical; Lynch SS: Precautions with over-the-counter drugs. In *The Merck manual home health handbook.* http://www.merckmanuals.com/home/drugs/over-the-counter_drugs/precautions_with_over-the-counter_drugs.html. Accessed January 16, 2017.

- Side effects from OTC drugs are relatively uncommon, but read the label to know what they are.
- Responses to drugs vary from person to person.
- OTC drugs often interact with other drugs, and with food or alcohol, or they might have an effect on other health problems you may have. Ask a pharmacist if you are not sure about interactions.
- If you do not understand the label, check with the pharmacist.
- Do not take the drug if the package does not have a label on it.
- Throw away drugs that have expired (i.e., are older than the date on the package).
- Do not use drugs that belong to a friend.
- Buy products that treat only the symptoms you have.
- If cost is an issue, generic OTC products may be cheaper than brand name items.
- Avoid buying these products online, outside of well-known Internet insurance company sites, because many OTC preparations sold through the Internet are counterfeit products. These may not be what you ordered and may be dangerous.

Parents should know the following special information about using OTC drugs for children:

- Never guess about the amount of drug to give a child. Half an adult dose may be too much or not enough to be effective. This is very true of drugs such as acetaminophen (Tylenol) or ibuprofen (Advil), in which repeated overdoses may lead to poisoning of the child, liver destruction, or coma.
- If the label says to take 2 teaspoons and the dosing cup is marked with ounces only, get another measuring device. Do not try to guess about how much should be given.
- Always follow the age limits listed. If the label says the product should not be given to a child younger than 2 years, do not give it.
- Always use the child-resistant cap, relock the cap after use, and keep drugs in a safe place away from children.
- Throw away old, discolored, or expired drugs, or any drug that has lost its label instructions.
- Do not give to children a drug that contains alcohol.

HERBAL PRODUCTS AND COMPLEMENTARY AND ALTERNATIVE MEDICINE

According to data from the National Institutes of Health (NIH), 4 out of 10 adults and 1 out of 9 children use some form of CAM. CAM practices, which include dietary supplements (botanicals and herbs), acupuncture, massage, mind-body medicine, and traditional Chinese medicine, have been used by people in the search for health and wellness for thousands of years. Evidence-based research for many CAM therapies is often absent, and the safety and efficacy of many CAM therapies are unclear. The NIH Center for Complementary and Integrative Health (NCCIH) sponsors and publishes research based on scientific evidence regarding many CAM therapies. You can better educate yourself and your patients using current evidenced-based research by doing a search on the NIH NCCIH website (https://nccih.nih.gov).

> **Bookmark This!**
>
> NCCIH: https://nccih.nih.gov.

It is important to have up-to-date, balanced, and scientific materials to help you understand herbal therapies. Such scientific materials can help you know more about the strengths, weaknesses, clinical indications, proper dosages, toxicities, and interactions of different alternative drug therapies so you are able to accurately answer patient questions.

PRODUCT LABELING

The federal government has regulated dietary supplements through the FDA since 1994. A dietary supplement is one that contains one or more ingredients such as vitamins, herbals, botanicals, or amino acids. However, regulations for dietary supplements are not the same as those for prescription or OTC drugs.

According to the FDA, a dietary supplement must be labeled as a dietary supplement and be intended to be taken only as a dietary supplement. Labeling information must not be deceptive. Producers of dietary supplements are responsible for ensuring that products are safe; however, they do not have to provide the FDA with information that demonstrates the safety of the product before it is marketed. Prescription and OTC drugs are FDA regulated to demonstrate that drugs are both safe and effective before marketing.

If a claim is made about the effects of a dietary supplement, the producer must have data to support the claim. Any claims about how a supplement may affect the body must have this statement on the label: "This statement has not been evaluated by the US Food and Drug Administration (FDA). This product is not intended to diagnose, treat, cure, or prevent any disease."

The FDA has the authority to remove a product from the market, but this happens only after the agency can prove that the product is unsafe or ineffective. Ephedra is such an example. Ephedra was an ingredient in some dietary supplements used for weight loss, increased energy, and enhanced athletic performance. The FDA banned its use from all products in 2004 because of increased heart problems and serious side effects when combined with caffeine.

Labeling on herbal products is generally designed to promote sales and product use, and not necessarily to educate the consumer. Health professionals with a general understanding of popular herbs and supplements can talk to patients about efficacy, common side effects, risks, and interactions. Ask about the patients' use of alternative herbal or Chinese medicines, so the healthcare prescriber can explore the products in detail to avoid drug interactions with drugs ordered in the hospital or clinic.

Patients with medical problems should not use herbs and dietary supplements without medical supervision. When patients rely on themselves for diagnosis and treatment, they may delay the essential diagnosis of serious medical problems, and this delay may worsen their condition. In addition, some herbal products have adverse effects, and many herbal products interact with prescribed drugs.

PROS AND CONS

Safety, purity, and effectiveness are the major issues in evaluating herbal products. Many important issues and questions must be considered in looking at herbal products.

Herbal products are made by grinding up parts of the plant and making them into pills, capsules, or liquids. One of the major criticisms of herbal products is that the plants vary so much in concentration or dosage because plants make different amounts of chemicals depending on the soil, water, and sun where they were grown. So the weight of one leaf may be the same as that of another, but the amount of biologically active chemical in each leaf may vary according to the amount of sunlight, the nutrition in the soil, and the extent of watering. The plants may also contain harmful pesticides or other chemicals.

Hormone replacement therapy has become a hot market for the use of "natural" products. Natural estrogens are really estrogen-like chemicals called *phytoestrogens*. Examples of plants that contain natural estrogens or phytoestrogens are flaxseed, red clover sprouts, and soy flour. These supplements have not been clearly shown to improve the symptoms of menopause. In addition, the evidence does not support claims that custom-mixed bioidentical hormones are more effective than conventional hormone therapy.

Many nonprescription products are advertised to have the same function as prescription drugs. For example, there are herbal preparations that are supposed to act like sildenafil (Viagra) to treat erectile dysfunction. Herbal products for weight loss, depression, high cholesterol level, and asthma are also for sale. Some products may include amphetamine-like compounds that can cause high blood pressure, heart rate irregularities, stroke, and death.

St. John's wort has been shown to improve mild-to-moderate depression but has potentially dangerous interactions if taken with selective serotonin reuptake inhibitors, benzodiazepines, warfarin, statins, verapamil, digoxin, cyclosporine, antiviral HIV drugs, and oral contraceptives. Goldenseal has a high potential for herb–drug interactions, and ginseng may affect the blood levels of drugs with narrow therapeutic ranges because it increases liver enzyme activity.

> **Memory Jogger**
>
> St. John's wort, ginseng, and goldenseal are common herbal products most likely to cause dangerous interactions with many prescription drugs.

The Council for Responsible Nutrition is a trade association that represents dietary supplements. Companies that are members are expected to comply with not only federal and state regulations but also additional voluntary guidelines, as well as to a code of ethics. They also provide news releases on dietary supplements and government recommendations. For more information, check out their website (https://www.crnusa.org).

> **Bookmark This!**
>
> Council for Responsible Nutrition: https://www.crnusa.org.

Some European countries have more extensive experience than the United States with selected herbal products. Many of the products now gaining attention in the United States have been used for years in other countries, either as OTC products or by prescription. A lot of information has been learned not only about the effects of these products but also about how they interact with other foods and drugs. For example, natural products that reduce blood glucose level or blood pressure, or have a sedating effect may be dangerous when taken along with prescription drugs with the same actions. Be sure to use the NIH website (https://nccih.nih.gov) to check on specific herbal preparations.

A few nonherbal natural remedies in common use are considered both safe and effective. Sometimes the products themselves, such as calcium, may be of proven use. However, if the calcium comes from oyster shells taken from polluted waters, the shells may be filled with lead, zinc, or arsenic. A similar problem occurs with melatonin, a hormone extracted from the pineal gland of the cow. If the drug maker does not make sure that the cow is disease free, the consumer may be at risk for Creutzfeldt-Jakob disease or what is known as *mad cow disease,* which can be fatal.

VITAMINS

Vitamins are chemical compounds that are found naturally in plant and animal tissues, but most are not made in the human body. Some are available in their active form; others come from food as a *precursor* or *provitamin* that is later converted to the active form. People take vitamins to maintain health or to correct specific nutritional deficiencies. Most people who take vitamins decide to do so on their own without the advice of a healthcare professional.

Vitamins are necessary for life and essential to normal metabolism. They can act as coenzymes to regulate the creation of compounds in the body. Vitamins are classified into two types. *Fat-soluble* vitamins are found primarily in various plant and animal oils or fats and can be stored in the body so that daily intake is not essential. *Water-soluble* vitamins are readily excreted in the urine and are not stored in the body. Water-soluble vitamins are destroyed by heat, and deficiencies are quickly seen in patients who have a deficient diet. Normally if a well-balanced, nutritious diet is followed, vitamin supplements are not necessary. However, when certain conditions prevent eating solid food or when vitamins are poorly absorbed as in ulcerative colitis, increased vitamin intake is needed. Vitamin supplements are also advised in conditions in which metabolism increases, such as hyperthyroidism, pregnancy, and burns, to name a few.

> **Memory Jogger**
>
> To remember the fat-soluble vitamins, think "the fat cat is on ADEK."

If a variety of healthy foods are eaten, the necessary vitamins can likely be obtained from diet alone. The government has determined the usual vitamin levels that are needed daily to maintain health. This is known as the recommended dietary allowance (RDA). Table 19.2 shows the RDA for common vitamins. When patients are deficient for one or more vitamins, supplements are needed. For supplementation vitamins should have 50% to 150% of the RDA.

There are known dangers to vitamin use, especially high-dose use. When megadoses of water-soluble vitamins are taken, the excess amount is quickly excreted in the urine with no additional benefit to the patient. However, excesses of fat-soluble vitamins (e.g., vitamins A, D, E, and K) can be stored, and levels can cause toxic side effects. Most vitamins can be toxic to children when accidentally exposed to high levels, and iron can be deadly to small children.

Advertisers suggest that natural products are better than synthetic vitamins. However, current research concludes that vitamins are probably the same whether they are natural or synthetic, costly or cheap. The most important differences are that some preparations may dissolve better than others or contain the active product in amounts that increase the absorption of other vitamins and minerals taken at the same time. Some vitamins contain fillers that may cause stomach upset if taken on an empty stomach. All vitamins should be kept in airtight dark containers out of the reach of children.

Table 19.2	Function, Deficiency, and Recommended Daily Intake of Vitamins			
VITAMIN	FUNCTION	DEFICIENCY	RDI	RDI PREGNANT AND LACTATING WOMEN
Vitamin A	Stabilizes skin membrane and eye health	Sprue, colitis, night blindness	Adults: 5000 IU Children: 2500 IU Infants: 1500 IU	800 IU
Vitamin D	Promotes calcium and phosphorous absorption	Rickets, osteomalacia, hypoparathyroidism	Adults: 400 IU Children: 400 IU Infants: 400 IU	400 IU
Vitamin E	Prevents damage to cell membranes	Unknown	Adults: 30 IU Children: 10 IU Infants: 5 IU	30 IU
Vitamin K	Formation of blood clotting factors	Blood clotting disorders	Adults: 80 mcg Children: 2.5 mcg Infants: 2 mcg	90 mcg
Vitamin C	Formation of collagen, healing, absorption of iron, protective	Scurvy	Adults: 60 mg Children: 40 mg Infants: 35 mg	60 mg
Vitamin B_{12} Cyanocobalamin	DNA synthesis and red blood cell maturation	Pernicious anemia	Adults: 6 mcg Children: 3 mcg Infants: 2 mcg	8 mcg
Vitamin B_9 Folic acid/folate	Red blood cell formation	Folic acid anemia	Adults: 400 mcg Children: 200 mcg Infants: 100 mcg	800 mcg
Vitamin B_3 Niacin	Amino acid metabolism and energy release	Pellagra	Adults: 20 mg Children: 9 mg Infants: 8 mg	20 mg
Vitamin B_6 Pyridoxine	Metabolism of CHO, proteins, and fats	B_6 anemia	Adults: 2 mg Children: 0.7 mg Infants: 0.4 mg	2.5 mg
Vitamin B_2 Riboflavin	Metabolism of CHO, proteins, and fats	Discomfort eating, swallowing	Adults: 1.7 mg Children: 3 mg Infants: 2 mg	2.0 mg
Vitamin B_1 Thiamine	Carbohydrate metabolism	Beriberi	Adults: 1.5 mg Children: 0.7 mg Infants: 0.5 mg	1.7 mg

Adult: older than age 4 years; child: age 1–4 years; infant: age 0–1 years.
RDI, Recommended daily intake.
Modified from US Food and Drug Administration: Guidance for industry: A food labeling guide (14. Appendix F: Calculate the percent daily value for the appropriate nutrients). Published January 2013. Updated August 20, 2015. http://www.fda.gov/Food/GuidanceRegulation/GuidanceDocumentsRegulatoryInformation/ LabelingNutrition/ucm064928.htm; and US Food and Drug Administration: Guidance for industry: A food labeling guide (15. Appendix G: Daily values for infants, children less than 4 years of age, and pregnant and lactating women). Published January 2013. Updated December 16, 2014. http://www.fda.gov/Food/ GuidanceRegulation/GuidanceDocumentsRegulatoryInformation/LabelingNutrition/ucm064930.htm.

VITAMIN A

Action and Uses

Vitamin A is important for vision, gene characteristics, reproduction, embryo growth and development, and healthy immune system function. Vitamin A supplementation is used to treat diagnosis associated with fat malabsorption, such as celiac disease and colitis. It is also used for the treatment of specific eye diseases and night blindness. This vitamin may be given orally, intravenously (IV), or IM, depending on how fast replacement is needed.

If vitamin A is given in high doses for a long time, **hypervitaminosis** can occur. Any patient who is receiving 25,000 International Units (IU) or more should be closely supervised. Pregnant women should not receive more than 6000 IU daily, or they may risk fetal abnormalities.

Women who are taking oral contraceptives often show elevated plasma vitamin A levels and should be closely monitored for hypervitaminosis. Giving cod-liver oil and vitamin A together is contraindicated.

❖ Nursing Implications and Patient Teaching

Common food sources of vitamin A include dairy products, fish, liver, spinach, broccoli, and dark orange vegetables.

Women who are using oral contraceptives should only take prescribed amounts of vitamin A to avoid hypervitaminosis. Vitamin A can cause birth defects in women who are pregnant, and excess vitamin A ingestion during pregnancy can cause birth defects of the central nervous system.

An early indication of vitamin A overdose is anorexia, abdominal pain, malaise, and yellowing of the skin, especially on the nose and ears.

VITAMIN B₁ (THIAMINE)

Action and Uses

Vitamin B₁, or thiamine, is water soluble and is a coenzyme needed in many physiologic pathways for carbohydrate metabolism and energy production. It also is thought to assist in nervous system function. Thiamine is excreted in the urine.

Vitamin B₁ is used to treat beriberi, which is a rare disorder in North America. Other conditions that lead to vitamin B₁ deficiency include alcoholism, gastric lesions, or hyperemesis of pregnancy. Symptoms include anorexia (lack of appetite), vomiting, fatigability, aching muscles, ataxia (poor coordination) of gait, and emotional disturbances such as moodiness, depression, or excess alcohol use.

Usual reactions to thiamine are mild itching, sweating, and nausea. However, adverse reactions can be severe and include anaphylactic shock and death when given IV. Sensitivity tests are performed before parenteral doses are started if sensitivity is suspected. IV doses must be given very slowly. If giving thiamine to an alcoholic or thiamine-deficient patient, IV glucose should also be given to prevent precipitation or worsening of Wernicke's encephalopathy.

> ### ⌖ Top Tip for Safety
>
> When giving parenteral thiamine, assess the patient continually for indications of allergic reactions: feelings of warmth, pruritus (itching), urticaria (hives), nausea, angioedema (lip and facial swelling), shortness of breath, sweating, tightness of the throat, and cyanosis (blue color to the skin). If these occur, stop the infusion and notify the emergency team.

❖ Nursing Implications and Patient Teaching

Common food sources of thiamine include meats, whole grains, peas, dried beans, and peanuts. Thiamine in food is destroyed when food is boiled, fried, or cooked for a long time under pressure.

VITAMIN B₂ (RIBOFLAVIN)

Action and Uses

Vitamin B₂, or riboflavin, is water soluble and is important in the metabolism of proteins, fats, and carbohydrates. It combines with proteins to form enzymes that are important for tissue metabolism. Riboflavin is used to prevent or treat riboflavin deficiency. Symptoms of deficiency may include cracks in the corner of the mouth, soreness and burning of the tongue and lips, and sore throat.

Riboflavin levels in the body can be decreased by oral contraceptives, even in low doses, increasing the risk for a deficiency in women who have been taking oral contraceptives for 3 years or longer.

❖ Nursing Implications and Patient Teaching

Teach patients that common food sources of riboflavin include dairy products, eggs, green leafy vegetables, organ meats, and peanuts. Warn patients that these supplements can turn urine a deeper yellow color.

NIACIN

Action and Uses

Niacin, previously called vitamin B₃, is water soluble and is an essential part of two compounds that are important in generating cellular energy. It is used to prevent or treat deficiency states that can cause pellagra or as a nutritional supplement caused by limited dietary intake. Niacin is also used to treat high blood fat level conditions such as hyperlipidemia, hypertriglyceridemia, and atherosclerosis.

Symptoms of deficiency include *glossitis* (smooth, swollen, beefy-red tongue), *stomatitis* (inflammation of the mouth), and diarrhea. Dermatitis of different body parts exposed to sun or trauma may develop, as well as lesions on the skin that result from sun, fire, or heat. Mental changes that are mild early in deficiency may progress to disorientation, loss of memory, confusion, hysteria, and, sometimes, manic outbursts.

Expected side effects of niacin supplementation are skin warmth, flushing, and itching that can be relieved when giving niacin with aspirin. Adverse reactions to niacin include allergies or anaphylactic reaction.

❖ Nursing Implications and Patient Teaching

Food sources of niacin include lean meats, peanuts, yeast, cereal (especially bran and wheat germ), eggs, liver, red meat, whole grains, and enriched bread.

When taken with beta-blocking drugs and calcium channel blockers for hypertension, the side effects of niacin increase, especially the skin warmth and flushing and blood vessel dilation. This effect may lead to *postural hypotension* (low blood pressure when a person suddenly stands up). If dizziness occurs with niacin, tell the patient to sit or lie down.

Taking niacin with cerivastatin or red yeast rice may cause rhabdomyolysis (muscle breakdown that can cause kidney dysfunction).

VITAMIN B₆

Action and Uses

Vitamin B₆, or pyridoxine hydrochloride, is water soluble and functions as a coenzyme in the metabolism of protein, carbohydrates, and fat. It is used to treat pyridoxine deficiency, vitamin B₆–responsive chronic anemia, neuritis, and other rare vitamin problems.

Pyridoxine deficiency is most likely to develop in the older adult population and in women of childbearing age, especially those who are pregnant or breast-feeding. Women who are taking oral contraceptives, individuals who are alcoholics, and those whose diets are of poor protein quality and quantity or are high in refined foods are also at risk.

Symptoms of deficiency include malaise, nervousness, irritability, and difficulty in walking. There may also be personality changes in adults, such as depression and a loss of sense of responsibility. High doses of pyridoxine may produce neurotoxicity, with symptoms of ataxia (loss of control of body movements), numb feet, and clumsiness.

Oral contraceptives may induce pyridoxine deficiency. Pyridoxine may prevent chloramphenicol-induced optic neuritis. Some drugs interfere with vitamin activity enough to block action and produce symptoms of deficiency. Pyridoxine should never be given with levodopa.

❖ Nursing Implications and Patient Teaching

Good food sources of vitamin B_6 include yeast, wheat, corn, egg yolk, liver, kidney, muscle meats, soybeans, cereals, whole grain bread, and soybeans. Limited amounts are available from milk and vegetables.

Appropriate food preparation is important in preserving this vitamin. Freezing of vegetables results in a 20% loss of pyridoxine, and the milling of wheat results in a 90% loss.

FOLIC ACID

Action and Uses

Folic acid (also known as vitamin B_9) is required for normal *erythropoiesis*, or red blood cell formation, and DNA synthesis. It is metabolized in the liver, where it is changed to its more active form. Folic acid is used to treat anemias caused by folic acid deficiency. It is also used in alcoholism, hepatic disease, hemolytic anemia, infancy (especially for infants receiving artificial formulas), lactation, oral contraceptive use, and pregnancy. Folic acid supplements may be needed in low-birth-weight infants, infants nursed by mothers who are deficient in folic acid, or infants with infections or prolonged diarrhea.

Recent guidelines emphasize the importance of increased folic acid intake by all women of childbearing age, especially in those women who are intending to get pregnant and during early pregnancy to help prevent spinal cord malformations in the fetus (neural tube defects). The folic acid additives in commercial bread and grain products have been increased in an attempt to provide more adequate supplies of this important vitamin.

Low levels of vitamin B_6, vitamin B_{12}, and folate are associated with high levels of homocysteine, which is a common amino acid in the blood. High levels of homocysteine are linked to the early development of heart disease.

Folic acid interacts with several drugs. It may decrease the anticancer effect of methotrexate. Antiseizure drugs reduce folic acid levels, and sulfasalazine (a sulfa drug used to treat the pain and swelling of arthritis) inhibits intestinal absorption of folate.

❖ Nursing Implications and Patient Teaching

Proper nutrition is essential, and dietary measures are preferable to drug therapy. Vegetables and fruits are good sources of folate. In the United States, bread, cereal, flour, pasta, rice, and cornmeal are fortified with folic acid. Beef liver, peas, beans, nuts, and eggs are also sources of folate.

VITAMIN B_{12}

Action and Uses

Vitamin B_{12} or cyanocobalamin is water soluble and contains cobalt. It functions in many processes for protein, fat, and carbohydrate metabolism. The coenzymes of B_{12} also take part in red blood cell maturation and are needed to make DNA in new cells. Vitamin B_{12} is needed to form red blood cells, and it is essential for growth, cell reproduction, and making the myelin sheath that surrounds nerve cells. Intrinsic factor must be present in the stomach and small intestine to absorb B_{12}. Vitamin B_{12} interacts with folate in metabolic functions, and a deficiency in vitamin B_{12} makes folate useless in the body.

Vitamin B_{12} is used to treat all B_{12} deficiency conditions, including pernicious anemia, megaloblastic and macrocytic anemias, malabsorption syndromes, hemorrhage, intestinal bacterial overgrowth, chronic liver disease complicated by deficiency of vitamin B_{12}, malignancy, pregnancy, and thyrotoxicosis (in which deficiency is seen because of increased metabolic rate), and kidney disorders.

Symptoms of deficiency occur mainly in people on strict vegetarian diets, because although vitamin B_{12} is water soluble, it is found only in animal products. Symptoms of B_{12} deficiency include constipation, upset stomach, tiredness, palpitations, shortness of breath, pale skin, smooth tongue, numbness, tingling, muscle weakness, and behavioral changes.

Most patients with vitamin B_{12} deficiency have a malabsorption problem in the GI tract, pernicious anemia, alcoholism, or are on vegan diets. Vitamin replacement is injected to bypass the GI tract. Parenteral, nasal, or oral therapy may be used to maintain normal B_{12} levels.

Cyanocobalamin (vitamin B_{12}) comes as a nasal spray or nasal gel and can be used as a maintenance drug for persons in remission after undergoing IM therapy for pernicious anemia. The dose is usually 500 mcg intranasally once weekly. If the patient develops adverse effects such as infection, headache, glossitis, nausea, and rhinitis after taking the nasal spray, it is often necessary to start IM vitamin B_{12} again. The maintenance dose of cyanocobalamin is 100 mcg IM every month. Cyanocobalamin is also packaged as a sublingual tablet.

Allergy to vitamin B_{12} is rare. The patient may report pruritus, a feeling of swelling of the entire body, or a severe anaphylactic reaction. A few patients may experience mild pain, localized skin irritation, or mild transient diarrhea after an injection of cyanocobalamin.

Alcohol, colchicine, and para-aminosalicylic acid (antibiotic for tuberculosis) lower the absorption of vitamin B_{12}. Some antibiotics lower the response to vitamin B_{12} therapy.

❖ Nursing Implications and Patient Teaching

The best food sources of vitamin B_{12} include organ meats; clams and oysters; nonfat dry milk; fermented cheese such as Camembert and Limburger; and seafood such as lobster, scallops, flounder, haddock, swordfish, and tuna.

VITAMIN C

Action and Uses

Vitamin C, or **ascorbic acid**, is necessary for formation of collagen in connective tissue, cartilage, tooth dentin, skin, and bone matrix and tissue repair. It is essential in energy-producing reactions and in metabolizing some neurotransmitters, hormones, carbohydrates, and amino acids. It helps maintain the integrity of blood vessels and may promote resistance to infection. Vitamin C regulates iron distribution and plays a role in antioxidant renewal. It may be used therapeutically to treat severe burns, chronic iron intoxication, and acidification of urine.

The use and dosage of vitamin C in the prevention and treatment of diseases, other than scurvy, is uncertain. Recent research indicates a possible positive role for vitamin C in prevention of coronary heart disease (especially in women), diabetes mellitus management, stroke reduction, osteoporosis prevention, reducing the risk for Alzheimer's disease in combination with vitamin E, and cataract prevention.

With modern refrigeration and processing methods of citrus fruits, scurvy is rarely seen in the United States, but it may be found when other vitamin deficiencies are present. Symptoms include tender, painful muscles, joints, and bones; muscle cramps; anorexia; fatigue; malaise; and sore gums. Wound healing is impaired, and excessive bleeding symptoms manifestations are demonstrated by petechial hemorrhages. Bruising, faulty bone and tooth development, loosened teeth, and gingivitis also may develop.

Vitamin C may be given by oral, IM, IV, and subcutaneous dosage to treat scurvy. The dosage ranges from 100 to 250 mg orally, IM, or IV twice a day in adults, but larger doses may be given.

The patient may experience mild, brief soreness at injection sites if the drug is given IM or subcutaneously. Patients may also experience brief episodes of faintness or dizziness when IV injections are given too rapidly. Excessive doses are usually rapidly excreted into the urine. Doses in excess of 1 to 3 g daily may result in GI problems, glycosuria, and development of kidney stones, especially in patients prone to these problems.

Ascorbic acid may have varying effects on anticoagulants, blocking the action of some and prolonging the intensity and duration of others. Ascorbic acid increases the effect of salicylates through increased kidney reabsorption. There is also an increased chance of crystallization of sulfonamides in the urine when ascorbic acid is given at the same time as sulfa drugs. Ascorbic acid decreases the effect of tricyclic antidepressants by decreasing kidney reabsorption. Calcium ascorbate may cause *cardiac dysrhythmias* (irregular heartbeats) in patients receiving digoxin. Ascorbic acid is chemically incompatible with potassium penicillin G and should not be mixed in the same syringe. Smoking may lead to an increased need for vitamin C by decreasing ascorbic acid serum levels. Intermittent use of ascorbic acid in patients who are taking ethinyl estradiol (a compound in many birth control pills) may increase the risk for contraceptive failure.

❖ Nursing Implications and Patient Teaching

Vitamin C comes in three major forms that may be given orally or parenterally: ascorbic acid, sodium ascorbate, and calcium ascorbate. The recommended daily intake is 60 mg for adults.

Vitamin C is easily destroyed by air, heat, and light. This drug should be kept tightly capped in its own container. Foods high in vitamin C should not be boiled for long periods or left uncovered in the refrigerator.

Good food sources of vitamin C include oranges, grapefruit, strawberries, cauliflower, cantaloupe, beef liver, asparagus, green leafy vegetables, and potatoes.

VITAMIN D

Action and Uses

Vitamin D is a label used for a group of fat-soluble, chemically similar *sterols* (plant steroids). The three main categories within this group are:

1. *ergocalciferol* (vitamin D_2), which is very limited in nature in both distribution and concentration but can be artificially manufactured by ultraviolet irradiation on ergot and yeasts;
2. *cholecalciferol* (vitamin D_3), which occurs naturally in fish liver oils and can be formed in animals and humans by ultraviolet irradiation on the skin; and
3. other lesser compounds such as vitamins D_4, D_5, D_6, and D_7.

The main action of this group of vitamins is the movement of calcium and phosphorous ions into three main sites: the small intestine (to promote absorption of calcium and phosphorus from the gut), the kidneys (to cause phosphate reabsorption and, to a lesser extent, to stimulate calcium and sodium reabsorption), and bone (to help increase the mineralization of newly formed bone). Vitamin D_3 contributes to skin growth and repair. It is used in the treatment of some skin disorders.

Vitamin D preparations are used to treat childhood rickets and adult osteomalacia, hypoparathyroidism, and familial hypophosphatemia. In childhood the first symptoms of rickets are excessive sweating and GI disturbances. These may appear before any obvious changes in bone have occurred. In adult cases of osteomalacia, patients may have skeletal pain and progressive muscular weakness.

Symptoms of vitamin D toxicity include anorexia, nausea, malaise, weight loss, vague aches and stiffness, constipation, diarrhea, convulsions, anemia, mild acidosis, and impairment of kidney function. The kidney effects are usually reversible. A variety of more serious systemic effects may be seen in adults. Dwarfism may be present in infants and children. Most toxic effects persist for several months in adults at doses of 100,000 IU or more daily or in children at doses of 20,000 IU or more daily. Reactions gradually disappear if treatment is discontinued at the first sign of symptoms.

Mineral oil and some of the antihyperlipidemic (blood fat-lowering) drugs may interfere with the absorption of fat-soluble vitamins. Thiazide diuretics and vitamin D together contribute to hypercalcemia. There is a possible connection between phenytoin (Dilantin) and phenobarbital use leading to hypocalcemia, which, in turn, may contribute to rickets or osteomalacia.

❖ Nursing Implications and Patient Teaching

The dosage of vitamin D must be planned for each patient and given under close supervision, because the range between the therapeutic and the toxic levels is narrow. Calcium intake should be enough to give a serum calcium level between 9 and 10 mg/dL. In rickets 12,000 to 500,000 IU/day can be taken. In hypoparathyroidism the initial dose is typically 50,000 to 200,000 IU/day, with a maintenance dosage of 50,000 to 400,000 IU/day. Other than sun exposure, natural sources of vitamin D are few, so the majority of vitamin D is obtained from fortified sources. Fortified foods high in this vitamin are milk, evaporated milk, infant formula, and powdered skim milk. Cereals, margarine, and diet foods also contain vitamin D supplements. Breast milk is usually already vitamin D rich. Vitamin D should be protected from light in a light-resistant container.

VITAMIN E

Action and Uses

Vitamin E is fat soluble and consists of naturally occurring tocopherols. Vitamin E is considered an essential nutrient for humans, even though its specific functions are not yet understood. Vitamin E may function as an antioxidant to prevent damage to cell membranes. It stabilizes red blood cell walls and protects them from breakage or destruction. It may also increase vitamin A use and stop platelet aggregation.

Many suggested uses of vitamin E are controversial and unproved. The only established use is to prevent or treat vitamin E deficiency. Vitamin E has been touted as a powerful antioxidant. New evidence suggests that vitamin E supplements do not reduce the risk for cancer or major cardiovascular disease and may even increase the risk for heart failure.

Vitamin E appears to be the least toxic of the fat-soluble vitamins. No signs and symptoms of toxicity or hypervitaminosis have been identified as yet in humans. However, results of a 2004 meta-analysis of research studies suggest that doses greater than 150 IU/day increase the risk for all-cause mortality. The higher the dose taken, the higher the mortality rate. The most commonly marketed dose in the United States is 400 IU.

❖ Nursing Implications and Patient Teaching

Food sources of vitamin E are primarily from plants. The highest amounts are found in vegetable oils, such as soybean and corn, and in nuts, wheat germ, rice germ, and green leafy vegetables. Meat and dairy products provide less vitamin E. An accurate assessment of tocopherol levels in food is difficult to obtain. The amount in the body depends on the initial concentration of vitamin E and the processing, storage, and preparation of the food. Vitamin E products should be stored in tightly closed, light-resistant containers.

VITAMIN K

Action and Uses

Vitamin K helps liver formation of factors II, VII, IX, and X, which are essential for normal blood clotting. The exact mechanism is unknown. K_3 and K_1 are synthetic lipid-soluble forms of vitamin K.

Vitamin K is used to treat or prevent various blood clotting disorders that result in damaged formation of factors II, VII, IX, and X. The American Academy of Pediatrics recommends routine phytonadione (K_1) injection at birth to prevent hemorrhagic disease of the newborn. Vitamin K does not counteract the anticoagulant activity of heparin, although it is helpful in reversing the effects of warfarin (Coumadin) overdosage.

Specific adverse reactions to phytonadione (K_1) are transient flushing, dizziness, a strange taste in the mouth, sweating, hypotension, and pain or swelling at injection site. Severe hypersensitivity reactions can occur. Anaphylactic shock including cardiac arrest, respiratory arrest, and death have occurred during and immediately after IV injection.

Use of vitamin K along with oral anticoagulants, especially warfarin, may decrease the effects of the anticoagulant. Mineral oil and cholestyramine inhibit GI absorption of oral vitamin K.

❖ Nursing Implications and Patient Teaching

The preferred routes of administration of vitamin K are subcutaneous or IM. IV administration is not recommended because of the risk for anaphylaxis. Naturally occurring vitamin K is found in liver and green leafy vegetables.

MINERALS

Nineteen **minerals** are present in the body, at least 13 of which are essential to normal metabolism and function. These minerals are present in body fluids as *ions* with positive and negative charges, leading to the formation of salts. They act as catalysts to speed up various biochemical reactions. Minerals are obtained from a diet that includes a variety of animal and vegetable products, and meets the energy and protein needs of the body. The Food and Nutrition Board of the National Research Council has established recommended daily intakes for calcium and iron. Calcium, iron, and iodine are the three elements most frequently missing in the diet. Zinc, iron, copper, magnesium, and potassium are the five minerals most frequently involved in disturbances of metabolism. As electrolytes, these preparations are commonly infused to critically ill patients who are unable to take food orally.

CALCIUM

Action and Uses

Calcium is a major mineral in the body and is essential for muscular and neurologic activity, especially in the cardiac system. Calcium is important in these actions:

- assists in the formation and repair of skeletal tissues (bones and teeth),
- activates several enzymes that influence cell membrane permeability and muscle contraction,
- aids in blood clotting by stimulating the release of thromboplastin and the conversion of fibrinogen to fibrin,
- activates pancreatic enzymes for digestion,
- increases the intestinal absorption of cobalamin,
- is involved in the transmission of neurotransmitters and in metabolic processes, and
- helps regulate some white blood cell functions.

Calcium is used as a supplement when dietary levels of calcium are not adequate. Calcium requirements may be increased during adolescence, pregnancy, and breast-feeding, and for postmenopausal women. Calcium is also used to treat neonatal hypocalcemia and to prevent and treat postmenopausal and senile osteoporosis. It may also be used as a supplement to parenterally given vitamin D in cases of hypoparathyroidism, pseudohypoparathyroidism (a relatively rare condition in which the body fails to respond to parathyroid hormone), rickets, and *osteomalacia* (a condition resulting in the formation of soft bones).

Signs of *hypocalcemia* (low blood calcium levels) are muscle spasms; numbness and tingling of the lips and fingers; weak, brittle nails; and fractures. Symptoms of hypercalcemia are polyuria (excretion of a large amount of urine), constipation, abdominal pain, dryness of mouth, anorexia, nausea, and vomiting.

Vitamin D is essential for the absorption of calcium in the body. Calcium status is affected by the calcium-to-phosphorous ratio in the body and by the level of protein in the diet. Phytic acid (found in bran and whole-grain cereals) and oxalic acid (found in spinach and rhubarb) may interfere with calcium absorption by combining with calcium to form insoluble salts in the intestine. Calcium compounds and calcium-rich substances such as milk interfere with the absorption of oral tetracycline, so their use together should be avoided. Use of corticosteroids may also decrease the absorption of calcium.

❖ Nursing Implications and Patient Teaching

In patients with low calcium levels, hand (carpal) spasm may be elicited by compressing the upper arm with a blood pressure cuff, causing ischemia (decreased blood supply) to the distal nerves. The patient may report a tingling sensation and may inadvertently flex the arm. This is called *Trousseau's sign*. Excessive amounts of calcium may lead to hypercalcemia and hypercalciuria, especially in hyperthyroid patients. Calcium should not be given to patients who already have kidney stones.

Calcium products come in combination with various other chemicals, with a concentration between 6% and 40%. Preparations come in both parenteral and oral forms. OTC antacids containing calcium (e.g., Tums) are composed of calcium carbonate, the most elemental form of calcium. It is better absorbed than many calcium products and is a smaller tablet than many other calcium products, making administration easier.

The recommended daily intake of calcium is 1200 mg/day for adults and adolescents, 800 mg/day for children, 360 to 540 mg/day for infants from birth to 1 year, and 1500 mg/day for nursing mothers. Milk, cheese, yogurt, bok choy, tofu, okra, broccoli, almonds, and fish canned with bones are the richest sources of calcium. Egg yolks and most dark green leafy vegetables are also good sources.

IRON

Action and Uses

Iron is an essential mineral for the body to make myoglobin and hemoglobin. It stimulates the hematopoietic system and increases the production of hemoglobin to correct iron deficiency. Iron from cellular hemoglobin is recycled and most is used again. During pregnancy the reabsorption of iron increases to 15% as the body's way of adapting to physiologic anemia.

Iron is used to treat symptomatic iron deficiency anemia only after the cause of the anemia has been identified, and it is used to prevent hypochromic anemia during infancy, childhood, pregnancy, and breast-feeding; in patients recovering from other anemias; and after some GI surgeries.

Expected reactions to iron supplements include constipation and cramping. Adverse reactions such as diarrhea or epigastric or abdominal pain may occur. Symptoms of overdosage may occur after 30 minutes to several hours and include *lethargy* (sleepiness), nausea, vomiting, abdominal pain, diarrhea, *melena* (blood in stools), and *dyspnea* (uncomfortable breathing). Coma and metabolic acidosis may occur, as well as symptoms of systemic absorption. Children who mistake vitamins for candy are particularly sensitive to large amounts of iron and may die of overdoses.

> ### ⚠ Drug Alert
> Fatal anaphylactic reactions can occur with iron dextran IV or IM administration. Hypersensitivity reactions include rash, itching, joint pain, muscle aches, and fever.

Large iron doses may cause a false-positive test result for occult blood using the toluidine test (Hematest, Occultist, Clinistix). Absorption of oral iron is inhibited by tannic acid in tea, antacids (particularly magnesium-containing antacids), milk, and eggs. Patients who are receiving chloramphenicol concurrently with iron may show a delayed response to iron therapy. Absorption of iron increases when given with orange juice or ascorbic acid (vitamin C) in doses of 200 mg per 30 mg of iron. Iron interferes with absorption of oral tetracycline. Vitamin E decreases the response to iron therapy. Many other drugs have interactions with iron.

❖ Nursing Implications and Patient Teaching
Replacement of iron in iron deficiency anemia requires 90 to 300 mg of elemental iron daily in divided doses (6 mg/kg/day). Symptoms usually go away within 2 weeks, and laboratory studies are normal within 2 months, if treatment is adequate. Therapy for 4 to 6 months after the anemia has been corrected is advised to replenish iron stores.

More iron is absorbed if the iron is taken on an empty stomach with water or in an acid environment, although taking it after meals can reduce stomach irritation. Taking iron after a meal can reduce the absorption by 40% to 50%. Liquid iron preparations can discolor teeth and should be taken through a straw after dilution with liquid.

All simple oral iron preparations are available OTC. The absorption of iron taken orally or through dietary foods is generally about 10%. The body does have the capability to increase iron absorption during times of physiologic stress, such as pregnancy and severe blood loss.

The recommended daily intake of elemental iron in adult men is 10 mg; in adult women, 18 mg (with an additional 10 mg during pregnancy or lactation); and in children, 10 to 15 mg. A diet high in natural iron should be encouraged to meet these needs. Fish, red meat, spinach, and dried fruits are the best sources of dietary iron.

Iron supplements can cause dark green or black stools. Tell patients to report constipation, diarrhea, nausea, or abdominal pain to the healthcare provider.

MAGNESIUM
Action and Uses
Magnesium is an electrolyte that is essential to several enzyme systems. It is important in maintaining osmotic pressure, ion balance, bone structure, muscular contraction, and nerve conduction. This mineral has been determined to be especially important in cardiac function, and only slight deficiencies may prolong the QT interval and lead to a very dangerous form of *ventricular tachycardia* (rapid heartbeat) called *torsades de pointes*. Excessive magnesium intake may produce diarrhea.

❖ Nursing Implications and Patient Teaching
Magnesium deficiencies are seen primarily when malabsorption syndromes are present. Magnesium is usually used with other vitamins as a general dietary supplement when multiple deficiencies are suspected. Deficiency states have been associated with convulsions, slowing of growth, digestive disturbances, spasticity of muscles and nerves, accelerated heartbeat, dysrhythmias, nervous conditions, and vasodilation (opening of blood vessels). Magnesium is available in adequate quantities in meat, milk, fruits, and vegetables, and special dietary planning is unnecessary. Large amounts of magnesium are present in spinach, chard, and pumpkin seeds.

POTASSIUM
Action and Uses
Potassium is the principle intracellular positive ion (*cation*) of most body tissues, acting in the maintenance of normal kidney function, contraction of muscle, and transmission of nerve impulses. It is found in the body within a very narrow range.

Potassium may be taken *prophylactically* (for prevention) when the patient has nephrotic syndrome, in patients with liver cirrhosis with ascites, and in patients with hyperaldosteronism who have normal kidney function. Potassium products are used prophylactically or to replace potassium that may be lost as a result of long-term diuretic therapy, digoxin intoxication, or low dietary intake of potassium. Supplementation may be necessary for deficits resulting from vomiting and diarrhea, diabetic acidosis, metabolic alkalosis, or corticosteroid therapy, or to counteract increased kidney excretion of potassium because of acidosis, certain kidney tubular disorders, or diseases that produce increased secretion of glucocorticoids or aldosterone.

Either an excess or a deficit of potassium causes symptoms. Adverse reactions to potassium supplements include nausea, vomiting, diarrhea, abdominal discomfort, and GI bleeding. Potassium intoxication or *hyperkalemia* (increased potassium in the blood) may result from overdosage of potassium or from a change in the patient's underlying condition, which may make potassium buildup possible. Signs and symptoms of potassium intoxication include flaccid paralysis, *paresthesias* (numbness and tingling) of the hands and feet, mental confusion, restlessness, listlessness, malaise, and heaviness of the legs. Hypotension and cardiac dysrhythmias leading to heart block may also develop. Potentially fatal dysrhythmias may develop if potassium cannot be excreted (or if it is given too rapidly IV). When it is detected, hyperkalemia requires immediate treatment because lethal levels of potassium may be reached in a few hours in untreated patients. Potentially fast and irregular lethal dysrhythmias may also occur with *hypokalemia* (decreased potassium in the blood).

Potassium should not be used in patients who are receiving potassium-sparing agents such as aldosterone antagonists or triamterene, because overdosage may develop.

❖ Nursing Implications and Patient Teaching

All potassium supplements must be diluted properly or taken with plenty of liquid to avoid producing GI ulcers. The usual adult dietary intake of potassium ranges between 40 and 60 mEq/day. The loss of 200 or more mEq of potassium from the total body store is enough to produce hypokalemia.

The dosage must be *titrated* (increased or decreased slowly) based on the patient's needs, and he or she must be closely watched during therapy, especially in the initial stages of therapy. For patients who are receiving diuretic therapy, 20 mEq/day is usually adequate for the prevention of hypokalemia. In cases of potassium depletion, 40 to 100 mEq/day or more may be required for replacement. Blood levels must be closely monitored.

Potassium comes in various salt combinations; potassium chloride is the form most frequently prescribed. It may be ordered either by percentage of potassium chloride or in milliequivalents of potassium chloride, with 10 mEq KCl per 15 mL equivalent to 5% KCl. Other salt combinations are potassium gluconate, potassium citrate, potassium acetate, and potassium bicarbonate.

A potassium-rich diet includes foods such as bananas, citrus fruits (especially tomatoes and oranges), apricots, and dried fruits such as raisins, prunes, and dates. Fresh cantaloupe and watermelon, nuts, dried beans, beef, and fowl also contain ample quantities of potassium.

> **Memory Jogger**
>
> Both low blood potassium levels and high blood potassium levels can cause fatal heart dysrhythmias.

ZINC

Action and Uses

Zinc is a part of many enzymes and is essential for normal growth and tissue repair. Zinc functions in the mineralization of bone and in the detoxification of methanol and ethylene glycol. It plays a role in the creation of DNA and the synthesis of protein from amino acids. It is important in wound healing and functions in moving vitamin A from liver stores.

Zinc supplements are used to prevent zinc deficiency and to treat delayed wound healing. There is some evidence to support the use of zinc OTC products in reducing the severity of symptoms of the common cold.

Patients who are taking zinc may report abnormalities of taste and smell, rough skin, and anorexia with profound disinterest in food. Patients who lack zinc may demonstrate sexual immaturity, delayed wound healing, and decreased absorption of dietary folate.

Adverse reactions to zinc supplements include gastric ulceration, nausea, and vomiting. Doses in excess of 2 g produce *emesis* (vomiting). Acute zinc intoxication produces drowsiness, lethargy, light-headedness, staggering gait, restlessness, and vomiting leading to dehydration.

Calcium competes with zinc for absorption. Phytates form insoluble complexes with zinc and interfere with its absorption. Zinc impairs the absorption of tetracycline derivatives.

❖ Nursing Implications and Patient Teaching

Seafood and meats are rich sources of natural zinc; cereals and legumes also have significant amounts of this mineral.

Get Ready for the NCLEX® Examination!

Key Points

- Patients think herbals and OTC products are safe. Ask patients to bring all herbals and OTC drugs with them to every appointment.
- Some OTC, herbal, and complementary therapy drugs can interact and interfere with a patient's prescribed therapy.
- St. John's wort, goldenseal, and ginseng are the top three herbals that people take and they are likely to have dangerous interactions with many prescribed drugs.
- Almost all vitamins can be destroyed by air, light, and heat. Keep vitamins in a tightly capped bottle away from the light and heat.
- Fat-soluble ADEK vitamins, if not taken as prescribed or recommended, can have toxic effects called *hypervitaminosis*.
- If giving vitamin B$_1$ (thiamine) to alcoholics or thiamine-deficient persons, IV glucose needs to be given to prevent Wernicke's encephalopathy.
- Vitamin B$_{12}$ requires intrinsic factor to be absorbed. In pernicious anemia give vitamin B$_{12}$ via nasal, sublingual, or IM route.
- Use of vitamin K may decrease the effectiveness of oral anticoagulants.
- Vitamin D is essential for calcium absorption.
- A deficit or excess of potassium can lead to fatal cardiac dysrhythmias.

Review Questions for the NCLEX® Examination

1. Which class of over-the-counter drug should be avoided by recovering alcoholics?
   1. Analgesics
   2. Decongestants
   3. Cough syrups
   4. Antacids
2. A label of a liquid vitamin preparation says to take 10 mL of syrup every 4 hours. The patient asks if 2 teaspoons of the drug is the right amount. What is the nurse's best response?
   1. Yes, one teaspoon is the same amount as 5 mL.
   2. I will call your prescriber to see if that is the right dosage.
   3. No, you will need to take 3 teaspoons to cover that amount.
   4. The measurement is not the same. I will give you a marked syringe to use.
3. The nurse learns a patient is taking both the herbal drug St. John's wort and an antidepressant. What is the nurse's most appropriate advice based on this information?
   1. You will be able to decrease your dose of antidepressant because the St. John's wort has the same effect.
   2. Notify your prescriber to increase your dose of antidepressant.
   3. Stop the St. John's wort immediately because a dangerous interaction can occur.
   4. St. John's wort is an effective antidepressant so you can taper off your antidepressant now.
4. When purchasing nonprescription products, what is the advantage of looking for a company that is a member of the Council for Responsible Nutrition?
   1. The companies provide lists of dietary supplements at discount prices.
   2. The companies comply with federal and state regulations, as well as a code of ethics.
   3. The companies use only organic supplements approved by the FDA.
   4. The companies conduct evidenced-based research and provide information.
5. Which individual is most likely to have a vitamin deficiency?
   1. A breast-fed infant
   2. A patient with ulcerative colitis
   3. A moderately overweight patient who is on a Weight Watchers diet
   4. A patient who is NPO for 24 hours
6. A new nurse asks why thiamine and glucose have been ordered together for a severely malnourished patient. What is the best explanation?
   1. The patient's blood sugar was likely low because of the malnourished state.
   2. The glucose helps the thiamine enter the cell.
   3. The glucose will help prevent precipitation of an encephalopathy.
   4. Glucose helps with thiamine-deficient symptoms such as poor coordination.
7. What precaution is important to give to patients on antihypertensive drugs who are also taking niacin?
   1. The itching caused by the combination can be relieved with antihistamines.
   2. You should slowly get up from a sitting position to prevent hypotension.
   3. The drug combination can cause disorientation and memory loss.
   4. You should stay out of the sun to prevent dermatitis.
8. A patient with pernicious anemia asks the nurse why she must get an injection of vitamin B$_{12}$ every month. What is the best response given by the nurse?
   1. The injection works in the fastest way to cure the anemia.
   2. The health professional you are seeing prefers this route of administration.
   3. Your body cannot absorb the vitamin B$_{12}$ orally because your stomach does not secrete a necessary protein.
   4. I will ask the prescriber to order the vitamin B$_{12}$ in a tablet you can swallow.
9. Which statement about vitamin D preparations are true?
   1. They are used to treat rickets and adult osteomalacia.
   2. They are used to treat beriberi.
   3. They are used to treat pellagra.
   4. They must be given with calcium for the vitamin to be absorbed.

Bibliography

American Diabetes Association. (2016). Approaches to glycemic treatment. Sec. 7. In standards of medical care in diabetes, 2016. *Diabetes Care*, *39*(Suppl. 1), S52–S59.

American Gastroenterological Association, Bharucha, A. E., Dorn, S. D., et al. (2013). American Gastroenterological Association medical position statement on constipation. *Gastroenterology*, *144*(1), 211–217. doi:10.1053/j.gastro.2012.10.029.

American Heart Association. (2017). *Heart disease and stroke statistics at-a-glance*. https://www.heart.org/idc/groups/ahamah-public/@wcm/@sop/@smd/documents/downloadable/ucm_491265.pdf.

American Psychiatric Association (APA). (2010). *Practice guideline for the treatment of patients with major depressive disorder* (3rd ed., p. 152). Arlington (VA): American Psychiatric Association (APA). https://guideline.gov/summaries/summary/24158/Practice-guideline-for-the-treatment-of-patients-with-major-depressive-disorder-third-edition. [1170 references] [Retrieved from AHRQ National Guideline Clearinghouse].

Armstrong, P. W., & Collen, D. (2001). Fibrinolysis in acute myocardial infarction. *Circulation*, *103*, 2987–2992. https://doi.org/10.1161/01.CIR.103.24.2987.

Ashjian, E., & Tingen, J. (2017). Sodium-glucose co-transporter 2 inhibitors. *Nurse Practitioner*, *42*(4), 9–15.

Asthma Treatment. (2014). http://acaai.org/asthma/asthma-treatment.

Bittle, P. A. (2017). Use of dipeptidyl peptidase-4 inhibitors in patients with type 2 diabetes and chronic kidney disease. *Nurse Practitioner*, *42*(6), 31–38.

Bravo, K., & Cochran, G. (2016). Nursing strategies to increase medication safety in inpatient settings. *Journal of Nursing Care Quality*, *31*(4), 335–341.

Bureau of Labor Statistics United States Department of Labor. (Dec. 17, 2015). *Occupational outlook handbook: Licensed practical and licensed vocational nurses*. https://www.bls.gov/ooh/healthcare/licensed-practical-and-licensed-vocational-nurses.htm.

Centers for Medicare & Medical Services. (2005). *Commonly prescribed medications by category by brand (generic)*. Retrieved from https://www.cms.gov/Medicare/Quality-Initiatives-Patient-Assessment-Instruments/NursingHomeQualityInits/downloads/MDS202005AppendixE.pdf.

Chamberlain, J. J., Herman, W. H., Leal, S., et al. (2017). Pharmacologic therapy for type 2 diabetes: Synopsis of the 2017 American Diabetes Association Standards of Medical Care in Diabetes. *Annals of Internal Medicine*, *166*(8), 572–578. PMID: 28288484.

Clinical Pharmacology. (2017). https://www.clinicalpharmacology.com/Forms/login.aspx?ReturnUrl=%2fdefault.aspx.

Cohen, M. R. (2016). Medication errors. *Nursing*, *16*(12), 72.

Cookson, K. (2013). Dimensional analysis: Calculate drug dosages the easy way. *Nursing*, *43*(6), 57–62.

Council for Responsible Nutrition. (2017). http://www.crnusa.org/.

Current Treatment for Alzheimer's Disease. (2017). http://www.alz.org/research/science/alzheimers_disease_treatments.asp.

De Villiers, T. J., Pines, A., Gambacciani, M., et al. (2013). Updated 2013 international menopause society recommendations on menopausal therapy and preventive strategies for midlife health. *Climacteric: The Journal of the International Menopause Society*, *16*, 316–337.

Del Vecchio, L., & Locatelli, F. (2016). An overview on safety issues related to erythropoiesis stimulating agents for the treatment of anaemia in patients with chronic kidney disease. *Expert Opinion on Drug Safety*, *15*(8), 1021–1030. doi:10.1080/14740338.2016.1182494. [Epub 2016 May 13].

Emani, S., Hamishehkar, H., Mahmoodpoor, A., et al. (2012). Errors of oral medication administration in a patient with enteral feeding tube. *Journal of Research in Pharmacy Practice*, *1*(1), 37–40.

Farkouh, A., Frigo, P., & Czejka, M. (2016). Systemic side effects of eye drops: A pharmacokinetic perspective. *Clinical ophthalmology*, *10*, 2433–2441.

Feng, Y., & Yang, H. (2017). Metformin - a potentially effective drug for gestational diabetes mellitus: A systematic review and meta-analysis. *Journal of Maternal-Fetal & Neonatal Medicine*, *30*(15), 1874–1881. PMID: 27549367.

Fischer, B., Russell, C., Sabioni, P., et al. (2017). Lower-risk cannabis use guidelines: A comprehensive update of evidence and recommendations. *American Journal of Public Health*, *107*(8), e1–e12.

Flemming, S., Brady, A. M., & Malone, A. M. (2014). An evaluation of the drug calculation skills of registered nurses. *Nurse Education in Practice*, *14*, 55e61.

Fletcher, C. E. (2000). Accurate data: An essential component in reducing needlestick injuries. *Policy, Politics & Nursing Practice*, *1*(4), 316–324.

González-Pérez, A., Sáez, M. E., Johansson, S., et al. (2015). Incidence and predictors of hemorrhagic stroke in users of low-dose acetylsalicylic acid. *Journal of Stroke and Cerebrovascular Diseases*, *24*(10), 2321–2328.

Hadaway, L. (2004). Closing the case on the keep vein open rate. *Nursing*, *34*(8), 18. PMID: 15286486. NLM UID: 7600137.

Haw, C., & Stubbs, J. (2010). Administration of medicines in food and drink: A study of older inpatients with severe mental illness. *International Psychogeriatrics*, *22*(3), 409–416.

Hennessey, J. V., & Espallat, R. (2015). Diagnosis and management of subclinical hypothyroidism in elderly adults: A review of the literature. *Journal of the American Geriatrics Society*, *63*, 1663–1673.

HIV Basics. (2017). https://www.cdc.gov/hiv/basics/index.html.

Hseih, C. (2005). Treatment of constipation in older adults. *American Family Physician*, *72*(11), 2277–2284.

Institute for Safe Medication Practices. (2015). *ISMP's list of confused drug names*. http://www.ismp.org/Tools/confuseddrugnames.pdf.

Institute for Safe Medication Practices. (2015). *ISMP's list of error-prone abbreviations, symbols, and drug designations*. http://www.ismp.org/Tools/errorproneabbreviations.pdf.

Institute for Safe Medication Practices. (2016). *FDA and ISMP lists of look-alike drug names with recommended tall man letters*. https://www.ismp.org/Tools/tallmanletters.pdf.

Institute for Safe Medication Practices. (2017). *ISMP's list of high-alert medications*. https://www.ismp.org/Tools/highAlert-MedicationLists.asp.

James, P. A., Oparil, S., Carter, B. L., et al. (2014). Evidence-based guideline for the management of high blood pressure in adults: Report from the panel members appointed to the Eighth

Joint National Committee (JNC 8). *JAMA: The Journal of the American Medical Association, 311*(5), 507–520. doi:10.1001/jama.2013.284427.

Kahrilas, P. J., Shaheen, N. J., & Vaezi, M. F. (2008). American gastroenterological association medical position statement on the management of gastroesophageal reflux disease. *Gastroenterology, 135*(4), 1383–1391.e1385.

Kansagra, S. M., McCudden, C. R., & Willis, M. S. (2010). The challenges and complexities of thyroid hormone replacement. *Labmedicine, 41*(6), 338–348.

Kirkevold, O., & Engedal, K. (2010). What's the matter with crushing pills and opening capsules? *International Journal of Nursing Practice, 16*, 81–85.

Koharchik, L., & Flavin, P. (2017). Teaching students to administer medications safely. *The American Journal of Nursing, 117*(1), 62–66.

Lanas, A., & Gargallo, C. J. (2015). Management of low-dose aspirin and clopidogrel in clinical practice: A gastrointestinal perspective. *Journal of Gastroenterology, 50*(6), 626–637.

Lilley, L., Collins, S., & Snyder, J. (2014). *Pharmacology and the nursing process.* St. Louis: Elsevier.

Liu, D., Ahmet, A., Ward, L., et al. (2013). A practical guide to the monitoring and management of the complications of systemic corticosteroid therapy. *Allergy, Asthma, and Clinical Immunology : Official Journal of the Canadian Society of Allergy and Clinical Immunology, 9*(1), 30. http://doi.org/10.1186/1710-1492-9-30.

Manza, P., Amandola, M., Tatineni, V., et al. (2017). Response inhibition in Parkinson's disease: A meta-analysis of dopaminergic medication and disease duration effects. *NPJ Parkinson's Disease, 3*, 23. http://doi.org/10.1038/s41531-017-0024-2.

Marmur, J. D. (2002). Direct versus indirect thrombin inhibition in percutaneous coronary intervention. *The Journal of Invasive Cardiology, 14*(Suppl. B).

McAnich, E. A., & Bianco, A. C. (2016). The history and future of treatment of hypothyroidism. *Annals of Internal Medicine, 164*, 50–56.

McCance, K., & Huether, S. (2006). *Pathophysiology, the biological basis for disease in adults and children.* St. Louis: Elsevier Mosby.

McCuistion, L. E., DiMaggio, K., Winton, M. B., et al. (2018). *Pharmacology: A patient-centered nursing process approach* (9th ed.). St. Louis: Elsevier.

Mestre, T., & Ferreira, J. J. (2010). Pharmacotherapy in Parkinson's disease: Case studies. *Therapeutic Advances in Neurological Disorders, 3*(2), 117–126. http://doi.org/10.1177/1756285609352366.

National Center for Complementary and Integrative Health. (2016). https://nccih.nih.gov/.

National Council of State Boards of Nursing. (2005). *Practical nurse scope of practice white paper.* https://www.ncsbn.org/Final_11_05_Practical_Nurse_Scope_Practice_White_Paper.pdf.

National Council of State Boards of Nursing. (2015). *2015 LPN/VN practice analysis: Linking the NCLEX-PN examination to practice* (Vol. 67). https://www.ncsbn.org/16_2015LPN_Practice_Analysis_vol67.pdf.

National Eye Institute. (nd). *Eye disease facts for health professionals.* https://nei.nih.gov/sites/default/files/health-pdfs/Health_Professional_Handout.pdf.

National Institute of Health. *Nutrient recommendations: Dietary reference intakes.* https://ods.od.nih.gov/Health_Information/Dietary_Reference_Intakes.aspx.

National Institute of Health. *Herbs at a glance.* https://nccih.nih.gov/health/herbsataglance.htm.

National League for Nursing Board of Governors. (2014). *A vision for recognition of the role of licensed practical/vocational nurses in advancing the nation's health.* http://www.nln.org/docs/default-source/about/nln-vision-series-%28position-statements%29/nlnvision_7.pdf.

Potter, P., Perry, A., Stockert, P., et al. (2013). *Fundamentals of nursing.* St. Louis: Elsevier.

Powers, M. A., Bardsley, J., Cypress, M., et al. (2015). Diabetes self-management and support in type 2 diabetes. A joint position statement of the American Diabetes Association of Diabetes Educators, and the Academy of Nutrition and Dietetics. *The Diabetes Educator, 43*(1), 40–53.

Preston, S., & Drusano, G. (2017). *Penicillins. Antimicrobe.* http://www.antimicrobe.org/d24.asp.

Registered Nurses' Association of Ontario. (2011). *Prevention of constipation in the older adult: Guideline supplement.* http://rnao.ca/sites/rnao-ca/files/Constipation_supplement_2011.pdf.

Revankar, S., & Sobel, J. (2014). *Antifungal drugs. Merck manual.* http://www.merckmanuals.com/professional/infectious-diseases/fungi/antifungal-drugs.

Riddle, M. C. (2017). Modern sulfonylureas: Dangerous or wrongly accused? *Diabetes Care, 40*(5), 629–631. PMID: 28428320.

Rojo, L. E., Gaspar, P. A., Silva, H., et al. (2015). Metabolic syndrome and obesity among users of second generation antipsychotics: A global challenge for modern psychopharmacology. *Pharmacological Research, 101*(Suppl. C), 74–85.

Sexton, K., Lindauer, A., & Harvath, T. (2016). Administration of subcutaneous injections. *The American Journal of Nursing, 116*(12), 49–51.

Shastay, A. (2016). Evidence-based practice guidelines for I.V. push medications. *Nursing, 46*(10), 38–44.

Silvestri, L. (2013). *Saunders comprehensive review for the NCLEX-PN examination.* St Louis: Elsevier.

Stolic, S. (2014). Educational strategies aimed at improving student nurse's medication calculation skills: A review of the research literature. *Nurse Education in Practice, 14.*

Tanga, H. Y. (2011). Nurse drug diversion and nursing leaders' responsibilities: Legal, regulatory, ethical, humanistic and practical considerations. *JONA's Healthcare Law, Ethics, and Regulation, 13*(1), 13–16.

Umanath, K., Greco, B., Jalal, D. I., et al. (2017). The safety of achieved iron stores and their effect on IV iron and ESA use: post-hoc results from a randomized trial of ferric citrate as a phosphate binder in dialysis. *Clinical Nephrology,* doi:10.5414/CN108924. [Epub ahead of print].

Vrbnjak, D., Denieff, S., O'Gorman, C., et al. (2016). Barriers to reporting medication errors and near misses among nurses: A systematic review. *International Journal of Nursing Studies, 63*, 162–178.

Welliver, M. (2016). Cannabinoid agonists for nausea and vomiting. *Gastroenterology Nursing, 39*(2), 137–139.

Whelton, P. K., Carey, R. M., Aronow, W. S., et al. (2017). A guideline for the prevention, detection, evaluation, and management of high blood pressure in adults: A report of the American College of Cardiology/American Heart Association Task Force on Clinical Practice Guidelines. *Journal of the American College of Cardiology,* [Epub ahead of print].

Workman, M., & Ignatavicius, D. (2016). *Medical surgical nursing: A collaborative approach.* St. Louis: Elsevier.

Workman, M., & LaCharity, L. (2016). *Understanding pharmacology essentials for medication safety.* St. Louis: Elsevier.

World Health Organization. (2014). *Mental health: A state of well-being.* [Retrieved from] http://www.who.int/features/factfiles/mental_health/en/.

Yin, H. S. (2016). Parents often give the wrong dose of medication to their children. *The American Journal of Nursing, 166*(12), 18.

Glossary

A

absorption Drugs enter the body and pass into the circulation to reach the part of the body it needs to affect through the processes of diffusion, osmosis, and filtration.

acquired immunity A long-acting and "learned" protective response by lymphocyte production of antibodies that are directed against specific microorganisms.

active immunity Acquired immunity in which your body makes specific antibodies to antigens. Can be natural or artificial.

acute pain Pain that is usually related to an injury, such as recent surgery, trauma, or infection, and ends within an expected time frame.

addiction A psychological dependence in which there is a desperate need to have and use a drug for a nonmedical reason. The addicted person has a limited ability to control this drug craving or use.

additive effect When two drugs are given together and either make one drug stronger or make the action of the two drugs more powerful.

adrenergics A category of drugs that affects nervous system control of various organs and tissues by activating or blocking receptors that respond to the body's natural adrenergic substances, epinephrine and norepinephrine.

adverse effect A drug effect that is more severe than expected and has the potential to damage tissue or cause serious health problems. It may also be called *adverse effect, toxic effect,* or *toxicity,* and it usually requires intervention by the prescriber.

adverse reactions Severe symptoms or problems that can cause great harm.

agonist Drug that works by activating or unlocking cell receptors, causing the same actions as the body's own chemicals.

AIDS The later stage of HIV disease that causes a breakdown in the immune system, leaving the patient unable to fight infection.

aldosterone A hormone secreted by the adrenal cortex that regulates sodium and water balance.

allergy An excessive reaction that leads to an inflammatory response when a person comes into contact with a substance (allergen) to which he or she is sensitive. It is a common immune response to substances such as pollen, animal dander, food, or dust. Also known as hypersensitivity.

alpha-adrenergic agonists These drugs bind to receptor sites in the eye and reduce the amount of aqueous humor produced.

alpha$_1$-adrenergic antagonists A type of adrenergic drug that lowers blood pressure by blocking the adrenergic receptor sites in blood vessel smooth muscle that, when activated, cause constriction and raise blood pressure.

alpha$_2$-adrenergic agonists A type of adrenergic drug that works centrally (in the brain) to turn on special alpha$_2$ receptors that, when normally activated, actually cause vasodilation and decrease blood pressure.

alpha-glucosidase inhibitors A category of oral noninsulin antidiabetic drug that lowers blood glucose levels by preventing enzymes in the intestinal tract from breaking down starches and more complex sugars into glucose.

alternative medicine Medical therapies such as herbalism, homeopathy, and acupuncture that are not considered mainstream.

ampules Small, breakable glass containers that contain one dose of drug for IM or intravenous injection.

amylin analog A category of injectable noninsulin antidiabetic drugs similar to natural amylin, which is a hormone produced by pancreatic beta cells that works with and is cosecreted with insulin in response to blood glucose elevation. It prevents hyperglycemia by delaying gastric emptying and making the patient feel full so he or she eats less.

anabolic steroids Synthetic drugs with the same use and actions as androgens.

analgesic Drugs that have the specific purpose of relieving pain either by changing the patient's perception of pain or by reducing painful stimulation at its source.

anaphylactic reaction A severe, life-threatening form of an allergic reaction.

androgens Synthetic or natural hormones that help to develop and maintain the male sex organs at puberty and develop secondary sex characteristics in men (i.e., facial hair, deep voice, body hair, body fat distribution, and muscle development).

angiotensin-converting enzyme inhibitor (ACE-I) A type of renin-angiotensin-aldosterone system drug that reduces high blood pressure by stopping the conversion of angiotensin I to angiotensin II (the hormone that causes the vasoconstriction and increased aldosterone).

angiotensin II receptor blockers (ARBs) A type of renin-angiotensin-aldosterone system drug that actually blocks the vasoconstrictor and aldosterone-secreting effects of angiotensin II to lower blood pressure by selectively blocking the binding of angiotensin II at receptor sites found in many tissues.

antacids A category of drugs used to help neutralize gastric acid and reduce symptoms of indigestion and heartburn.

antagonist Drug that attaches at a drug receptor site but does not activate or unlock the receptor.

antibacterial Antimicrobial drug that kills or slows the reproduction of bacteria only. Often used interchangeably with antibiotics.

antibiotic Any drug that has the ability to destroy or interfere with the development of a living organism. Often used interchangeably with antibacterials.

antibody A blood protein that is produced in response to and binds with any substance that the body's white blood cells consider foreign, such as bacteria, viruses, and foreign substances in the blood.

antibody titer A test that detects and measures the amount of antibodies in the blood to help determine the strength of a person's immunity against a specific microorganism.

anticoagulants Drugs that interfere with one or more steps in the blood-clotting process that either reduce or prevent new clots from forming, or prevent existing clots from getting larger.

antidiarrheal Drug that reduces or stops loose, watery stools (diarrhea) and helps restore normal bowel movements.

antidysrhythmic Drug that works to make heart rhythm more regular and reduces serious dysrhythmias.

antiemetic drugs A category of drugs used to prevent and treat nausea and vomiting.

antiepileptics drugs (AEDs) Drugs that reduce or prevent seizures.

antifungal drugs Any drug used to treat a fungal infection, also called a *fungicide* or *fungistatic*.

antigen Any substance your body's white blood cells recognize as foreign that will cause lymphocytes to produce an antibody against it.

antihistamine Drug that stops histamines from attaching to histamine receptors in the tissues and producing inflammatory and allergic symptoms. This action counteracts the response of histamine in causing smooth muscle contraction and dilation and leakage of capillaries.

antihyperlipidemics Drugs that lower blood cholesterol levels.

antihypertensive Drug that has the main purpose of lowering blood pressure.

anti-inflammatory drug Drug that has as its primary purpose to prevent or limit the tissue and blood vessel responses to injury or invasion.

antimicrobial drug A general term for any drug that has the purpose of killing or inhibiting the growth of pathogenic microorganisms.

antimicrobial resistance The ability of an organism to resist the killing or growth-suppressing effects of anti-infective drugs.

antiproliferative drugs Drugs that slow the growth of those lymphocytes most responsible for autoimmune diseases and for transplant rejection.

antirejection drugs Drugs that suppress the cells and factors of the immune system responsible for the receiving patient's rejection of transplanted tissues and organs.

antiretrovirals Drugs that are a subset of antiviral drugs and specifically suppress the reproduction of retroviruses.

antithyroid drugs Thyroid-suppressing drugs that work directly in the thyroid gland to stop production of new hormones by preventing an enzyme from connecting iodine (iodide) with tyrosine to make active thyroid hormones.

antitussive Drug that works to prevent and/or relieve coughing.

antiviral Drug capable of interfering with the ability of the virus to carry out its reproductive functions.

anxiolytic A description for any drug that can reduce anxiety.

artificial acquired active immunity The type of immunity that a person develops against a specific microorganism when a form of it is deliberately injected into his or her body as a vaccination or immunization.

artificial acquired passive immunity The type of immunity that is transferred as "premade" antibodies from one person or persons and even from animals into another person to provide immediate protection against a specific dangerous infection.

as-needed or PRN drug order An order for a drug to be given PRN based on a nurse's judgment of safety and patient need.

ascorbic acid Vitamin C.

aseptic technique Manipulation that does not contaminate the sterility of the drug and drug delivery system.

assessment The first step in the nursing process that involves gathering information about the patient that will be used in planning care.

asthma controller drug Drug that has the main purpose of preventing an asthma attack. Also known as asthma prevention drugs. This drug must be taken daily even when no asthma symptoms are present. Also known as *prevention* drug.

asthma reliever drug Drug that has the main purpose of stopping an asthma attack once it has started. Also known as asthma *rescue* drug.

attenuated vaccine A vaccine that contains live organisms that have been weakened and rendered harmless so that they are not capable of causing disease but are still able to produce an immune response.

atypical antidepressants Drugs that affect the neurotransmitters dopamine, norepinephrine, and/or serotonin to help reduce depression.

atypical antipsychotics Drugs that are usually a combination of dopamine and serotonin (5-HT) blockers used to reduce positive symptoms and improve negative symptoms of some types of psychosis without causing severe extrapyramidal side effects.

B

bacteria Microscopic living organisms that exist everywhere and are both beneficial and dangerous. They are capable of both preventing and causing infection.

bactericidal Drug with mechanism of action that kills bacteria.

bacteriostatic Drug with mechanism of action that only suppresses or slows bacterial growth.

benzodiazepines A class of sedating-hypnotic drugs that depresses the CNS by binding to benzodiazepine receptors, which then act with gamma-aminobutyric acid (GABA) receptors to enhance GABA effects. The results of these effects can reduce anxiety, induce sleep, and relax skeletal muscles depending on drug dose and concentration.

beta-adrenergic blocking agents Drugs that inhibit adrenergic receptor sites in the eye and decrease production of aqueous humor.

beta blocker Drug that works as antagonist and blocks the activity of beta-adrenergic receptors. Its main actions lower blood pressure and slow heart rate.

biguanides A category of oral noninsulin antidiabetic drug that lowers blood glucose levels by reducing the amount of glucose the liver releases and by reducing how much and how fast the intestines absorb the glucose in food.

bioequivalent Drug products that are chemically the same or identical.

biological response modifier (BRM) Drug that modifies the patient's immune response to abnormal triggers for immunity and inflammation.

biosynthetic vaccine A vaccine composed of human-made substances that are very similar to the parts of a virus or bacterium that cause disease.

biotransformation The transformation or altering of a drug into either active or inactive chemicals after it has been absorbed.

bisphosphonates Calcium-modifying drugs that both prevent bones from losing calcium and increase bone density by moving blood calcium into the bone, binding to calcium in the bone, and preventing osteoclasts from destroying bone cells and resorbing calcium.

black box warning A special designation from the US Food and Drug Administration that the drug has a higher-than-normal risk for causing serious and even life-threatening problems in addition to its positive benefits for some people.

body surface area (BSA) The total tissue area (including height and weight) of a patient's body.

brand name The proprietary name that a manufacturer gives to a specific drug. Also known as a trade name.

bronchodilators Drugs that relax the airway smooth muscles allowing the lumen of the airways to widen.

buccal route Drug placement against the cheek.

C

calcineurin inhibitors A class of drugs that works by forming a complex around the normal calcineurin present inside T lymphocytes preventing the calcineurin from activating those cells.

calcium channel blockers A class of antihypertensive drugs that lower blood pressure by reducing the effect of calcium in the heart muscle and in the smooth muscles of arteries.

cannabinoids Drugs that are either natural or synthetic forms of tetrahydrocannabinol that reduce nausea and vomiting by binding to both cannabinoid receptors in the chemoreceptor trigger zone (CTZ) and by preventing serotonin (5-HT$_3$) from binding to its receptors in the CTZ.

capsules Gelatin containers that hold powder or liquid drug.

carbonic anhydrase inhibitor (CAI) A type of diuretic that also can lower intraocular pressure by decreasing production of aqueous humor by 50% to 60%.

cART A combination of antiretroviral drugs that must be taken every day to combat the progression of HIV disease from becoming AIDS or to prevent HIV infection after exposure.

catechol-O-methyltransferase (COMT) inhibitor Drug that suppresses the activity of the COMT enzyme so that both naturally occurring dopamine and dopamine agonist drugs remain active in the body longer, helping to restore the acetylcholine–dopamine balance in the brain.

cerumenolytics Drugs that soften earwax.

chemical name The names of the chemicals that actually form the drug.

cholinergic agents Drugs that increase the availability of acetylcholine to activate specific receptors. This leads to decreased production of aqueous humor and improving outflow of aqueous humor to decrease intraocular pressure.

cholinergic antagonist Drugs that block the action of acetylcholine thereby inhibiting the parasympathetic nervous system response. Also known as cholinergic blockers, parasympatholytics, or anticholinergic drugs.

cholinesterase inhibitors Drugs that delay memory loss by binding to the enzyme acetylcholinesterase and slowing its action, which allows any acetylcholine produced to remain functional longer.

chronic pain Any pain that continues beyond the expected time frame of an acute injury process and that does not trigger the stress response.

chronotropic drug A drug that affects heart rate. A positive chronotropic drug increases heart rate; a negative chronotropic drug decreases heart rate.

Clark's rule A method for determining pediatric drug dosage calculated by ratio and proportion, based on the child's body weight.

clot A semisolid amount of coagulated (thickened) blood that blocks blood flow in a blood vessel. May also be referred to as a thrombus.

complementary medicine Alternative medicine therapies used in conjunction with a conventional or mainstream approach.

contraindication A health-related reason for not giving a specific drug to a patient or a group of patients.

controlled substances Drugs that are highly regulated because they are commonly abused. Also known as "scheduled drugs."

corticosteroid Drugs built on the structure of cholesterol that are able to prevent or limit inflammation and allergy by slowing or stopping production of the mediators histamine and leukotriene.

cytoprotective drugs A class of drugs that protects the lining of the stomach and prevents further damage to the lining from stomach acid.

D

decongestant Drug that reduces the swelling of nasal passages by shrinking the small blood vessels in the nose, throat, and sinuses so breathing is easier.

deep vein thrombosis (DVT) A clot lying in a deep vein, usually in the legs.

delirium A distressed state of mind that causes irrational beliefs characterized by illusions and paranoia.

dependence A state in which the body shows withdrawal symptoms when the drug is stopped or a reversing agent is given.

desired action The drug does what it is supposed to do.

diabetes mellitus (DM) A common chronic endocrine problem in which either the lack of insulin or poor function of insulin impairs glucose metabolism, which then leads to problems in fat metabolism and protein metabolism.

diagnosis A name (or label) for the patient's disease or condition.

direct thrombin inhibitor (DTI) Anticoagulant drug that prevents the formation of blood clots by interfering with the activity of the enzyme thrombin (factor II).

disease-modifying antirheumatic drug (DMARD) Drug that reduces the progression and tissue destruction of the inflammatory disease process, especially rheumatoid arthritis, by inhibiting tumor necrosis factor.

distribution Movement of a drug in the body to reach its site of action by way of the blood and lymph system.

diuretic Drug that has the main action of decreasing fluid volume by increasing urine output.

dopamine agonist Drug that has the same chemical structure of natural dopamine and is used to increase the levels of dopamine in the brain and restore balance between acetylcholine and dopamine action.

dopamine system stabilizers (DSSs) Drugs that affect dopamine and serotonin receptors slightly differently than other atypical antipsychotics. They partially activate dopamine 2 and 5-HT$_{1A}$ receptors and block 5-HT$_{2A}$ receptors. As a result, they have fewer motor side and adverse effects.

DPP-4 (dipeptidyl peptidase-4) inhibitors A category of noninsulin antidiabetic drugs that helps prevent hyperglycemia by reducing the amount of the enzyme (DPP-4), which inactivates the normal incretins, glucagon-like peptide and gastric inhibitory polypeptide. These actions allow the naturally produced incretins to be present and work with insulin to control blood glucose levels.

drop factor The number of drops per mL of fluid.

drug interaction When one drug changes the action of another drug.

dyskinesia An abnormality and distortion in performing voluntary movements. It results in jerky motions and looks much like uncoordinated dance movements.

dystonia Abnormal involuntary movements such as chewing, grinding of the teeth, protrusion of the tongue, opening and closing the mouth, head bobbing, or jerky, constant movements of the feet or hand.

E

embolism A blockage in an artery by a blood clot or air bubble.

emergency or "stat" drug order A one-time drug order to be given immediately.

enteral (route) Giving a drug by way of the GI system; oral, feeding tube, sublingual and rectally.

entry inhibitor Antiretroviral drug that prevents cellular infection with HIV by blocking the CCR5 receptor on CD4$^+$ T cells.

erythropoiesis-stimulating agent (ESA) Drug that is a synthetic form of the hormone *erythropoietin,* which stimulates the bone marrow to make more red blood cells at a faster rate.

estrogen agonists/antagonists Drugs for osteoporosis that activate (agonize) estrogen receptors in the bone to promote calcium retention in the bone and block (antagonize) estrogen receptors in breast tissue and uterine tissue.

evaluation The process of determining the right response looking at what happens to the patient when the nursing care plan is put into action. It is an appraisal of the treatment effectiveness.

F

fibrin A protein formed from fibrinogen that is a netlike substance in the blood with the function of trapping blood cells and platelets to form the matrix, or frame, of a clot during the clotting process.

fibrinogen A protein found in the blood's plasma that is converted to fibrin to help form a blood clot.

fibrinolytic drug Drug that uses enzymes to dissolve the fibrin in a clot. Also known as thrombolytic drugs or "clot busters."

first-pass (effect) After they are consumed, drugs are inactivated in the liver before being distributed to other parts of the body.

flow rate The rate at which intravenous fluids are given.

fungus A group of microorganisms that is everywhere and exists by absorbing nutrients from a host organism. Includes yeasts and molds. A fungal infection is called a *mycosis*.

fusion inhibitor Antiretroviral drugs that prevent cellular infection with HIV by blocking the ability of HIV's surface protein *gp41* to fuse with the host cell's CD4 receptor.

G

generation A new group of drugs developed from other similar drugs is called a *drug generation*. Each new generation of antibiotics manufactured from the original generation has significantly greater antimicrobial properties than the preceding generation.

generic name The most common drug name used by the manufacturer in all countries. Also known as the nonproprietary name.

glucagon A hormone produced by alpha cells of the pancreas that works to raise the concentration of glucose and fat in the bloodstream.

glucose A sugar-based nutrient critically important for energy production in cells and organs.

H

half-life The time it takes the body to remove 50% of the drug from the body.

healthcare setting Any setting in which the LPN/VN practices nursing.

hepatotoxic Adverse drug effects that can result in liver damage.

herbal Plants used in cooking and medicine.

high-alert drugs Drugs that have the potential to cause significant harm to patients.

histamine H$_2$-receptor antagonists A class of drugs that inhibits the binding of histamine to H$_2$-receptors on the parietal cells in the stomach, thereby decreasing gastric acid secretions.

HIV The specific retrovirus responsible for the immune system problems associated with destruction of helper T cells (CD4 cells) when the infection results in HIV disease and progresses to AIDS.

hormonal contraception The use of hormones to suppress ovulation for the intentional prevention of pregnancy.

hormone A protein secreted by an endocrine gland that changes the action of another gland or tissue, known as its target tissue.

hormone replacement therapy (HRT) Temporary or permanent therapy with drugs that perform the function of natural endocrine hormones.

hydroxymethylglutaryl-coenzyme A (HMG-CoA) reductase inhibitors (statins) Antihyperlipidemic drugs that lower blood low-density lipoprotein levels by slowing liver production of cholesterol.

hyperglycemia A condition of higher-than-normal blood glucose levels.

hypersensitivity An exaggerated response to a drug. An allergy is an example of a hypersensitive response.

hypervitaminosis High storage levels of vitamins (notably ADEC) that can lead to toxic symptoms.

hypnotics Drugs that have the main purpose of promoting sleep by changing signals in the CNS and reducing responses to stimulation. Same as sedative.

hypoglycemia A condition of lower-than-normal blood glucose levels.

I

identifiers Information used to reliably prove an individual is the person for whom the drug treatment was intended. Identifiers may be person's full name, his or her medical record identification number, birthdate, or even the telephone number.

idiosyncratic response Responses to a drug that are peculiar and unpredicted.

IM Giving a drug by way of an injection deep into the muscle.

IM route Injections that deposit drugs past the dermis and subcutaneous tissue, deep into the muscle mass.

immunity The body's physical resistance to becoming ill every time it comes into contact with pathogenic (disease-causing) microorganisms.

immunization The result of successful vaccination that causes a person to develop his or her own antibodies for immunity against the substance in the vaccine. Often used in the same way as the term *vaccination*.

immunosuppressant drugs Drugs that subdue or decrease the strength of the body's immune system.

implementation The act of carrying out the planned interventions.

inactivated vaccine A vaccine in which the organisms have been killed or inactivated by heat, radiation, or chemicals to prevent them from reproducing and causing disease, but that can still trigger antibody production and immunity. Also called a *killed* vaccine.

incretin mimetics A category of noninsulin antidiabetic drugs that acts like the natural gut hormones (e.g., glucagon-like peptide-1) that are secreted in response to food in the stomach. They work with insulin to prevent blood glucose levels from becoming too high after meals by slowing the rate of gastric emptying.

indirect thrombin inhibitor Anticoagulant drug that reduces clot formation by increasing the protein antithrombin III.

inflammation A predictable set of tissue and blood vessel actions caused by white blood cells (*leukocytes*) and their products as a response to injury or invasion.

innate immunity The body's intact protective barriers and the cellular responses of inflammation.

inotropic drug A drug that affects contractility of the myocardium. A positive inotrope drug increases contractility; a negative inotropic drug decreases contractility of the myocardium.

insulin A protein hormone produced by the pancreas or injected as a drug that binds to insulin receptors on many cells, which then promotes the movement of glucose from the blood into the cells.

insulin sensitizers A category of oral noninsulin antidiabetic drugs that lowers blood glucose levels by making insulin receptors more sensitive to insulin, which increases cellular uptake and use of glucose.

insulin stimulators A category of oral noninsulin antidiabetic drugs that lowers blood glucose levels by triggering the release of insulin stored in the beta cells of the pancreas. The sulfonylureas and the meglitinides are the two classes of drugs in this category.

integrase inhibitor Antiretroviral drug that inhibits the HIV enzyme *integrase,* which the virus uses to insert the viral DNA into the host cell's human DNA.

integrative practices Complementary and conventional approaches to healthcare that mainly focus on health and wellness.

intradermal injection Injection that is given into the dermis, just below the epidermis, most often used for allergy testing and tuberculosis testing.

intravenous Giving a drug by way of an injection into a vein or giving the drug into tubing that is connected to a catheter that is inserted into a vein.

intravenous (IV) route The administration of drugs directly into the bloodstream.

L

laxatives A class of drugs that promotes bowel movements by stimulating peristalsis, increasing the bulk of the stool, or softening the stool. They are typically used to relieve constipation.

legal responsibility The nurse's authority as defined by the state Nurse Practice Act. It involves the nurse's judgment and actions while performing professional duties. Each nurse must know what is legal in regard to drugs in the state where he or she practices.

leukotriene inhibitor Drug that blocks the leukotriene response and lessens or prevents the symptoms of allergy and asthma.

long-acting beta-adrenergic agonist Orally inhaled drug that binds over time to beta$_2$-adrenergic receptors and is used as an asthma controller drug that must be taken on a daily schedule to prevent bronchospasms and asthma attacks even when symptoms are not present.

loop diuretic Drug that increases urine output by blocking active transport of chloride, sodium, and potassium in the thick ascending loop of Henle.

M

mast cell stabilizer (cromone) Drug that works on the surface of mast cells and prevents them from opening to release the inflammatory mediators.

minerals Substances found in food that are necessary for normal body function.

miscellaneous analgesic Drugs that have specific purposes and actions for other health problems but can help provide relief for certain types of pain.

Mix-o-Vial A two-compartment vial that contains a sterile solution in one compartment and the powdered drug in the second compartment, separated by a rubber stopper. The solution and drug powder are mixed together immediately before use.

monoamine oxidase inhibitors (MAOIs) Drugs that inhibit the enzyme monoamine oxidase that is responsible for breaking down certain neurotransmitters including dopamine, norepinephrine, and serotonin. Blocking this enzyme increases the available neurotransmitters and results in reduction of depressive symptoms.

monoamine oxidase type B (MAO-B) inhibitor Drug that suppresses the action of MAO-B, which allows dopamine levels to increase and reduce the symptoms of PD.

mood stabilizers Drugs used in treating patients with bipolar illness. They have a variety of actions that help to reduce the symptoms associated with mania, as well as improve the symptoms of depression. Several drugs in this category are also used as antiseizure drugs.

mucolytics Drugs that decrease the thickness of respiratory secretions and aid in their removal. Also called *expectorants.*

N

9 Rights of Drug Administration A series of nursing actions to protect the patient from medication error.

nasogastric (NG) tube An enteral route of drug administration and oral feeding that bypasses the mouth by use of a tube going through the nose and esophagus into the stomach.

natural acquired active immunity The type of immunity a person develops to a microorganism that invades his or her body, usually making him or her sick, and triggering his or her immune system to make antibodies against it.

natural acquired passive immunity The immunity provided by the antibodies that a woman transfers to her fetus during pregnancy and to her infant during breast-feeding.

***N*-methyl-D-aspartate (NMDA) blocker** Drug that slows the progression of Alzheimer's disease by blocking the entrance of calcium into neurons, which reduces or slows neuronal damage.

nephrotoxic Adverse drug effects that can result in kidney damage.

neurotransmitter Chemical that is released from the end of one nerve, crosses a space (cleft), and then binds to receptors on the beginning of the next nerve in the line (or a skeletal muscle) to transmit the electrical signal from one nerve to the next.

niacin Vitamin B$_3$ or nicotinic acid helpful in lowering triglycerides and preventing pellagra.

nitrates A category of drugs that relaxes (dilates) peripheral veins and reduces resistance to blood flow in the arteries.

nomogram A chart that displays the relationships between two different types of data so that complex calculations are not necessary.

nonbenzodiazepine Drug that has a different chemical structure from the benzodiazepines (BNZs) but still binds strongly to BNZ receptors and acts in the same ways as BNZs to initiate sleep and promote longer sleep with less risk for dependence.

noninsulin antidiabetic drugs Oral and injectable drugs that use a variety of mechanisms other than binding to insulin receptors to help lower blood glucose levels back to the normal range.

nonnucleoside reverse transcriptase inhibitor (NNRTI) Antiretroviral drug that works by binding directly to the HIV-1 enzyme *reverse transcriptase,* preventing viral cell DNA replication, RNA replication, and protein synthesis.

nonopioid centrally acting analgesic Drug that works in the CNS to help manage pain but does not interact with opioid receptors to do so.

nonphenothiazines Drugs that are chemically different from the phenothiazines but have similar actions, side effects, and adverse effects.

normal flora Organisms of many different types that are usually present on the skin, mouth, intestinal tract, and vagina of a healthy individual and do not cause infection unless the person has reduced immunity or the organisms are located in the wrong body area.

NSAID Drug that is not based on the chemical structure of cholesterol but is able to prevent or limit the tissue and blood vessel responses to injury by slowing the production of one or more inflammatory mediators.

nucleoside reverse transcriptase inhibitors (NRTI) Antiretroviral drug that has a similar structure to the four nucleoside bases of DNA, making them "counterfeit" bases. When these counterfeit bases are used by the HIV enzyme *reverse transcriptase,* viral DNA synthesis and reproduction are suppressed.

Nurse Practice Act The state law that licenses LPN/LVN, registered nurses, nurse anesthetists, nurse practitioners, and nurse midwives. It describes the minimal educational preparation and professional requirements needed to perform specific functions, including drug administration, to protect the public safety.

nursing process A system to guide the nurse's work in a logical way. Consists of five major steps: (1) assessment, (2) diagnosis, (3) planning, (4) implementation, and (5) evaluation.

O

objective data Information that can be seen, heard, felt, or measured by someone other than the patient.

ophthalmic drugs Liquid or ointment drugs prepared to place on the eye or the conjunctiva.

opioid Any substance either derived from natural opium or that is chemically similar to opium that alters the perception of pain and has the potential to induce dependence and addiction.

opioid agonist Any drug that "turns on" (activates) the opioid receptors to change a patient's perception of discomfort and pain.

opioid agonist-antagonist analgesics Pain-management drugs that have mixed actions at opioid receptor sites.

osteoporosis The gradual loss of bone density and strength, which leads to spinal shortening and increased risk for bone fractures.

otic drugs Drugs prepared for delivery into the external ear canal.

over-the-counter (OTC) drugs Actual drugs approved by the US Food and Drug Administration that do not require a prescription to purchase.

P

pain An unpleasant sensation or emotion that produces or might produce tissue damage.

pain threshold The smallest amount of tissue damage that makes a person aware of having pain.

parasite An organism that lives on or in a human and relies on the human for its food and other functions.

parenteral route Administration of a drug by injection directly into the dermal, subcutaneous, or IM tissue; epidurally into cerebrospinal fluid; or through intravenous injection into the bloodstream.

partial agonists Drugs that attach to the receptor site but produce only a partial effect rather than a full effect (agonist).

passive immunity Acquired immunity in which antibodies made in another person or animal are given to you, and your body had no part in making them. Can be natural or artificial.

pathogen An organism that is expected to cause infection even among people with a strong immune system.

percutaneous route Administration of a drug through topical (skin), sublingual (under the tongue), buccal (against the cheek), or inhalation (breathing) methods.

pharmacodynamics The effects of a drug on body function (what a drug does to the body).

pharmacokinetics The metabolism of a drug within the body (what the body does to a drug).

pharmacotherapeutics The use of drugs in the treatment of disease.

phenothiazines A type of antiemetic drug that reduces nausea and vomiting by blocking dopamine receptors in the chemoreceptor trigger zone. These drugs are also called *dopamine antagonists*.

phenytoins Antiepileptic drugs that reduce or prevent seizures by binding to sodium channels on nerve membranes in the brain and making them less active, which prevents the spread of neuron excitation.

physical dependence The actual physical symptoms that occur with drug withdrawal (e.g., shaking, increased heart rate, pain, confusion, and seizures).

piggyback infusion A second or secondary intravenous (IV) fluid bag or bottle containing drugs or solution that is connected to the main IV line rather than directly to the patient.

platelet inhibitors Drugs that prevent platelets from clumping together (aggregating), which then interferes with blood clotting within arteries.

potassium-sparing diuretics Drugs that increase the excretion of water and sodium through increased urine output without the loss of potassium in the urine.

prescription drugs Category of drugs regulated by federal legislation because they are dangerous and their use must be controlled; may be purchased only when prescribed. Examples are antibiotics or oral birth control pills.

prescriptive authority The authority designated by an individual state that determines who is legally permitted to write an order or prescription for drugs.

prodrug Drugs that must be metabolized before they are active.

professional responsibility The obligation of nurses to act appropriately, ethically, and to the best of their ability as a healthcare provider.

promotility drugs A class of drugs that increases contraction of the upper GI tract, including the stomach and the small intestines, to move contents more quickly through the tract. They do this by blocking dopamine 2 receptors in the chemoreceptor trigger zone and the intestinal tract.

prostaglandin agonists Drugs that bind to specific prostaglandin receptor sites in the eye, causing an increased outflow of aqueous humor.

protease inhibitor (PI) Antiretroviral drug that suppresses the formation of infectious virions by inhibiting the retroviral protease enzyme.

proton pump inhibitors A class of drugs that binds to the proton pump of the parietal cells in the stomach, which blocks acid secretion into the stomach.

pseudomembranous colitis An abnormal intestinal reaction to a strong antibiotic that causes excessive watery, bloody diarrhea, abdominal cramps, and low-grade fever, and can lead to dehydration and damage to the walls of the intestinal tract.

psychological dependence Feelings of anxiety, stress, or tension when a patient does not have a drug.

R

receptor site Small "locklike" area of cell membrane that controls what substances either enter the cell or change its activity.

renin-angiotensin-aldosterone system (RAAS) drugs Drugs that include angiotensin-converting enzyme inhibitors and angiotensin II receptor blockers that have the effect of interfering with the action of angiotensin.

retrovirus Viral organisms that carry special enzymes (reverse transcriptase, integrase, and protease) with them and use RNA instead of DNA as their genes to reproduce.

riboflavin Vitamin B_2 used in riboflavin deficiency.

S

sedatives Drugs that have the main purpose of promoting sleep by changing signals in the CNS and reducing responses to stimulation. Same as hypnotic.

selective serotonin reuptake inhibitors (SSRIs) Drugs that act by inhibiting the cellular reuptake of serotonin, increasing the concentration of active serotonin that is available to bind to postsynaptic receptors and improve a patient's sense of well-being and reduce depression.

serotonin (5-HT$_3$) receptor antagonists A class of antiemetic drugs that reduces or halts nausea and vomiting by blocking (5-HT$_3$) receptors in the intestinal tract and the chemoreceptor trigger zone so serotonin cannot activate these receptors.

serotonin norepinephrine reuptake inhibitors (SNRIs) This class of drugs inhibits the reuptake of both serotonin and norepinephrine, increasing the concentration of both neurotransmitters available to postsynaptic receptors. These actions can improve a patient's sense of well-being and reduce depression.

short-acting beta-adrenergic agonist (SABA) Orally inhaled drug that binds rapidly to beta$_2$-adrenergic receptors and can start smooth muscle relaxation within seconds to minutes. Also known as asthma reliever or rescue drugs.

side effect Mild but annoying response to the drug. Nausea and headache are common and usual side effects to many drugs.

single drug order A one-time order to be given at a specified time.

skeletal muscle relaxants Drugs that depress the CNS to reduce muscle spasms.

sodium-glucose cotransport inhibitors A category of noninsulin antidiabetic drugs that lowers blood glucose levels by preventing the kidney from reabsorbing glucose that was filtered from the blood into the urine. This glucose then remains in the urine and is excreted rather than moved back into the blood.

solubility The ability of a drug to dissolve in body fluids.

spectrum The number of different specific organisms the drug is effective against.

standing drug order A drug order that indicates that the drug is to be given until discontinued or for a certain number of doses.

subcutaneous Drug placement into fatty tissue.

subcutaneous injection Injection that places no more than 2 mL of drug solution into the loose connective tissue between the dermis of the skin and muscle layer.

subjective data Reports of what the patient says he or she is feeling or thinks.

sublingual Drug placement under the tongue.

sublingual route Application of a drug to the mucous membranes under the tongue.

substance P/neurokinin$_1$ (NK$_1$) receptor antagonists A class of antiemetic drugs that blocks the substance P/neurokinin$_1$ (NK$_1$) receptors in the chemoreceptor trigger zone (CTZ), preventing the substance P and neurokinin that are released from cells exposed to chemotherapy and from tissues that are damaged during surgery from binding to and triggering the CTZ.

sympathomimetics Drugs that mimic the sympathetic nervous system and have the same actions as the body's own adrenaline. Also called *beta-* and or *alpha-adrenergic agonists.*

synergistic effect The effect of two drugs taken at the same time is greater than the sum of the effects of each drug given alone.

T

tablet Dried, powdered drug compressed into a small shape.

therapeutic effect The intended action of the drug, also known as a drug's beneficial outcomes.

thiamine Vitamin B$_1$ used to treat beriberi.

thiazides and thiazide-like sulfonamides diuretics Drugs that increase urine output by preventing water, sodium, potassium, and chloride from being reabsorbed into the blood through the walls of the nephron.

thrombin An enzyme that acts on *fibrinogen* (a protein found in the blood plasma) to convert it to fibrin, which then helps clots to form.

thyroid hormone agonist Drug that mimics the effect of thyroid hormones, T$_3$ and T$_4$, helping to regulate metabolism.

tolerance A drug-related metabolism problem that causes the same amount of drug to have less effect over time.

topical route Drugs applied directly to the area of the skin that requires treatment; most common forms are creams, lotions, and ointments.

toxoid A pathogenic microorganism that is modified chemically so it is no longer toxic and can be used as a vaccine.

trade name The proprietary name that a manufacturer gives to a specific drug. Also known as a brand name.

transdermal Drugs are applied to the skin for absorption into the bloodstream.

tricyclic antidepressants (TCAs) Older drugs used to reduce depression. Precise action is not known, but they are thought to interfere with the reuptake of norepinephrine and serotonin.

typical antipsychotics These drugs are thought to block dopamine 2 (D2) receptors in the brain. The blocking of dopamine receptors can help treat the positive symptoms of psychosis such as with schizophrenia (such as hallucinations and delusions). Blocking dopamine can also result in a variety of side and adverse effects including pseudoparkinsonism and other extrapyramidal symptoms.

U

urinary antispasmodics Drugs that reduce overactive bladder symptoms by relaxing the bladder muscle.

V

vaccination An injection or ingestion of a harmless form of bacteria or virus to stimulate antibody production against a certain disease.

vaccine A preparation of a synthetic, killed, or weakened form of a bacteria or virus that can be injected or ingested to stimulate antibody production against certain diseases.

vasodilators A class of drugs that acts directly on the smooth muscle in the blood vessel walls to cause them to dilate (widen or relax).

vial Small, single- or multiple-dose glass drug container.

virion New viral particle reproduced in cells infected with retroviruses that can leave the cell and infect more human body cells.

virus A small infectious agent that can reproduce only inside other living cells, including human cells.

vitamin A Beta-carotene used in vitamin A deficiency.

vitamin K antagonist Anticoagulant drug that interferes with blood clotting by reducing the amount of vitamin K available to help the liver form clotting factors.

vitamins Substances found in food that are necessary for body functions.

W

withdrawal symptoms Changes in the body or mind, such as nausea or anxiety, that occur when a drug is stopped or reduced after regular use.

Z

Z-track technique A type of IM injection technique used to prevent tracking (leakage) of the medication into the subcutaneous tissue (underneath the skin).

Index

Page numbers followed by "*f*" indicate figures, "*t*" indicate tables, and "*b*" indicate boxes.

A

Abacavir, 100*t*–101*t*
Abilify. *see* Aripiprazole.
Absence seizures, 171
Absorption, drug, 24, 25*b*, 25*f*–26*f*
  in older adult, 30
  in pediatric patients, 30
Acarbose, 315*t*
Accolate. *see* Zafirlukast.
Accupril. *see* Quinapril.
ACE-Is. *see* Angiotensin-converting
  enzyme I.
Acebutolol, 142*t*–144*t*
Acetaminophen, 219–220
  action of, 219
  adverse reactions to, 219
  drug interactions with, 220, 220*b*
  nursing implications and patient
    teaching on, 220
  side effects of, 219
  uses of, 219, 219*b*
Acetazolamide, 342*t*
Acetylcholine, 185*t*
Acetylsalicylic acid (ASA, aspirin), 228*t*,
  267*t*–268*t*
AcipHex. *see* Rabeprazole.
Acquired immunity, 281, 281*b*, 281*f*
Activase. *see* Alteplase.
Active immunity, 281
Actos. *see* Pioglitazone.
Acute angle closure glaucoma, 335
Acute dystonia, 190–192, 192*f*
Acute pain, 211, 211*b*, 212*t*
Acyclovir, 95*t*
Adalimumab, 235*t*
Addiction, 216
Additive effect, in drug interactions, 28
Adjuvant therapy, 174, 176*t*
Adrenal gland hyperfunction,
  298–299
  action and uses of, 298, 299*t*
  adverse effects of, 299
  patient teaching, 299, 299*b*
  side effects of, 299
Adrenal gland hypofunction, 297–298,
  298*f*
Adrenal gland problems, drugs for,
  297–299
Adrenal suppression, 232, 233*f*
Adrenergic drugs, 141–145, 142*t*–144*t*
Adult-onset diabetes, 311

Adverse reaction/effects, 9, 27, 28*b*, 39
  anaphylactic, 27
  hepatotoxic, 27
  idiosyncratic, 27
  nephrotoxic, 27
  paradoxical, 27
Advil. *see* Ibuprofen.
Afrin. *see* Oxymetazoline.
Age, drug therapy and, 32
Agonists, 23–24, 24*b*
  definition of, 141
Agranulocytosis, 194
AIDS. *see* HIV/AIDS.
Akathisia, 190–192, 192*f*
Akinesia, 164
Albendazole, 90
Albenza. *see* Albendazole.
Albiglutide, 317*t*
Albuterol, 117*t*
Alcohol, drug interactions with,
  28–29
Aldactone. *see* Spironolactone.
Aldomet. *see* Methyldopa.
Aldosterone, 297–298
Aleve. *see* Naproxen.
Alfuzosin, 131*t*
Allegra. *see* Fexofenadine.
Allergic reactions, 27
Allergy, 27, 27*b*, 107, 108*f*
  drug therapy for, 107–114, 107*b*,
    109*t*–110*t*
Allopurinol, for gout, 237, 237*t*
Alogliptin, 319*t*
Aloprim. *see* Allopurinol.
Alpha-adrenergic agonists, 340–341,
  341*t*
Alpha-glucosidase inhibitors, 315–316,
  315*t*
Alpha$_1$-adrenergic antagonists, 141–144,
  145*f*
Alprazolam, 186*t*–187*t*
Alteplase, 275*t*
Alternagel. *see* Aluminum hydroxide.
Alternative medicine. *see*
  Complementary and alternative
  medicine.
Aluminum-based antacids, 238
Aluminum hydroxide, 249*t*–250*t*
Alzheimer's disease, 166–169
  cholinesterase inhibitors for, 167–169
  drugs for the management of, 168*t*

Alzheimer's disease *(Continued)*
  N-methyl-d-aspartate blockers for,
    169
  neurons of, 167*f*
  warning signs of, 167*b*
Alzheimer's Disease Assessment Scale,
  168, 169*b*
Alzheimer's Foundation of America,
  167*b*
Amantadine, 95*t*
Amaryl. *see* Glimepiride.
Ambien. *see* Zolpidem.
American Diabetes Association,
  311*b*
American Heart Association, 138*b*
Amikacin, 75*t*
Amiloride, 128*t*–129*t*
Aminoglycosides, 76
Aminopenicillins, 69
Amitriptyline, for depression,
  198*t*–199*t*
Amlodipine, 142*t*–144*t*
Amnesia, 222
Amoebiasis, 87
Amoxicillin, 70*t*–71*t*
Ampules, 46, 47*f*
Amylin analogs, 317–318, 317*t*, 318*b*
Anabolic steroids, 304
Analgesics, 213
  nonopioid centrally acting, 218–219,
    218*b*
  opioid agonist, 214–217, 214*b*. *see also*
    Opioid agonists.
  opioid agonist-antagonist, 217–218,
    217*b*
  for pain management, 212–220
Anaphylactic reaction, to drug, 27, 28*b*
Anaphylaxis, 69–72
Anaprox. *see* Naproxen.
Androgens, 304–305
  actions and uses of, 304–305
  adverse reactions, 305
  drug interactions with, 305
  nursing implications and patient
    teaching on, 305
  side effects, 305
Angina, 134
  acute, 148*b*
  antianginals for, 147, 149*t*
  drugs used for, 147–155
  nitrates for, 147–149

Angioedema, 69–72, 145f
Angiotensin-converting enzyme I
    (ACE-Is), 140–141, 141b, 142t–144t
Anorexia, 268
Antacids, 249t–250t
    action of, 251
    adverse reactions to, 251
    drug interactions with, 251
    nursing implications and patient
        teaching on, 251–252
    side effects of, 251
    uses of, 251
Antagonistic effect, in drug interactions,
    28
Antagonists, 24, 24b, 141, 141b
Anti-infectives, 66
Antianginals, 147, 149t
Antianxiety drugs, 187–189
    action of, 188
    adverse reactions to, 188
    drug interactions with, 188
    nursing implications and patient
        teaching on, 188–189
    side effects of, 188
    uses of, 188
Antiarthritis drugs, 225–239
Antibacterial agents, 64–92
Antibiotics, 66–78, 68f
    aminoglycosides, 75t, 76
    cephalosporins as, 70t–71t, 72–73
    fluoroquinolones as, 77–78, 78t
    macrolides, 74, 75t
    penicillins as, 68–72, 68f, 70t–71t
    sulfonamides as, 76–77, 78t
    tetracyclines as, 73–74, 75t
Antibody, 281
Antibody titer, 284–285
Anticholinergic drugs, 257t–258t
Anticoagulants, 266–275, 266b,
    267t–268t, 269b
Anticonvulsants, 223, 223b
Anticytomegalovirus drugs, 96t
Antidepressants, 195–196, 198t–199t,
    222–223, 223b
    categories of, 197b
    tricyclic, 196, 198t–199t. see also
        Tricyclic antidepressants.
Antidiabetic drugs, 311–324
    categories of, 312b
Antidiarrheals
    action of, 259–260
    adverse reactions to, 260
    nursing implications and patient
        teaching on, 260
    side effects of, 260
    uses of, 259–260
Antidysrhythmics, 149–153,
    151t–153t
    action of, 150
    adverse reactions to, 151b
    evaluation of, 153
    nursing implications and patient
        teaching on, 151–153

Antidysrhythmics (Continued)
    patient and family teaching on, 153
    uses of, 150
Antiemetic drugs, 242–248, 242b–243b,
    242f, 243t–244t, 245b
Antiepileptic drugs (AEDs), 170–174,
    170b. see also Anticonvulsants.
    children and, 173b
    drug interactions with, 174b
    newer, 174–178, 174b, 175t
    nursing considerations for, 171b
    patient and family teaching points
        on, 171b
    pregnancy and, 173b
    traditional, 172t
Antifungals, 83–87
    action and use of, 84, 84b, 85t, 86b
    drug interactions with, 84
    nursing implications and patient
        teaching on, 84–87, 86b–87b
    side effects and adverse reactions to,
        84, 84b
Antigen, 107, 281
Antigout drugs, 237–238, 237t
    actions of, 237
    adverse reactions to, 238
    drug interactions with, 238
    nursing implications and patient
        teaching on, 238
    side effects of, 238
    uses of, 237
Antihelmintics, 90
Antihistamine, 107–111
    actions of, 107–110
    adverse effects to, 110
    drug interactions with, 110
    nursing implications and patient
        teaching on, 110–111
    side effects of, 110, 110b
    use of, 110
Antihyperlipidemics, 134–138, 135b
Antihypertensives, 138–147, 142t–144t,
    146b
    action of, 140–145
    adverse reactions to, 146
    drug interactions with, 146–147
    drug uses, 145
    nursing implications of, 139b,
        146–147, 146b
    patient and family teaching on, 147
    side effects of, 145
    sites of action of, 140f
Antiinflammatory drugs, 119, 120t,
    225–239
Antimalarials, 89t
Antimicrobial drug, 66
Antimicrobial resistance, 66
Antiparasitic drugs, 87–90, 89t
    anthelmintics as, 90
Antiproliferative drugs, 287, 288t, 290b
Antiprotozoal drugs, 87–90
    action and use of, 87–88, 89t
    drug interaction of, 88

Antiprotozoal drugs (Continued)
    nursing implications and patient
        teaching on, 88–90
    side effects and adverse reactions to,
        88
Antipsychotics, 189–195, 190t–191t
    atypical, 193–195, 194b
    typical, 190–193
Antirejection drugs, 287
Antiretroviral drugs, 99–103, 100t–101t,
    102b
    actions of, 102
    adverse effects to, 102
    pre-exposure prophylaxis, 103,
        103b
    side effects of, 100t–101t, 102
Antispasmodic drugs, 257t–258t
Antithyroid drugs, 294t, 296–297
    actions and uses of, 296, 296b
    adverse effects to, 297
    drug interactions with, 297
    nursing implications and patient
        teaching on, 297, 297b
    side effects of, 296
Antitubercular drugs, 78–83, 79b, 79f
    action and use of, 81, 81b, 82f
    adverse interactions of, 82
    drug interactions with, 82
    nursing implications and patient
        teaching on, 82–83
    side effects of, 81–82
Antitussives, 121–122, 121t
Antivirals, 94–98
    actions and use of, 95–96
    nursing implications and patient
        teaching on, 95t–96t, 97–98, 98b
    side effects, adverse reactions, and
        drug interaction with, 95t–97t, 97
Anxiety
    drugs for, 184–189, 186t–187t. see also
        Antianxiety drugs.
    Parkinson's disease and, 160–161
Anxiolytics, 188
Apixaban (Eliquis), 267t–268t
APOE-e4 gene, Alzheimer's disease
    and, 166–167
Apraclonidine, 341t
Aprepitant, 243
Aqueous humor, 332–333
Arachidonic acid (AA) cascade, 226,
    226f
Areflexia, 173
Arformoterol, 117t
Aripiprazole, 190t–191t
Arrhythmia, 150
Artificial acquired active immunity,
    282
Artificial acquired passive immunity,
    282, 282b
As needed or "prn" drug order, 16
ASA. see Acetylsalicylic acid.
Ascending loop of Henle, 127, 127f
Ascorbic acid, 351t, 354

Aseptic technique, 41, 41*b*
Aspirin, 228*t. see also* Acetylsalicylic acid.
Assessment
  on corticosteroids, 233–234
  on disease-modifying antirheumatic drug, 236, 236*b*
  factors to consider in, 3
  on nonsteroidal anti-inflammatory drug, 229–230
  in nursing process, 2–3, 2*f*, 3*b*
Asthma, 114, 114*b*–115*b*, 114*f*
  drug therapy for, 114–119, 115*t*
Asthma controller drug, 115
Asthma reliever drug, 115
Atazanavir, 100*t*–101*t*
Atenolol, 142*t*–144*t*
Atherosclerosis, 134, 134*f*
Atorvastatin, 136*t*
Attenuated vaccines, 283
Atypical antidepressants, 196
Atypical antipsychotic drugs, 190*t*–191*t*, 193–195, 194*b*
  action of, 193–194
  adverse reactions to, 194
  drug interactions with, 194
  nursing implications and patient teaching on, 194–195
  side effects of, 194
  uses of, 193–194
Auscultation, 3
Availability, drug, 29
Azathioprine, 288*t*
Azithromycin, 75*t*
Azoles, 85*t*

B
Bacteria, 65
Bactericidal agents, 66, 66*b*
  sites of action of, on bacterial pathogens, 68*f*
Bacteriostatic agents, 66, 66*b*
  sites of action of, on bacterial pathogens, 68*f*
Beclomethasone, 120*t*
Bedaquiline, 81
Benign prostatic hyperplasia (BPH), drugs for, 130
Benzodiazepine agonists, 185, 186*t*–187*t*
Benzodiazepines, 185
  for anxiety, 186*t*–187*t*
  pregnancy and, 185*b*
  for sleep, 186*t*–187*t*
Benzonatate, 121*t*
Beta-adrenergic antagonists, 336–340, 336*b*, 339*t*, 340*b*
Beta blockers, 141, 142*t*–144*t*
  sites of action for, 144*f*
Betamethasone, 231*t*
Betaxolol, 339*t*
  for hypertension, 142*t*–144*t*
Biguanides, 313*t*, 314
Bile acid sequestrants, 137

Bimatoprost, 339*t*
Bioequivalence, 28
Biological response modifiers (BRMs), 179
Biosynthetic vaccines, 283
Biotransformation, of drug, 25–26
Bisacodyl, 257*t*–259*t*
Bismuth subsalicylate, 249*t*–250*t*
Bisphosphonates, 306–307
Black box warning, 20, 20*f*
Bladder anesthetics, 130
Bleb, 47
Blood-brain barrier, 32
Blood clotting, 265–266, 266*f*
Blood thinners, 266
Body surface area (BSA), 38–39
Bony ossicles, 329
Brain, function of, 159
Brand name, of drug, 23
Brinzolamide, 342*t*
Broad-spectrum drugs, 67
Brompheniramine, 109*t*–110*t*
Bronchodilator, 115–118
  action of, 115–116
  adverse reactions to, 116
  drug interactions with, 117
  nursing implications and patient teaching on, 116*b*, 117–118, 118*f*–119*f*, 119*b*
  side effects of, 116
  use of, 116, 117*t*
Buccal (route) administration, 24, 57–58, 59*b*
Budesonide, 120*t*
Bulk-forming laxatives, 255, 257*t*–259*t*. *see also* Laxatives.
Bullous pemphigoid, 319*f*
Bumetanide, 128*t*–129*t*
Buprenorphine, 218*t*
Bupropion, 198*t*–199*t*
Buspirone, 187
Butorphanol, 218*t*
Byetta. *see* Exenatide.

C
Calcineurin inhibitors, 283, 287, 288*t*
Calcium, 356
Calcium carbonate, 249*t*–250*t*
Calcium channel blockers, 141, 142*t*–144*t*
Canada
  drug importation from, 15
  drug regulations in, 15
Canadian drug legislation, 15
Canagliflozin, 319*t*
Cancer pain, 212*t*
Candesartan, 142*t*–144*t*
Cannabinoids, 243*t*–244*t*
  action of, 247
  adverse reactions to, 247
  drug interactions with, 247
  nursing implications and patient teaching on, 247–248

Cannabinoids *(Continued)*
  side effects of, 247
  uses of, 247
Capsule, 41
Captopril, 142*t*–144*t*
Carbachol, 341*t*
Carbamazepine, 171, 172*t*, 198*t*–199*t*
Carbamide peroxide, 332*t*
Carbidopa/levodopa, 161, 162*t*–163*t*
Carbonic anhydrase inhibitors, 342–343, 342*t*, 343*b*
Carboxypenicillins, 69
Cardiovascular system, 133*f*–134*f*
  antihyperlipidemics and, 134–138. *see also* Antihyperlipidemics.
  antihypertensive drugs and, 138–147. *see also* Antihypertensives.
  drugs affecting, 132–155, 134*b*, 150*b*
  nonstatin antihyperlipidemic drugs and, 137–138
Carteolol, 339*t*
Cascade, 266
Catechol-*O*-methyltransferase (COMT) inhibitor, 161, 162*t*–163*t*, 165
Cefaclor, 70*t*–71*t*
Cefazolin, 70*t*–71*t*
Cefdinir, 70*t*–71*t*
Cefepime, 70*t*–71*t*
Ceftriaxone, 70*t*–71*t*
Cefuroxime, 70*t*–71*t*
Celecoxib, 228*t*
Cell wall synthesis inhibitors, 70*t*–71*t*, 73
  drug interactions with, 73, 73*b*
  side effects and adverse reactions to, 73
Centers for Disease Control and Prevention, 196*b*
Central nervous system
  catechol-O-methyltransferase inhibitors and, 165
  cholinesterase inhibitors and, 167–169
  dopamine agonists and, 161–165
  drug therapy for, 158–182
  functions of, 159–160, 159*f*
Centrally acting alpha₂-adrenergic agonists, 144–145
Cephalexin, 70*t*–71*t*
Cephalosporins, 72–73
  action of, 70*t*–71*t*, 72
  adverse reactions to, 72
  drug interactions with, 72
  nursing implications and patient teaching on, 70*t*–71*t*, 72–73, 73*b*
  side effects of, 72
  use of, 72, 72*b*
Cerumen, 329
Ceruminolytic drugs, 331, 332*t*, 341*b*
Chemical name, of drug, 23
Child(ren). *see* Pediatric patient(s).
Chlorothiazide, 128*t*–129*t*
Chlorpromazine, 190*t*–191*t*
Cholecalciferol, 354

Cholelithiasis, 137
Cholinergic antagonist, 116, 117t
Cholinergic drugs, 341–342, 341t, 342b
Cholinesterase inhibitor, 167–169
    adverse effects to, 168b
Chronic bronchitis, 114
Chronic obstructive pulmonary disease
    (COPD), 114
    drug therapy for, 114–119
Chronic pain, 211, 211b, 212t
Cidofovir, 96t
Cilostazol, 267t–268t
Ciprofloxacin, 78t
Clarithromycin, 75t
Clark's rule, in pediatric dosage
    calculation, 38
Clavulanic acid, 70t–71t
Clindamycin, 75t
Clonidine, 142t–144t
Clopidogrel, 267t–268t, 268
Clot, 265–266. see also Blood clotting.
Cochlea, 329–330
Codeine-containing antitussives, 121t
Cogwheel rigidity, 160
Collecting-duct, 127, 127f
Columbia Suicide Severity Rating Scale,
    200t
Combination agent, 97t
Combination antiretroviral therapy
    (cART), 99
Complementary and alternative
    medicine (CAM), 347–350, 349b
    product labeling of, 349
Conjugated estrogens, 302t
Conjugated female sex hormones, 302t
Constipation, 254f
    drugs for, 253–260, 256b, 257t–258t
    nursing considerations for, 256b
    signs and symptoms of, 254b
Continuation phase, 79
Continuous aerosol therapy, 58
Continuous pain, 212t
Contraindication, definition of, 5
Controlled substances
    classification of, 13t
    definition of, 12–14, 14b
    distribution for, 14
Controlled Substances Act, 12
Convulsion, 169–170
COPD (chronic obstructive pulmonary
    disease), 114
    drug therapy for, 114–119
Corticosteroid nasal sprays, 112
Corticosteroids, 112, 220, 230–235, 231t,
    233f, 297–298
    action and uses of, 230, 298
    adverse effects of, 298
    adverse reactions to, 232–233, 233b
    drug interactions with, 233
    nursing implications and patient
        teaching on, 233–235, 234b, 298
    side effects of, 231–232, 232t, 298
    uses of, 231

Cortisol, 232
Council for Responsible Nutrition, 350,
    350b
Cozaar. see Losartan.
Cromones, 109t–110t, 112
Cross-sensitivity, 72
Cryptorchidism, 304–305
"Cushingoid" appearance, 232f
Cushing's disease, 298
Cyanocobalamin, 351t
Cyclobenzaprine, 222b
Cyclooxygenase (COX), 226
Cyclooxygenase-1 inhibitors (COX-1),
    for inflammation, 228t
Cyclooxygenase-2 (COX-2) inhibitors,
    for inflammation, 228t
Cyclosporine, 288t
Cytochrome P-450 system, 26
Cytomegalovirus (CMV), antiviral
    drugs for, 94–96, 96t
Cytoprotective drugs, 253

D

Dabigatran, 267t–268t
Dalfopristin, 75t
Dalteparin, 267t–268t
Dapagliflozin, 319t
Darunavir, 100t–101t
Data
    objective, 3
    subjective, 2–3
Decongestants, 112–114, 113t
Deep vein thrombosis (DVT), direct
    thrombin inhibitors for, 270
Delavirdine, 100t–101t
Delirium, 189
Dementia, 166
Dependence, 216
    physical, 12b
    psychologic, 12b
Depression, 195, 196f
    Parkinson's disease and, 160–161
    symptoms of, 195b
Desired action, 27
Desirudin (Iprivask), 267t–268t
Dexamethasone, 231t
Dextromethorphan, 121t
Diabetes mellitus (DM)
    blood glucose control in, 310, 310t
    classification of, 311
    definition of, 310
    drugs for, 311–324. see also
        Antidiabetic drugs.
    management of, 309–328
Diagnosis, in nursing process, 4
Diamox. see Acetazolamide.
Diarrhea
    causes of, 254b, 259b
    drugs for, 253–260, 257t–258t
    nursing considerations for, 260b
    pathophysiology of, 254f
Diazepam, 186t–187t
Dicyclomine, 257t–258t

Didanosine, 100t–101t
Dietary supplement, 349
Digestion, 241
Digestive enzymes, 242
Digestive system, 241–242, 241f. see also
    Gastrointestinal tract.
Digital nasolacrimal occlusion, 336–340
Digoxin, 150, 154b
Dihydrotestosterone inhibitors, 131t
Diltiazem, 142t–144t
Dimensional analysis method, in
    pediatric dosage calculation, 36–37
Dimetapp. see Brompheniramine.
Dimethyl fumarate, 179
Dipeptidyl peptidase-4 inhibitors
    (DPP-4), 318–320, 319t
Diphenhydramine, as antihistamine,
    109t–110t
Diphenoxylate, with atropine, 257t–258t
Dipivefrin hydrochloride, 341t
Direct-acting stimuli, 242
Direct thrombin inhibitors (DTIs),
    270–271. see also Anticoagulants.
    action of, 267t–268t, 270
    adverse reactions to, 270
    drug interaction of, 270, 270b
    evaluation of, 272, 272b
    nursing implications and patient
        teaching on, 270–271, 271b
    side effects of, 270
    use of, 270
Disease-modifying antirheumatic drugs
    (DMARDs), 235–237
    actions of, 235, 235t
    adverse reactions to, 236, 236b
    drug interactions with, 236
    nursing implications and patient
        teaching on, 236–237
    side effects of, 236
    uses of, 236
Displacement, in drug interactions, 28
Distal convoluted tubule, 126–127, 127f
Distribution, drug, 25, 26f
    in older adult, 31
    in pediatric patients, 30
Diuretics, 126–130, 142t–144t
    action of, 126–127, 127b, 127f
    adverse effects of, 129
    assessment of, 129–130
    categories of, 126b
    common, 128t–129t
    drug interactions with, 129, 129b
    loop, 127
    nursing implications and patient
        teaching on, 129–130
    older adults and, 127b
    patient and family teaching on, 130,
        130b
    planning and implementation of, 130
    potassium-sparing, 127
    pregnancy and, 127b
    side effects of, 129
    uses of, 129

DMARDs (disease-modifying antirheumatic drugs), 235–237
DNA polymerase inhibitors, 96t–97t
Documentation. *see also* Patient charts.
   of drug administration, 8–9
Docusate, 257t–259t
Dolasetron, 243t–244t
Dolutegravir, 100t–101t
Donepezil, for Alzheimer's disease, 167, 168t
Dopamine, 160, 185t
Dopamine agonist, 161–165, 162t–163t
Dopamine system stabilizers (DSSs), 190t–191t
   as atypical antipsychotic, 194
Dorzolamide, 342t
Dosage drug calculation, 36–39, 37b
   for children, 38–39
   dimensional analysis method for, 36–37
   fraction method for, 36
   for infants, 38–39
   ratio and proportion method for, 36
Doxazosin, 142t–144t
Doxycycline, 75t
Dronabinol, 243t–244t
Drop factor, in IV infusion calculation, 39, 40b
Drug(s)
   absorption of, 24, 25f–26f
   administration of. *see* Medication administration.
   adverse reactions to, 27. *see also* Adverse reaction/effects.
   allergic reactions to, 27
   anaphylactic reaction to, 27
   attachment of, 23–24
   availability of, 29
   bioequivalence, 28
   distribution of, 25, 26f
   diversion, 12
   elimination of, 26–27
   errors, 18–20, 19b
   excretion of, 26–27, 26f
   high-alert, 19, 20b
   hypersensitivity to, 27
   idiosyncratic responses to, 27
   long-acting or extended-release, 27b
   metabolism of, 25–26, 26f
   names of
      brand, 23
      chemical, 23
      generic, 23
      trade, 23
   nephrotoxic, 27
   over-the-counter, 12
   paradoxical response to, 27
   prescription, 12, 14–15
   processes involving, 24–27
   receptor sites for, 23–24, 24f

Drug(s) *(Continued)*
   regulation of, 12–15
      in Canada, 15
      in United States, 12, 13t
         federal laws in, 12–15
         health care agency policies in, 16–17
         state law in, 16–17, 16b
   side effects of, 27. *see also* Adverse reaction/effects.
   topical, 56, 56b, 57f
Drug action(s), 27–29, 28b
   adverse, 27
   desired, 27
Drug calculation, 35–63
   for insulin, 37–38, 38b
   for IV infusions, 39–40
   using units, 37–38
Drug cards, 32, 33t
Drug generation, 67–68
Drug interaction, 28–29
   with alcohol, 28–29
   with food, 28–29
Drug names, 23
Drug order(s), 16–17
   legal prescriptions, 16
   tip for safety in, 5b
   types of, 16
Drug systems, electronic, 18, 18b, 18f
Drug therapy
   for mental health, 183–209
   in older adult, 30–31
   patient teaching considerations in, 31–32
   in pediatric patients, 30
   personal factors influencing, 29
   pregnancy and lactation and, 32
   special populations and, 29–32
Dry-powder inhaler, 58, 58f
Ductless glands, 292–293
Dulaglutide, 317t
Duloxetine, 198t–199t
Duodenum, 242
Dutasteride, 131t
Dyskinesia, 163
Dyspepsia, 268
Dysrhythmias, 134, 150
Dystonia, 164

E
Ear
   eardrops for, 331b, 331f
   external, 330f
   inner, 330f
   middle, 330f
   problems, 329–345
      drug management of, 330–331
   structure and function of, 329–330, 330f, 331b
Ear canal, 329
Ear drops, 58, 59b
Education. *see* Patient and family teaching.

Efavirenz, 100t–101t
Electronic drug systems, 18, 18b, 18f
Electronic medical record (EMR), 17
Elimination, drug, 26–27
   in older adult, 31
   in pediatric patients, 30
Elvitegravir, 100t–101t
Embolism, direct thrombin inhibitors for, 270
Emergency or stat drug order, 16
Emotional liability, 247
Empagliflozin, 319t
Emtricitabine, 100t–101t
Enalapril, 142t–144t
Endocrine system, 293f. *see also* Corticosteroids; Hormone(s).
   drug affecting, 292–308
Enfuvirtide, 100t–101t
Enoxaparin, 267t–268t
Entacapone, 162t–163t
Enteral route of administration, 24, 41–43
   nasogastric, 42–43
   oral, 41–42
Entry inhibitor, 99f, 100t–101t, 102
Enzymes, digestive, 242
Epilepsy
   antiepileptic drugs for, 170–174
   definition of, 169–170
   drugs for, 169–179. *see also* Anticonvulsants.
Epistaxis, 201
Equivalency ratios, 36
Ergocalciferol, 354
Ertapenem, 70t–71t
Erythema, 69–72
Erythromycin, 75t
Erythropoiesis, 276
Erythropoiesis-stimulating agents (ESAs), 276–277
   action of, 276, 277t
   adverse reactions to, 276
   nursing implications and patient teaching on, 277
   side effects of, 276
   use of, 276
Escherichia coli, 65
Escitalopram, 198t–199t
Esomeprazole, 249t–250t
Estazolam, for insomnia, 186t–187t
Estrogen agonist/antagonist, 307
Eszopiclone, 186t–187t
Etanercept, 235t
Ethambutol, 80t–81t
Ethosuximide, 171, 172t
Etravirine, 100t–101t
Eunuchism, 304–305
Euphoria, 177
Evaluation
   in nursing process, 9, 9b
   response to drug, factors to consider in, 9

Everolimus, 287, 288t
Excitatory neurotransmitters, 159
Excretion, drug, 26–27, 26f
Exenatide, 317t
Expected side effects, 9
Expectorants, 119–120
Extrapyramidal symptoms (EPSs), 190
  characteristics of, 193b
Eye
  drug, self-administration of, 339b–340b
  ointment for, instilling, 337f, 338b
  posterior segment of, 333–334
  problems, 331–343
  structure and function of, 332–334, 332f–333f
Eye drops, 58, 59b
Ezetimibe, 137

F

Famciclovir, 95t
Family teaching. *see* Patient and family teaching.
Famotidine, 249t–250t
Famvir. *see* Famciclovir.
Fat-soluble vitamins, 350, 350b
Febuxostat, 237, 237t
Federal laws, on medications, 12–15
Feldene. *see* Piroxicam.
Felodipine, 142t–144t
Fenofibrate, 137
Fexofenadine, 109t–110t
Fibrates, 137
Fibric acid derivatives, 137
Fibrin, 266
Fibrinogen, 266
Fibrinolytic drug, 275–276, 276b
  action of, 275, 275t
  adverse reactions to, 276
  drug interactions with, 276
  nursing implications and patient teaching on, 276
  side effects of, 276
  use of, 275
Fight-or-flight response, 211
Finasteride, 131t
First-generation antihistamines, 109t–110t
First generation antipsychotics, 190
First-line TB drug therapy, 79, 80t–81t
First-pass (effect), metabolism, 26
FLACC pain rating scale, 213f
Flovent. *see* Fluticasone.
Flow rate, 39
  calculation of, 39
  factors influencing, 40
  IV calculation of, 54, 55b
Fludrocortisone, 298
Fluid retention, 141b
Flumazenil, 187b
Flunisolide, 120t

Fluoroquinolones, 77–78, 78t
  action of, 77
  adverse reactions to, 78
  drug interactions with, 78
  nursing implications and patient teaching on, 78
  side effects of, 77–78
  use of, 77
Fluoxetine, 198t–199t
Fluphenazine, 190t–191t
Flurazepam, 186t–187t
Fluticasone, 113t
Fluvastatin, 136t
Folic acid, 351t, 353
Fondaparinux sodium, 267t–268t
Food(s), drug interactions with, 28–29
Formoterol, 117t
Fosamprenavir, 100t–101t
Foscarnet, 96t
Fraction method, for dosage calculation, 36
Fragmin. *see* Dalteparin.
Fungus, 65
Furosemide, 128t–129t
Fusion inhibitor, 100t–101t, 102

G

Galantamine, for Alzheimer's disease, 167, 168t
Gamma-aminobutyric acid (GABA), 185t
Gastric reflux, 242
Gastroesophageal reflux disease (GERD)
  drugs for, 248–253
  pathophysiology of, 249f
Gastrointestinal problems, drugs for, 240–264
Gastrointestinal tract
  antacids and, 249t–250t, 251–252. *see also* Antacids.
  antiemetic drugs and, 242–248, 242b–243b, 242f
  protective substance in, 241–242
  proton pump inhibitors and, 249t–250t, 252–253. *see also* Proton pump inhibitors.
  serotonin (5-HT₃) receptor antagonists and, 243–245
  stimulants of, 257t–258t
Gemfibrozil, 137
Generic equivalent drug, 28
Generic name, of drug, 23
Gentamicin, 75t
Giardiasis, 87
Glaucoma, 334–343, 334f, 335b
  drugs for, 335b
  prostaglandin agonist therapy for, 335–336, 335f
Glimepiride, 313t
Glipizide, 313t
Glucagon, definition of, 310, 310b

Glucophage. *see* Metformin.
Glucose
  control, blood, 310
  definition of, 310
  loss of, 310–311
Glyburide, 313t
Glycemic control, 310
Glycerin suppository, 259t
Goiter, 296
Gout
  antigout drugs, 237–238
  management of, 237
Gram-negative bacteria, 65b
Gram-positive bacteria, 65
Grapefruit juice, in drug absorption, 26b
Griseofulvin, 85t
Guaifenesin, 120, 121t
Gynecomastia, 305

H

Half-life, of drugs, 26–27
Hallucinations, Parkinson's disease and, 160–161
Haloperidol, 190t–191t
Health care agency policies, in medication regulation, 16–17
Health care setting, 2
Health care workers, protection of, 20, 21b
Healthcare practices, in documenting patient, 346–347
Heart failure, 134
Helicobacter pylori infection, 251
Hematologic system, drugs affecting, 265–278
Hepatitis B virus, antiviral drugs for, 96–98, 97t
Hepatitis C virus, antiviral drugs for, 96–98, 97t
Hepatotoxic drug, 27
Hepatotoxicity, 135
Herbal products, 348–350
Herd immunity, 283
Herpes simplex virus type 1 (HSV-1), antiviral drugs for, 94, 95t
High-alert drugs, 19, 20b
High blood pressure (HBP), 138, 138t, 139b
High-density lipoproteins (HDLs), 135, 135b–136b
High-tyramine foods, to avoid if taking monoamine oxidase inhibitors, 203b
Histamine H₂-receptor antagonists, 249t–250t, 252b
  action of, 252
  adverse reactions to, 252
  drug interactions with, 252
  nursing implications of, 252
  patient teaching on, 252
  side effects of, 252
  uses of, 252

HIV/AIDS, 98, 99f
Hormonal contraception, drugs for, 301f, 302–304, 303t, 304b
Hormone(s), 292–293
    conjugated female sex, 302t
    sex
        of female, 299–304, 300f
        of male, 304–305
Hormone replacement therapy (HRT), 293, 349
Hydralazine, 142t–144t
Hydrochlorothiazide, 128t–129t
Hydrocortisone, 231t
Hydrocortisone sodium succinate, 231t
Hydroxymethylglutaryl coenzyme A reductase inhibitors, 135–137, 136b, 136t
Hypercholesterolemia, 134
Hypercortisolism, 298
Hyperglycemia, 310–311, 311b
Hyperhidrosis, 201
Hyperlipidemia, 134–135
Hypersensitivity, drug, 27
Hypertension, 138
Hypertensive crisis, MAOIs and, 203b
Hyperthyroidism, 296, 296f
Hypertriglyceridemia, 194
Hypervitaminosis, 351
Hypnotics (defined), 185
Hypoglycemia, 310
    indications of, 312b
Hypothyroidism, 293, 293b

I
Ibuprofen, 228t
Identifiers, 6
Idiosyncratic response, to drug, 27
Illnesses, drug therapy and, 30
Imipenem, 70t–71t
Imipramine, 198t–199t
Immunity, 280–282
Immunization, 282
    drugs for, 279–291
Immunomodulating therapy, 287–290
Immunosuppressant drugs, 287
Implementation, in nursing process, 5
Inactivated vaccines, 283
Incompatibility, in drug interactions, 28
Incretin mimetics, 316–317, 317t
Indapamide, 128t–129t
Indinavir, 100t–101t
Indirect-acting stimuli, 242
Indirect thrombin inhibitors, 267t–268t
Infants
    calculating drug dosages for, 38–39
    flow rates for, 40
Infection, 65–66
    anti-infectives, 66
    determination of, 65–66
    drug susceptibility and resistance, 66, 66b

Infection (Continued)
    general considerations for anti-infective drug therapy, 66, 66b–68b
    normal flora, 65
    pathogens, 65
Inflammation, 280
    action of, 225–226, 226b
    causes of, 225–226, 225b
    management of, 226–237
Inflammatory chemical mediators, 225–226
Influenza, antiviral drugs for, 94, 95t
Inhaled corticosteroids, 120t
Inhalers
    continuous aerosol therapy, 58
    dry-powder, 58, 58f
    pressurized metered-dose, 58
    types of, 58f
Inhibitory neurotransmitters, 159–160
Innate immunity, 280–282, 280f, 281b
Inotropic drugs, 153–155, 153b
Insomnia, 185
Insulin
    actions and uses of, 320–322, 321b, 321f, 324b
    definition of, 310, 310b
    dosage of, calculation of, 37–38, 38b
    injection sites for, 324, 326b, 326f
    lack of, 310–311
    pump, 322f
    regimen, 321
    sensitizers, 314–315, 315t
    side effects of, 322
    stimulators, 312–314, 313b, 313t
    syringe for, 37, 38f
    types of, 38, 322, 323t, 324f–325f
    units of, 37, 38f
Insulin-dependent diabetes mellitus (IDDM), 311
Insulin pen injector, 323f
Integrase inhibitor, 99f, 100t–101t, 102
Intensive insulin therapy, 321
Intermittent insomnia, 185
Intermittent pain, 211, 212t
Intradermal injections, 47–48, 48f
Intramuscular (IM) route of administration, 24, 49–51, 49f, 50b
    advantages and disadvantages of, 50t
    deltoid, 50f
    vastus lateralis (thigh), 51f
    ventrogluteal, 50f
Intraocular pressure (IOP), 332–333, 334b, 334f
Intravenous (IV) drugs, 51–55, 51b
    adding drugs to solution container, 52
    fluid regulation, 53–54, 54f
    infusion, 52–53, 53f, 54b
    by intermittent (piggyback) infusion, 52
    peripheral IV locks, 52
    push, 52

Intravenous (IV) infusion
    administration time for, 39
    calculations for, 39–40
    flow rate for, 39
    infection in, 39
    total infusion time in, 39–40
Intravenous (IV) route of administration, 24
Intravenous (IV) therapy
    allergic reactions in, 55
    completion of, 54–55
    evaluation for complications of, 55, 55t
    fluid overload, 55
    infection and, 55
    infiltration, 55
Ipratropium, 117t
Irbesartan, 142t–144t
Iris, 333
Iron, 356–357, 357b
Irritant laxatives, 254–255
Ischemia, 134
Isocarboxazid, 198t–199t
Isoniazid, 80t–81t

J
Jaundice, 135
Juvenile diabetes, 311

K
Kardex, 18, 18f
Ketoacidosis, 311
Ketorolac, 228t

L
Labetalol, 142t–144t
Lacosamide, 175t, 176–177
β-Lactamases, 66
Lactation, drug therapy and, 32
Lactic acidosis, signs and symptoms of, 103b
Lactulose, 259t
Lamictal XR, 175t
Lamivudine, 100t–101t
Lamotrigine, 174–176, 175t, 176b
Lansoprazole, 249t–250t
Lantus, 324
Lantus insulin, 38
Laryngeal edema, 69–72
Latanoprost, 339t
Laxatives, 258b, 259t
    action of, 255–256, 255f
    adverse effects to, 256
    drug interactions with, 256
    nursing implications and patient teaching on, 256–259
    side effects of, 256
    uses of, 255–256
Legal responsibility, 13–14
Lennox-Gastaut syndrome, 174–175

Leukotriene inhibitors, 109t–110t, 111–112
  action of, 111
  nursing implications and patient teaching on, 111–112
  side effects, adverse reactions, and drug interactions, 111
  use of, 111
Leukotriene modifiers, 111
Levalbuterol, 117t
Levemir, 324
Levemir insulin, 38
Levobunolol, 339t
Levocetirizine, 109t–110t
Levodopa, 161–163
Levofloxacin, 78t
Levothyroxine sodium, 294t
Licensed practical or vocational nurses. *see* LPNs/LVNs.
Linagliptin, 319t
Linezolid, 75t, 76, 76b
Liothyronine sodium, 294t
Lipid pneumonia, 256
Lipoproteins, 135
Liraglutide, 317t
Lisinopril, 142t–144t
Lithium, 205, 205b
  levels, elevated, 205t
  toxicity, 205b
Lithium carbonate, 198t–199t
Live virus vaccines, 283
Lixisenatide, 317t
Long-acting β-adrenergic agonist (LABA), 117t
Loop diuretics, action of, 127
Loperamide, 257t–258t
Lopinavir/ritonavir, 100t–101t
Loratadine, 109t–110t
Lorazepam
  for anxiety, 186t–187t
  for insomnia, 186t–187t
Losartan, 142t–144t
Lovastatin, 136t
Low-density lipoproteins (LDLs), 135, 135b
Low-molecular-weight heparin (LMWH), 271, 272f
LPNs/LVNs
  role of, nursing process and, 1–9
  substance abuse by, 13
Lubiprostone, 259t
Lubricant laxatives, 255, 259t
Lymphocytes, 107

M

Macrodrip, 39
  calculation of, 54
  chamber, 53f
Macrolides, 74
  actions of, 74
  adverse effects of, 74
  drug interactions with, 74

Macrolides (Continued)
  nursing implications and patient teaching on, 74, 75t
  side effects of, 74
  use of, 74
Magnesium, 357
Magnesium hydroxide, 249t–250t, 259t
Malaria, 87
Mania, symptoms of, 204, 204b
"Manic-depressive" illness, 204
Maraviroc, 100t–101t
Masklike facial expression, 160, 161f
Mast cell stabilizer (cromones), 109t–110t, 112
Mediators, 107
Medication administration
  ear drops, 58, 59b
  enteral, 24, 41–43
  evaluation in, 9, 9b
  eye drops and ointments, 58, 59b
  intradermal, 47–48
  intramuscular, 49–51
  legal, regulatory, and ethical aspects of, 11–21
  nasogastric, 42–43, 43b
  nine "rights" of, 5–9, 5b–6b, 9b, 17t
  in older adults, 42b
  parenteral, 43–55
  percutaneous, 56–60
  percutaneous endoscopic gastrostomy tube, 42–43, 43b
  principles of, 40–41
  rectal, 60, 60b–61b
  regulation of, 12–15
    federal, 12–15
  respiratory mucosa, 58, 58t
  right documentation in, 8–9
  right dose in, 8
  right drug in, 6–7, 6t–7t, 7b
  right patient in, 6, 6f, 8b
  right route in, 8
  right time in, 7, 8b
  right to refuse in, 9
  subcutaneous, 48–49, 49b
  systems, nursing process in, 17–18
  through mucous membranes, 57–60
  topical, 56, 56b
  transdermal, 56, 56b
  vaginal, 58–60, 60b
Medication cup, for drug administration, 41–42, 42f
Medication reconciliation, 20
Medroxyprogesterone, 302t
Meglitinide analogs, 312, 313t
Meloxicam, 228t
Memantine, 168t
Menopause, 300, 300b, 301f
  relief of, drugs for, 300–302, 302b, 302t
Mental health
  drug therapy for, 183–209
  and mental illness continuum, 184f

Mental health (Continued)
  neurotransmitters and their function in, 185t
Meropenem, 70t–71t
Metabolism, drug, 25–26, 26f
  in older adult, 31
  in pediatric patients, 30
Metformin, 313t, 314b
Methazolamide, 342t
Methimazole, 294t
Methocarbamol, 222b
Methylcellulose, 257t–258t
Methyldopa, 142t–144t
Methylprednisolone, 231t
Metipranolol, 339t
Metoclopramide, 243t–244t
  dopamine agonists and, 163–164
Metolazone, 128t–129t
Metoprolol, 142t–144t
Metronidazole, 87–88
Microdrops, 39
  calculation, 54
  chamber, 53f
Miglitol, 315t
Mineralocorticoid, 297–298
Minerals, 356–358
Minocycline, 75t
Minoxidil, 142t–144t
Miosis, 173, 215, 333, 333b, 333f
Miscellaneous analgesics, 220, 220b
  corticosteroids as, 220
  NSAIDS, 221
  skeletal muscle relaxants, 221–222
Miscellaneous protein synthesis inhibitors, 76, 76b
Misoprostol, 249t–250t, 253
Mitotane (Lysodren), 298
Mix-o-vial, 46, 47f
Mometasone, 120t
Monoamine oxidase inhibitors (MAOIs), 188
  action of, 203
  adverse reactions to, 203
  for depression, 198t–199t, 203–204
  drug interactions with, 203
  high-tyramine foods to avoid, 203b
  hypertensive crisis, 203b
  nursing implications AND patient teaching on, 204
  serotonin syndrome, 203b
  side effects of, 203
  uses of, 203
Monoamine oxidase type B (MAO-B) inhibitor, 161, 165–166
Monoclonal antibodies, 179
Montelukast, 109t–110t, 111
Mood stabilizers
  action of, 205
  adverse reactions to, 205
  for depression, 195–206, 198t–199t
  nursing implications and patient teaching on, 206

Mood stabilizers (Continued)
  side effects of, 205
  uses of, 205
Mucolytics, 119–121, 120b, 121t
Multiple-dose vials, 46
Multiple sclerosis
  early symptoms of, 179b
  monoclonal antibodies for, 179
  neurologic drugs for, 179
  nonspecific antiinflammatory drugs
    for, 179
  pathogenesis of, 178f
  relapsing-remitting, 180t
  specific drugs for, 179
Mycophenolate, 287, 288t
Mycosis, 65
Mydriasis, 333, 333b, 333f
Myelin, 178–179
Myocardial infarction, 134, 268
  antianginals for, 147
  drugs for, 147–155
  nitrates for, 147–149
Myocardial oxygen demand, 147

N
Nabilone, 243t–244t
Nabumetone, 228t
Nadolol, 142t–144t
Nalbuphine, 218t
Naproxen, 228t
Narrow-spectrum drugs, 67
Nasal corticosteroids, 113t
Nasogastric (NG) tube, 42
Nateglinide, 313t
National Alliance for Mental Illness,
  184b
National Eye Institute, 334b
National Institute of Mental Health,
  193b
National Institutes of Health, 147b
Natural acquired active immunity,
  281–282
Natural acquired passive immunity,
  282
Natural penicillins, 69
Nelfinavir, 100t–101t
Nephrotoxic drug, 27
Nephrotoxicity, in cephalosporins, 72
Neuraminidase inhibitors, 95t
Neuroleptic malignant syndrome
  (NMS), 163, 192, 192b
Neuropathic pain, 212t
Neurotransmitters, 159, 160f
Niacin, 137, 351t, 352
Nicardipine, 142t–144t
Nicotinic acid, 137
Nifedipine, 142t–144t
Nitrates, 147–149
Nitroglycerin, 147
  patient education for taking, 148b
Nizatidine, 249t–250t
N-methyl-d-aspartate (NMDA) blocker,
  166, 168t, 169

Nociceptive pain, 212t
Nomogram, 38–39
Non-benzodiazepines, 185
Non-insulin-dependent diabetes
  mellitus (NIDDM), 311
Non-nucleoside reverse transcriptase
  inhibitors (NNRTIs), 99, 99f,
  100t–101t, 102, 102b
Nonopioid centrally acting analgesics,
  218–219, 218b
  action of, 218–219
  adverse reactions to, 219
  drug interactions with, 219
  nursing implications and patient
    teaching on, 219
  side effects of, 219
  uses of, 219
Nonpathogens, 65
Nonphenothiazines, 190, 190t–191t
Nonproprietary name, 23
Nonselective COX inhibitors, 227
Nonsteroidal anti-inflammatory drugs
  (NSAIDs), 221, 227–230
  actions of, 227, 227f, 228t
  adverse reactions to, 229
  drug interactions with, 229
  nonselective, 227, 229b
  nursing implications and patient
    teaching on, 229–230
  selective, 227
  side effects of, 229
  uses of, 227–228
Norepinephrine, 185t
Normal flora, 65
NPH insulin, 37
Nucleoside reverse transcriptase
  inhibitors (NRTIs), 100t–101t, 102,
  102b
Nurse Licensure Compact, 16
Nurse Practice Act, 16
Nurses
  licensed practical/vocational. see
    LPNs/LVNs.
  registered, responsibility of, 16
  substance abuse by, 13–14
Nursing process
  assessment in, 2–3, 2f, 3b
  definition of, 2
  diagnosis in, 4
  in drug administration systems,
    17–18
  evaluation in, 9, 9b
  implementation in, 5
  LPN practice and, 1–10
  planning in, 4, 4b
Nystatin, 85t

O
Objective data, 3
Observation, 3
Older adults
  antianxiety for, 188b
  antihypertensives and, 146b

Older adults (Continued)
  digoxin and, 154b
  drug therapy for, 30–31
    absorption as, 31
    distribution as, 31
    elimination as, 31
    metabolism as, 31
  histamine H₂ receptor antagonists for,
    252b
  lithium for, 206b
  NSAIDs for, 229b
  opioid agonist analgesics for, 216b
  risk for problems with prescription
    drugs, 15
  selective serotonin reuptake
    inhibitors for, 200b
Oligospermia, 304–305
Omeprazole, 249t–250t
Omnibus Budget Reconciliation Acts,
  15
Ondansetron, 243t–244t
Ophthalmic drugs, 331–332
  nursing considerations for, 337b,
    337f
Opioid, 214
Opioid agonist analgesics, 214–217,
  214b, 214t–215t
  action of, 214–215, 215b
  adverse reactions to, 215–216, 216b
  drug interactions with, 216, 216b
  nursing implications and patient
    teaching on, 216–217
  side effects of, 215
  uses of, 215
Opioid agonist-antagonist analgesics,
  217–218
  action of, 217, 217b, 218t
  adverse reactions to, 218
  drug interactions with, 218
  nursing implication and patient
    teaching on, 218
  side effects of, 218
  uses of, 217–218
Opioid agonists, 214, 257t–258t
Opportunistic infection, 98
Opportunistic infections, 83–84
Oral contraceptives, 302–303
Oral drugs, 41–42
  for infant or child, 41–42, 42f
  liquid-form, 41–42, 42f
  tablets or capsules, 41
Oral hypoglycemic agents, 312
Oral sympathomimetic decongestants,
  112
Oseltamivir, 95t
Osmotic laxatives, 255, 257t–259t
Osteoclast monoclonal antibodies,
  307
Osteoporosis, 305–306
  drugs for, 305–307, 305f, 306t
Otic drugs, 330, 330b
Otitis media, 329
Outbreaks, 94

Over-the-counter (OTC) drugs, 12, 15, 347–348
  common active ingredients in, 348t
  patient teaching in, 347–348
  product labeling of, 347
Overactive bladder
  drugs for, 132, 132t
  pathophysiology of, 132f
Overactive thyroid, 296
Oxcarbazepine, 174, 175t
Oxtellar XR, 175t
Oxymetazoline, 113t

P
Pain
  acute, 211, 211b, 212t
  assessment, 216b
  cancer, 212t
  chronic, 211, 211b, 212t
  classification of, 212t
  continuous, 212t
  definition, 210–211, 211b
  intermittent, 211, 212t
  measurement scales, 213f
  neuropathic, 212t
  nociceptive, 212t
  perception, 211–212, 211f
  visceral, 212t
Pain management
  analgesic drugs for, 212–220
  drugs for, 210–224, 213b
  miscellaneous drugs for, 220–223
  principles of, 212
Pain threshold, 211
Palonosetron, 243t–244t
Palpation, 3
Pancreatitis, 317b
  signs and symptoms of, 103b
Pantoprazole, 249t–250t
Paradoxical response, to drug, 27
Parasite, 65
Parenteral route of administration, 24, 43–55
  mixing, 46, 46b
  needles for, 44–45, 45f, 45t
  preparation of, 45–47, 45b
  principles for, 43–55, 45b
  procedure for, 45–55
  syringes for, 44, 44f, 45t
Parkinson's disease
  catechol-O-methyltransferase inhibitors for, 165
  clinical trials and research into, 161b
  dopamine agonists for, 161–165
  drugs for, 160–166, 161b
  neurotransmitter abnormality in, 160f
  symptoms of, 161b
Paroxetine, 198t–199t
Partial agonist, 24, 24b
Passive immunity, 281
Pathogen, 65

Patient and family teaching
  on acetaminophen, 220
  on antacids, 252
  on antianxiety drugs, 189
  on antidiarrheals, 260
  on antigout drugs, 238
  on atypical antipsychotic, 195
  on cannabinoids, 247–248
  on corticosteroids, 234–235
  on disease-modifying antirheumatic drugs (DMARDs), 237
  on histamine H_2-receptor antagonists, 252
  on laxatives, 258–259
  on monoamine oxidase inhibitors (MAOIs), 204
  on mood stabilizers, 206
  on nonsteroidal anti-inflammatory drugs (NSAIDs), 230
  on opioid agonist analgesics, 217
  on phenothiazines, 247
  on promotility drugs, 248
  on proton pump inhibitors, 253
  on sedative-hypnotics, 187
  on selective serotonin reuptake inhibitors, 200
  on serotonin norepinephrine reuptake inhibitors, 201
  on serotonin (5-HT_3) receptor antagonists, 245
  on skeletal muscle relaxants, 222
  on substance P/neurokinin$_1$ (NK_1) receptor antagonists, 246
  on typical antipsychotic drugs, 193
Patient charts, 14
Pediatric patient(s)
  acetaminophen in, 220b
  aspirin for, 229b
  dosage calculations for, 38–39
  drug therapy for, 30
    absorption as, 30
    distribution as, 30
    elimination as, 30
    metabolism as, 30
  flow rates for, 40
  NSAIDS for, 221b
  pain assessment for, 216b
Penciclovir, 95t
Penicillinase-resistant penicillins, 69
Penicillin G benzathine, 70t–71t
Penicillin G procaine, 70t–71t
Penicillins, 68–72, 68f
  action of, 69
  adverse reactions to, 69–72
  drug interactions, 72, 72b
  natural, 69
  nursing implications and patient teaching on, 70t–71t, 72, 72b
  penicillinase-resistant, 69
  side effects of, 69
  use of, 69, 70t–71t
Penicillin VK, 70t–71t

Pentazocine, 218t
Peptic ulcer disease, 248–253, 248b, 249t–250t, 251b
  nursing consideration for, 251b
  therapies for, for older adults, 252b
Percutaneous drugs, 56–60, 56b
Percutaneous endoscopic gastrostomy (PEG) tube administration, 42–43, 43b
Percutaneous route of administration, 24
Perimenopause, 300
Peripheral nervous system (PNS), 159
Pharmacodynamics, 23
Pharmacokinetics, definition of, 23
Pharmacology, 1–10
  drug attachment in, 23–24
  drug names in, 23
  principles of, 22–34
Pharmacotherapeutics, definition of, 23
Phenazopyridine, 130–131, 131b
Phenelzine, 198t–199t
Phenobarbital, 171–173, 172t
Phenothiazine, 190, 190t–191t, 243t–244t
  action of, 246
  adverse reactions to, 246
  drug interactions with, 246
  nursing implications and patient teaching on, 246–247
  side effects of, 246
  uses of, 246
Phenylephrine, 113t
Phenytoin, 172t
  adverse reaction of, 173b
  dopamine agonists and, 163–164
Physical dependence, 12b
Phytoestrogens, 349
Piggyback infusion, 52
Pill, 41
Pilocarpine, 341t
Pioglitazone, 314, 315t
Pirbuterol, 117t
Piroxicam, 228t
Planning
  to give drug, factors to consider in, 5
  in nursing process, 4, 4b
Platelet inhibitors, 267t–268t, 268–270
  action of, 268
  adverse reactions to, 268–269
  drug and food interactions with, 269, 269b
  nursing implications and patient teaching on, 269–270, 269f
  side effects of, 268
  use of, 268
Plavix. *see* Clopidogrel.
Pletal. *see* Cilostazol.
Polydipsia, 311
Polyethylene glycol, 257t–259t
Polyphagia, 311
Polypharmacy, 30
Polyuria, 311
Potassium, 357–358, 358b

Potassium-sparing diuretics, action of, 127
Pradaxa. *see* Dabigatran.
Pramipexole, 161, 162*t*–163*t*
Pramlintide, 317, 317*t*
Pravastatin, 136*t*
Praziquantel, 90
Prazosin, 142*t*–144*t*
Prednisolone, 230*b*, 231*t*
Prednisone, 230*b*, 231*t*
Pregnancy
   benzodiazepines and, 185*b*
   drug therapy and, 32
   statins and, 135*b*
Prescription drugs, definition of, 12, 14–15
Prescriptive authority, 16
Pressurized metered-dose inhaler, 58, 58*f*
Primidone, 172*t*
Prochlorperazine, 243*t*–244*t*
Prodrugs, 25–26
Professional responsibility, 17
Prokinetic drugs, 248
Promethazine, 243*t*–244*t*
Promotility drugs, 243*t*–244*t*
   action of, 248
   adverse reactions to, 248
   drug interactions with, 248
   nursing implications and patient teaching on, 248
   side effects of, 248
   uses of, 248
Proportion method, in calculating drug dosages, 36
Propranolol, 142*t*–144*t*
Propylthiouracil, 294*t*
Prostaglandin agonists, 335–336, 336*b*, 339*t*
Prostaglandin, protecting GI tract, 241–242
Prostate gland, 131*f*
Protease inhibitors (PIs), 97*t*, 99*f*, 100*t*–101*t*, 102, 102*b*
Prothrombin, 266
Proton pump inhibitors (PPIs), 249*t*–250*t*, 253*b*
   action of, 252–253
   adverse reactions to, 253
   drug interactions with, 253
   nursing implications and patient teaching on, 253
   side effects of, 253
   uses of, 252–253
Protozoa, 87, 87*b*
Pruritus, 268
Pseudoephedrine, 113*t*
Pseudomembranous colitis, 67*b*
Pseudoparkinsonism, 190–192, 192*f*
Psychologic dependence, 12*b*
Psychosis, 189
Psyllium, 257*t*–259*t*

Punctal occlusion, 336–340, 337*f*
Purpura, 268
Pyrantel, 90
Pyrazinamide, 80*t*–81*t*
Pyridoxine, 351*t*

Q
Quetiapine, 190*t*–191*t*
Quinapril, 142*t*–144*t*

R
Rabeprazole, 249*t*–250*t*
Rabies, and artificial acquired passive immunity, 282
Raltegravir, 100*t*–101*t*
Ranitidine, 249*t*–250*t*
Rasagiline, 162*t*–163*t*
Ratio method, in calculating drug dosages, 36
Receptor site, drug, 23–24, 24*f*
Recommended dietary allowance (RDA), 350
Rectal drug administration, 60, 60*b*–61*b*
Registered nurse, responsibility of, 16
Renal system, drugs affecting, 125–157
Renin, 140–141
Renin-angiotensin-aldosterone system (RAAS) drugs, 140–141
Repaglinide, 313*t*
Respiratory problems, drugs for, 106–124
Respiratory syncytial virus (RSV), 95
Retina, 333–334
Retrovirus, 98–99
Reye syndrome, 229
Rhabdomyolysis, 135
Ribavirin, 96*t*
Riboflavin, 351*t*, 352
Rifampin, 80*t*–81*t*
Rilpivirine, 100*t*–101*t*
Rimantadine, 95*t*
Risperidone, 163*b*, 190*t*–191*t*
Rivaroxaban (Xaretto), 267*t*–268*t*
Rivastigmine, for Alzheimer's disease, 167, 168*t*
Rolapitant, 243*t*–244*t*
Ropinirole, 161, 162*t*–163*t*, 163*b*
Rosiglitazone, 314, 315*t*
Rosuvastatin, 136*t*
Rotigotine, 161, 162*t*–163*t*
Route of administration
   enteral, 24, 41–43
      nasogastric, 42–43
      oral, 41–42
   intramuscular (IM), 24, 49–51, 49*f*, 50*b*
      advantages and disadvantages of, 50*t*
      deltoid, 50*f*
      vastus lateralis (thigh), 51*f*
      ventrogluteal, 50*f*

Route of administration (*Continued*)
   intravenous (IV), 24
   parenteral, 24, 43–55
      mixing, 46, 46*b*
      needles for, 44–45, 45*f*, 45*t*
      preparation of, 45–47, 45*b*
      principles for, 43–55, 45*b*
      procedure for, 45–55
      syringes for, 44, 44*f*, 45*t*
   percutaneous, 24
   subcutaneous, 24
   sublingual, 24, 57–58, 59*b*

S
Safinamide, 162*t*–163*t*
Saline laxatives, 255
Salmeterol, 117*t*
Saquinavir, 100*t*–101*t*
Saxagliptin, 319*t*
Scheduled drugs, 12
Schizophrenia, 189*b*, 190
Seasonal influenza vaccination, 285, 285*b*–286*b*
   adverse reactions to, 286, 286*b*
   nursing implications and patient teaching, 285*b*, 286–287
   side effects of, 286
Second-generation antihistamines, 109*t*–110*t*
Second-generation antipsychotics, 193, 194*b*
Secretogogues, 312–314
Sedatives, 185
Sedatives-hypnotics, 184–187
   action of, 185
   adverse reactions to, 185
   drug interactions with, 187
   nursing implications and patient teaching on, 187
   side effects of, 185
   uses of, 185
Seizures, 169–170, 170*b*
Selective cholesterol absorption inhibitors, 137
Selective immunosuppressants
   for autoimmune diseases, 287
   transplant rejection prevention, 287–290
      action of, 287, 288*t*
      adverse effects to, 289
      drug interactions with, 289
      nursing implications and patient teaching on, 289–290
      side effects of, 287–288
Selective MAO-B inhibitors, 162*t*–163*t*
Selective serotonin reuptake inhibitors (SSRIs), 198*t*–199*t*, 200*b*
   action of, 196–197, 197*f*
   adverse reactions to, 197
   for anxiety, 188
   for depression, 196–200
   drug interactions with, 197

Selective serotonin reuptake inhibitors (SSRIs) *(Continued)*
nursing implications and patient teaching on, 197–200
serotonin syndrome, 203*b*
side effects of, 197
uses of, 196–197
Selegiline, 162*t*–163*t*, 198*t*–199*t*
Semicircular canals, 329–330
Serotonin, 185*t*
Serotonin norepinephrine reuptake inhibitors (SNRIs)
action of, 201
adverse reactions to, 201
for anxiety, 188
for depression, 198*t*–199*t*, 201
drug interactions with, 201
nursing implications and patient teaching on, 201
side effects of, 201
uses of, 201
Serotonin (5-HT₃) receptor antagonists, 243*b*, 243*t*–244*t*
action of, 243
adverse reactions to, 243
drug interactions with, 244
nursing implications and patient teaching on, 244–245
side effects of, 243
uses of, 243
Serotonin syndrome, 194*b*
Sertraline, 198*t*–199*t*
Sex hormone
of female, 299–304, 300*f*
of male, 304–305
Short-acting β-adrenergic agonist (SABA), 116, 116*b*, 117*t*
Side effect, 27
SIGMA spectrum infusion system, 54*f*
Silodosin, 131*t*
Simvastatin, 136*t*
Single drug order, 16
Sirolimus, 288*t*
Sitagliptin, 319*t*
Skeletal muscle relaxants, 221–222
action of, 221
adverse reactions to, 222
drug interactions with, 222
nursing implications and patient teaching on, 221*t*, 222
side effects of, 222
uses of, 222
Skeletal muscle spasm, 221
Sleep, drugs for, 184–189, 186*t*–187*t*
Sodium-glucose co-transport inhibitors, 319*t*, 320, 320*b*
Sodium phosphate, 259*t*
Sodium phosphate monobasic monohydrate, 257*t*–258*t*
Solubility, of medications, 24
Spectrum, 67
Spironolactone, 128*t*–129*t*
St. John's wort, 349–350, 350*b*

Standing drug order, 16
State law, on medications, 16–17, 16*b*
Stavudine, 100*t*–101*t*
Stimulant laxatives, 255–256, 257*t*–259*t*
Stool softeners, 255, 257*t*–259*t*
Streptomycin, 75*t*
Subcutaneous heparin, 271–272, 272*b*
Subcutaneous injections, 48–49, 48*f*–49*f*, 49*b*
Subcutaneous route of administration, 24
Subjective data, 2–3
Sublingual route of administration, 24, 57–58, 59*b*
Substance abuse, by nurses, 13–14
Substance P/neurokinin₁ (NK₁) receptor antagonists, 243*t*–244*t*
action of, 245
adverse reactions to, 245–246
drug interactions with, 246
nursing implications of, 246
patient teaching on, 246
side effects of, 245
uses of, 245
Sucralfate, 249*t*–250*t*, 253
Sulfamethoxazole, 78*t*
Sulfonamide diuretics, 126–127
Sulfonamides, 76–77
action of, 76–77
adverse reactions to, 77
drug interactions with, 77
nursing implications and patient teaching on, 77, 78*t*
side effects of, 77
use of, 77
Sulfonylureas, 312, 313*b*, 313*t*
Sustained-release drug, 42*b*
Sympathomimetic nasal decongestants, 112
Sympathomimetics, 112, 113*t*
Synergistic effect, in drug interaction, 28
Syringe
insulin, 37, 38*f*
for oral administration, 42*f*
for parenteral drugs, 44, 44*f*, 45*f*
prefilled, 47, 48*f*

T
Tablet, 41
Tacrolimus, 288*t*
Tamsulosin, 131*t*
Tardive dyskinesia, 164, 192, 192*f*
Target tissue, 292–293
Temazepam, 186*t*–187*t*
Tenofovir, 100*t*–101*t*
Terazosin, 131*t*, 142*t*–144*t*
Tetracyclines, 73–74, 75*t*
action of, 73
adverse effects of, 74, 74*b*
drug interactions with, 74
side effects of, 73
use of, 73

The Joint Commission (TJC), official "do not use" list, 19, 20*t*
Therapeutic effects, 9
Thiamine, 351*t*, 352, 352*b*
Thiazide diuretics, 126–127
Thiazolidinediones, 314
Thrombin, 266
Thrombophlebitis, 266
Thromboplastin, 266
Thrombus, 266
Thyroid crisis, 296
Thyroid hormone agonists, 294–295
action and uses of, 294, 294*t*
adverse effects to, 294
drug interactions with, 294
nursing implications and patient teaching on, 295, 295*b*–296*b*
side effects of, 294
Thyroid problems, drugs for, 293–297, 293*f*
Thyroid storm, 296
Ticagrelor (Brilinta), 267*t*–268*t*
Ticlopidine (Ticlid), 267*t*–268*t*
Timolol, 339*t*
Tinzaparin (Innohep), 267*t*–268*t*
Tiotropium, 117*t*
Tipranavir, 100*t*–101*t*
Tolcapone, 162*t*–163*t*
Tolerance, 216
Topical drugs, 56, 56*b*, 57*f*
Topical eye drug therapy, 338*b*
Topiramate, 175*t*, 177–178, 178*b*
Torsades de pointes, 167–168, 357
Toxoids, 283
Toxoplasmosis, 87
Trade name, of drug, 23
Transcriptinase, 98
Transdermal patches, 56, 56*b*, 57*f*
Travoprost, 339*t*
Triamcinolone, 113*t*, 231*t*
Triamterene, 128*t*–129*t*
Trichomoniasis, 87
Tricyclic antidepressants (TCAs), 196, 198*t*–199*t*
Trimethobenzamide, 243*t*–244*t*
Trimethoprim, 78*t*
Tuberculosis, 78–79
Tympanic membrane, 329
Typical antipsychotic drugs, 190–193, 190*t*–191*t*
action of, 190
adverse reactions to, 190–192
drug interactions with, 192
nursing implications and patient teaching on, 192–193
side effects of, 190–192
uses of, 190
Tyramine, foods that contain, 166*b*

U
U-100 and U-50 syringes, for diabetes, 322*f*

Ulcer, peptic, 248–253, 248b, 249t–250t, 251b
  nursing consideration for, 251b
  pathophysiology of, 249f
  therapies for, for older adults, 252b
Uncoating inhibitors, 95t
Unit-dose system, 18
United States, drug regulations in, 12, 13t
  federal laws, 12–15
  health care agency, 16–17
  state laws, 16–17, 16b
Ureidopenicillins, 69
Urgency, 132
Uric acid synthesis inhibitors, for gout, 237t
Urinary antispasmodics, 132, 132t
Urinary incontinence, 132
Urinary system, 126f
  bladder anesthetics and, 130–131
  diuretics and, 126–130
  drugs affecting, 126–132

V

Vaccination, 282–287, 282b
  boosting schedule and, 283–284, 283b–284b, 284f
Vaccine, 282
  administration of, 285b
  types of, 283, 283b
Vaginal drugs, 58–60, 60b
Valproic acid, 172t, 173, 198t–199t
Valsartan, 142t–144t

Vancomycin, 70t–71t
Vasodilators, 140, 145
Venlafaxine, 198t–199t
Verapamil, 142t–144t
Verbal order, 16
Vials
  insulin, 37, 38f
  multiple-dose, 46
  for parenteral drugs, 45–46, 46f
Viral DNA polymerase inhibitors, 95t
Virion, HIV and, 99f
Virus, 65, 94
Visceral pain, 212t
Vitamin A, 351–352, 351t
Vitamin B$_1$, 351t, 352, 352b
Vitamin B$_2$, 351t, 352
Vitamin B$_3$, 351t
Vitamin B$_6$, 351t, 352–353
  carbidopa/levodopa and, 163–164
Vitamin B$_9$, 351t, 353
Vitamin B$_{12}$, 351t, 353–354
Vitamin C, 351t, 354
Vitamin D, 351t, 354–355
Vitamin E, 351t, 355
Vitamin K, 351t, 355, 356b
Vitamin K antagonist, 267t–268t, 273–275
  actions of, 273
  adverse reactions to, 273, 273b, 273f
  drug and food interactions with, 273–274
  nursing implications and patient teaching on, 274–275, 274b–275b

Vitamin K antagonist (Continued)
  side effects of, 273
  use of, 273
Vitamins, 350–355
  function, deficiency, and recommended daily intake of, 351t
Vitreous humor, 333–334

W

Warfarin (Coumadin), 267t–268t
Water-soluble vitamins, 350
Weight, body, drug therapy and, 30
Withdrawal symptoms, 216
Wong-Baker FACES pain rating scale, 213f

X

Xanthine-based drugs, 116

Z

Z-track technique, 51, 51f
Zafirlukast, 109t–110t, 111
Zaleplon, 186t–187t
Zanamivir, 95t
Zidovudine, 100t–101t
Zileuton, 109t–110t, 111
Zinc, 358
Ziprasidone, 190t–191t
Zolpidem, 186t–187t